Imaging in Clinical Oncology

Athanasios D. Gouliamos
John A. Andreou · Paris A. Kosmidis
Editors

Imaging in Clinical Oncology

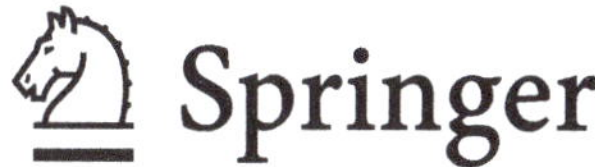

Editors
Athanasios D. Gouliamos
Aretaieion Hospital, National and
Kapodistrian University of Athens
Athens
Greece

Paris A. Kosmidis
Medical Oncology Department
Hygeia Hospital
Athens
Greece

John A. Andreou
Imaging Department
Hygeia and Mitera Hospitals
Athens
Greece

ISBN 978-88-470-5384-7 ISBN 978-88-470-5385-4 (eBook)
DOI 10.1007/978-88-470-5385-4
Springer Milan Heidelberg New York Dordrecht London

Library of Congress Control Number: 2013948442

Printed on acid-free paper

Springer is part of Springer Science+Business Media (www.springer.com)

This book is dedicated to all cancer patients and their families.
We are grateful to our teachers and thankful to our staff.

Preface

Over the past four decades, Radiology has seen tremendous growth. Similarly, the progress that Oncology has made recently is exceptional and the multidisciplinary approach for each cancer patient is mandatory to ensure a longer and better life.

Radiologists may consider that without their contribution, timely detection of tumors and hence effective therapeutic intervention would be deemed impossible. Oncologists should understand the potential applications, limitations and advantages of imaging techniques and the radiologist should have adequate knowledge of the pathology, prognosis, clinical information, and treatment options for different types of tumors.

Improved survival rates are attributable to a great extent to the transformation of both disciplines. Medical imaging is nowadays an integral and indispensable part of the approach to oncologic patients. The clinician and the radiologist are complementary and, as such, they should interact and comprehend each other's language. The aforementioned evolution has rendered medical imaging a clinical specialty, and clinical oncology an imaging-dependent discipline.

These key points are elucidated and elaborated in an all-inclusive oncology imaging textbook that will be beneficial for radiologists and clinicians alike, integrating a language comprehensible to both.

New technological advances in Radiology along with the progress that has been made in Molecular Oncology and personalized treatment have brought together the physicians of the two specialties to work in the multidisciplinary team against cancer.

Similarly, collaboration of the radiologist and the radiotherapy oncologist is mandatory. All technically sophisticated radiotherapy treatments are safe and effective, provided an accurate assessment of the gross tumor volume has been made.

This book, *Imaging in Clinical Oncology*, is written with the purpose of highlighting the benefit that arises as a result of the radiologist–oncologist communication within the multidisciplinary team providing cancer care.

The book begins with general principles such as molecular imaging, imaging criteria for tumor response, oncologic imaging in radiotherapy, interventional radiology in oncology, and imaging in pediatric oncology.

The great majority of tumors are then presented in a uniform fashion. The clinical oncologist begins with an introduction of each type of tumor. All relevant imaging techniques necessary for the prevention, diagnosis, staging, response evaluation, and follow-up of the particular tumor are then assessed by expert radiologists. Finally, the clinical oncologist provides an analysis of the treatment implications, usefulness, sequence, and combination of the imaging techniques presented. Quantitative imaging data combined with laboratory biomarkers can help the clinical oncologist to recognize at the earliest possible time whether the applied treatment is ineffective so that therapy can be modified.

It is our sincere hope that that this book will serve as a guide through which radiologists and clinicians can rapidly acquire the basic knowledge essential to oncologic daily practice.

Athens, November 2013

Athanasios D. Gouliamos
John A. Andreou
Paris A. Kosmidis

Acknowledgements

The editors would like to express their gratitude to the authors of this book for their enthusiasm and commitment to the text's completion, as well as the staff of Springer Verlag Italia, Milan for their continuous support. We offer our thanks especially to Antonella Cerri who has guided this edition from the first steps. Our sincere thanks also go to Juliette Ruth Kleemann and Corinna Parravicini for their contribution in the preprint process. L. Sundari and R. Nalini Gyaneshwar provided outstanding book production services.

Also we are indebted to the technical staff, of the Radiology Departments of "Aretaieio" University Hospital and "Hygeia" Hospital for their tireless devotion to excellence in their daily work.

Finally we would like to thank Stella Voudouri, Sofia Kelekidou and Vivi Triantaphilou for their secretarial assistance.

Contents

Part VII Gynecologic Cancer

Part VIII Breast Cancer

Part IX Gastrointestinal Cancer

Esophagus, Stomach

Solid Organs (Liver, Pancreas)

Peritoneal Cavity

Large Bowel

Prostate Cancer

Part XII Melanoma

Part I
Introduction to Oncologic Imaging

Molecular Imaging in Oncology

Hybrid Imaging and Personalized Therapy of Cancer

1

George N. Sfakianakis

(Diagnosis—Staging—Response to Therapy—Restaging of the Tumors).

1.1 Introduction

It has been proposed that the "telomeres" of the chromosomes, their four endpoints, determine our future: Harbingers of mortality, the telomeres at the chromosome tips glow brightly with appropriate color dying; they influence vulnerability, mortality, longevity, and survival. The longer the telomeres, the longer the person lives. If their length decreases, the person dies sooner. However, the utilization of telomeres in clinical practice for patient evaluation is still in the distant future. At the present time, we can report that substantial advances have recently been achieved with the applications of **Molecular Imaging (MI)** in the evaluation of oncologic patients.

1.1.1 Molecular Imaging: The Principle and its Historical Development

In searching recent literature one will find many definitions of Molecular Imaging (MI).

Sanjiv S. Gambir, one of the leading experts on this topic, defines MI as follows [1]:

"MI of living subjects is an Emerging Field that aims to study molecular and cellular events in the intact living animal and human. These events can be as simple as location(s) of a specific population of cells or levels of a given protein receptor on the surface of cells (or) more complex events, such as the interaction of two intracellular proteins, cellular metabolic flux, or transcription of a set of genes when a cell type comes into contact with another cell type."

Other definitions stress the point that MI is not just an emerging field but a new field:

"MI is a New Field of Imaging, which includes the following:

- Clinical Multimodality MI with Molecular Probes
- Laboratory Cellular and Molecular Biology and Research
- Chemistry/Pharmacology for Molecular Probes
- Medical Physics for MI
- New Biomathematics/Bioinformation/Biomechanics" [2].

However, based on our knowledge and experience, the correct definition of MI ought to be:

"MI is a New Name for an Old Imaging Field", because in nuclear medicine (NM) we were practicing MI since the beginnings of the NM Specialty.

G. N. Sfakianakis (✉)
Radiology/Nuclear Medicine, 1611 NW 12th Avenue, JMH West Wing 279, Miami, Florida 33136, USA
e-mail: gsfakian@med.miami.edu

A. D. Gouliamos et al. (eds.), *Imaging in Clinical Oncology*,
DOI: 10.1007/978-88-470-5385-4_1, © Springer-Verlag Italia 2014

In his new book "A Personal History of Nuclear Medicine", Henry N. Wagner Jr., a NM guru, specifies in the introduction: "...MI had been the hallmark of Nuclear Medicine since its beginning" and later "The tracer principle was invented in 1913 by George Hevesy" [3].

1.2 General Methods of Molecular Imaging

MI promises significant progress in the clinical practice of oncology. It is usually performed after injecting the patient with a **Molecular Probe**, (the **Tracer**, or **Biomarker**), a biologic molecule, most of the time labeled with a radioactive atom (e.g., ^{99m}Tc, or ^{18}F etc.). This Probe is selected after detailed biological research of the target to be studied (normal cells, or abnormal cells, e.g., cancer cells), and helps to study molecular events by participating in the molecular reactions taking place within that target cell. The Probe, like a natural molecule, participates in the biological functions of the studied cells, but having been carefully and purposefully chemically altered before injection, it is not fully metabolized, like the physiologic molecules it mimics, but, instead, it finally accumulates within the cells under study, and leads finally to MI, when its concentration is high enough, by utilizing the radioactive decay of its radioactive labels.

MI of living organisms is an expanding field, which by using specific harmless biologically active molecular indicators, as explained above, tries to study specific molecular and cellular functions with imaging of normal or abnormal tissues, in living humans or animals, without danger, as well as in cell cultures. Thus, sensitivity and specificity of imaging are substantially improved and discovery of molecular characteristics of tumors and their sensitivities to drugs is enabled to improve results of diagnosis and eventually therapy of cancers.

1.2.1 External Probes

Most applications of MI are based on the introduction into the body of a living organism (usually intravenously) of a molecular Probe (the Biologic Marker or Biomarker), usually a radiolabeled diagnostic molecule of great biologic significance for the case. This Probe is specifically selected to react biologically with the target (tumor, etc.), to accumulate within the target cells at higher quantities than in the normal cells and, since it is (radio)-labeled, to allow the MI of the target with the current imaging equipment.

This Probe must not have a pharmacologic effect on the living organism and, of course, it must not be toxic in either the acute or chronic phase.

The External Probes, prior to injection, undergo specific chemical modification of their molecules. These specific modifications maintain the useful properties of the Probes while altering them in such ways that they are not completely metabolized and they accumulate locally, thus allowing imaging. The External Probes are also labeled. There are different methods of labeling these molecules, therefore there are different methods of MI: Radioisotopes = Nuclear Studies, Magnetic = MRI, Light = Optical.

After their injection, the modified and labeled External Probes enter the metabolism/function of the cell and participate to the point the modification allows, with imaging performed at the most appropriate time point for MI techniques.

1.2.2 Internal Probes

These are normal or pathologic molecules in the body that may be imaged in vivo utilizing their magnetic or other properties, or properties of the cells that carry them (fMRI, optical, etc.).

The selection and the study of the diagnostic molecular Probes currently constitute the most important effort in research for MI and Cancer therapy.

1.3 Clinical Applications of Molecular Imaging

1.3.1 Traditional Clinical Applications of MI

Single Photon and **Positron Imaging** in Oncology (Planar and Tomographic, SPECT and PET)

As mentioned above MI has been applied in oncology since the advent of Nuclear Medicine, first utilizing **Rectilinear Scanners** and later **Gamma Cameras** for planar and tomographic studies and eventually **Positron Emission Tomography (PET)**. Some work had also been done with MRI. For the nuclear studies the probes are external; for the fMRI usually internal. Characteristic examples are shown in Figs. 1.1, 1.2, 1.3.

1.3.2 Current Clinical Applications of MI

Multifunctional/Multimodality/Hybrid Imaging in Oncology (PET/CT, SPECT/CT, PET/MRI, SPECT/MRI, fMRI, etc.)

The Old In Vivo Imaging Methods (X-rays/US/MRI) are based on imaging differences in water content and differences in tissue densities or magnetic properties of Body Tissues and Tumors. They were amplified by contrast enhancement and tomography (CT) and they provide excellent anatomical images of the body and its anomalies and diseases including tumors.

Molecular Imaging begins with molecular biology, that is the study and understanding of the biological problem to be evaluated (e.g., the study of tumors). This is followed by the selection, development, and production of the **Probes**, the biologic markers. The new MI utilizes these probes for studies in vitro or in vivo (PET-SPECT-fMRI-Optical).

Despite the fact that clinically MI provides very useful information, on its own it is suboptimal in identifying the anatomic localization of the lesions. This generated the Multimodality Imaging.

A Multimodality (Hybrid) Imaging perspective, that is the combination of the old and the new imaging methods by simultaneously or sequentially performing MI and CT or MRI, is currently used to identify the exact location of the accumulation of the Molecular Probes (PET/CT, SPECT/CT, PET/MRI, etc.). This approach

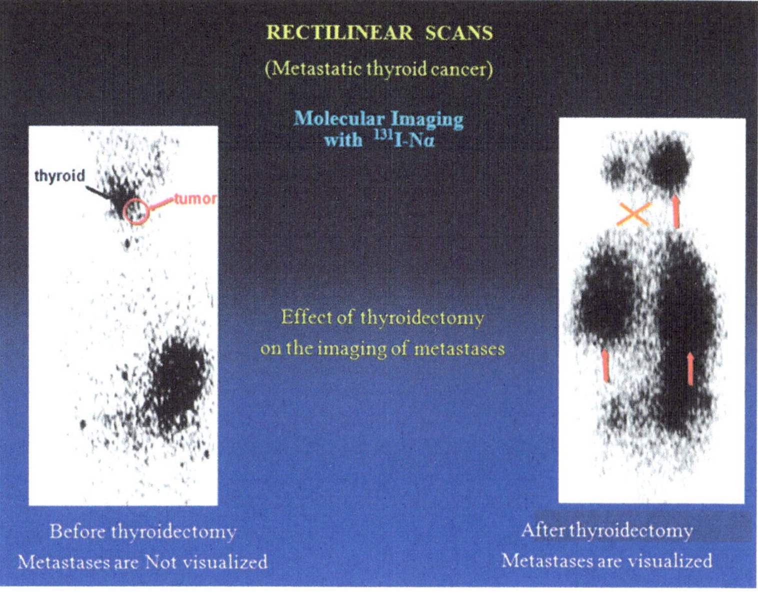

Fig. 1.1 Rectilinear scans for metastatic thyroid cancer with ^{131}I–Na. The studies were performed before and after thyroidectomy to evaluate for metastasis

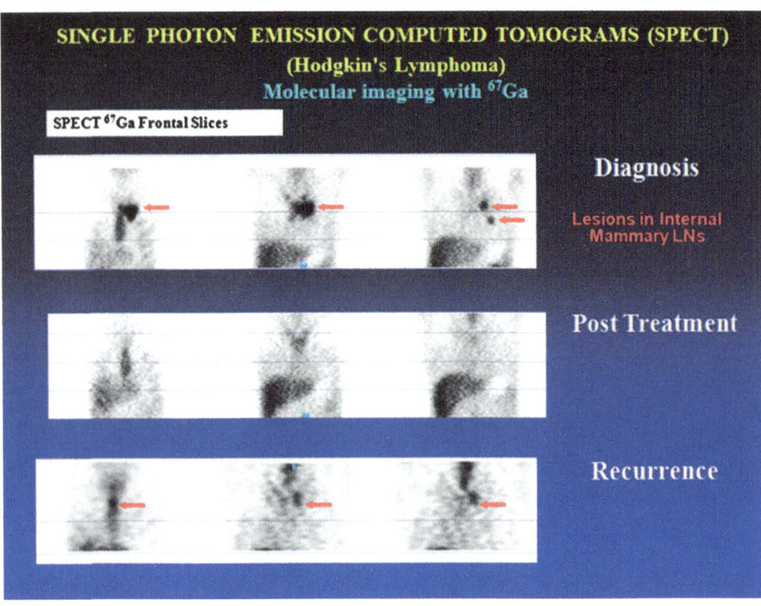

Fig. 1.2 SPECT studies with ^{67}Ga citrate in Hodgkin's lymphoma, coronal views. The studies were performed for diagnosis, treatment effect, and for recurrence

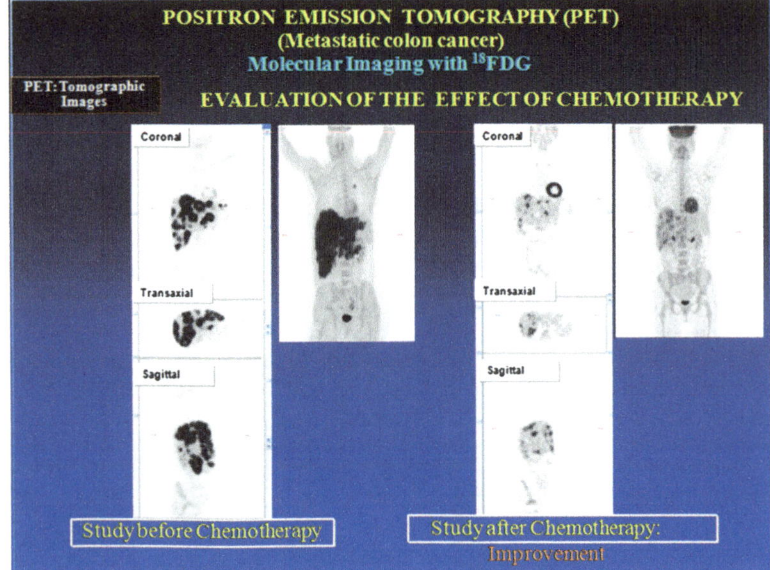

Fig. 1.3 FDG-PET studies in metastatic colon cancer. The studies were performed before and after partially effective therapy of lesions in the liver and lungs

improves the diagnosis, staging, treatment response, and restaging, by providing excellent anatomical localization of the PET findings.

Although Molecular and Hybrid Imaging can be applied to study many benign conditions, their most common clinical application is the study of malignant tumors.

Contemporary Hybrid Imaging of Cancer

1. **Morphologic Characteristics of Tumors**
The old imaging of tumors (X-rays/CT-US-MRI) is based on their size and X-ray attenuation: Masses of a specified size, orthotopic or ectopic, and destructive of organs in their vicinity.

2. **Molecular Characteristics of Cancer Cells** MI is based on molecular/biologic characteristics of the tumors as follows:

(a) Blood Flow: ^{15}O-Water
(b) Metabolism: Metabolism of Glucose (^{18}FDG-PET) and other metabolic molecules
(c) Proliferation: ^{11}C-Thymidine
(d) Hypoxia: ^{18}F-FMISO
(e) Angiogenesis: ^{18}F-Galacto-RGD
(f) Receptor Binding: Somatostatin, PSA, Transporter Imaging of cerebral cells (^{18}F-DOPA)
(g) Specific Atom or Molecule Binding Iodine ^{131}INa, ^{123}INa, ^{124}INa
(h) Mitochondrial Binding ^{201}Thallium/^{99m}Tc-Agents/^{82}Rubidium/^{67}Gallium
(i) Tumor Antigen Binding in Receptors (Antibodies)
(j) Senile Plaques ^{18}F-FDDNP
(k) Gene Expression: ^{18}F-FHBG

In clinical practice PET and SPECT were initially compared with CTs acquired at different times using the "Side by Side" approach (Fig. 1.4). The "Multimodality Imaging" or "Hybrid Imaging" emerged later and it is currently utilized for both PET/CT (Fig. 1.5), and SPECT/CT (Fig. 1.6) and it is advancing for the PET/MRI and SPECT/MRI.

The selection of the Probe for MI is based on the molecular characteristics of tumor cells.

A more detailed table of Probes is in the Seminars in Nuclear Medicine July 2011 [4].

1.3.3 Personalized Therapy of Cancer [5]

Cancer as a Genomic Problem

Cancer is a DNA aberration, a gene mutation, which leads to the genesis of the cancer cell. Same histologic tumors may be the result of different gene mutations. In the same tumor, there may originally be multiple aberrations, multiple gene mutations, which may lead to genomic differences in primary tumors of the same histology. There can also be tumor genomic changes later in the history of the specific tumor, additional gene mutations, as the tumor increases in size, metastasizes, or it is treated. These may lead to:

(a) Differences in tumor cell genomics in extensions of the (same) tumor in the same or other parts of the body

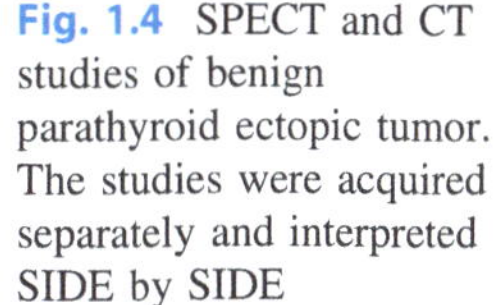

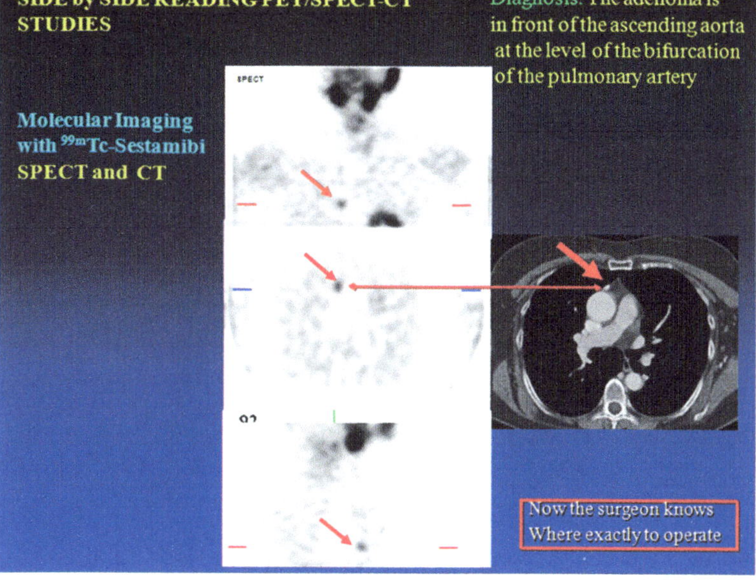

Fig. 1.4 SPECT and CT studies of benign parathyroid ectopic tumor. The studies were acquired separately and interpreted SIDE by SIDE

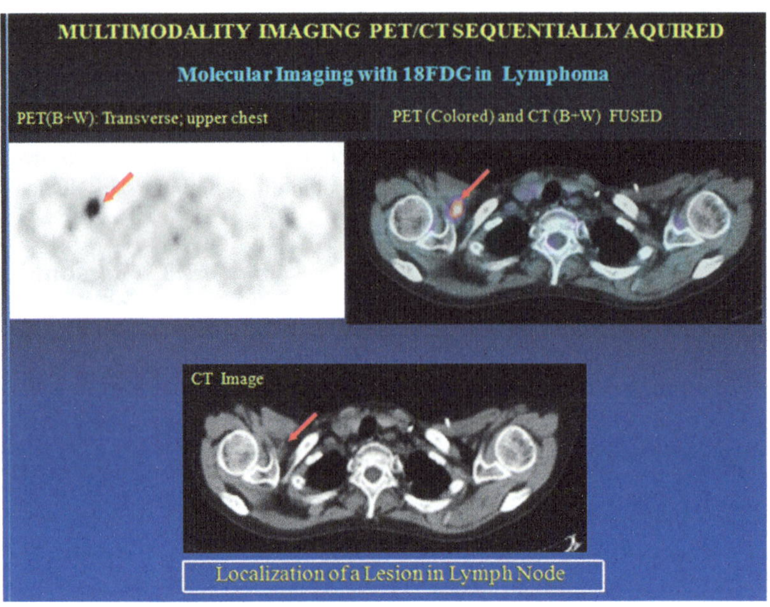

Fig. 1.5 PET/CT studies, Multimodality imaging, of malignant tumor (lymphoma). This study enabled the characterization of activity (right axilla) as due to an abnormal, enlarged (lymphomatous) lymph node

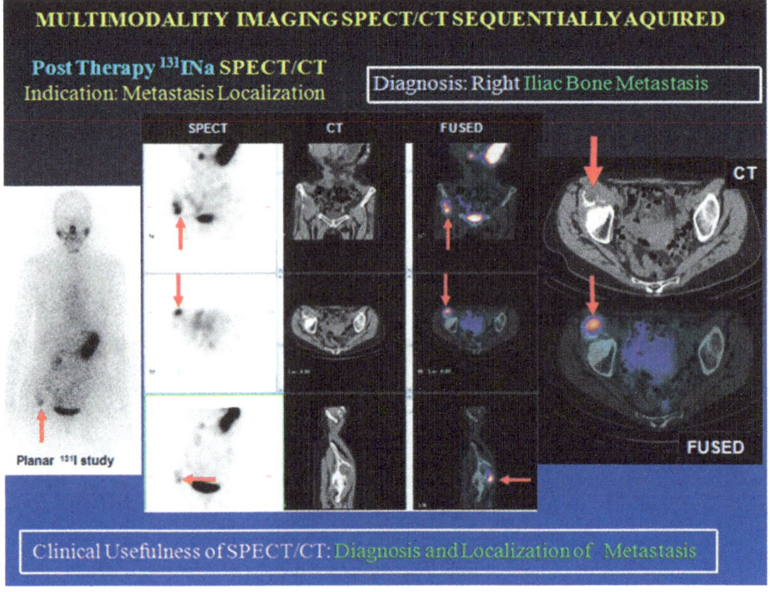

Fig. 1.6 SPECT/CT studies, Multimodality imaging of malignant metastatic thyroid tumor. This study enabled the localization of metastasis in the iliac bone

(b) Differences in genomics of metastases of same tumor to different organs and
(c) Differences in genomics of tumors as a result of therapy

Differences in cancer genomics lead to therapy issues, such that patients with the same histologic cancer may need different therapy and patients responding to therapy originally may need to change therapy for additional treatments (if there is another medicine now or discovered later).

Current Therapeutic Issues of Cancer

MI in clinical oncology progressed from the simple SPECT, PET, and fMRI to hybrid imaging (SPECT/CT, PET/CT, PET/MR, etc.), which improved substantially sensitivity and specificity of imaging tumors. However, at present oncology faces important therapeutic problems, which demand further advances in MI and the other diagnostic tests. These issues include the following:

(a) Most histologic types of cancer cannot be treated successfully.
(b) The responses of patients with the same histologic cancer to the same therapy differ.
(c) Histology by itself cannot foresee the response of the neoplasms to treatment or retreatment.

Potential solutions for these problems include the following:

(a) Continuing research for new effective therapeutic medications for cancers in general.
(b) The development of cancer genomics and new biomarkers for in vitro/vivo tumor analysis to find explanations for the differences in response to therapy of the same histologic types of tumors in different patients and in the same person/tumor.
(c) This requires the development of **Personalized Therapy** for same/different cancers.

Personalized Cancer Therapy (PCT)

Personalized Therapy was described by Sir William Osler in 1892. The current ideal is "right drug and right dose, for the right patient, the first time of therapy." The understanding of tumor biology and genomics indicates that tumors are heterogeneous: "No one size fits all." Patients with the same histologic diagnosis are not the same and the same histologic tumors cannot be treated as a single disease. The M.D. Anderson Hospital Research Experience [5] is important, as they created and built a Center for Personalized Cancer Therapy and they try to finance its function, but they foresee many difficulties.

They applied successful targeted therapies based on specific genetic aberrations that require targeted therapies: The general current basic concept is that since therapy depends on the exact molecular characteristics of the tumor, or its metastasis, as analyzed above, molecular profiling must be repeatedly performed before each therapy [6]. Tissue availability for biomarker discovery leads to core needle biopsy (CNB) of the primary tumor for molecular profiling, before deciding on the type of therapy. CNB is repeated for the metastases and if there is progression of the tumor after the original treatment. Certainly there is a need to verify with biomarkers the uniform existence inside the tumor and its metastasis of the molecular profiling as well as its uniform persistence in vivo. This is usually performed with MI. For this reason it is necessary to develop agents for specific biomarker imaging.

Personalized Cancer Therapy Requirements

Cancer Centers should develop and repeatedly offer to their patients the following applications:

(a) The ability to perform and obtain the diagnosis of the genomic characteristics of cancer cells, originally and repeatedly.
(b) To be able to verify with biomarkers their uniform existence inside the tumor and their uniform persistence in vivo (MI).

This way personalized therapy of cancers of the same histology will develop and (due to differences in tumor cell genomics in the same cancer, even in the same patient) repeated treatments of the same histologic cancer may need to be different.

On the basis of the above, the following should be developed:

(a) Establish the clinical necessity for personalized therapy.
(b) Discover biomarkers for in vitro/in vivo MI.
(c) Integrate imaging (PET-SPECT/CT-MRI, Other)

Tasks for Molecular and Hybrid Imaging

The effort should commence by identifying the differences in tumor DNA in patients with the same histologic tumor and between the primary and metastatic tumors as well as tumors post-therapies in each individual patient and by studying the genomics of multiple biopsies of the tumors. Next it should be found how these differences in genomics are expressed as molecular/cellular structural/functional characteristics of the cells of the tumor in each biopsy

(a) Membrane receptor specific characteristics
(b) Nucleus different structure/functions
(c) Protoplasm protein characteristics
(d) Organelle specific activators or suppressors

Probes should be developed to study those differences, first in vitro and later in vivo with MI.

Research should be performed for effective therapies, which can be preselected with the probes and MI, for the primary tumor and for metastases.

Finally, for clinical and financial reasons, it should be proven that these therapies are preferable to traditional cancer treatments.

Current Experience in Applying PCT

The experience in clinical practice regarding PCT is thus far good but not very impressive. Very little progress has been achieved in identifying individual patient tumor genomics and only a small number of patients have so far benefited from PCT.

However, PCT is promising and needs support and continuing research. It has great potential in the therapy of many types of cancer, yet many promising drugs have produced disappointing results. There are many challenges that must be addressed to advance the field. There are proposals for future trials:

1. Perform clinical trials requiring biopsies to obtain relevant tumor specimens for tumor genomic findings.
2. Adapt novel statistical designs.
3. Develop appropriate Biomarkers (BMs, that is Probes) to help guide the selection of the best treatment for each case with MI or other approach.
4. Go beyond BMs based on single mutations:
   (a) Use BMs based on gene expression or protein expression signatures
   (b) Use new imaging technologies for new improved BMs.
   (c) Resolve existing challenges impeding the rapid identification and translation of validated BMs with clinically acceptable sensitivity and specificity, from the in vitro laboratory to the clinic (human trials, MI), like limitations of current BM development methodologies and regulatory and reimbursement (funding) policies and practices.

Current Specific Studies in Applying PCT

Clinical research and experience using PET-SPECT/CT-MRI Imaging with Radiolabeled old and new Biomarkers is currently active [7], including the following:

1. Membrane receptor-based imaging
2. Glucose metabolism
3. DNA synthesis
4. Hypoxia
5. Integrins.

Future Directions

There are Hopes, Expectations, and Progresses to emerge from these efforts but also new and unforeseen Problems.

References

1. Massoud TF, Gambir SS (2003) Molecular imaging in living subjects: seeing fundamental biological processes in a new light. Genes Dev 17(5):545–580

2. Gambir SS (2008) Molecular Imaging of Cancer: From Molecules to Humans. J Nucl Me (49). Suppl 2:1–4
3. Henry N, Wagner Jr (2006) A Personal History of Nuclear Medicine. Springer-Verlag, London
4. Vallabhajosula S, Solnes L, Vallabhajosula B et al (2011) A broad overview of PET Radiopharmaceuticals and clinical applications: What is new? Sem Nucl Med 4:246–264
5. Homer Macapinlac (2011) MI in Clinical Oncology (Imaging guided Personalized Therapy): iiCME: Multimodality Imaging: PET/CT and SPECT/CT
6. Wistuba II, Gelovani JG, Jacoby JJ et al (2011) Methodological and practical challenges for personalized cancer therapies. Nat Rev Clin Oncol 8(3):135–141
7. Sohn HJ, Yang YJ, Ryu JS et al (2008) Clin Cancer Res 14:7423–7429

Imaging Criteria for Tumor Treatment Response Evaluation

2

Arkadios Chr. Rousakis and John A. Andreou

The evaluation of the tumor response to therapy represents a significant and continuously expanding part of the radiological practice, especially in services with oncological departments. The modern imaging modalities are valuable tools for objective quantitative assessment of the result of new antineoplastic therapeutic schemes. The standardization of criteria provides common endpoints for clinical trials, permits comparisons between different studies, facilitates the formation of more effective therapies and accelerates the procedure of approval of new drugs by the authorized organizations. The most widely used imaging criterion of a successful therapy is the shrinkage of the neoplastic lesions in a certain patient. It represents the typical endpoint in phase II trials, targeted to the preliminary evaluation of the effectiveness of new antineoplastic drugs in order to decide if these have to be further tested in wider clinical studies. Also, the objective criterion of "tumor shrinkage" and the duration of "progression free survival " (PFS) represent the commonest endpoints for phase III clinical trials, aiming to assess the benefit of applying one or more therapeutic schemes in specific patient populations.

In parallel, the degree of shrinkage of the total tumor burden is widely used in the routine oncological practice in order to assess the therapeutic result in every patient and guide decisions for further clinical management. However, it has to be noted that the most important proof of an effective antineoplastic therapy is the improvement of clinical symptoms and overall survival.

2.1 The Response Evaluation Criteria of the World Health Organization

The first organized attempt for introducing standardized criteria for assessing tumor response, mostly for use in phase II trials, appeared in 1981 through a working group of experts under the auspices of the World Health Organization (WHO). According to the methodology proposed by the "WHO guidelines", in a patient with neoplastic disease the maximum diameter and the greater diameter perpendicular to the previous had to be measured on each neoplastic lesion, providing a numeric product. The sum of the products of all the neoplastic lesions represents the objective criterion of the measurable tumor burden, and its changes during and at the end of therapy permit the assessment of tumor response [1].

During the following two decades, the WHO criteria were adopted by many research groups and pharmaceutical companies and used in

A. Chr. Rousakis (✉) · J. A. Andreou
Radiology, Hygeia Hospital, 4 Erythrou Stavrou, 15123 Marousi, Attica, Greece
e-mail: a.rousakis@hygeia.gr

A. D. Gouliamos et al. (eds.), *Imaging in Clinical Oncology*,
DOI: 10.1007/978-88-470-5385-4_2, © Springer-Verlag Italia 2014

numerous phase II and III trials. However, the remarks that arose from their use and the wide application of new imaging modalities imposed the need for modifications, in order to overcome some imperfections and ambiguities of the initial guidelines. An international working group of experts was constituted in 1994, in order to reevaluate and modify the WHO criteria.

2.2 The Response Evaluation Criteria in Solid Tumors

Based on the proposals of the previously mentioned working group, finally the WHO, the National Cancer Institute of USA and the European Organization for the Research and Therapy of Cancer (EORTC), adopted in 2000 new guidelines, named Response Evaluation Criteria In Solid Tumors (RECIST) [2]. They incorporated the use of new imaging technologies that have appeared, matured, and gained wide clinical application, such as spiral computed tomography (CT) and Magnetic Resonance Imaging (MRI).

With RECIST, the terms of "measurable" and "non-measurable" disease were more clearly defined. Also, the procedure for selecting the most representative neoplastic lesions that have to be measured and followed ("target lesions") was better described. Specifically, it was defined that the "target lesions" must be selected among the largest, be representative of all the organs affected by the neoplasia and should not be more than ten (10) in total and five (5) per organ. The measurement of the size of "target lesions" was simplified, by taking into account only the greater transverse diameter of each lesion and not the product of two perpendicular diameters as with WHO criteria. Additionally, the term of "non target lesions" was introduced and the way of evaluating their changes was described. Finally, the methodology of assessing the "overall response" to therapy was more clearly defined.

The RECIST has been widely adopted by academic institutions, medical research groups, and pharmaceutical companies and were applied in trials where the main endpoints were the "objective response to therapy" or the "time-to-progression" of the disease. The simplification of the measurement methodology did not seem to influence the reliability of RECIST, compared to WHO criteria. However, together with the wider acceptance and application of RECIST, problems and imperfections were noted regarding their use for evaluation of specific neoplasms, such as pleural mesothelioma and tumors of childhood. Also, the decrease of the number of target lesions, the evaluation of abnormally enlarged lymph nodes, the substitution of unidimensional by three-dimensional (3D) measurement, and the incorporation of newer imaging modalities (providing molecular and "functional" imaging), were proposed.

In order to address all these issues, a new RECIST working group was constituted, including clinical doctors experienced in the development and evaluation of new drugs, representing academic sites, state health organizations, and the pharmaceutical industry, together with imaging specialists and statisticians. The group evaluated the database of EORTC, including more than 6,500 patients with more than 18,000 target lesions, and its work resulted in the first revision of RECIST 1.1, published in 2009.

2.3 The Revision 1.1 of RECIST [3]

2.3.1 Aim of Guideline RECIST 1.1

It was defined as the introduction of a new standardized procedure of measuring the extent of solid tumors and a methodology of objective evaluation of its changes, for use in clinical trials concerning neoplasias both of adulthood and childhood. It was, also, stated that it may be applied in trials for brain gliomas, although there are other criteria in wider use [4] (see Sect. III-CNS Tumors). Additionally, it was clarified that this guideline is not proposed for use in trials assessing the response of malignant lymphomas, where other widely accepted guidelines are considered to be more appropriate [5] (see section VI-Lymphoma).

Although there were proposals of incorporating the use of 3D volumetric measurements of the neoplastic lesions and of functional techniques (such as ^{18}F-FDG-PET, dynamic contrast-enhanced CT, dynamic, and functional MRI techniques), it was judged that there is still not efficient standardization nor wide availability of these modalities in order to be adopted into the frame of a general official guideline. However, ^{18}F-FDG-PET has been officially accepted as a complementary method of assessing the extent and progression of some specific neoplasias, in terms of special therapeutic protocols (see Sects. I, IV, VI, IX, XII).

2.3.2 Assessment of Measurable Tumor Burden

A neoplastic disease affecting a specific patient is defined as "measurable" if it includes at least one "measurable lesion". To consider a lesion as measurable, it must be possible to define with accuracy its greatest diameter and this should be at least 10 mm on the transverse CT or MRI slices (given that the slice thickness is ≤5 mm) (Fig. 2.1a, b). Although conventional radiographs are nowadays very rarely used for therapy assessment (e.g., in lung tumors), RECIST guideline implies that a measurable lesion on them has to be ≥20 mm. Regarding the lymph nodes (its measurement was first introduced in the RECIST 1.1 edition), in order to be characterized as abnormally enlarged and "measurable", their short axis diameter must be ≥15 mm on transverse CT slices (given the slice thickness is ≤5 mm). It has to be noted that only the short axis diameter of the affected lymph nodes has to measured, since it has been shown that it offers more reproducible measurements than the long axis (Fig. 2.1c).

All measurements should be performed using the "metric system", in centimeters (cm) or millimeters (mm), and on the transverse plane, with the exception of some neoplasias where, due to their growth pattern, the measurement is more representative when performed on the sagittal or coronal plane (as in cases of paraspinal tumors). In any case, repeat measurements during follow-up studies should always be performed on the same imaging plane.

As "non-measurable" are considered all the remaining lesions, including those with a maximum long axis transverse diameter <10 mm, enlarged lymph nodes with a short axis diameter ≥10 mm but <15 mm and, also, all the tiny and difficult-to-be-measured foci. The latter include: leptomeningeal disease, ascites, pleural or pericardial effusion, inflammatory breast cancer, carcinomatous lymphangitis of the lung or skin, abdominal masses which are clinically detectable but not amenable to reproducible measurements with the currently recommended imaging techniques (Fig. 2.1d).

According to the RECIST 1.1 guidelines, secondary deposits to the bones cannot be reliably measured by means of bone scanning, ^{18}F-FDG-PET or radiographs. However, it is estimated that these imaging modalities can be used to assess the presence or elimination of the bone lesions. It is, also, clarified that secondary deposits to the bones of lytic or mixed type which are accompanied by CT or MRI detectable soft tissue masses, may be considered as "measurable" lesions if the accompanying soft tissue mass fulfills the definition described above (Fig. 2.1e). Sclerotic bone lesions are by definition "non-measurable".

Neoplastic lesions previously treated (e.g., with radiotherapy), may be considered as measurable, only if the presence of active disease in them was previously established with biopsy or cytology.

2.3.3 Evaluation of Response to Therapy [3, 6–8]

During the first (baseline) examination, which has to be performed within 4 weeks before starting therapy, it is imperative to assess accurately the total tumor burden, in order to have a reference of comparison for the new measurements during follow-up.

After assessing the presence of "measurable disease" (as defined previously) in a certain patient, the next step is to define "target" and

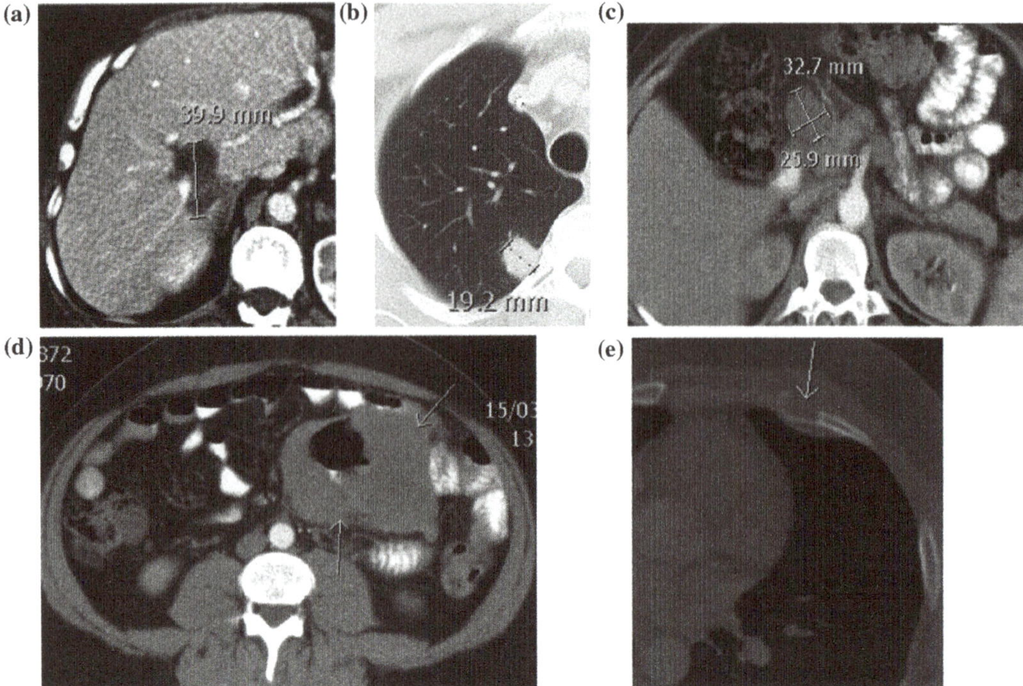

Fig. 2.1 Measurable disease: "target" and "non-target" lesions. Selected images from a CT scan of thorax and abdomen, performed in terms of the baseline examination of a patient with metastatic melanoma of the skin, before the initiation of chemotherapy. Two secondary deposits at the *right* hepatic lobe (**a**) and *right* upper pulmonary lobe (**b**) are shown, which have a maximum transverse diameter >1 cm and, hence, they fulfill the criteria to be defined as "measurable lesions" and be selected as "target lesions". The maximum diameters of these two lesions (4 cm and 1.9 cm, respectively) will be incorporated in the "total sum of diameters" of all target lesions. Also, an abnormally enlarged lymph node is depicted in the abdomen (**c**) which has a short axis transverse diameter of 2.6 cm (>1.5 cm); consequently, it can also be selected as a "target-lesion". In the "total sum of diameters" of target lesions, the short axis diameter of 2.6 cm (not the long axis diameter of 3.3 cm!) of the lymph node must be encountered. On image (**d**), the largest secondary deposit in this patient is shown, located in the small bowel wall. However, despite its large size, this lesion is not recommended to be selected as "target-lesion", since its location on the bowel wall makes its appearance on transverse slices unstable and, hence, the corresponding measurements of its diameter during the follow-up studies will lack reproducibility. On the image (**e**), a small lytic secondary deposit in the anterior part of a left rib is depicted (*arrow*), with a small accompanying soft tissue mass <1 cm, which is considered as a "non-measurable" lesion

"non-target" lesions. According to RECIST 1.1 guidelines, as "target lesions" are selected up to five measurable lesions per patient (while in the initial RECIST guideline they could be up to 10). These must be selected in order to be representative of all the organs affected by the neoplasia and, generally, should not exceed two lesions per organ (while in the initial RECIST, they could be selected up to five target lesions per organ). The selection criteria of target lesions are their size (the larger lesions in each organ should be chosen) and their suitability for reproducible repetitive measurements (Fig. 2.1a, b, d). It is advised to prefer non-cystic lesions, instead of cystic or necrotic. Also, they have to be representative of all organs affected by the tumor. In each follow-up (CT or MRI) examination, the longest diameter of each target lesion has to be measured on the transverse slice and with the direction that reflects better its size (Fig. 2.1a, b). If a target lesion separates during follow-up into more than one fragments, the sum of the longest diameters of these fragments has to be measured (Fig. 2.2). In the case that two adjacent target lesions coalesce (without leaving a plane of normal tissue between them), then the longest diameter of the new lesion has to be measured (Fig. 2.3). If a target lesion becomes, during follow-up, too small to be measured accurately, its diameter that will be added to the sum is advised to be, by default, 5 mm.

Enlarged lymph nodes with a short axis diameter ≥15 mm can also be selected as target lesions (Fig. 2.1c). On follow-up studies, if the maximum short-axis diameter of a "target nodal lesion" reduces below 10 mm, this is no longer considered pathologic but it still has to be measured on future studies in order to assess a possible progression.

After selecting and recording the target lesions, the sum of the largest long axis diameters of all the non-nodal lesions and the short axis diameters of the selected lymph nodes, has to be calculated. During follow-up, the changes of this "sum of diameters" provide the measure for assessing the objective response of the neoplastic disease to therapy. It is important that the same target lesions (initially selected on the baseline examination) have to be measured on every follow-up examination. For all the remaining measurable lesions, which were not selected as target lesions (including, also, all the enlarged lymph nodes with a short-axis diameter 10–15 mm), there is no need to measure their diameters during follow-up, but simply to record on each examination their presence or absence or any "unequivocal increase of their extent". Based on these changes, the response of the "non-target" lesions is assumed. The final judgment concerning the "overall response" must take into account both the "target" and "non-target" lesions and, also, the appearance or not of new lesions during follow-up. It has to be noted that, in order to categorize a patient case as "stable disease" (SD) or "progressive disease" (PD), one must not use as reference the measurements of the baseline examination but, instead, the measurements of the examination where the smallest "sum of diameters" was encountered (occasionally, this examination could be the baseline one).

There are not strict guidelines regarding the frequency of follow-up examinations. However, it is generally recommended to perform follow-up studies at the end of each chemotherapy cycle (usually every 6–8 weeks), at least

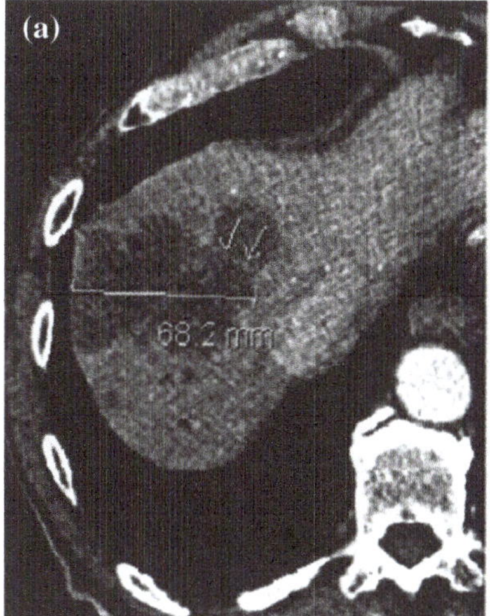

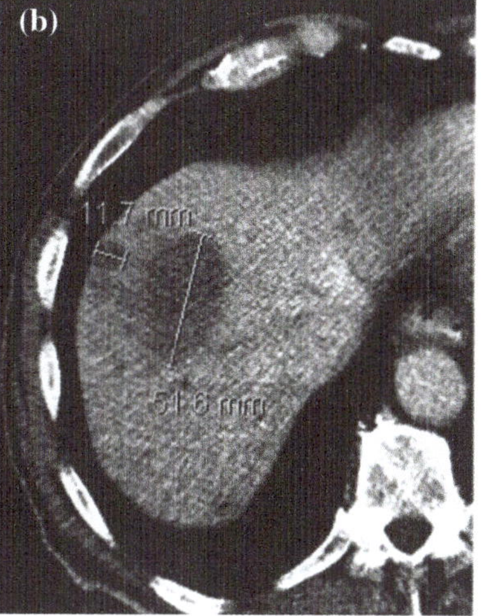

Fig. 2.2 Splitting lesions. On a CT image (**a**) a metastatic "target" lesion in the liver is shown, with a maximum diameter of 68.2 mm, which is separated from another adjacent lesion by a thin line of normal-appearing liver parenchyma (*arrows*). On follow-up CT (**b**), after effective chemotherapy, the previous lesion has split in two smaller adjacent lesions, clearly separated by normal-appearing liver tissue. Eventually, the longest transverse diameters of the two resulting lesions (51.6 and 11.7 mm) must be added in the sum of diameters of target lesions

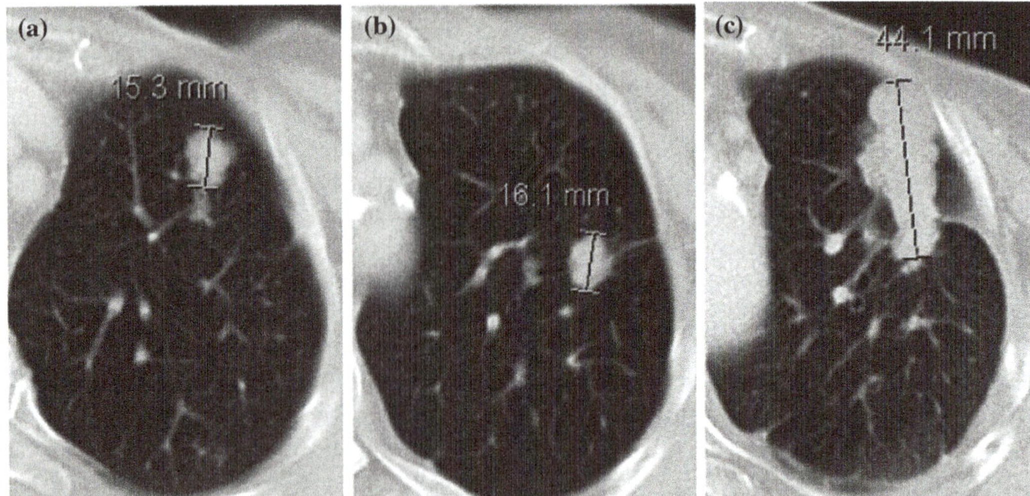

Fig. 2.3 Coalescent lesions. Two secondary deposits, selected as target lesions, in the *left upper* pulmonary lobe (**a**, **b**) have increased in size on the follow-up CT (**c**) and merged in a larger lesion. The largest transverse diameter of the latter must now be added in the sum of diameters of target lesions

in terms of phase II trials where the benefit of the therapy is unknown. The assessment of the "overall response to therapy" is performed on the results of the final examination at the end of therapy.

Evaluation of the Response of "Target-Lesions'

According to RECIST 1.1, the definitions on which the response evaluation is based are as follows:

Complete Response (CR): disappearance of all target-lesions. Additionally, every previously enlarged lymph node must have a decreased short axis diameter not exceeding 10 mm.

Partial Response (PR): decrease of the baseline "sum of diameters" of the target-lesions ≥30 %.

Progressive Disease (PD): increase of the "sum of diameters" of the target lesions of at least 20 % in comparison to the smallest value of this sum that was encountered during the whole period of the study (including the baseline sum). Additionally, the "sum of diameters of target lesions" must have shown an absolute increase of at least 5 mm (this criterion was not included in the first RECIST guideline).

Stable Disease (SD): changes of the "sum of diameters of target lesions" which do not fulfill the criteria for PR or PD (Fig. 2.4).

It must be noted that RECIST 1.1 includes detailed instructions concerning the methodology of measurement of target lesions, on the baseline and the follow-up imaging studies.

Evaluation of the Response of "Non-Target" Lesions

Non-target lesions must be evaluated only qualitatively (present, absent, or unequivocally larger), even if their diameters seem to be measurable. The corresponding criteria and definitions for response evaluation are as follows:

Complete Response (CR): disappearance of all the non-target lesions. All lymph nodes must have a short-axis diameter <10 mm. Additionally, tumor marker levels must be within normal limits.

Progressive Disease (PD): unequivocal increase of the size/extent of preexisting non-target lesions (Fig. 2.5).

Non-CR/non-PD: residual one or more non-target lesions and/or tumor markers measured above the normal levels.

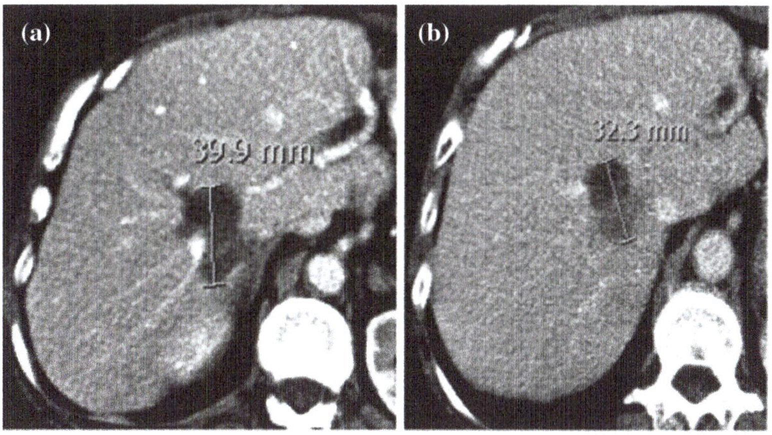

Fig. 2.4 Stable disease. Secondary deposit to the liver, from skin melanoma. On a transverse image from a baseline contrast-enhanced CT, performed before chemotherapy, the maximum diameter of the hepatic lesion is measured 4 cm (**a**). On the corresponding image of the follow-up CT study, performed after one cycle of chemotherapy (**b**), the maximum diameter of this "target lesion" is measured 3.2 cm. The 20 % decrease of the maximum diameter of the lesion does not accomplish the definition of partial response (it should be at least 30 %). Consequently, the status of this specific lesion has to be assessed as "stable disease"

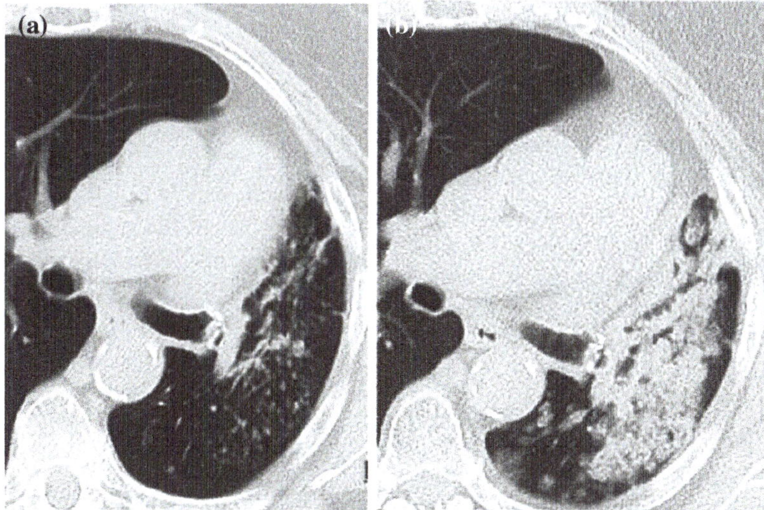

Fig. 2.5 Non-measurable disease, unequivocal progression. A slice from a thorax CT scan (**a**) of a patient with previous left upper lobectomy (due to lung cancer), shows multiple micronodular secondary deposits measuring only a few mm each, at the left lower lobe. Due to their tiny size, they are classified as "non-measurable disease". On the corresponding CT slice of the follow-up examination (**b**) a significant increase of the number and size of the lesions is observed, many of which coalesce, forming a large ill-defined mass. This change obviously represents an "unequivocal progression" of the disease

The RECIST 1.1 includes clarifications concerning the "unequivocal progression" of non-target lesions and guidelines for the methodology of evaluating response in patients with only "non-measurable" disease, since such patients may be included in the population of phase III clinical trials. In cases where non-target lesions show unequivocal increase (PD), while target lesions show PR or SD, the overall response is assessed as PD only if the progression of non-target lesions seems to increase substantially the overall tumor burden. A mild to moderate increase of only few non-target lesions, while the other lesions (target and non-target) show SD or PR, is not considered sufficient to change the overall response assessment to PD.

Evaluation of New Lesions

The appearance of new malignant lesions indicates PD, given that these are unequivocal, meaning not depended on the imaging modality and its technique and do not represent a false diagnosis. All the previous are very important, especially when the lesions (target and non-target) of baseline examination show PR or CR.

A lesion detected during follow-up at an anatomic area that was not included in the baseline study, it has to be considered by definition as "new lesion" indicating PD. For that reason, the protocol of each trial must provide to include in the baseline study all the anatomic areas that may be potentially affected by the specific neoplasia. If it is not certain that a new lesion represents neoplasia, its nature must be clarified during the follow-up.

Although ^{18}F-FDG-PET is not included in the basic imaging modalities proposed by RECIST 1.1, it could be used in selected cases as an additional method to confirm new lesions and verify cases of PD. According to the algorithm defined by this guideline, if a ^{18}F-FDG-PET scan performed during follow-up becomes positive while a baseline ^{18}F-FDG-PET was negative, this represents PD. If there is no available baseline ^{18}F-FDG-PET scan, but such a study performed during follow-up is positive for new sites of the disease, this situation is determined as PD only in the case that the new lesions are detectable by CT either at the same time-point (but not at baseline CT) or later during the following imaging studies [3, 7].

Assessment of the Best Overall Response

Best Overall Response (BOR) is defined as the best response encountered since the beginning of the evaluated therapy, till its completion. It is influenced by the changes of target and non-target lesions and by the appearance or not of new lesions. The methodology of evaluating BOR is described in detail in RECIST 1.1 guideline. As previously stated, depending on the type of the trial and the demands of its protocol, there may be a need for confirmation of this evaluation. Specifically, confirmation of a PR or CR with new imaging studies after at least 4 weeks, is required only in non-randomized trials in which objective response is the primary endpoint. It has to be noted that, according to RECIST 1.1, lesions must show larger increase to be categorized as PD, compared to WHO and RECIST 1.0 guideline [7, 8].

2.3.4 Recommendations and Guidelines for Performing Imaging Examinations

The recent RECIST 1.1 edition includes an appendix, where basic guidelines for the standardization of performing imaging studies, mainly CT and MRI, are offered. According to these guidelines, it is preferable to use systems of latest technology (such as multi-slice CT scanners), adequate and standardized scanning technique, protocols with reduced radiation dose and appropriate contrast media at the proper dose and way of administration [3, 6].

Computed Tomography (CT)

It is defined as the basic imaging study for the follow-up of patients with most types of neoplastic disease and for the assessment of therapeutic result. Significant issues are the full coverage of the possible anatomic extent of the disease, the slice thickness, the slice gap and the proper use of contrast media.

The baseline CT examination should cover all the anatomic areas of possible spread of the specific tumor. It is noted that the maximum diameter of a target lesion must be measured only on the transverse plane. In case of using a CT scanner of spiral of multislice technology, which is the common practice nowadays, a target lesion must have a minimum transverse diameter of at least 10 mm, given that the CT slices are reconstructed with a slice thickness ≤5 mm and without gap. The aim of this rule is to reduce the effect of "partial volume averaging" which may lead to underestimation of the size of a lesion. All the above are applicable to most anatomic areas and specifically to thoracic, abdominal, and pelvic lesions. Regarding the anatomic areas where the typical thickness of CT slices is less than 5 mm (e.g., the neck) and, also, patients with small size and children, the smaller transverse diameter of a measurable lesion in order to be selected as "target lesion" may vary according to the rule of "twice the slice thickness".

According to RECIST 1.1, the administration of diluted contrast medium per os is recommended in all CT scans of abdomen and pelvis.

The intravenous (IV) administration of iodinated contrast medium is recommended even in types of neoplasia where the data from studies do not favor such use. However, it is also noted that the IV contrast medium (CM) can be avoided when only a specific lesion in the lung is followed. It is obvious that IV use of CM must be avoided in cases of patients with allergy to iodine or renal insufficiency. However, RECIST 1.1 does not include specific guidelines concerning the optimal dose, the way of IV administration (with power injector or manually) and the flow rate of the CM. It is simply stated that this must be performed with adequate manner. The recent RECIST 1.1 edition incorporates additional recommendations concerning the examination protocol of liver and solid viscera of the abdomen after bolus IV injection of CM. Specifically, in most neoplasias a single post-contrast scanning at portal venous phase is considered to be efficient. A triphasic study (one scan before and two scans after bolus IV injection of CM, at arterial and portal venous phase) is recommended specifically for the hepatocellular cancer and the neuroendocrine tumors. If the IV use of iodinated CM is contraindicated in a patient, usually due to allergy or renal insufficiency that were previously known or appeared during the survey, it must be decided if the follow-up studies will be performed with noncontrast-enhanced CT or, alternatively, with MRI.

Magnetic Resonance Imaging (MRI)

According to RECIST 1.1, MRI may be used as an alternative to CT for measurements in most neoplasias, excluding those involving the lungs. It is well known that the clinical applications of MRI in oncological imaging are continuously expanding since the first edition of RECIST, while it is also considered as examination of choice or first-line in some specific neoplasias, like in children and young adults. Specifically, in childhood neoplasias, MRI offers better estimation of the extent of the disease (paraspinal/intracanalicular neuroblastoma is a typical example) and it does not involve the use of potentially harmful radiation.

It has to be noted that the measurements must always be performed on the same imaging plane (preferably on the transverse) and, if possible, the serial examinations must be done in magnets of the same type and with the same or similar pulse sequences. In general, the use of magnets of different power must be avoided during follow-up studies. The recent RECIST 1.1 edition does not include detailed guidelines regarding the specific parameters of the pulse sequences. It is simply recommended to use standardized T1-W and T2-W sequences, with and without fat suppression, before and after IV injection of paramagnetic contrast medium, which have to be suitable for each anatomic area studied and also, for the type of MR system used.

The size criteria for selecting "measurable" and "target" lesions depend on the slice thickness of the images as it is previously described in detail in the section for CT.

Ultrasonography (US)

According to RECIST 1.1 guideline, US must not be systematically used for evaluating the response of tumors to therapy, with the exception of superficially located lesions. This guideline is based on the fact that US is not an objective examination, since it is operator-dependent. Additionally, US do not provide reproducible images, adequate for future reevaluation.

Positron Emission Tomography (PET)

Although the use of PET in some types of neoplasia (such as lymphomas, non-small cell lung cancer-NSCLC- and melanoma) is already established and continuously expanding, the expert authors of RECIST 1.1 guideline estimated that there are still no standardized criteria which can permit the full incorporation of this modality (usually performed in combination with CT, in terms of the "hybrid" examination PET/CT) in the protocols of phase II clinical trials. However, it is a fact that PET/CT is frequently used in studies evaluating the effectiveness of new antineoplastic drugs. For that reason, RECIST 1.1 authors accept the use of FDG-PET as a complementary tool for assessing PR or PD.

2.3.5 Limitations of RECIST 1.1

The measurement of the size of a neoplastic lesion is a time-consuming procedure, susceptible to systematic and statistical errors, mainly due to interobserver and intraobserver variability regarding the estimation of the lesion borders. This may be particularly difficult in cases of lesions with irregular shape and spiculated borders or in small lesions and may eventually lead to a false categorization of the response (Fig. 2.6). Although RECIST 1.1 revision has addressed many of these issues, there are still sources of discrepancies in clinical practice. In terms of phase II trials, these causes of variability and inaccuracy may be counterbalanced or even eliminated through the use of independent evaluators, who reassess the data of measurements that were performed by the radiologists of the centers included in such studies.

Single center studies have shown that 3D volumetric measurements, using semi-automated or automated software, permit more accurate and reproducible assessment of the size of neoplastic lesions and its changes, compared to unidimensional measurements of RECIST and bidimensional measurements of WHO criteria. However, due to the variety and limited availability of such software tools which preclude their wide use, they were not incorporated in the RECIST 1.1 guideline [6, 9].

Some tumors, due to their growth pattern and shape, may be practically impossible to be measured with a reproducible manner. Malignant mesothelioma of the pleura represents a typical example of a neoplasia where the previously described methodology of RECIST 1.1 is not suitable. According to relative studies, it has been shown that the particular growth pattern and anatomical extension of this neoplasia can be more accurately assessed by measuring, on the selected transverse CT slices, the maximum diameter of the pleural lesions that is perpendicular to the adjacent part of the pleura, instead of the maximum longitudinal diameter according to RECIST 1.1 (Fig. 2.7). The evaluation of the size of other measurable lesions of the mesothelioma except of pleural lesions, including infiltrated lymph nodes, is performed according to the guidelines of RECIST 1.1 and the corresponding measurements are added to the sum of diameters of pleural lesions. The total sum of these diameters is counted and its changes, during the follow-up studies and at the end of therapy, represent the criterion for evaluating the response of mesothelioma to therapy. However, there are still problems and inconsistencies regarding the standardization of the methodology of measuring the lesions of pleural mesothelioma, which impose the need for accurate description of the way of selecting and evaluating measurable and target lesions in the protocol of each study targeted on this type of neoplasia [10].

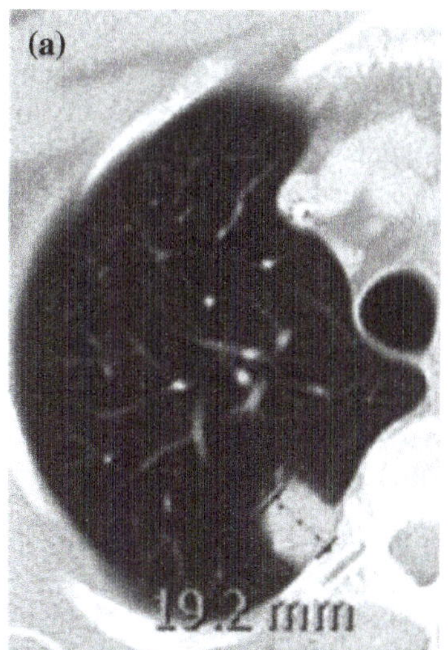

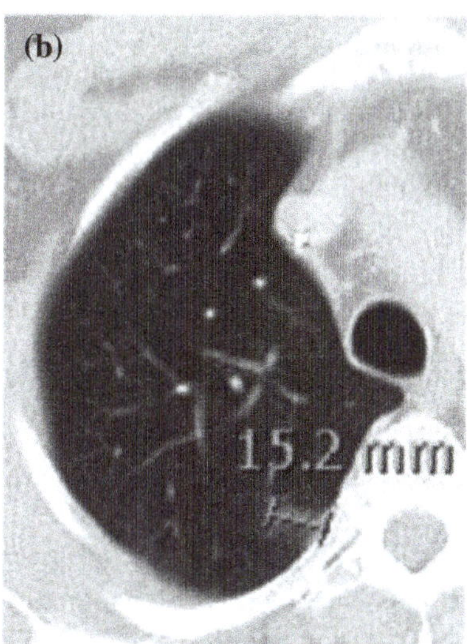

Fig. 2.6 Limitations of RECIST 1.1. CT of the thorax of a patient with metastatic melanoma at the right upper pulmonary lobe. Before initiation of the therapy (**a**) the maximum transverse diameter of this ovoid solid lesion is 19.2 mm. After completion of chemotherapy, on the corresponding CT slice the lesion shows almost complete regression, with only a faint ill-defined soft tissue lesion remaining. This has a maximum transverse diameter of 15.2 mm and could be attributed to scar tissue, not necessarily residual disease. By strictly implementing the measurement methodology of RECIST 1.1, the maximum diameter of the lesion has decreased by 21 % (from 19.2 to 15.2 mm) a change that typically corresponds to "stable disease". However, taking into account the overall appearance and 3D dimensions of the lesion, the decrease of its volume is obviously very significant, almost reaching the limits of Complete Response, especially if the absence of active disease in it could be verified

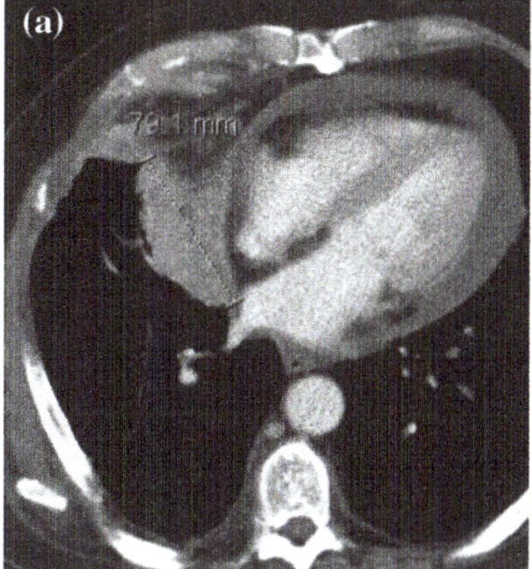

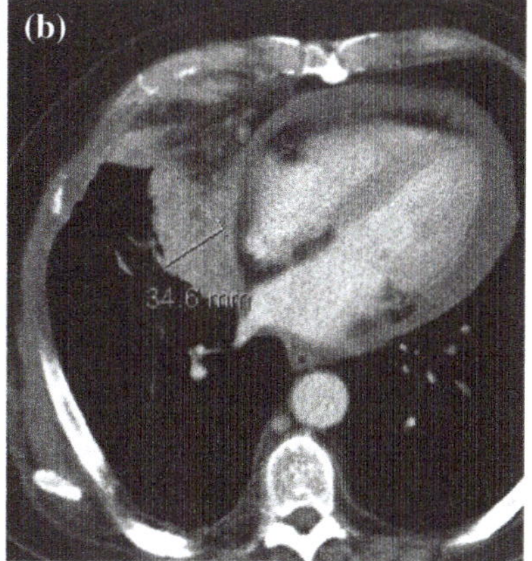

Fig. 2.7 Methodology for measuring on CT images the size of lesions of malignant mesothelioma. According to the general RECIST 1.1 guideline, on each area of pleural thickening that is selected as "target lesion" the longest transverse diameter should be measured (**a**). However, according to the modified RECIST criteria for mesothelioma (mRECIST), on each lesion the maximum diameter being perpendicular to the adjacent pleural segment has to be measured (**b**)

Another issue is the differentiation of neoplastic lesions from surrounding fibrosis or normal tissue, which in some cases may be difficult or even impossible based only on CT and MRI findings. If this differentiation is crucial for assessing CR, the ambiguous tissue must be sampled by core biopsy or fine needle aspiration and then characterized with histopathological or cytological examination, respectively. In this effort, ^{18}F-FDG-PET may be helpful in selected cases [3, 6–8]. However, both procedures have limitations regarding sensitivity and overall accuracy.

It is important to note that RECIST 1.1 are based on the assessment of the size change of neoplastic lesions, in order to evaluate the overall response of the disease to therapy. However, it is known that the shrinkage of a tumor is not always representative of the effect of therapy, especially when new antineoplastic drugs are used, which have rather a cytostatic than a cytotoxic action. Through several studies, it has been validated that, in such cases, the RECIST methodology often underestimates the objective response, while there may be clinical response and improved survival. Today, there are enough data imposing the use of modified criteria for assessing response in specific tumors and/or therapies, like hepatocellular carcinoma, gastrointestinal stromal tumors (GISTs) treated with imatinib mesylate, and hepatic metastases treated with antiangiogenic drugs. Also, the RECIST criteria are not reliable for assessing the therapeutic effect of radiofrequency ablation and cryoablation of liver lesions [6–8] (see Section I-chap. 4 and section IX).

As previously mentioned, RECIST guidelines do not incorporate the use of US for response assessment, although they accept and propose the clinical palpation, the endoscopic studies and the histopathological examination [3]. These latter cannot be considered as objective examinations since they are also highly operator-dependent. It worths consideration the fact that, in cases of patients with breast cancer, the evaluation of the size of the breast lesions by palpation is officially acceptable and recommended, while US evaluation is not. Also, US is a valuable tool in the daily practice of paediatric oncology, where the avoidance of radiation exposure is of major concern. Finally, recent studies confirm the usefulness of contrast-enhanced US in the evaluation of the therapeutic result after ablation of liver tumors or after the use of newer antiangiogenic therapies. These facts impose the need to reconsider the use of US in the aim of assessing the therapeutic result.

According to RECIST 1.1, ^{18}F-FDG-PET or PET/CT may be used selectively as a complementary tool for detecting active disease in residual masses and confirming the appearance of new neoplastic lesions [3]. Despite the validated usefulness of this modality in lymphomas and its growing use in NSCLC, breast cancer and colorectal cancer, the lack of standardization of data acquisition and evaluation criteria, precluded its incorporation in RECIST methodology. Recently, new guidelines for assessing solid tumors response to treatment, fully incorporating the use of ^{18}F-FDG-PET, have been proposed [11, 12].

New imaging techniques of dynamic contrast-enhanced CT and MRI and diffusion-weighted MRI, have shown promising results for assessing response of various tumors to new targeted therapies. However, they need further standardization and validation in order to be suitable for wider application and be incorporated in a future revision of RECIST guideline [12].

In conclusion, RECIST guidelines, including the last version 1.1 of 2009, are based on the assessment of the size changes of neoplastic lesions, in order to evaluate objectively the degree of response to therapy. Regarding the definition of different categories of response, there were not any essential changes, in comparison to the previous WHO guidelines. What has changed is the recognition of the importance of using newer imaging technologies as CT and MRI and the methodology of measuring the size of lesions (unidimensional instead of bidimensional measurements). Also, the estimation of the overall response to therapy is based on the change of all neoplastic lesions (target, measurable and non-measurable) and on the appearance or not of new lesions during follow-up. Finally, according to

RECIST 1.1, a larger increase of the total tumor burden is needed in order to categorize the case of a patient with neoplasia as "progressive disease".

References

1. World Health Organization (1979) WHO Handbook for reporting results of cancer treatment. WHO Publication No. 48, Geneva
2. Therasse P, Arbuck SG, Eisenhauer EA et al (2000) New guidelines to evaluate the response to treatment in solid tumors (RECIST Guidelines). J Natl Cancer Inst 92:205–216
3. Eisenhauer EA, Therasse P, Bogaerts J et al (2009) New response evaluation criteria in solid tumors: revised RECIST guideline (version 1.1). Eur J Cancer 45:228–247
4. Wen PY, Macdonald DR, Reardon DA et al (2010) Updated response assessment criteria for high-grade glioma: response assessment in neuro-oncology working group. J Clin Oncol 28911:1963–1972
5. Cheson BD, Pfistner B, Juweid ME et al (2007) Revised response criteria for malignant lymphoma. J Clin Oncol 10:579–586
6. van Persijn van Merten EL, Gelberblom H (2010) RECIST revised: implications for the radiologist. A review article on the modified RECIST guideline. Eur Radiol 20(6):1456–1467.
7. Nishino M, Jagganathan JP, Ramayia NH et al (2010) Revised RECIST guideline version 1.1: what oncologists want to know and what radiologists need to know. AJR Am J Roentgenol 195(2):281–289
8. Chalian H, Tore HG, Horowitz JM et al (2011) Radiologic Assessment of Response to Therapy: comparison of RECIST versions 1.1 and 1.0. RadioGraphics 31:2093–2105
9. Mantatzis M, Kakolyris S, Amarantidis K et al (2009) Treatment response classification of liver metastatic disease evaluated on imaging: are RECIST unidimensional measurements accurate? 19(7):1809–1816.
10. Nowak AK, Armato SG 3rd, Ceresoli GL et al (2010) Imaging in pleural mesothelioma: a review of imaging research presented at the 9th international meeting of the International Mesothelioma Interest Group. Lung Cancer 70(1):1–6
11. Wahl RL, Jacene H, Kasamon Y (2009) From RECIST to PERCIST: evolving considerations for PET response criteria in solid tumors. J Nucl Med 50:122S–150S
12. Desar IM, van Herpen CM, van Laarhoven HW et al (2009) Beyond RECIST: molecular and functional imaging techniques for evaluation of response to targeted therapies. Cancer Treat Rev 35(4):309–321

3 Imaging in Radiation Therapy

Despina M. Katsochi, Panayiotis Ch. Sandilos and Chryssa I. Paraskevopoulou

3.1 Introduction

Since their discovery, at the end of the nineteenth century, both diagnostic and therapeutic use of X-rays have followed a parallel course in development and have had direct interaction with each other.

In the past few decades, a new era arose. Imaging has passed from radiographs to computer development. The parallel development of high energy treatment machines, (linear accelerators) and treatment planning softwares established radiotherapy (RT) as a standard treatment option for a wide range of malignancies. Imaging is not only useful for pretreatment evaluation (diagnosis-staging) but it is also an important Radiation Therapy treatment planning tool. Undoubtedly, imaging serves both treatment monitoring and post-treatment evaluation of the disease outcome.

3.2 Pretreatment Evaluation

Clinical imaging techniques can be classified in those that measure various anatomical and physical characteristics of tissue, such as their density, and biological imaging techniques which measure functional characteristics, such as metabolism. The goal is to get as much information about the anatomical or functional details of the tumor as possible, using the appropriate imaging method based on sensitivity and specificity.

Computer Tomography (CT) (Fig. 3.1), which represents the principal tumor diagnostic method and a very important treatment planning tool, mainly due to its ability to offer:

1. very fast image acquisition of the whole body
2. various slice thicknesses with excellent spatial resolution
3. instant picture availability
4. a comfortable environment/position for the patient.

Magnetic resonance imaging (MRI) offers a new perspective improving organ anatomy imaging, especially in the central nervous system (Fig. 3.2). Additionally, in several parts of the body, such as pelvic region, MRI (compared

D. M. Katsochi (✉)
Department of Radiation Oncology, Diagnostic & Therapeutic Center of Athens Hygeia, 4 Erythrou Stavrou Street & Kifissias Avenue, 15123 Athens, Greece
e-mail: dkatsochi@aktinotherapeia.com

P. Ch. Sandilos
Department of Radiology, School of Medicine, National & Kapodistrian University of Athens, Aretaieion Hospital, 76 Vassilissis Sofias Avenue, 11528 Athens, Greece
e-mail: p.sandilos@hygeia.gr

C. I. Paraskevopoulou
Department of Medical Physics, Diagnostic & Therapeutic Center of Athens Hygeia, 4 Erythrou Stavrou Street & Kifissias Avenue, 15123 Athens, Greece
e-mail: c.paraskevopoulou@hygeia.gr

A. D. Gouliamos et al. (eds.), *Imaging in Clinical Oncology*,
DOI: 10.1007/978-88-470-5385-4_3, © Springer-Verlag Italia 2014

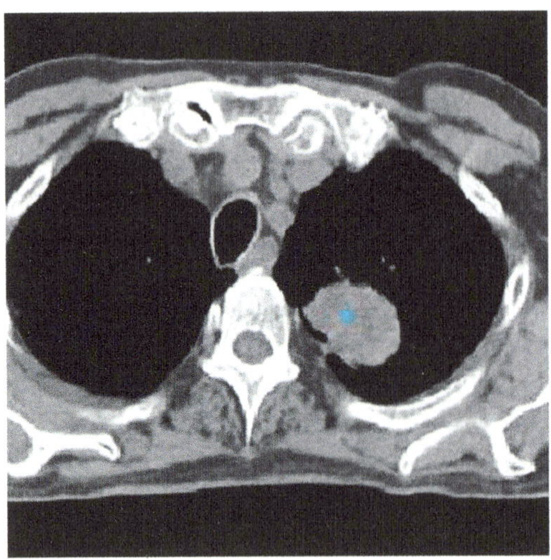

Fig. 3.1 CT image, lung tumor to the *left* upper lob

to CT) provides information regarding tumor extension or tumor infiltration to the adjacent organs (Fig. 3.3).

Furthermore, the advances in nuclear medicine led to new imaging protocols for oncological patients. The combination of positron emission tomography and computed tomography (PET/CT) offers metabolic mapping in addition to anatomic information of the primary lesion, nodal, and distant metastases and PET/CT staging improves patient selection by 20 % [1] (Figs. 3.4, 3.5). Therefore, it has emerged as an important tool in pretreatment evaluation and RT planning [2]. The combination of biological and anatomical information leads to a much more accurate target definition improving tumor coverage.

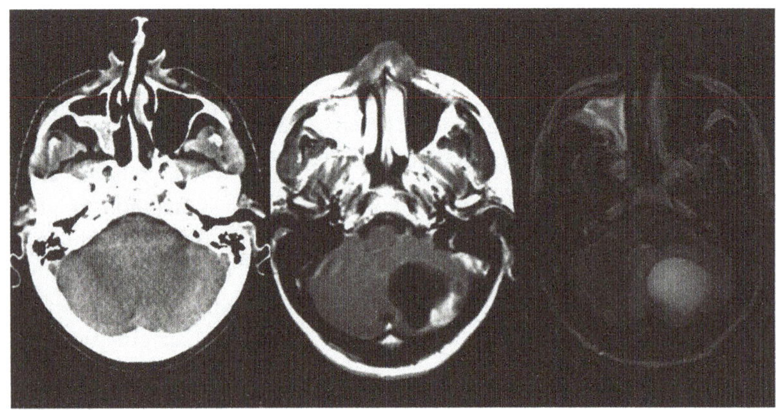

Fig. 3.2 Single metastasis in *left* cerebellum hemisphere. Comparison of CT and MR (T1, T2) images

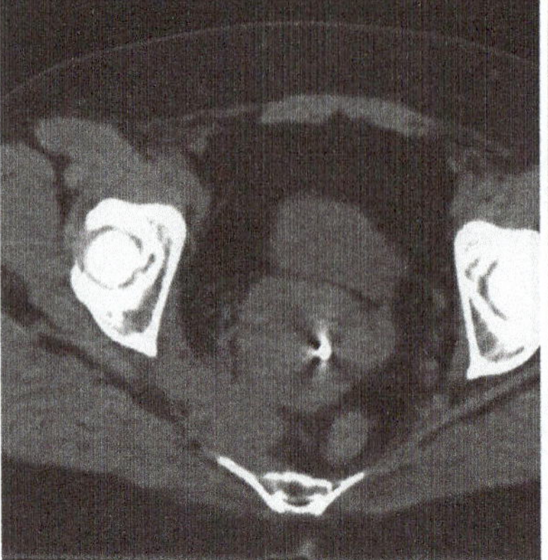

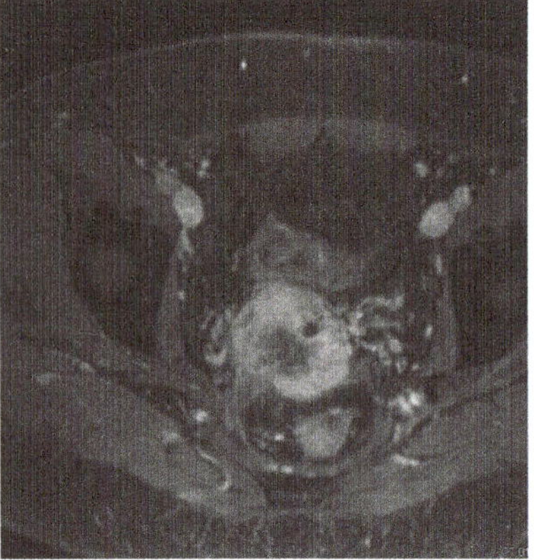

Fig. 3.3 Cervix cancer infiltration to the adjacent tissue. Comparison of CT and MR images

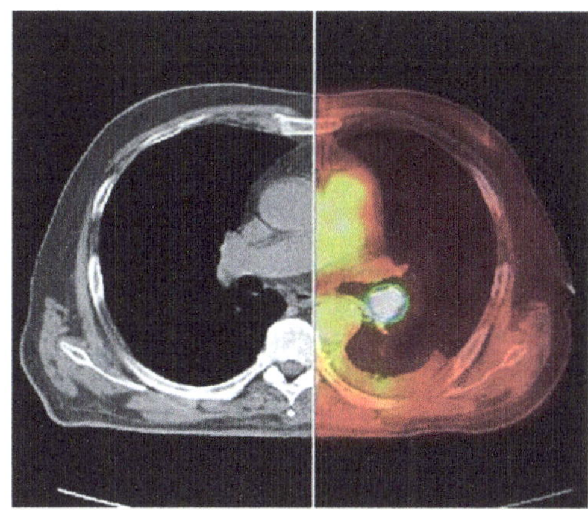

Fig. 3.4 PET/CT image, tumor at the hila of the *left* lung

3.3 Treatment Planning

RT has a dominant role in the treatment of cancer. Today, more than half of all cancer patients receive radiation therapy during the course of their treatment. The main aim of RT is to deliver the maximum dose to the tumor with minimal toxicity on neighboring healthy tissues. For this reason, the precise determination of the target and its spatial relation to critical surrounding organs is of main importance.

The modern developments in radiology (CT, MRI, and PET/CT scans) improved not only the diagnostic part in cancer patients, but also the overall treatment decision making. The recent advances in radiation imaging offer high accuracy in target delineation and ensure safe dose escalation.

Treatment planning is a complicated procedure. One of the most important steps which affect the whole treatment strategy is target determination. The definition of the extension of the infiltrated tissue is often an interdisciplinary procedure where the surgeon, pathologist, radiologist, and radiation oncologist have to cooperate to decide the most appropriate treatment plan.

The target volume includes the gross tumor volume (GTV) and the possible region of microscopical disease (clinical treatment volume, CTV). The planning target volume (PTV) is defined according to ICRU 62 report and includes GTV , CTV and takes into account internal organ motion and set up errors [3] (Fig. 3.6).

The reference imaging modality for radiation therapy treatment planning is CT because it provides information about tissue density and thus it is the only modality that can be used for accurate treatment planning dosimetric calculations. Although CT-based planning is the standard approach, it only provides anatomical information. In addition, the best imaging modality is chosen according to the anatomical site of the primary tumor for the delineation of the target volume and the surrounding organs at risk.

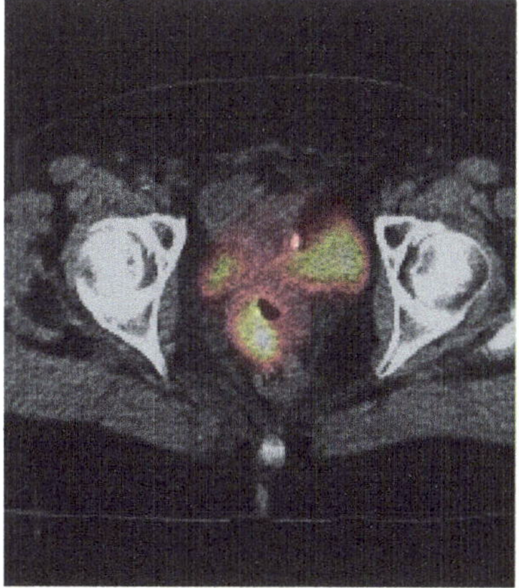

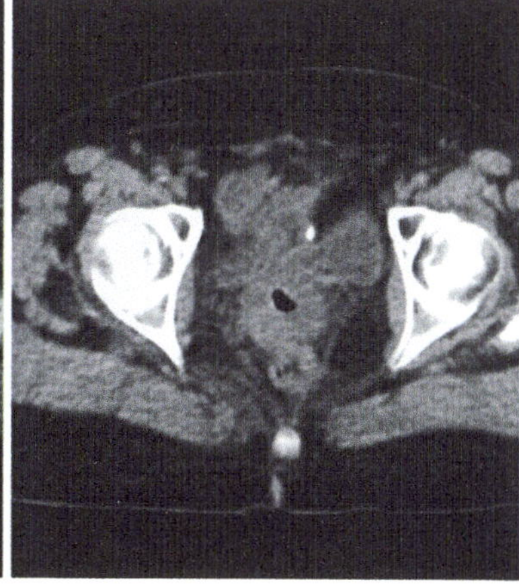

Fig. 3.5 PET/CT and CT images comparison in patient with cervical cancer

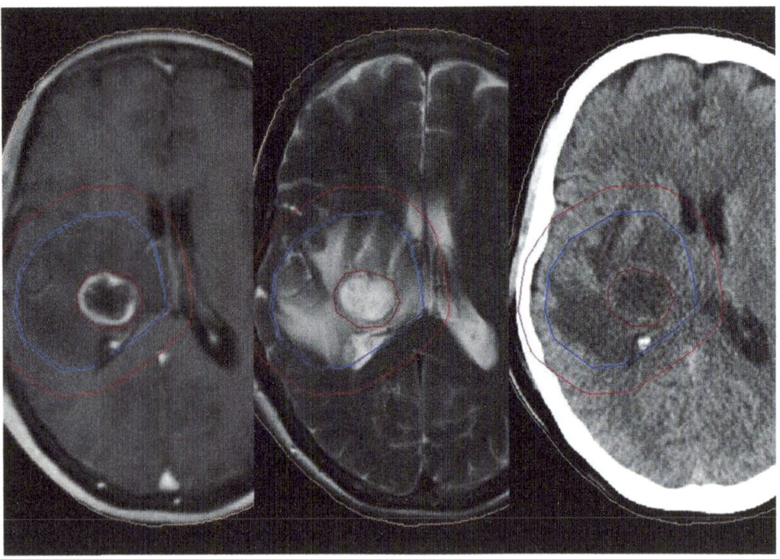

Fig. 3.6 Brain tumor MR and CT images co-registered. Delineation of GTV (tumor), CTV (edema), PTV (planning tumor volume)

Combined PET/CT imaging has been proposed as an integral part of RT treatment planning procedure because it provides biological information for the accurate delineation of GTV and the involved nodal disease, that is, accurate target definition between tumor and atelectasis in lung cancer [1, 4]. GTV delineation based on hypermetabolic tumor has shown to be significantly different from GTV drawn on CT only. In 35–60 % cases, target volume was reduced using PET/CT images [4, 5]. These patients showed a better treatment outcome (31 vs. 16 months) and increase 1 year survival from 8 to 17 % [6] (Figs. 3.7, 3.8).

An important step in the procedure of tumor and organs at risk delineation is the alignment of medical images, which results from the spatial placement of two or more sets of data in a way that the common structures coincide. This procedure is called image fusion and combines different image modalities to provide the maximum diagnostic information.

Three-dimensional conformal radiation therapy (3DCRT) is the standard treatment technique using static radiation fields and allows the delivery of highly conformed radiation to the PTV, while significantly reducing the amount of radiation received by surrounding healthy tissue. Randomized controlled trials using this technique have demonstrated improved tumor control with dose escalation but at the cost of increasing toxicity. Recent advances in technology have resulted in more sophisticated treatment planning techniques. Intensity-

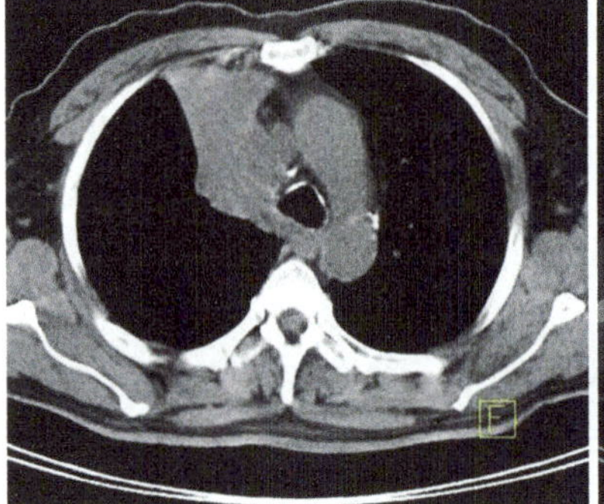

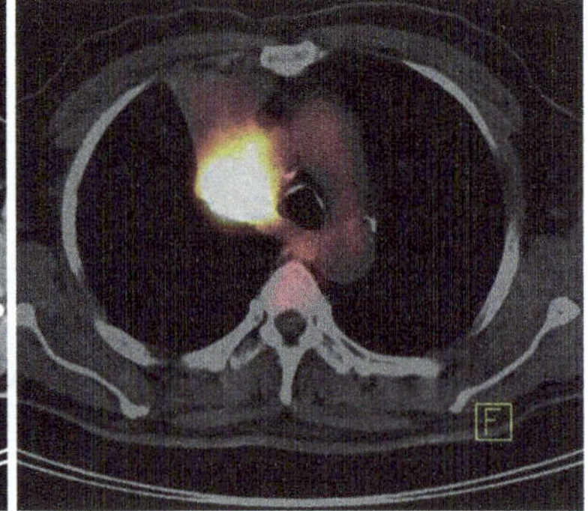

Fig. 3.7 Lung cancer patient, PET/CT shows the active metabolic part of the tumor and distinguishes it from atelectasis

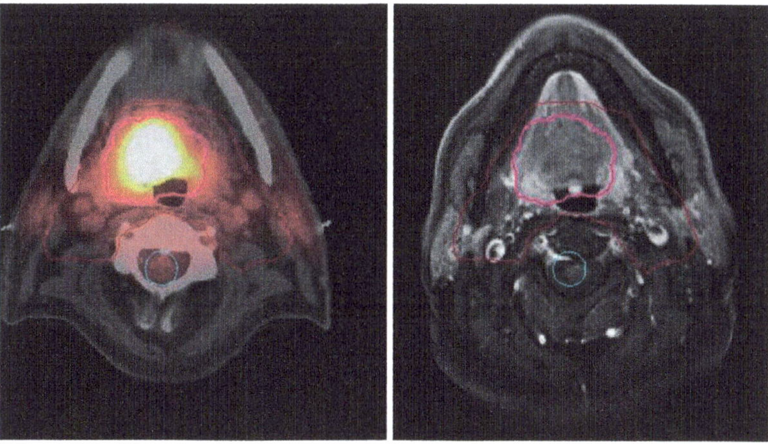

Fig 3.8 PET/CT and MR images for accurate delineation of GTV in patient with oropharygeal cancer

modulated radiotherapy (IMRT), volumetric modulated arc therapy (VMAT), and stereotactic body radiotherapy (SBRT), in combination with image-guided radiotherapy (IGRT) have enabled higher radiation doses to be delivered to tumors which increases the rate of tumor control while also decreasing side effects [7]. Higher conformity in combination with smaller PTV allows 25 % RT dose escalation and increases the effectiveness of therapy [8].

IMRT optimizes the radiation intensity distribution within each beam in order to achieve a higher rate of conformity and target coverage especially for irregularly shaped tumors. VMAT is a novel form of IMRT optimization that allows the radiation dose to be accurately and efficiently delivered in a single or multiple gantry arcs. IMRT/VMAT requires accurate target delineation and produces tightly conformal doses and dose gradients next to normal tissues improving target coverage due to high conformity and allows dose escalation along with better sparing of surrounding normal tissues. These techniques have been shown to reduce toxicity and potentially may lead to improved local tumor control [8] (Fig. 3.9).

Stereotactic radiosurgery (SRS) and SBRT are techniques for delivering very high doses in a single or in a few fractions (hypofractionation) in order to shorten treatment duration and escalate the biological equivalent dose. SRS and SBRT require high precision in target determination [9] (Fig. 3.10).

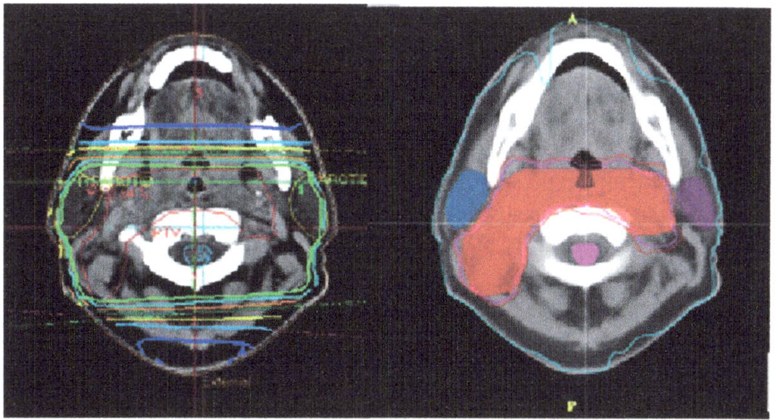

Fig. 3.9 Comparison of 3DRT and IMRT in patients with nasopharynx cancer

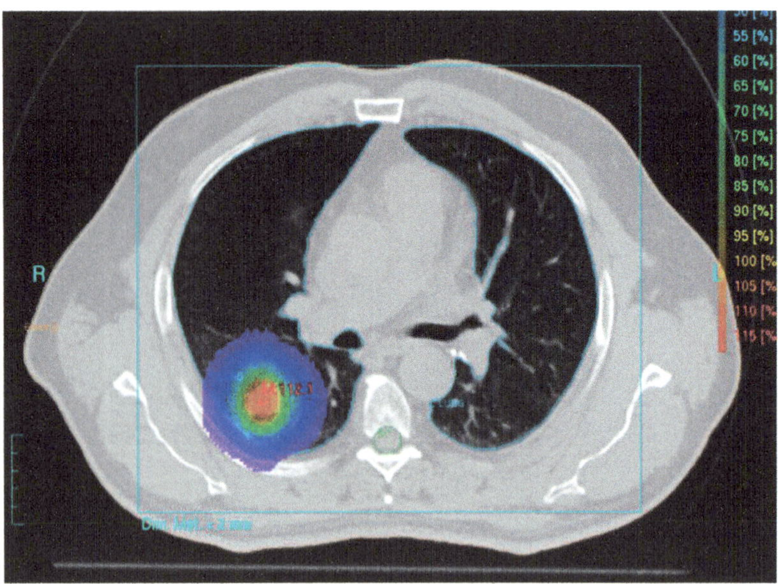

Fig. 3.10 SBRT, 3 fractions × 12 Gy at 65 % isodose for single lung metastasis

The three main factors that contribute to local treatment failure after RT are.

1. Geographic misses due to inadequacy of imaging tools for staging and RT planning.
2. Geographic misses due to respiration-induced tumor motion and anatomic changes during radiation delivery.
3. Inadequate radiation dose due to concerns about toxicity.

Control of locoregional disease, locally advanced or postoperatively, remains a great challenge for the radiation oncologist. There is a direct relationship between the probability of achieving tumor control and delivered radiation dose. Lung cancer patients treated with 3D-CRT a dose escalation of 10 Gy is correlated with 36 % decrease in local failure rates [10].

3DCRT and, recently, SRS and SBRT, IMRT, and VMAT, using dose-escalated treatment, appear to improve local disease control and possibly survival. One of the main challenges is to individualize treatment adaptation based on changes in anatomy and tumor motion during the course of RT.

3.4 Image-Guided Radiation Therapy: Adaptive Radiotherapy

Image-Guided Radiation Therapy (IGRT) refers to the use of patient imaging in the treatment room to ensure accurate dose delivery to the target [11]. In other words, IGRT is an important tool to monitor all treatment-relevant time-dependent factors for a complete treatment course and use this information to improve patient's therapy. The potential applications of the clinical IGRT range from fast corrections of interfractional errors in patient positioning to tumor response monitoring during a RT course [12].

The development of image-guidance tools and techniques in RT has been greatly motivated by the continual advances in external beam radiation delivery and tumor dose escalation. However, as the planned dose distributions conform more closely to the reference planning CT, the precision of dose delivery becomes

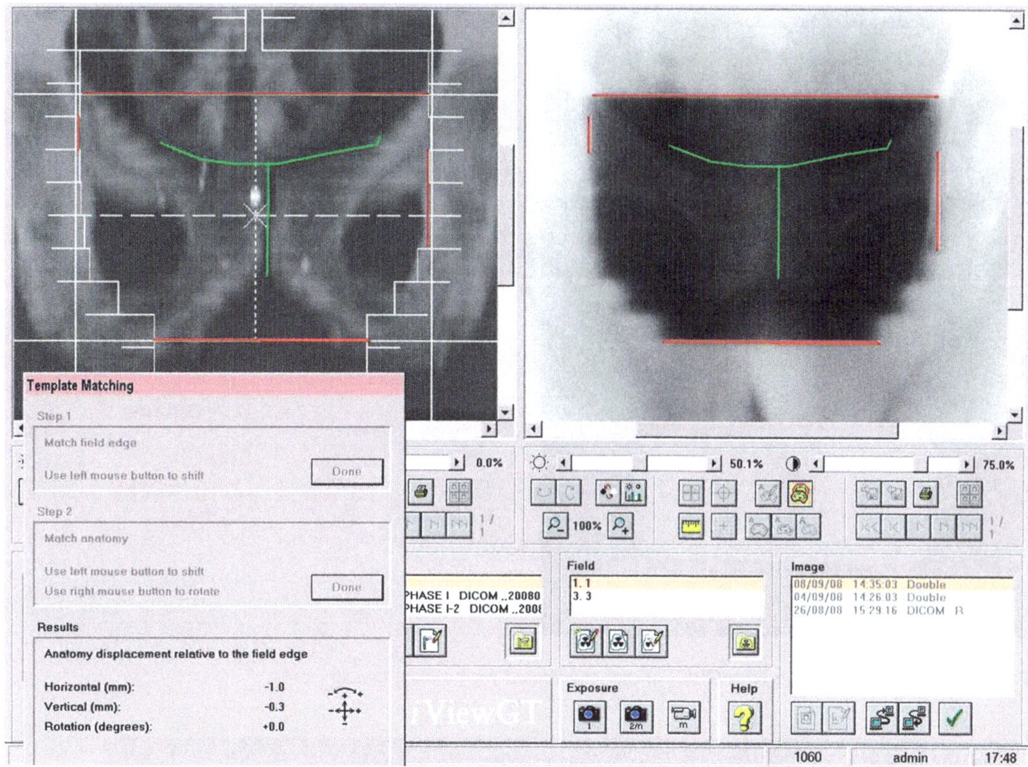

Fig. 3.11 Electronic portal image of anterior field prostate 3D conformal RT for the correct positioning of the patient prior to treatment

limited by the assumption that the planning CT represents the patient's anatomy on the treatment table throughout an extended course of treatment. Organs may change in size, shape, and position during treatment due to normal anatomical variability, as well as to tumor response to radiation therapy. Therefore, patient anatomical and positional information, that can be obtained immediately before treatment, is of great importance [11, 12].

Imaging has long played a key role in assuring the accuracy of radiation therapy delivery. Electronic portal imaging devices (EPIDs) have been the preferred tools for verification of patient positioning for RT in recent decades. Recent implementation of highly sensitive and automated on-board EPIDs enable daily low-dose portal imaging to verify and adjust the patient positioning. In addition, EPID images can be used to calculate the actual dose delivered to the patient as an in vivo dosimetry tool. However, the utility of portal imaging is limited because corrections applied to patient positioning are based on 2D planes and mainly on bone visualization and not on soft tissue (Fig. 3.11). This has motivated the development of 3D on-board imaging devices [11, 12].

Cone beam CT (CBCT) (Kilovoltage kV or Megavoltage MV) generates an accurate three-dimensional representation of the patient anatomy on the treatment table just before the treatment starts. CBCT images are registered with the planning CT for patient setup verification and correction online (Figs. 3.12, 3.13). The three-dimensional images provide additional information on the patient's treatment position and offer a wide range of opportunities to improve the delivery of radiation. Periodic acquisition of three-dimensional images allows monitoring of anatomical changes over the treatment course due to tumor response or weight loss (Figs. 3.14, 3.15). The CBCT

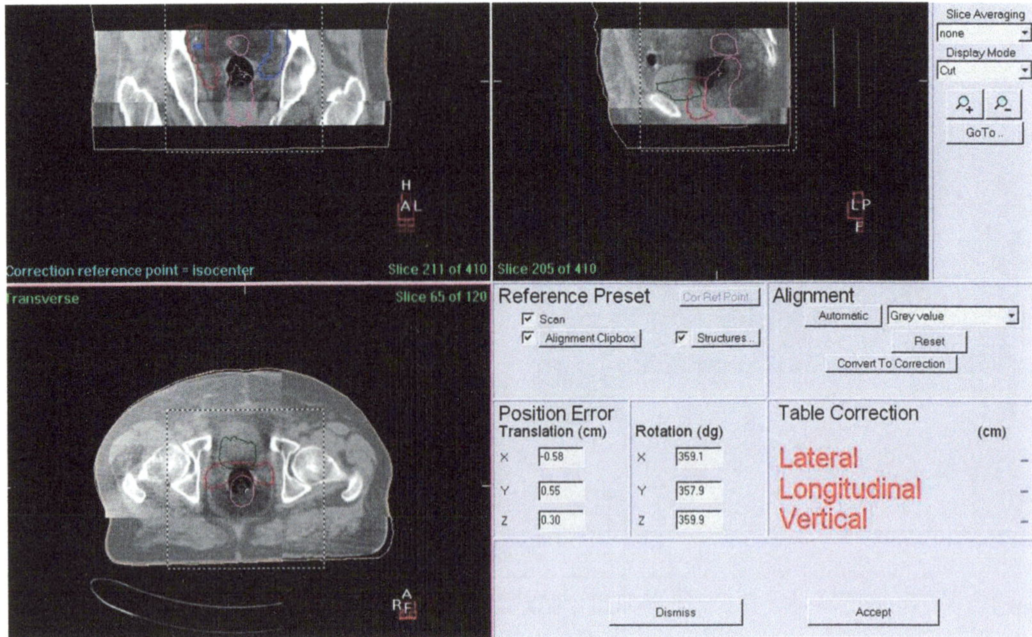

Fig. 3.12 Online correction with CBCT in patient treated for prostate cancer

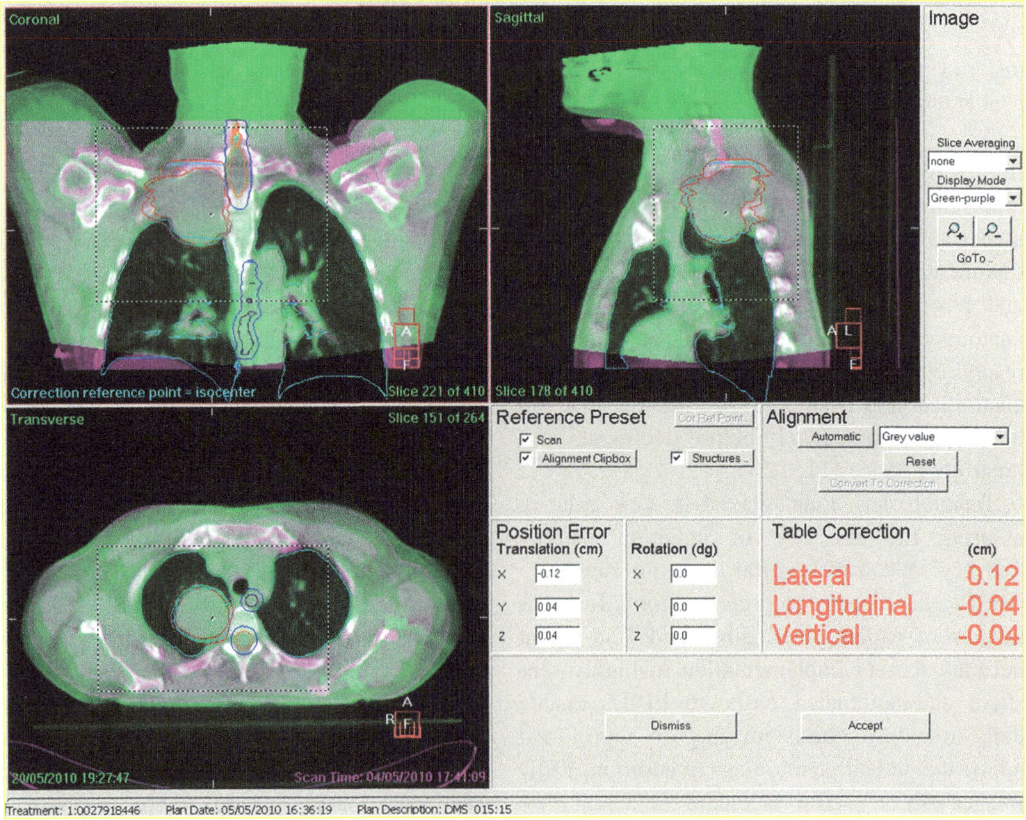

Fig. 3.13 Online correction with CBCT in patient treated for lung cancer

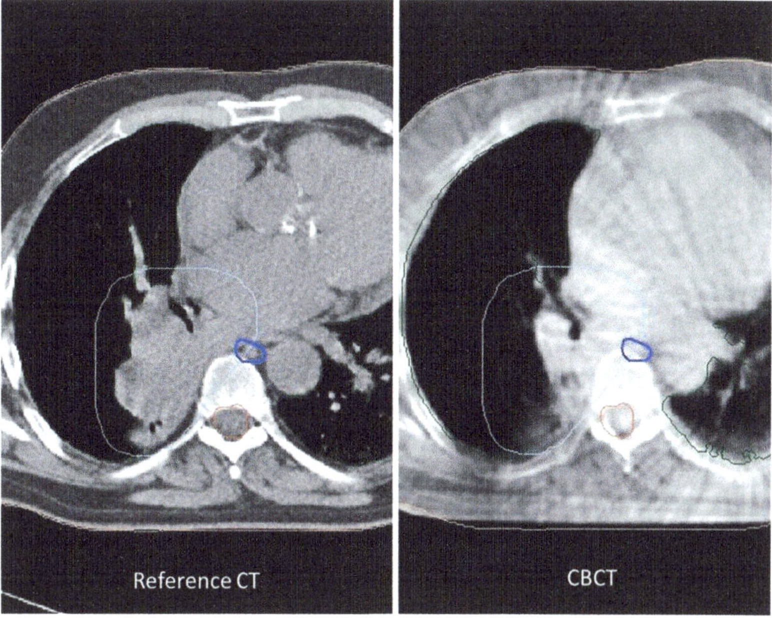

Fig. 3.14 Comparison of reference CT and CBCT. Tumor response during therapy and reevaluation of the target volume

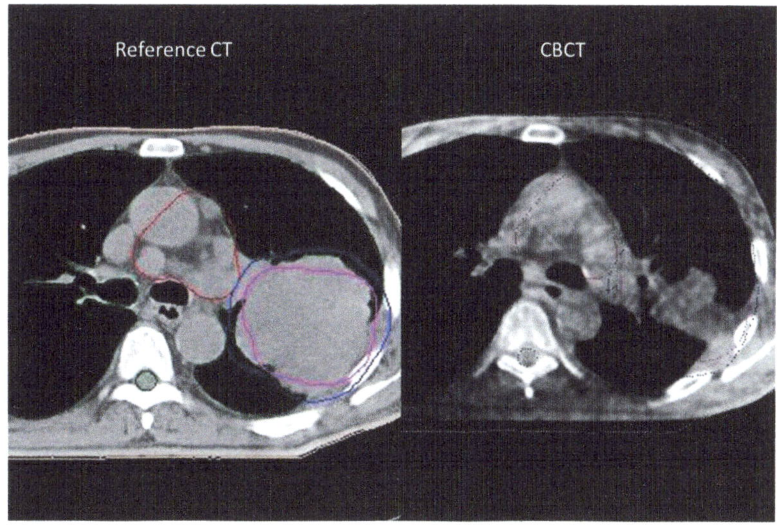

Fig. 3.15 Comparison of reference CT and CBCT. Tumor response during therapy and reevaluation of the target volume

images can also be imported into the treatment planning system. The reference images are fused with the CBCT images thus providing information about tumor changes and response. In addition, it is possible to measure the dosimetric impact of patient misalignment and anatomy modification on dose distribution.

Breathing-induced organ motion has been identified as a significant source of uncertainty in the treatment planning especially for pulmonary tumors (Fig. 3.16). The conventional approach is to apply typical site-specific motion amplitude of 1–2 cm to the GTV generated from a free-breathing CT data set to create the PTV. This increases the amount of irradiated normal tissue which could lead to increased toxicity, while it also limits dose escalation which is necessary to improve local control. Early methods to account for patient-specific tumor motion use multiphase CT scans taken during free-

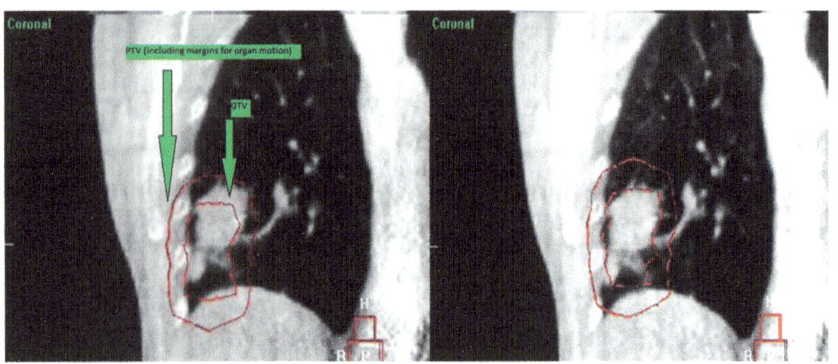

Fig. 3.16 Breathing-induced GTV motion in lung cancer

breathing, end-inspiration, and end-expiration breath-hold fused for treatment planning (Fig. 3.17). This approach assumes that images taken during the extremes of respiration define the extremes of target motion, thus accounting for tumor positioning during all respiratory phases. Recent advances in imaging technology provided more reliable tool to study patient-specific motion. Four dimensional (4D) CT has been proposed as a technique to avoid motion artifacts and to provide detailed information about breathing-induced motion of the tumor and the organs at risk. The 4DCT technique synchronizes image acquisition with respiratory phase. Sequence of 3D images is acquired at different phases of respiratory cycle. The reconstruction of the multiple CT series allows the calculation of the probability of how long the tumor remains at each phase of the breathing cycle. Using the 4DCT images, the iGTV (internal Gross Tumor Volume) is created which envelops the GTV motion throughout the respiratory cycle. On the other hand, 4DCT provides only a snapshot and a single stochastic sampling of the patient's breathing. Attention should be paid to irregular breathing and breathing pattern variations during each treatment session and over the entire treatment course and to the effects of these irregularities on the iGTV margin [7, 8, 13].

Several systems of motion control during treatment have been developed (gating or tracking). The most commonly employed form of respiratory gating involves tracking the motion of external fiducials using infrared imaging. The beam is then turned on only during

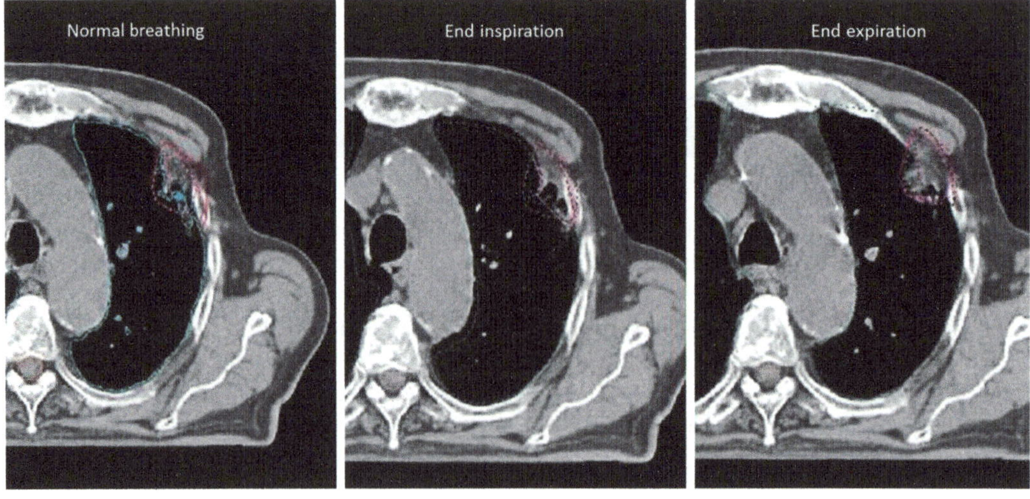

Fig. 3.17 GTV definition using CT taken in three phases (normal breathing, end inspiration, and end expiration)

a specified phase of the respiratory cycle. Some centers also use implanted fiducials within the tumor that are tracked with respect to externally placed fiducials and a correlative model is built. The correlation between tumor position and external fiducials is assumed to remain constant during the time course of radiation treatment. The beam position is then changed according to the position of these external fiducials in near 'real-time' during treatment. This approach is the closest to real-time tracking at the present time and is ideal for minimizing the effects of target motion not only between treatments but also during a treatment fraction [8].IGRT with CBCT incorporates volumetric imaging information to improve the accuracy of daily patient positioning but also provides information about the changes of target volume when the anatomy of the tumor and/or normal organs changes during therapy [14]. During treatment, variations or changes in tumor can occur caused by tumor shrinkage, changes in tumor biology (hypoxia), patient weight lost, or local edema. These are the major factors for target missing and/or overtreating normal tissues. As a result, the initial target delineation and treatment plan does not match the treatment delivered. In order to adapt changes in patient anatomy between treatment fractions, redefinition of the treatment volume and re-planning is needed. This procedure is called adaptive radiotherapy and enables dose escalation as well as minimization of normal tissue irradiation [15].

Imaging is central to radiation oncology practice, with advances in radiation oncology occurring in parallel to advances in imaging. CT, MR, and PET/CT images are used to delineate the PTV and the organs at risk in the planning process. Computer-assisted calculation of the radiation dose distribution ensures that the objectives for target coverage and avoidance of healthy tissue are achieved. The new robotic state-of-the-art radiation treatment units are capable of three-dimensional soft tissue imaging immediately before, during, or after radiation delivery, improving the localization of the target at the time of radiation delivery (IGRT). IGRT allows changes in tumor position, size, and shape to be measured during the course of RT. Adjustments are made to maximize the geometrical accuracy and precision of radiation delivery, reducing the volume of healthy tissue irradiated and permitting dose escalation to the tumor. These advantages increase the chance of tumor control, reduce the risk of toxicity after RT, and facilitate the development of shorter RT schedules [14].

3.5 Post-Treatment Outcome Evaluation

The objectives of post-treatment follow-up in oncology are to detect recurrence and second primary tumor and also evaluate acute and chronic treatment-related side effects. Other very important issues are to guide the rehabilitation process, manage pain and functional loss, and also restore nutritional status.

There are specific guidelines depending on tumor anatomy and biological characteristics. In order to achieve a complete and coherent surveillance and to evaluate treatment response, baseline imaging (computed tomography and magnetic resonance imaging) should be obtained within 2–6 months after definitive therapy. If indicated, PET/CT should be performed 3 months after the completion of curative-intent therapy. The imaging modalities chosen for post-treatment follow-up should always be the same with the pretreatment ones in order to have an accurate estimation about the current status of the disease. (Figs. 3.18, 3.19, 3.20, and 3.21).

3.6 Future Trends: Functional Image-Guided Dose Optimization or Dose Painting

PET/CT has come to the forefront of staging and overall treatment decision making while it provides physiological and functional information about tumor and their surroundings. Molecular imaging promises to reveal tumor biology. Based on biological principles, tumors are not homogeneous. Tumor subregions may

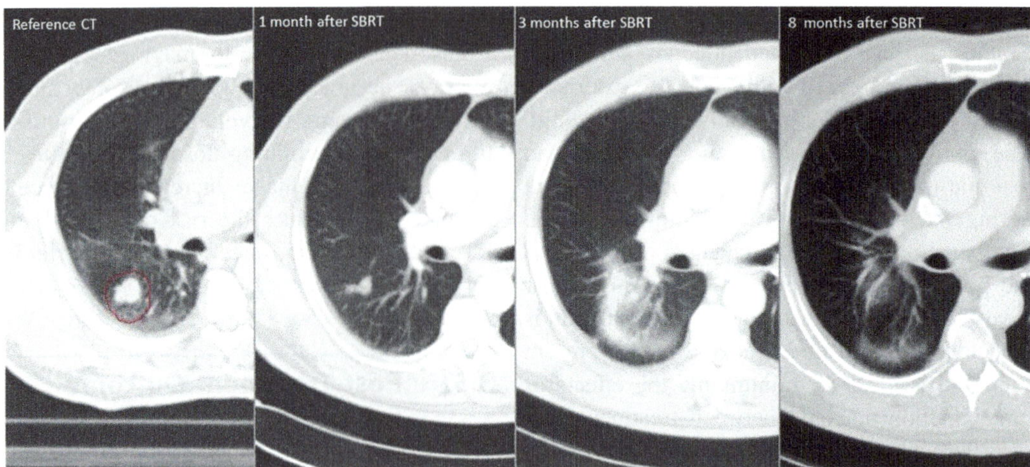

Fig. 3.18 Patient follow-up after SBRT 1, 3, and 8 months. Complete tumor response and regression of local pneumonitis

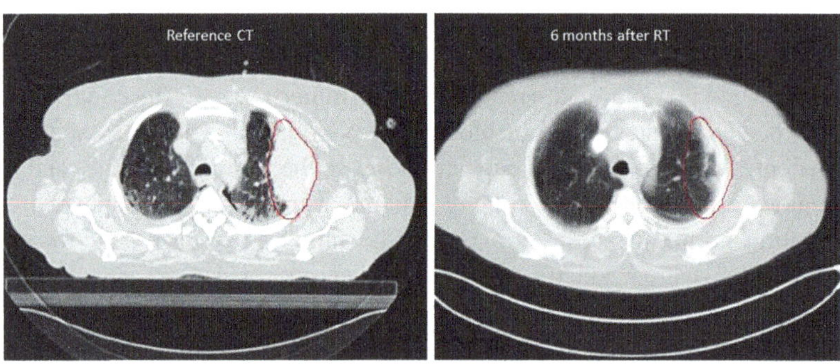

Fig. 3.19 Patient follow-up 6 month after 3D-CRT treatment for lung cancer

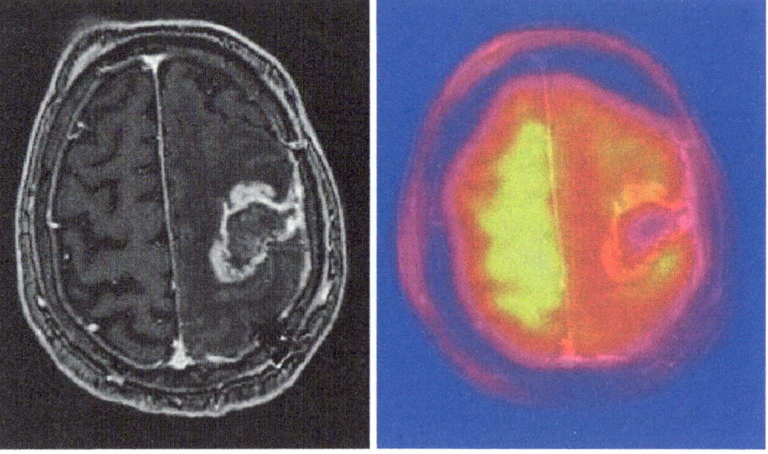

Fig. 3.20 Patient follow-up 3 months after γ-knife SRS. MRI positive, PET/CT negative proves necrotic tissue

selectively contain an enriched population of cancer stem cells that may be responsible for recurrence and distant metastasis. Tumor metabolic activity, estimated by Standard Uptake Value (SUV) in PET/CT images, provides important prognostic and predictive information

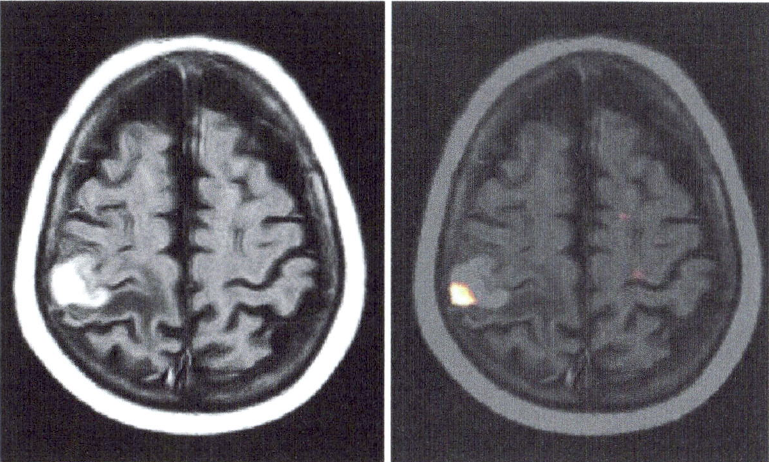

Fig. 3.21 Residual tumor showed in PET/CT and necrotic tissue after γ-Knife SRS

especially in patients with lung cancer. Meng X et al. [16] correlated microscopic extension of tumor on histopathology with GTV's SUV_{max} in NSCLC and found that microscopic extension is larger in tumors with higher SUV_{max} values. Klopp et al. 2007 and Ling et al. 2000 examined the utility of FDG-PET and hypoxic imaging as radiographic biomarkers for treatment failure. The studies have shown that high-SUV (SUV > 13.8) regions and hypoxic areas are more likely to have local recurrence after a standard dose of RT [17, 18].

These developments, in combination with new treatment planning techniques, provide great opportunities for enhancing RT success. IMRT and VMAT can deliver inhomogeneous dose distributions and thus selectively paint dose to subregions within the target. Dose painting or

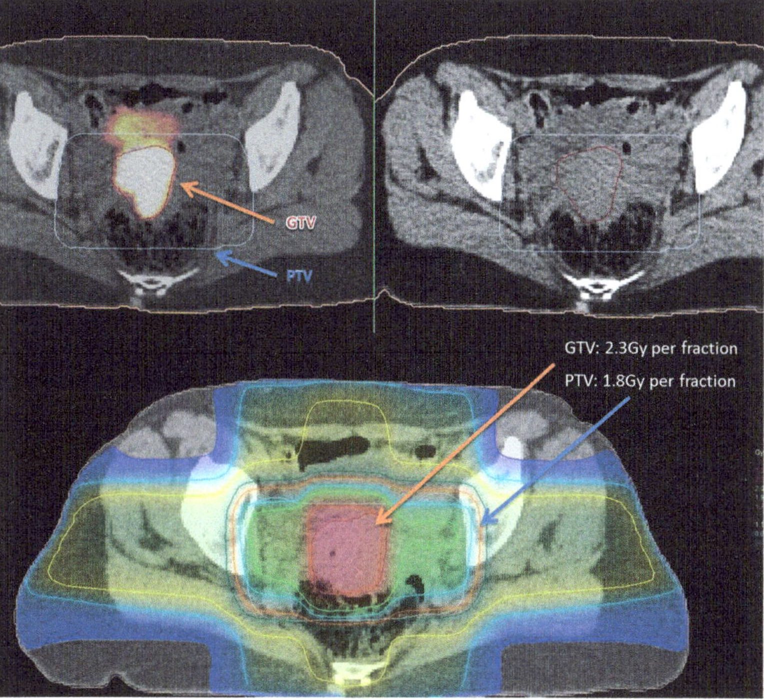

Fig. 3.22 Dose painting to the hypermetabolic part of the cervix tumor

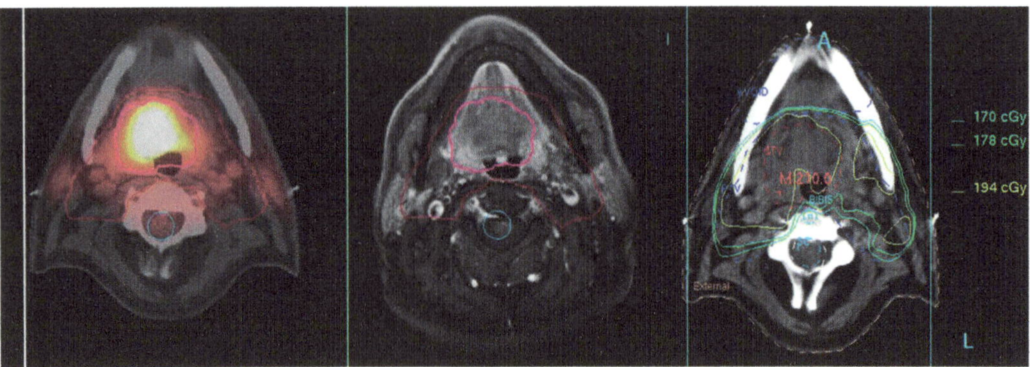

Fig. 3.23 Dose painting to the hypermetabolic part of the oropharynx tumor

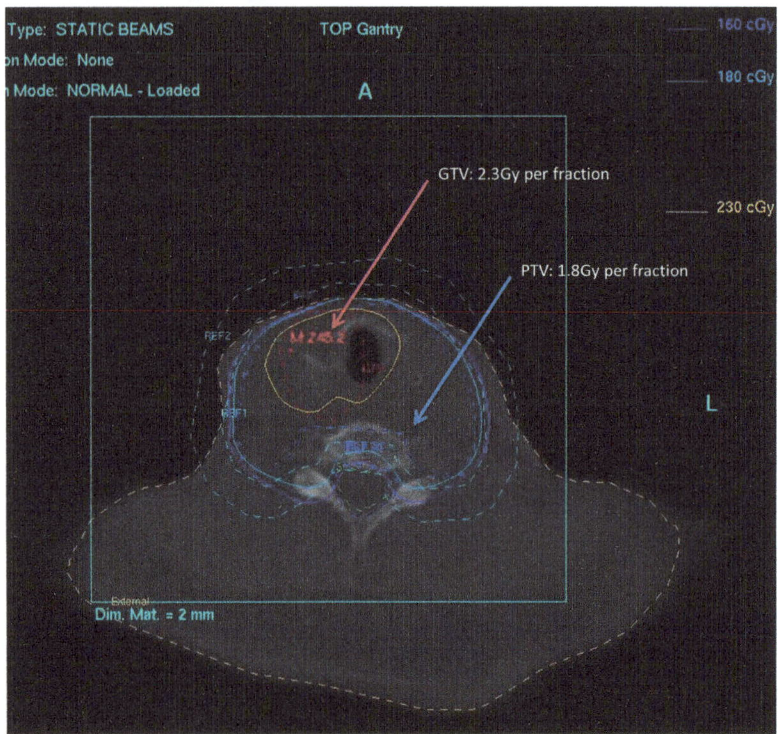

Fig. 3.24 Dose painting concomitant boost in patient with malignant neoplasm of larynx

delivery of higher doses to regions (concomitant boost) at high risk of tumor recurrence, may further improve local control and potentially survival, while protecting large areas of normal tissue from high-dose radiation (Figs. 3.22, 3.23, 3.24).

Whereas new treatment planning techniques (IMRT/VMAT) had significantly improved physical conformality in RT, functional imaging offers the ability to incorporate tumor biological information and has launched a new era of biological conformality. Combined, these two approaches could further improve the success of RT.

3.7 Conclusions

Since diagnosis and staging, two very important steps of the treatment plan, are both performed with radiological images, it is a natural consequence that radiation oncology follows a parallel development path with imaging methods. These advances have allowed radiation oncologists to better determine and target tumors, which have resulted in better treatment outcomes, organ preservation, and fewer side effects. These radiology advances have been joined by those in surgical and medical oncology so that organ preservation is now most probable in cancers of the prostate, breast, cervix, anus, larynx, and esophagus. This new team approach in oncology will continue to increase the number of cured patients with minimal side effects.

References

1. Erdi YE, Rosenzweig K, Erdi AK et al (2002) Radiotherapy treatment planning for patients with non-small cell lung cancer using positron emission tomography (PET). Radiother Oncol 62(1):51–60
2. Kolarova I, Vanasek J, Kandrnal V et al (2012) PET/CT significance for planning radiotherapy of head and neck cancer. Neoplasma 59(5):536–540
3. International Commission on Radiation Units and Measurements (1999) ICRU Report 62: Prescribing, recording, and reporting Photon Beam Therapy. IPEM Publications, New York
4. Hicks RJ, Kalff V, MacManus MP et al (2001) $^{(18)}$F-FDG PET provides high-impact and powerful prognostic stratification in staging newly diagnosed non-small cell lung cancer. J Nucl Med 42(11):1596–1604
5. Grégoire V, Haustermans K, Geets X et al (2007) PET-based treatment planning in radiotherapy: a new standard? J Nucl Med 48(Suppl 1):68–77
6. Mac Manus MP, Wong K, Hicks RJ et al (2002) Early mortality after radical radiotherapy for non-small-cell lung cancer: comparison of PET-staged and conventionally staged cohorts treated at a large tertiary referral center. Int J Radiat Oncol Biol Phys 52(2):351–361
7. Lee P, Kupelian P, Czernin J et al (2012) Current concepts in F18 FDG PET/CT-based radiation therapy planning for lung cancer. Front Oncol 2:71
8. Chang JY, Cox JD (2010) Improving radiation conformality in the treatment of non–small cell lung cancer. Semin Radiat Oncol 20(3):171–177
9. De Ruysscher D, Wanders S, van Haren E et al (2005) Selective mediastinal node irradiation based on FDG-PET scan data in patients with non-small-cell lung cancer: a prospective clinical study. Int J Radiat Oncol Biol Phys 62(4):988–994
10. Rengan R, Rosenzweig KE, Venkatraman E et al (2004) Improved local control with higher doses of radiation in large-volume stage III non-small-cell lung cancer. Int J Radiat Oncol Biol Phys 60(3):741–747
11. Oelfke U, Tücking T, Nill S et al (2006) Linac intergrated kV-cone beam CT: technical features and first applications. Med Dosim 31(1):62–70
12. Morin O, Gillis A, Chen J et al (2006) Megavoltage cone-beam CT: system description and clinical applications. Med Dosim 31(1):51–61
13. Vedam SS, Keall PJ, Kini VR et al (2003) Acquiring a four-dimensional computed tomography dataset using an external respiratory signal. Phys Med Biol 48(1):45–62
14. Guckenberger M, Sweeney RA, Flickinger JC et al (2011) Clinical practice of image-guided spine radiosurgery–results from an international research consortium. Radiat Oncol 6:172
15. Hansen EK, Bucci MK, Quivey JM et al (2006) Repeat CT imaging and replanning during the course of IMRT for head-and-neck cancer. Int J Radiat Oncol Biol Phys 64(2):355–362
16. Meng X et al (2012) Noninvasive evaluation of microscropic tumor extensions using standardized uptake value and metabolic tumor volume in non-small-cell lung cancer. Int J Radiat Oncol Biol Phys 82:960–966
17. Klopp AH, Chang JY, Tucker SL et al (2007) Intra-thoracic patterns of failure for non-small cell lung cancer (NSCLC) with PET/CT-defined target delineation. Int J Radiat Oncol Biol Phys 69:1409–1416
18. Ling CC, Humm J, Larson S et al (2000) Towards multidimensional radiotherapy (MD-CRT): biological imaging and biological conformality. Int J Radiat Oncol Biol Phys 47:551–560

4 Interventional Radiology in Oncology

Michael K. Glynos and Katerina S. Malagari

The contribution of interventional radiology in oncology was from its early years consisted of diagnostic procedures like percutaneous biopsy and palliative procedures as biliary drainage and stenting, nephrostomy and ureteral stenting, percutaneous gastrostomy, vascular, esophageal, or enteral stent insertion. Superior Vena Cava (SVC) stenting in malignant disease is now the standard treatment for malignant SVC obstruction and SVC syndrome [1], (Fig. 4.1). However, rapid technological evolution of new drugs, devices or materials along with developments within the discipline, upgraded interventional radiology to a strong partner in the area of management of cancer patients. Transarterial superselective embolization or chemoembolization and thermal tumor ablation are now listed among curative procedures in certain patients.

4.1 Thermal Tumor Ablation

Direct exposure of a living tissue to temperatures above or below certain degrees results in cell destruction and cell death. Since its first step, thermal tumor ablation has gained a significant role in the treatment of armamentarium for solid tumors, sometimes proven comparable success rates to surgery, as in cases of osteoid osteoma [2].

Excellent results have been reported for thermal tumor ablation bone tumors, either alone or in conjunction with cementoplasty. However, it is beyond the scope of this chapter to refer in details on thermal tumor ablation in every target organ. This chapter will focus on ablative techniques in liver, kidneys, and lung.

4.1.1 Radiofrequency Ablation (RFA)

RFA is based on the theory that appliance of alternative electric current in the RF wavelength (400–500 kHz) in the conductive human body, i.e., between an antenna in the tissue and a ground pad in another part of the body, causes the electric energy to create resistive heat (the Joule effect). In fact, a complete electric circuit is created [3]. After creation of direct heating in close proximity to the RF antenna, thermal energy is mediated by conduction in the surrounding tissue.

Temperature at 42–45 °C causes cell damage after 60 min. Above 45 °C it results in protein decomposition. At 60 °C immediate cell death occurs (coagulation necrosis), while above 105 °C leads to carbonization and vaporization.

M. K. Glynos (✉)
Department of Interventional Radiology, Hygeia Hospital, Erythrou Stavrou 4 & Kifisias, 15123 Marousi, Greece
e-mail: mglynos@gmail.com

K. S. Malagari
Second Department of Radiology, University of Athens, 19 Monis Kykkou, 15669 Athens, Greece
e-mail: kmalag@otenet.gr

A. D. Gouliamos et al. (eds.), *Imaging in Clinical Oncology*,
DOI: 10.1007/978-88-470-5385-4_4, © Springer-Verlag Italia 2014

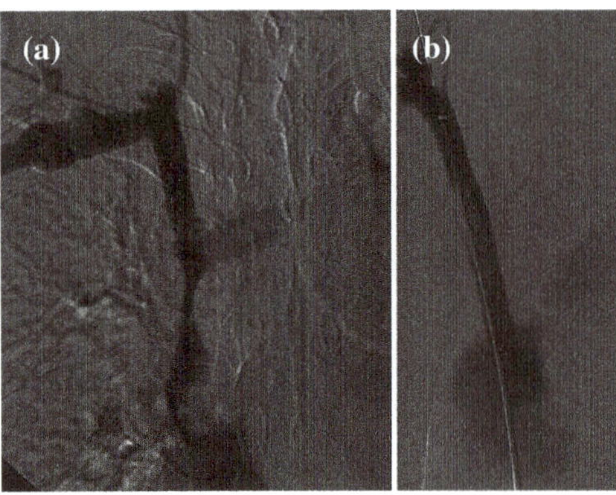

Fig. 4.1 **a** SVC stenosis from external compression **b** 16 × 80 mm self-expanding nitinol stent

Under vital signs, monitoring and conscious sedation or, in selected cases, under general anesthesia (GA), a 16–18 G needle (antenna) is inserted into the tumor. Ultrasound or CT guidance can be used. Single, triple coaxial or multitined probes are commercially available as well as bipolar devices which do not need grounding pads, as the circuit is completed between the two probes. The area of necrosis depends on the active part of the needle and on certain properties of the surrounding tissue. Ablation areas of 2–4 cm around the antenna are usually expected.

RFA has been successfully applied in tumors of liver, kidneys, lung, bones, and soft tissues.

4.1.2 Microwave Ablation (MWA)

Microwave ablation is based on the theory of dielectric heating. Alternative current in the 900–2,500 MHz frequency range causes oscillation of dipolic water molecules, thus converting electromagnetic energy into heat by agitation. Conclusively, lesions rich in water, as solid organs, convert more energy to heat, while areas with less percentage of water, such as fat, convert less [3, 4].

MWA advantages in comparison to RFA are: 1. Larger and more homogeneous ablation area, as it is much less affected by the heat-sink effect in the proximity to large vessels or the carbonization around the probe, 2. no need for ground pads which are associated with skin burns, and 3. decreased ablation time. On the other hand during RFA in contrast to MWA, air or vascular insulation protects surrounding organs from undesirable heating. Extreme care should therefore be taken when using MWA in close proximity to bile ducts, stomach, and bowel after previous surgery or air-filled biliary tree.

In general, complications of MWA are not significantly different from those of RFA. Livraghi et al. report a 2.9 % major and 7.3 % minor complications of MWA of liver tumors [5]. Of note is reports of portal vein thrombosis (PVT) after MWA, which is attributed to heating of portal endothelium with subsequent thrombosis [5, 6].

4.1.3 Cryoablation

Cryoablation is the result of inducing subfreezing temperatures into the tumor via thin (18 G) needles, killing cells by disruption and apoptosis. This is engineered with devices which are based on the argon gas decompression. An "iceball" encompasses target tissue and can be immediately seen on CT or MRI but not in ultrasound, as it creates acoustic shadow. Advantage of the method is reduced periprocedural pain as well as the ability to simultaneously use multiple probes, thus increasing the overall ablation volume. Increased risk of post-procedure hemorrhage, high cost, need of special infrastructure (argon and helium supply), and CT or MRI dependence are the main disadvantages.

Cryoablation is mostly applied in renal and prostate tumors with results similar or superior to thermal ablative methods. [7]. In the liver, cryoablation is reported to be of comparable results, but of 6.3–15 % complication rates [8, 9]. Cryoshock, a potentially fatal complication in about 1 % of cases, consists of thrombocytopenia, multiorgan failure, and disseminated intravascular coagulopathy [10].

Table 4.1 Indications and contraindications of RFA for HCC

Indications	Contraindications
Inoperable HCC	Coagulation disorders (INR > 1.2)
Absence of extrahepatic spread	Platelet count < 50,000/mm^3
Child-Pugh A-B	Extrahepatic dissemination
<5 lesions	Ascites (needs to be controlled before RFA)
<4 cm in diameter each	Bilioenteric anastomosis (high risk of sepsis)

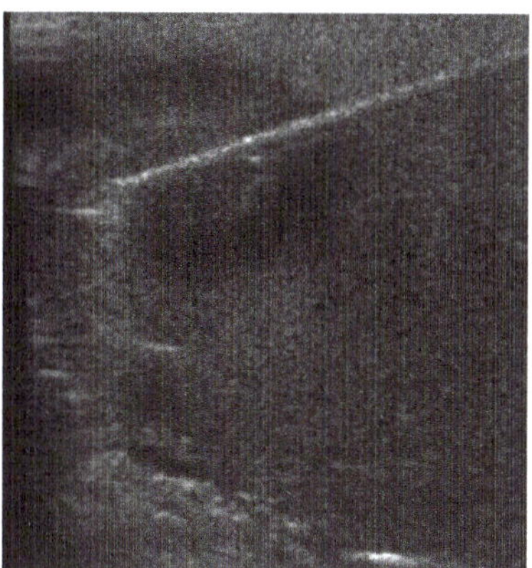

Fig. 4.2 Intraoperative RFA

4.2 Liver Tumors

4.2.1 Hepatocellular Carcinoma (HCC)

RFA is indicated in HCC patients who are not candidates for hepatic resection either because of unfavorable anatomy or inadequate hepatic reserve. According to BCLC 2003 treatment algorithm, RFA has been enlisted among curative options [11, 12]. In an analysis of 1,000 cases, Tateishi et al. [13] reported cumulative survival rates at 3 and 5 years of 77.7 and 54.3 %, respectively, for patients initially treated by RFA, while for those who had RFA for recurrent tumor after previous treatment the rates were 62.4 and 38.2 %, respectively.

Indications and contraindications for RFA of HCC are summarized in Table 4.1.

In cases of intraoperative change of treatment plan because of inoperability, intraoperative RFA can be performed under ultrasound guidance (Fig. 4.2).

Tumor dimensions are of great importance, as with current devices the ablation volume does not exceed 4 cm at its best. Excellent results have been reported in solitary HCC < 4 cm [13, 14]. The goal is to ablate the lesion plus a 1 cm surrounding hepatic tissue. For bigger tumors (5–6 cm), longer multitined needles or overlapping ablations can be of some benefit. Combination with transcatheter arterial embolization (TACE) has also been reported effective. Studies [15, 16] in early HCC have shown superiority of combined TACE and RFA over TACE or RFA alone. Moreover, comparable to the surgical resection results have been reported concerning the probability of overall survival (OS) at 1, 3, and 5 years, although inferior in terms of local recurrence rates.

Troubles during RFA

1. Heat-sink effect:

   Heat abduction by vessels close to ablated area result in suboptimal coagulation. Troubleshooting includes longer ablation times, MWA, or pre-ablative embolization [17].

2. Tumor seeding (1.5 %):

   Cancer cells' seeding is supposed to take place during RFA probe removal. Track ablation and keeping of punctures to a minimum are strongly suggested.

3. Adjacent organs penetration or ablation:

   Colon, duodenum (or small bowel after bilioenteric anastomosis), and stomach are at risk during RFA or MWA at the periphery of the liver. Pre-existing adhesions increase the risk [18]. Troubleshooting includes insulation by means of saline, and 5 % glycose solution or CO_2 injection between the liver and adjacent organs.

4. Bilioenteric anastomosis, sphincterotomy:
   Patients with bilioenteric anastomosis or recent sphincterotomy are prone to develop hepatic abscess post RFA or MWA.

Complications

RFA is associated with a considerably low mortality of 0.3 % [19]. Overall complication rates are reported in range of 1.9–4.5 % [19, 20]. Major complications include hemorrhage, abscess formation, hepatic infarction, tumor seeding, bilhemia, and gastrointestinal tract perforation. Other complications are portal venous thrombosis, hepatic venous thrombosis, arteriovenous fistula, hepatic artery pseudoaneurysm, biloma formation, hemobilia, bile duct stenosis, bilary peritonitis, diaphragmatic injury and grounding pad burns, pneumothorax, pleural effusion, and biliocutaneous or bronchobiliary fistula. Rare incidents of pulmonary embolism secondary to hepatic venous thrombosis and pulmonary hypertension due to RFA-produced microbubble accumulation in the pulmonary arteries have been reported [21].

Some of the complications could be treated by means of interventional radiologic procedures, as indicated in the Table 4.2.

Side Effects

Localized pain radiating to the ipsilateral shoulder, perihepatic or pleural effusion, epigastric discomfort, and nausea, are common postablation symptoms that are not considered as complications. Postablation syndrome is a flu-like condition which lasts 1–10 days and presents with mild fever (<38.5 °C), malaise, pain, and nausea [22]. The bigger area ablated, the more intense the manifestation of postablation syndrome. Special care must be taken not to misinterpret an abscess formation for postablation syndrome; persistence of symptoms beyond 2 weeks should alert the treating doctor to exclude abscess formation. Nearly one-third of the radiofrequency ablated patients will develop some degree of postablation syndrome.

4.2.2 Liver Metastases

RFA or MWA is among the treating procedures for hepatic metastases, mostly from colorectal cancer (CRC). Although most studies are not randomized and vary in inclusion criteria, surgical resection shows better results in terms of OS and disease-free survival [23]. However, about half of the CRC patients develops liver metastases, half of them are confined to the liver. From the remaining cohort only 10–25 % is eligible for metastasectomy or partial hepatic resection. For the patients with CRHM that cannot be rendered tumor-free by resection, a multimodality treatment is mandatory, ablative techniques having a pillar role. Resection combined with ablation can be applied in the following scenarios [24]: 1. Synchronous metastases which cannot be cleared by resection or in which resection is considered of high risk for the particular patient. 2. Rendering appropriate tumor-free liver segments for future hepatic resection. This scenario can be

Table 4.2 Complications of RFA and suggested treatment

Complications after RFA	Treatment
Arterial hemorrhage	Embolization of the bleeding source
GI tract penetration	Consider surgery
Abscess formation	Drainage, IV antibiotics
A-V fistula	Covered stent placement
Hepatic artery pseudoaneurysm	Covered stent, embolization
Hemobilia	Embolization of the bleeding source, biliary drainage if needed
Bile duct stenosis	Endoscopic or percutaneous dilation, plastic stent insertion
Biloma formation	Drainage
Subcapsular hematoma	Drainage
Pneumothorax	Drainage

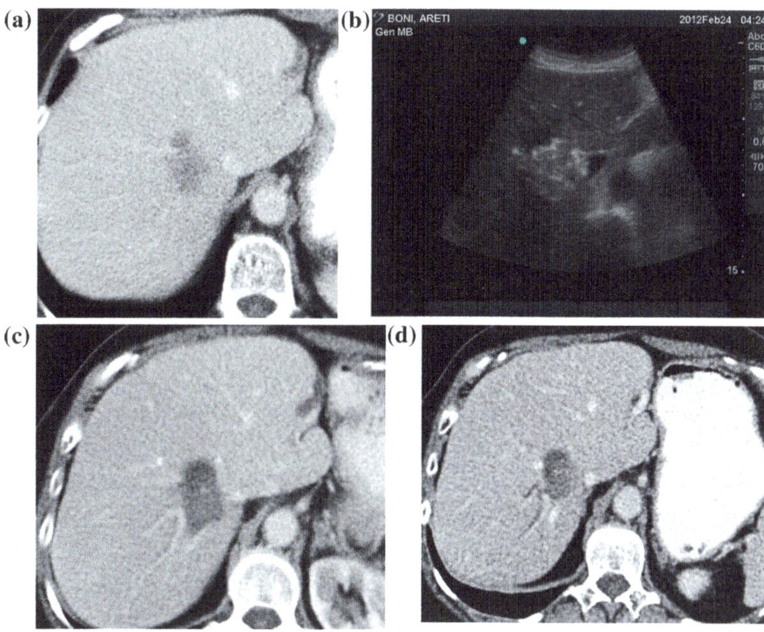

Fig. 4.3 Tumor ablation. **a** Solitary CRHM. **b** Ultrasound scan during RFA. **c** 1 month follow-up. **d** 2 years follow-up. Stable size, no peripheral enhancement

associated with portal vein branch embolization. 3. Treating intraoperatively discovered new lesions. 4. Small overall size CRHM with operable pulmonary metastases.

Standard care includes systemic chemotherapy, biologic therapy, and it almost invariably accompanies local treatment options. Combination of chemotherapy with ablation has shown to result in survival benefit compared to chemotherapy alone [25]. In a randomized phase II study, Ruers et al. reported progression-free survival (PFS) of 16.8 months in the RFA + chemotherapy arm versus 9.9 months in the chemotherapy alone arm. For 30 months, OS rates were 61.7 % and 57.6 %, respectively [26]. In a meta-analysis by Weng et al. [27], 5-year OS was reported 17.9–42 %, while the medium 5-year OS of untreated patients was <5 % [28].

In view of a 2 % risk of abscess development, prophylactic antibiotics could be administered. Several studies, however, do not report additional benefit [29]. In terms of safety, RFA shows morbidity rate 9.98 % (liver resection-LR 24.10 %) and mortality 0.34 % (LR 0.31 %), respectively.

Although there is no typical restriction as to the number of lesions that can be ablated, best results have been reported for single lesions, patients with CEA < 200 ng/ml or fewer than four lesions, smaller than 3 cm in diameter [30] (Fig. 4.3). Ablation of larger tumors leads in significantly increased tumor recurrence rate [31, 32].

Treatment assessment and follow-up imaging. Imaging of the liver after ablation techniques is mandatory in determining both treatment response and new lesions appearance. Since extensive tumor necrosis is not always associated by reduction in size, estimation of viable tumor volume is the goal of the imaging modalities. CT and MRI are the methods of choice. According to the EASL criteria [12], viable tumor is defined by increased contrast medium uptake during the arterial phase of dynamic CT or MRI. However, early CT scan could show a thick ring-like enhancement due to persisting postablative hyperemia and inflammatory reaction of the surrounding hepatic parenchyma. This, in turn, will vanish or give place to a thin, homogeneous ring-like enhancement in 4 weeks time, decreasing in size and intensity thereafter. Any inhomogeneity, partial thickness or reappearance of perilesional enhancement should be interpreted as recurrent lesion. RECIST criteria are listed in Chap. 2.

Apart from CRHM, thermal tumor ablation has been proved effective in treatment of neuroendocrine metastases by means of reducing both tumor load and hormonal symptoms [33–35], thus assisting the medical treatment.

4.2.3 Thermal Ablation of Renal Tumors

RFA and cryoablation are the two main ablative techniques in use in renal tumors, renal cell carcinoma in particular. The benefit of preserving renal function must not endanger the oncologic outcomes in these patients. Therefore, indications for ablative approach include :

- incidental finding of a small, <4 cm, RCC
- poor surgical candidates because of comorbidities
- patients with solitary kidney or bilateral tumors, in high risk for chronic dialysis.

Large tumors, presence of metastases, and unfavorable tumor location (e.g., in the hilum or adjacent to renal pelvis and proximal ureter) are relative contraindications, whereas coagulopathy or poor general condition are absolute ones.

Tumors 4–5 cm in diameter could be, instead of RFA, treated with cryoablation using multiple probes.

Complications of ablative procedures in the kidneys are 3.1 % [36] and consist mainly of hemorrhage, thermal injury of the proximal ureter with subsequent urinoma formation or delayed ureteral stenosis, infection, tumor seeding, and heat injury of adjacent structures. To avoid the latter, a 5 mm insulation space (fat, CO_2, and saline) between the ablation area and the adjacent organ is suggested.

Although usually self-retained, hemorrhage is more likely to complicate cryoablation than RFA. However, in a meta-analysis by Kunkle and Uzzo [37], cryoablation shows better results in terms of tumor recurrence, number of retreatments, and risk of metastatic progression compared to RFA, although the incidence of progression to metastatic disease was similar.

4.2.4 Thermal Ablation of Lung Tumors

Thermal tumor ablation (RFA or MWA) has been used in patients with primary or secondary lung tumors, either alone or in combination with other modalities [38]. Still not being an established treatment, ablation could be considered for patients with tumors ≤3.5 cm in diameter who cannot have a surgical resection due to impaired respiratory function or severe cardiopulmonary comorbidities (stage I–IIIa for NSCLC, I–II for SCLC) [39]. Concerning secondary depositions, thermal ablation should be decided by tumor board. Less than five lesions, <3 cm each as well as absence of concomitant extrapulmonary depositions are among the accepted inclusion criteria. *Contraindications* include irreversible coagulopathy, short life expectancy, and poor performance status. Lesions close to hilum, large vessels, trachea, main bronchi, or esophagus should be avoided due to increased risk of inadvertent life-threatening damage [40].

RFA is the most widespread ablation modality. MWA is less reported but has some theoretical advantages, as heating is not hampered by air insulation, heat sink, or charring around the probe. During and immediately after ablation, ground glass opacity is created encompassing the ablated lesion. This opacity is suggested to be up to four times the size of the lesion to ensure complete ablation [41].

Immediate or delayed pneumothorax is the usual *complication* of thermal lung tumor ablation, occurring in 30–40 % of the cases [39, 42]. Other complications include postprocedural pain, fever, bronchopleural fistula (extensive track ablation is a predisposing factor), thermal injury of phrenic nerve or brachial plexus, systemic air embolism (rare), and hemoptysis (usually transient). Pulmonary artery pseudoaneurysm has been reported complicating central lesion's RFA [43].

Encouraging results have been reported for both primary and secondary lung tumors in highly selected patient cohorts [44, 45]. A 5-year OS of

27 % for NSCLC and of 57 % for inoperable lung metastases was reported by Simon et al. in a cohort of 153 patients [46]. Gillams et al. reported overall median and 3-year survival of 41 months and 57 % in patients with lung metastases 1–8 in number, 0.5–4 cm in size [47]. Small, <3 cm lesions have a better prognosis post RFA, as the ablation is more likely to be complete in these cases.

4.3 Irreversible Electroporation (IRE)

IRE is a nonthermal ablation. The theory behind it is that AC under certain conditions (2,000–2,700 V, nanosecond exposure time) can create irreversible damage at the cell membrane leading to apoptotic death [48].

Under ultrasound or CT guidance, the electrodes are directed either to the center (bipolar) or to the periphery (multiple monopolar) of the lesion. The procedure needs GA and ECG synchronization, as the emission of the electric pulses must be given at the P peak.

Advantage of IRE is that it affects the cells only, sparing the connective tissue and the large vessels [49, 50]. Moreover, ablation margins are "clear-cut", without the transition zone seen by thermal ablation.

4.3.1 Chemoembolization

The intraarterially delivered targeted tumor therapies in the liver can be divided into four main categories: (a) Chemoembolization, (b) embolization, (c) drug eluting bead chemoembolization, and (d) radioembolization.

Percutaneous transarterial chemoembolization (TACE) or simply chemoembolization is a procedure during which infusion of a mixture of chemotherapeutic agent/s with or without iodized oil with an embolic agent such as gel foam or PVA is performed selectively in a hepatic artery feeding a tumor occluding the tumor vasculature.

Embolization is the blockade of hepatic arterial flow of a tumor with a vascular occlusion agent without a chemotherapeutic agent and is also called bland embolization.

Chemoembolization with drug eluting beads is the intraarterial administration of spheric particles containing a chemotherapeutic agent that is gradually released into the tumor in a predicted manner.

Radioembolization is defined as the infusion of radioactive substances including microspheres containing yttrium 90, iodine I131, or other similar agents in the hepatic artery.

The first three procedures are discussed collectively since they have several similarities, while radioembolization is discussed at the last and separately because the mechanisms and technique are substantially different.

Chemoembolization (conventional TACE; c-TACE).

The principle of lipiodol-based chemoembolization (conventional TACE; c-TACE) lies on the local effect of very high concentrations of chemotherapeutic agents in combination with the embolic effect of lipiodol enhanced by a final injection of particulate embolics after the administration of the emulsified chemotherapeutic agents. This technique is feasible in the liver due to its dual blood supply. In the normal liver, one-third of the blood supply comes from the hepatic artery and the other two-thirds from the portal vein. Conversely, both primary and secondary liver tumors derive 90 % of their blood supply from the hepatic artery with a smaller (10 %) percentage from the portal vein. However, the exact proportion of blood supply may differ depending on the differentiation, morphology, and growth patterns of the tumor/s since some nonencapsulated well-differentiated tumors may receive a significant component from the portal vein.

During TACE, the cytotoxic effect of the chemotherapeutic agents is enhanced by ischemia caused by the vascular blockade. Ischemia causes failure of transmembrane pumps in tumor cells, which results in increased absorption of chemotherapeutic agents by tumor cells. In addition, the reduction of the arterial flow after embolization leads to the prolongation of contact of the chemotherapeutic agents with the tumoral cells. Increased dwell time increases the cytotoxic effect. It has been reported that the tissue concentrations of chemotherapeutic agent within tumors are 40 times higher than in surrounding normal liver parenchyma several months after TACE. However, studies have shown that tumor ischemia and hypoxia up-regulate molecular factors such as vascular endothelial growth factor (VEGF) and hypoxia inducible factor-1(HIF-1), preventing sufficient cell apoptosis and stimulating tumor growth and neoangiogenesis [51]. Hypoxia-induced VEGF is elevated 7 days postchemoembolization [51]. For this reason, complete anoxia is preferred to hypoxia while when hypoxia is induced, it is expected that the role of the chemotherapeutic counteracts the deleterious effects of neoangiogenesis.

Iodized oil (lipiodol; Andre Guerbet, Aulnay-sous-Bois, France) is a lymphangiographic contrast media, with a predisposition to selectively accumulate in the neovasculature and extravascular spaces of liver tumors when injected into the hepatic artery. TACE based on lipiodol mixed with different chemotherapeutic agents or, more often, with an emulsion of iodized oil and anti-cancer drugs followed by gel foam embolization, has been the mainstay of palliative treatment for unresectable liver tumors and particularly HCC. Moreover, iodized oil has been considered not only as an embolic material but also as a carrier of the chemotherapeutic agents [52].

Pharmacokinetics of lipiodol-based chemoembolization have shown that when the chemotherapeutic agent is delivered with lipiodol within the hepatic artery, the intratumoral concentration and half-life of doxorubicin was higher, while doxorubicin concentration in plasma was lower compared when doxorubicin was administrated without the lipiodol. Doxorubicin is released slowly from the lipiodol mixture [53] prolonging the contact time with the tumor—a fact that enhances the cytotoxic effect. In addition, the embolization with gel foam at the end of the administration of the emulsified chemotherapeutic produces higher concentrations in tissue, prolonged half-life, and lower concentrations in plasma [52]. After injection into the hepatic artery, lipiodol remains in the tumor in high concentrations that range from 7 to 21 times more because of hemodynamic differences between hypervascular hepatic tumors and liver parenchyma, and the absence of Kupffer cells in tumors that in normal liver phagocytose lipiodol [53, 54]. Lipiodol injected in a segmental branch of the hepatic artery via the peribiliary plexus accumulates in the peripheral portal vein and also passes through the sinusoids causing in this way a further stasis in the tumor [55]. This distribution of lipiodol makes it an arterial and portal venous embolic material that is important for the tumors that have a significant portal venous component as mentioned above.

Embolization (Bland Embolization)

The principle is that oxygen deprivation can have a cytotoxic effect alone, while the chemotherapeutic used in the chemoembolization has not proven its particular value. Taking into account that both TACE and bland embolization may trigger angiogenesis the small sizes of particles are used. Centers that adopt this technique present good results. However, one randomized study and a study with pathology documentation showed that bland embolization has more recurrences, shorter time to progression, and less histologic necrosis compared with chemoembolization [56, 57].

Drug Eluting Bead Chemoembolization

The principle in drug eluting beads technology is that the membranes of the drug eluting agents are able to allow the high concentration and dose of the chemotherapeutic agents into the sphere and then allow release when the sphere is within the tumor environment for a prolonged and predicted manner. The advantage is the standardized technique and doses, high chemotherapeutic concentrations in the tumor and low in the peripheral circulation. The only loadable agents available today include DC Bead™ (Biocompatibles UK, Surrey, UK), Hepasphere/Quadrasphere (Biosphere, Merit), and Tandem (recently released by Celonova). DC Bead™ is a soft deformable device of spherical shape composed of a polyvinyl alcohol (PVA) and a hydrophilic ionic monomer known as AMPS that is able to be loaded with anthracycline drugs such as doxorubicin and irinotecan [58]. After in vitro loading in the angio room or the pharmacy, the chemotherapeutic is contained within the beads, and controlled drug elution occurs only within the tumor and in a gradual fashion. Doxorubicin loss on bead suspension and contrast agent mixture is about 0.2–2 % minimizing in this way the systemic release of doxorubicin, and hence the side effects are seen in conventional TACE [58]. Animal studies have shown that with drug eluting beads, the plasma levels of the chemotherapeutic agents are significantly lower than that of the c-TACE, while the intratumoral levels are four times higher. From a clinical point, the first published human study of Varela et al. showed that there was a 2-log reduction in plasma doxorubicin-loaded beads compared with TACE [59].

Hepasphere/quadrasphere is a nonbiodegradable superabsorbent polymer microsphere that absorbs fluid and swells when exposed to aqueous media. They are softer than DC Bead. Hepasphere is available in the dry form and it loads with doxorubicin or irinotecan in an ionic solution. Lee et al. showed that the loaded forms in rabbits caused significantly more extensive cell death compared to the nonloaded spheres, while the levels of doxorubicin and doxorubicinol in plasma were low [60]. Gupta et al. comparing intraarterial injection and TACE with embolization with Hepasphere loaded with doxorubicin found that the levels of the doxorubicin and metabolites were much lower with Hepasphere compared to TACE and intraarterial injection, while they found at least four times higher levels of doxorubicin in the tissue compared to chemoembolization [61].

Doxorubicin/irinotecan loading range: For DC Bead and Hepasphere the recommended dose range is 25–37.5 mg of doxorubicin per ml of hydrated beads/spheres (100–150 mg/patient). These concentrations should be achieved by the preparation of two vials of beads/spheres with 37.5 mg of hydrated beads (total 150 mg/patient) or, two vials of beads/spheres with 25 mg/ml of hydrated beads (total 100 mg/patient). Similarly for irinotecan, the dose should be 100 mg/patient—that is 50 mg/vial. For doxorubicin, this range achieves doses of 50–75 mg/m^2 that are considered safe treatment levels, with a maximum recommended life dose of 450 mg/m of body surface area to avoid cardiac toxicity.

Choice of beads. As a general rule, the choice of the bead diameter to load depends on the size and vascularity of the target lesion. The smaller particles penetrate deeper into the lesion. However, the small diameters can be more harmful to the adjacent liver and a versatile combination of bead diameters for each patient is needed. It has been proven that diameters of 100–300 μ are not associated with increased rate of complications [62]. No studies of safety have yet been done with loadable beads of <100 μ in diameter.

Common Considerations for Chemoembolization

Pre-embolization evaluation. For safe and efficient chemoembolization, MDCT or MRI of the liver is necessary to access accurately tumor stage. For metastatic disease MRI is clearly preferable. Contrast enhance ultrasound (CEUS) is also very useful to evaluate tumor vascularity. Liver function should be assessed along with tumor markers.

Patient selection. Chemoembolization is the preferred treatment for BCLC stage B HCC (Fig. 4.4), for BCLC, stage A HCC is not suitable for curative treatments such as RFA or surgery. Chemoembolization is indicated also for nonsurgical candidates with cholangiocarcinoma, neuroendocrine cell liver metastasis (carcinoid tumors and islet cell carcinomas), metastatic to the liver colon cancer, and

(a)
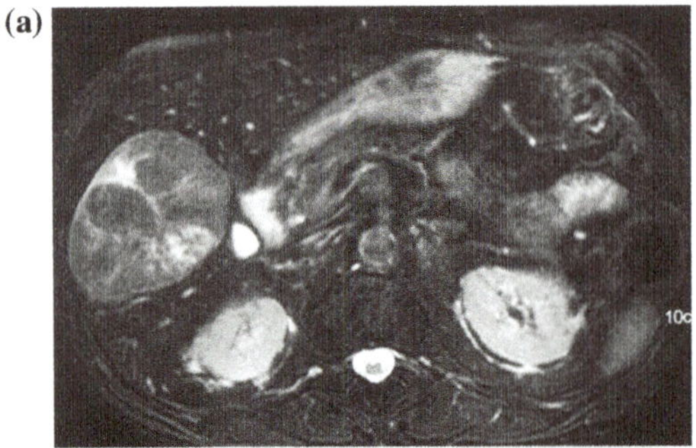
(b)
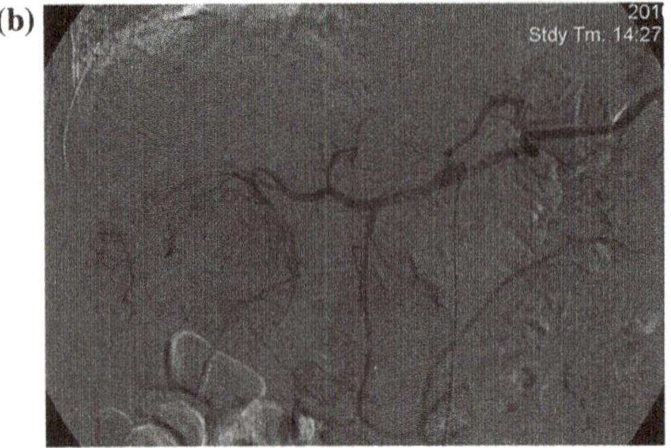

(c)
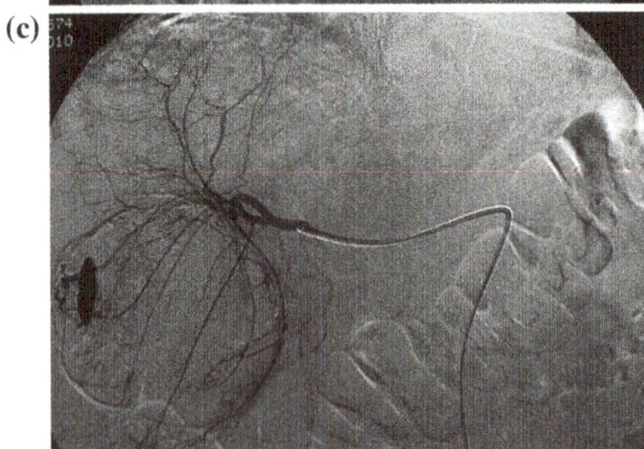

Fig. 4.4 **a** Solid hepatocellular carcinoma in T2 MRI sequence. **b** Angiography of haller tripod demonstrates a focal liver lesion with hypervascularity. **c** Image during selective chemoembolization shows intratumoral vascularity and a vascular lake

sarcomas metastatic to the liver. Parameters that are predictors of the outcome are related to tumor burden, liver functional status (Child-Pugh, bilirubin, and ascites), and performance status (Karnofsky score, Estern Cooperative Onclology Group—ECOG scale) and response to treatment. Absolute contraindications to TACE include Child Pugh C and patients suitable for curative treatments. Strong contraindications include: Serum bilirubin >2 mg/dL, lactate dehydrogenase >425 u/l, aspartate aminotransferase >100 u/l, tumor burden extending to more than 50 % of the liver, extrahepatic metastasis, cardiac, or renal insufficiency, intractable arteriovenous fistula, complete portal trunk thrombosis, and vascular invasion in the inferior vena cava or right atrium. The selective approach has limited the contraindications and can be performed now even in PVT, if hepatopetal collateral flow is present.

Patient preparation. Patients are fasted 8 h prior to the procedure and premedicated with good hydration, antiemetics, analgesia, antiedematous drugs, gastric protection, and antibiotics. In patients with compromised function of the sphincter of Oddi or prior hepatojejunostomy that are high risk for developing an hepatic abscess intense antibiotic prophylaxis and bowel preparation is indicated according to institutional protocols (common schemes: Patient-controlled analgesia, cefazolin 500 mg, IV q8 hr × 3d, metronidazole 500 mg, IV q8 × 3, ondansetron 8 mg, IC q12 hr prn, and dexamethasone 8 mg, IV q8). Informed consent is required.

Technique. A full arteriography of the tripod of Haller and superior mesenteric artery (SMA) is required to obtain information on regional vascular anatomy and variants and evaluate areas of arterial blush with hypervascularity. This is performed with a 5F Simmons or Cobra catheter. The SMA injection should extent to the full evaluation of retrograde flow through the gastroduodenal artery (GDA). The catheter should be advanced beyond the origin of the GDA and after the initial arterial mapping beyond the cystic artery that is the first branch of the proper hepatic artery. In tumor extending in the superior surface of the liver, intercostals arteries and inferior phrenic artery should also be interrogated, since they are common sources of parasitic feeding. Special focus is required to identify systemic arteries that originate from the liver arteries to avoid nontarget embolization. After the identification of the tumor feeders', selective or superselective catheterization with a use of a microcatheter is performed and the embolic material is injected slowly to avoid backflow. The infused material and the endpoint of the embolization are further discussed for each type of embolization specifically in the procedure specifics (below).

Postprocedural care. Patients should be medicated for pain, nausea, and vomiting and should be kept well hydrated. After 12–18 h a CT should be performed (IV contrast is not used if c-TACE with lipiodol has been performed), and in the absence of complications the patient can be discharged.

Follow-up and evaluation of results. The local response is evaluated with triphasic MDCT or MRI using the m-RECIST or RECIST criteria. Tumor markers and evaluation of the liver function complete the follow-up. In a patient in which the procedure was technically satisfactory, a failure of objective response in two successive embolizations or the development of a complication that consists a contraindication of the procedure or the development of nontreatable disease are indications for discontinuation of the procedures.

Procedure specifics for c-TACE. The emulsified chemotherapeutic agents mixture is injected slowly into the feeding vessel/s until stasis is induced. When embolizing tumors below 5 cm, it is recommended that the emulsion should be injected until small branches of the portal vein are visualized. In this way, a dual hepatic artery and portal vein embolization is achieved that enhances the embolic effect. The total volume of lipiodol used can be calculated with the following equation: 3/2d (d = diameter of tumor). Alternatively, the relative volumes of chemotherapeutics to lipiodol should be at a 1:1 or 2:1. Dry doxorubicin is preferred in order to achieve high concentrations locally and keep the total volume of the injected material to a minimum. For HCC and Intrahepatic Cholangiocarcinoma (ICC), the commonest combination is cisplatin 100 mg, doxorubicin 50 mg, and mitomycin C 10 mg. For colorectal metastasis 5 FU 1 gr, Mitomycin-C, 10 mg. For metastasis from neuroendocrine tumors bland embolization is used in many centers with particles 20–500 μ while others perform chemoembolization with 20 mg mitomycin C, 30 mg of doxorubicin and 50 mg lyophilized cisplatin. For metastasis from islet cell tumors doxorubicin alone at dosage of 50 mg/m^2 or cisplatin 100 mg with 50 mg adriamycin and 10 mg of mitomycin C are the two most commonly used combinations. The addition of 5–10 ml of intraarterial lidocaine 2 % may be used to reduce pain. Finally, the procedure is completed with the injection of 1–4 ml of a suspension of gel foam or embosphere or PVA of 100–500 μ in diameter.

In postprocedural CT, the lipiodol distribution can be studied and allows a good evaluation of the success of the embolization procedure. IV contrast is not used. The lipiodol does not preclude MRI evaluation and the follow up of these patients 3–6 weeks postprocedure should be done with this technique to evaluate residual disease and necrosis.

Procedure specifics for bland embolization. Bland embolization does not decrease the risk for patients with contraindications as listed above. Particles used for embolization are: Gelatin sponge (Gelfoam), polyvinyl alcohol (PVA-Contour), embospheres (Biosphere, Merit), embozene (Celonova), bead block (Biocompatibles), and lipiodol (Ethiodol). Postprocedural evaluation can be done either with triphasic MDCT or MRI since no lipiodol is used. However, to achieve anoxia rather than hypoxia to the tumor and avoid the cascade of neoangiogenesis, the smaller possible particles are advocated. However, the use of spheric particles well below 100 μ has been implicated with lung infarction and their use should not been preferred in tumors above 5–6 cm in diameter particularly if located in the upper surface of the liver. Bland embolization can be a safe alternative if embolization of parasitic collaterals in difficult cases.

Procedure specifics for drug eluting beads. There are plenty of evidences today for DC Bead and Hepasphere with large clinical series and these agents have proved to be safe and efficient. However, no clinical studies are available yet for Tandem. These agents can be easily loaded in vitro in the angiosuite in 20–60 min depending on the diameter. It is important to dilute these agents to large volumes immediately before injection (to 20 cc of contrast and saline per vial) and the injection should be slow and pulsatile to a rate of 1–3 cc/min depending on the size of the vessel injected. The microcatheter should not be wedged and preservation of some blood flow is necessary to carry the agents as distal to the lesion as possible. The maximum quantity of vials is two per session and no additional embolics are recommended to achieve stasis. Infact, the end point of the embolization is obliteration of the neovascularity within the tumor and not stasis. The rest of the procedure is similar to c-TACE. Postprocedural evaluation can be done either with triphasic MDCT or MRI since no lipiodol is used. For the first 3–4 h postembolization a noncontrast CT may allow to assess the distribution of the injected material from the dense vascular lakes that can be identified.

Complications and side effects. The postembolization syndrome is the commonest side effect of chemoembolization and is most frequent and more severe with c-TACE. However, postembolization syndrome requiring an extended hospital stay or readmission is reported in <4.6 %. Drug eluting bead chemoembolization causes frequent pain but is more limited and has duration of 1–3 days requiring only simple analgetic such as acetaminophen. Fever may occur in one-third of the patients and lasts for a few days. Differential diagnosis from an abscess formation, gallbladder infarction of cholecystitis, or septicemia is necessary. Liver failure is the most notorious complication especially in HCC patients due to the underlying cirrhosis and is reported in 2.3 % overall. Abscess formation is reported in 1–2.3 % overall, cholecystitis requiring surgical intervention in <2.1 %. According to the Quality Improvement Guidelines of the Society of Interventional Radiology, the accepted threshold of the commonest complications is as follows: For liver failure it should be <4 %, abscess <2 % in patients with a functional Oddi sphincter, abscess in a nonfunctional Oddi <10 %, postembolization syndrome requiring extension of hospitalization or readmission <10 %, surgical cholecystitis <1 %, biloma requiring drainage <2 % and pulmonary arterial embolus, gastrointestinal hemorrhage, iatrogenic dissection preventing treatment, and 30-day mortality should be <1 % [63].

Results

HCC. The results of chemoembolization can be assessed with local response and survival benefit. The studies of Lo and Llovet showed in randomized trials that the survival benefit of c-TACE over conservative treatment [64, 65]. Similar results were obtained by metanalysis studies; untreated BCLC B disease presents a median survival of 16 months that can be expanded with chemoembolization to 19–20 months (Bruix). Overall, Marelli et al. in their metanalysis found that in studies after 2,000 survival rates after c-TACE at 1, 2, 3, and 5 years are 71 ± 18 %, 48 ± 16 %, 34 ± 13 %, and 14 ± 10 %, respectively [66].

Recent reports of 5-year survival with drug eluting beads reached 23.5 and 27.6 % for Child A and B patients, respectively. However, the recurrences were not reported in these studies [67, 68].

Colorectal metastasis comparisons of FOLFIRI and DEBIRI (drug eluting beads loaded with irinotecan) showed a statistically significant difference between DEBIRI and FOLFIRI for OS (7 months), PFS (3 months), and quality of life (5 months). In addition, a clinically significant improvement in time to extrahepatic progression (4 months) was observed for DEBIRI [69, 70]. Martin et al. with DEBIRI found response rates 66 % at 6 months and 75 % at 12 months. OS was 19 months, with PFS of 11 months [70]. Overall, with c-TACE responses ranged from 14 to 87 % and median survivals from 7 to 29 months that are longer than the ones expected in patients who failed standard therapy [71]. In other studies median survival reached 24 months [71].

For intrahepatic cholangiocarcinoma (ICC). It has been shown that patients treated with c-TACE expanded median survival to 23 months compared to 6–8 months of nontreated patients [72]. However, chemoembolization is not the procedure of choice for the nonsurgical patients and local ablation is preferred if size and location are permitting.

Metastatic neuroendocrine tumors. Although not many studies have been performed, there is evidence that embolization prolongs survival in these patients with a 5-year survival of 50 % with embolization compared to medical treatment that presents a 5-year survival of only 25 % [73]. Most studies agree that there are no differences in response between c-TACE and bland embolization in metastatic carcinoid tumors while studies in neuroendocrine tumors show that with c-TACE there is a survival benefit with an OS of 31.5 months [74]. Roch et al. report a complete symptom relief in 53 % and a partial in 40 % of the patients [75], and result had been obtained after two sessions in 81 % of the patients. Regarding response, carcinoids have a better overall response as evaluated by local response and progression-free survival compared to islet cell tumors with an OS 33.8 months for carcinoids versus 23.2 months for islet cell carcinomas, respectively [76].

4.3.2 Radioembolization

Yttrium-90 (Y90) microspheres are radioactive particles which are used for the radioembolization. Y90 administered intraarterially directs the highly concentrated radiation to the tumor, while healthy liver parenchyma is relatively spared due to its preferential blood supply from portal venous supply. There are two available devices for Y90 administration: TheraSphere® (glass based) and SIR-Spheres® (resin based). Other radioisotopes are iodine-131 labeled iodized oil (I-131-Lipiodol), rhenium-188 HDD labeled iodized oil and milican/holmium-166 microspheres (HoMS) but they are not in clinical practice for liver embolization yet. For the Y90, the range of tissue penetration of the emissions is 2.5–11 mm. TheraSphere® (MDS Nordion, Ottawa, Canada) consists of nonbiodegradable glass microspheres that have a diameter between 20 and 30 microns. SIR-Spheres® (Sirtex, Lane Cove, Australia) consist of biodegradable resin microspheres. Each vial of SIR-Spheres® of 3 GBq contains 40–80 million microspheres ranging from 20 to 60 μm.

Patient selection/indications. Radioembolization has proven useful for the majority of patients with HCC as most of them present in advanced stage, beyond potentially curative options (resection/liver transplantation). Y90 microspheres can be used in downstaging large tumors to bring within transplantation criteria, in patients with portal venous thrombosis due to tumor invasion and as palliative therapy [77, 78]. It is suitable for patients with vascular invasion. ICC can be also treated with radioembolization. Radioembolization is also used for metastatic liver disease from colorectal cancer, neuroendocrine tumors, breast cancer, and other malignancies [79]. PVT is not a contraindication. Usually, more advanced tumors respond well to radioembolization compared to chemoembolization.

Technique: Several steps are required. (1) After arteriography of the celiac artery and SMA prophylactic embolization of the GDA and right gastric artery is recommended to minimize the risks of inadvertent deposition of microspheres in the gastrointestinal tract. Other vessels that may be needed to be embolized are the falciform, inferior esophageal, left inferior phrenic, accessory left gastric, supraduodenal, and retroduodenal arteries. (2) Technetium 99 m labeled macroaggregated albumin TAE and scan: To avoid shunting of Y90 microspheres to lungs that could result in radiation pneumonitis a technetium 99 m labeled macroaggregated albumin (99 mTc-MAA) scan is typically performed prior to embolization, since HCC is commonly associated with direct arteriovenous shunts that may be difficult to evaluate by the angiography. Since the 99 mTc-MAA has a similar molecule size with Y90, the scan simulates the distribution of Y90 post embolization. Lung shunt fraction (LSF) is used to calculate the dose delivered to the lungs and appropriate adjustments of the dose are made. The volume of the liver is calculated using 3-dimensional software and the dose that has to be injected in GBq is calculated by formulas given from the manufacturer and is different between SIR and

TheraSpheres. (3) The infusion of the radioactive particles is done in a lobar or a segmental fashion under fluoroscopic guidance.

Complications. The complications include nausea, fatigue, abdominal pain, hepatic dysfunction, biliary injury, fibrosis, radiation pneumonitis, GI ulcers, and vascular injury; however, these can be avoided by meticulous pretreatment assessment, careful patient selection, and adequate dosimetry. Hepatobiliary dysfunction from radiation-induced liver disease (RILD) occurs with an incidence ranging from 0 to 4 %. Liver radiation doses of 150 Gy in a single session are associated with liver toxicity. Biliary complications are reported in <10 % including bilomas, cholecystitis, and radiation-induced cholangitis. Radiation pneumonitis is reported in <1 %. Gastrointestinal complications from inadvertent embolization are reported in <5 %.

Results. The local response is evaluated with MRI and tumor markers. A comparative study with chemoembolization suggests response rates 49 and 36 % for radioembolization and chemoembolization, respectively, with longer time-to-progression (TTP) and reduced toxicities for patients treated with radioembolization 13.3 months versus 8.4 months, respectively (28). In a series with 291 HCC patients treated with Y90 response rates were 42 and 57 % based on WHO and EASL criteria, respectively. The overall TTP was 7.9 months and survival times for Child-Pugh A and B disease was 17.2 and 7.7 months, respectively. Patients with Child-Pugh B disease who had PVT survived 5.6 months indicating that the first patient group benefited best while the Child-Pugh B with PVT had a poor outcome. Kooby et al. comparing transarterial chemoembolization with radioembolization retrospectively for cases performed between 1996 and 2006 concluded that these therapies provided similar effectiveness and toxicity [80]. Similar results were published by Carr et al. [81]. Lewandowski et al. [82] compared the downstaging effectiveness of chemoembolization versus radioembolization in 86 patients with unresectable HCC and found that radioembolization was a better tool than chemoembolization for downstaging the disease from a size outside transplant criteria to a size within the Milan criteria for transplantation. Kennedy et al. [79] in 208 patients with chemorefractory colorectal metastases found a response rate of 35 % and a positron emission tomography (PET) response rate of 91 %. Survival rates were 10.5 months for responders and 4.5 months for nonresponders. In neuroendocrine tumor metastasis, a recent study has shown excellent results with 1, 2, and 3 years OS rates at 72.5, 62.5, and 45 %, respectively [77].

4.4 Palliative Procedures

Interventional radiology considerably contributes to palliative management of the cancer patients, targeting in symptomatic relief by means of drainage, decompression, or adjuvant procedures.

4.4.1 Indications for Esophageal Stent

Indications for esophageal stent insertion are malignant dysphagia due to esophageal carcinoma, external compression by lung or mediastinal tumor or anastomotic tumor recurrence postsurgery as well as tracheoesophageal fistula [83]. Contraindications are upper esophageal sphincter mechanism involvement, distal to esophagus obstruction of GI tract (e.g., peritoneal seeding), uncorrectable bleeding diathesis, and short life expectancy. Tracheal compression is a contraindication if it cannot be compensated by simultaneous tracheal stent insertion. Several self-expanding metallic stents are available in the market with dimensions varied from 18 to 24 cm in diameter and 60–170 cm in length (Fig. 4.5). Various designs have been tested to improve fixation and patency while avoiding distal migration and tumor ingrowth [84, 85]. Retrievable stents are also recently added to the list. Stents are inserted transorally under conscious sedation with continuous saliva aspiration to prevent aspiration. After crossing the obstruction with a guide wire, moderate balloon dilation facilitates accurate stent placement.

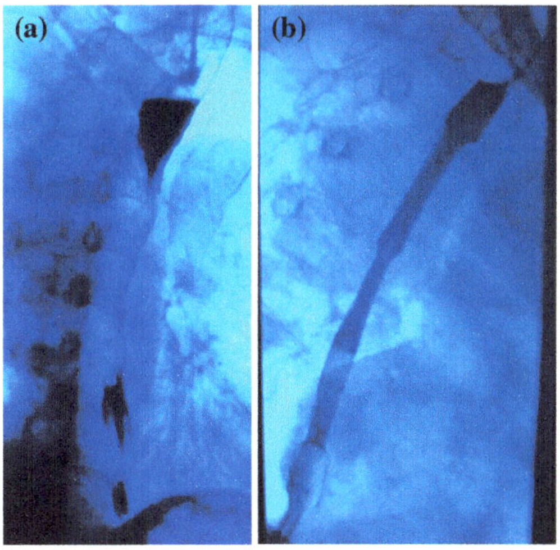

Fig. 4.5 **a** Malignant esophageal stenosis. **b** Self expanding Stent across the stenosis

Usually, a 60 % of the stent proximal and 40 % distal to the center of the lesion is indicated. *Complications* include postimplantation pain, hemorrhage, esophageal perforation, migration, food impaction, tumor ingrowth, tumor overgrowth, fistula development with mediastinitis, and sepsis [86, 87].

Self-expanding metallic stents can be deployed elsewhere in the GI tract as duodenum, proximal jejunum or colon, the latter usually as bridging procedure until surgical intervention, as acute colonic obstruction is associated with high operative mortality and morbidity [88]. Duodenal or jejunalstent insertion can be accomplished either transorally or via percutaneous gastrostomy. Uncovered stents are mostly in use for these sites.

Contraindications are perforation, <2 cm from the anal sphincters presence of malignancy (no landing zone), multiple obstruction locations (e.g., frozen pelvis), and uncorrectable coagulopathy. Guidance could be endoscopic, radiologic or a combination of two under fluoroscopy to ensure adequate guide wire negotiation with the obstruction and intraluminal position [89].

4.4.2 Percutaneous Biliary Drainage (PTBD) and Stent Insertion

Percutaneous transhepatic cholangiography (PTC) is performed to opacify the biliary tree in cases where ERCP or MRCP are inconclusive or inadequate for treatment plan. Beyond opacification, PTC is the first step in biliary drainage (PTBD).

Indication for PTBD is obstructive jaundice due to bile ducts occlusion of either internal (cholangiocarcinoma, ampullary cancer) or external origin (HCC, metastases, lymphadenopathy, and pancreatic carcinoma) (Fig. 4.6). Endoscopic drainage is usually the first choice as it carries less periprocedural risk. However, in case of unfavorable bowel anatomy (e.g., Billroth II gastrectomy), bile ducts are endoscopically inaccessible. Hilar or intrahepatic obstruction levels are troublesome for endoscopic approach while percutaneous drainage can almost always be effective.

Contraindications include: Uncorrectable coagulopathy (INR > 1.5, PLT < 50,000), multiple intrahepatic obstructions rendering drainage inadequate for functional liver, ascites (drainage is preliminary required).

All biliary procedures should be carried out under conscious sedation.

In case of bilateral hepatic duct obstruction, bilateral drainage is preferred, although in many cases unilateral drainage is sufficient for liver function. In case of bilateral approach, a PTC from the left hepatic lobe should also be performed under ultrasound guidance.

In case of PTBD, access through a peripheral bile duct is recommended to avoid inadvertent puncture of big portal vein or hepatic artery branches. Antibiotics are administered covering both gram-positive and gram-negative bacteria. Detailed PTBD procedure is described in several textbooks [90]. Self-expanding metallic endoprostheses are usually inserted. Mild (6–7 mm) balloon dilation could facilitate stent placement. Plastic stents do not provide as long patency as

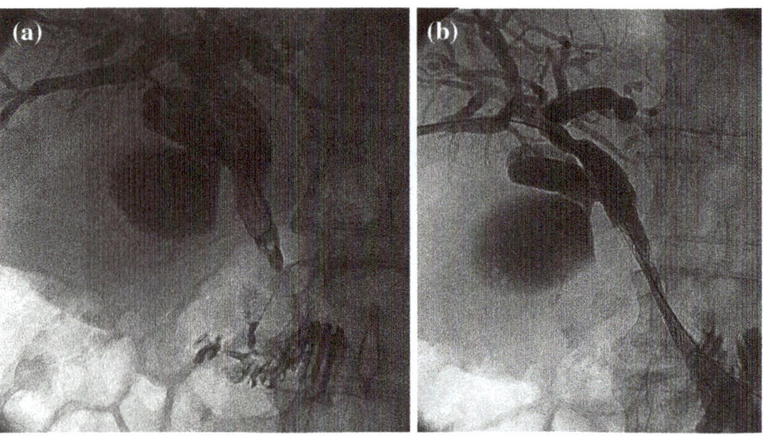

Fig. 4.6 **a** CBD stenosis from a pancreatic carcinoma. **b** Stent insertion

metallic ones. Indwelling internal–external drainage catheter could be an alternative solution, especially where operability has not been clarified. Failure to establish bile flow to the bowel leads to just an external drainage catheter placement for 3–4 days and retry after reduction of the bile ducts diameter.

Metallic stent patency is reported of approximately 4–7 months [91, 92]. Brountzos et al. reported primary patency of 120 days, restenosis rate 12 %, and secondary patency of 242.2 days [93]. Recently, covered stents have been compared to bare stents for palliation of malignant extrahepatic biliary obstruction and reported to be of better primary patency (87.6 vs. 69.8 % at 12 months) [94]. Major complications of PTBD as listed in the quality improvement guidelines for PTC and PTBD in CIRSE are sepsis (2.5 %), hemorrhage (2.5 %), localized inflammatory/infectious (1.2 %), pleural (0.5 %), and death (1.7 %). Portal and venous hemorrhage are usually self-retained, although tamponage with a large-bore catheter is advantageous. Coil filling of the access tract is of help too. Arterial hemorrhage should be treated with selective hepatic artery branch embolization.

Tumor ingrowth or overgrowth, bile sludge or debris due to enterobiliary reflux are common causes of stent dysfunction. Secondary stenting is then needed if the stent lumen cannot be cleared by means of balloon “sweeping”, i.e., partial inflation of an angioplasty balloon and push of it over a wire to the bowel.

4.4.3 Percutaneous Nephrostomy and Ureteral Stent Insertion

Malignant ureteric obstruction is a life-threatening condition because of inducing tubular atrophy and uremia as well as predisposing for infection and pyonephrosis. Decompression of hydronephrosis is therefore mandatory in the treating process. Endoscopic stent insertion is the first choice for drainage, followed by percutaneous approach. Urinary fistula or leakage is another indication for percutaneous nephrostomy alone or with a JJ stent insertion.

Terminal illness or irreversible coagulopathy are the main contraindications.

Preoperative assessment includes correction of any electrolytic imbalance, coagulation profile, and antibiotic prophylaxis. Detailed description of the related procedures can be found in several textbooks [95].

Major complications result in a mortality rate of 0.046–0.3 % [96] and consist of hemorrhage (1–3 %), sepsis (1–3 %, 7–9 % in case of pyonephrosis), and inadvertent puncture of adjacent organs (0.1–0.2 %). Marked bleeding should raise the suspicion of arterial puncture or pseudoaneurysm formation, thus angiographic evaluation and treatment is needed. In case of urine infection or pyonephrosis, every catheter or guide wire exchange add to the risk of hematogenous dissemination. All manipulations should be therefore kept to a minimum. Minor complications include minor hematuria, pain, urine extravasation, catheter dislodgement, or stent obstruction due to encrustation or blood clot.

JJ stents need a follow-up and replacement if occlusion is suspected. Monthly or bimonthly ultrasonographic check is advisable. Replacement of the JJ stent can be accomplished endoscopically; rarely, percutaneous removal and exchange can be performed.

4.5 Biopsy

Percutaneous biopsies under image guidance are the most common radiologic intervention to obtain tissue diagnosis. Endoluminal and transvascular biopsies are also feasible.

Indications. Include diagnosis of primary tumor, documentation of metastatic disease and staging of cancer, and treatment response monitoring.

Preparation and procedure. Full evaluation of patient records and informed consent are necessary. Patients who receive anticoagulative treatment should stop for 3–5 days and substitution with heparin should be considered. Patients should fast 4–6 h prior to the procedure and laboratory tests to evaluate hemostasis are first performed. PTT should be $< 1.5\times$ control, PT < 15 s, INR < 1.5, and platelets should be >100.000/ml. In biopsies with a high risk to bleeding Hgb and Hct should be obtained. In hypertensive patients suspected for a neuroendocrine tumor urine metanephrines, catecholamines, and vanillylmandelic acid (VMA) should be measured. In patients suspected for a hydatid cyst antiechinococcal serology should be obtained. If FNA (Fine Needle Aspiration) is going to be performed, it is better to have cytopathology evaluation "on site". Finally, the imaging modality that better demonstrates the lesion and the biopsy tools should be selected. The patients are draped and adequate anesthesia is given (usually local) and the biopsy is performed.

Biopsy needle selection. Fine needles 20–25 G are good for FNA and have a minimum tendency to cause bleeding. Larger needles are suitable for aspiration of viscous material. Cutting edge needles have various tip configurations and may be end-cutting type (with an acute bevel or 90 °bevel) and of side cutting needle type with a cannula cap or a stylet. Finally, spring loaded automated or semiautomated needles (side cutting) are also available and they are the most commonly used.

Postprocedural management. Check for pneumothorax, monitor of vital signs every 15 min for 1 h and every 30 min for 2 h and then every hour. Bed rest is recommended for 2–3 h. Patient can usually be discharged after 2–4 h.

Results. Biopsy yields diagnostic specimens in 80–95 % of cases [97]. Inadequate sampling is the most common cause of failure and the commonest cause of false negative biopsy. Inadequate sampling can be minimized when securing that the needle tip is in the center of the target lesion. However, difficult access, small lesions, and tissue inhomogeneities with necroses and areas of desmoplastic reactions are other well-known causes of inadequate sampling. In lesions with necrosis contrast enhancement prior to the biopsy facilitates avoidance of the necrotic areas and sampling from the solid part of the tumor/mass.

Complications. Overall, complications do not exceed 2 % [97, 98]. Bleeding is the most common in nonchest biopsies but clinically relevant hemorrhage is seen in <2 %. Pneumothorax is the most common in lung biopsies with an incidence from 12–22 %, however, in nonlung biopsies it is seen in <2 % [99]. Pancreatitis is seen in 2–3 % if normal pancreas is transgressed [98]. Needle tract tumor seeding is extremely rare and seen in <0.003–0.009 % [98]. Mortality rate is 0.006–0.031 % [98].

References

1. Uberoi R, Morgan R (2006) CIRSE quality assurance guidelines for superior vena cava stenting in malignant disease. CardioVasc Interv Radiol 29:319–322
2. Rosenthal DI, Hornicek FJ, Wolfe MW et al (1998) Percutaneous radiofrequency coagulation of osteoid osteoma compared with operative treatment. J Bone Joint Surg Am 80(6):815–821
3. Brace CL (2009) Radiofrequency and microwave ablation of the liver, lung, kidney and bone: what are the differences. Curr Probl Diagn Radiol 38:135–143
4. Simon CJ, Dupuy DE, Mayo-Smith WN (2005) Microwave ablation: principles and applications. Radiographics 25:S69–S83
5. Livraghi T, Meloni F, Solbiati L et al (2012) Complications of microwave ablation for liver tumors: results of a multicenter study. Cardiovasc Interv Radiol 35:868–874
6. Kojima Y, Suzuki S, Sakaguchi T et al (2000) Portal vein thrombosis caused by microwave coagulation therapy for hepatocellular carcinoma: report of a case. Surg Today 30:844–848
7. Kunkle DA, Uzzo RG (2008) Cryoablation or radiofrequency ablation of the small renal mass: a meta-analysis. Cancer 113:2671–2680
8. Yang Y, Wang C, Lu Y et al (2012) Outcomes of ultrasound-guided percutaneous argon-helium cryoablation of hepatocellular carcinoma. J Hepatobiliary Pancreat Sci 19(6):674–684. Accessed 24 May 2011
9. Smith MT, Ray CE (2006) The treatment of primary and metastatic hepatic neoplasms using percutaneous cryotherapy. Semin in Interv Radiol 23:39–45
10. Seifert JK, Morris DL (1999) World survey on the complications of hepatic and prostate cryotherapy. World J Surg 23:109–113
11. Llovet JM, Di Biseglie AM, Bruix J et al (2008) Design and endpoints of clinical trials in hepatocellular carcinoma. J Nat Cancer Inst 100:678–711
12. Bruix J, Sherman M, Llovet JM et al (2001) Clinical management of hepatocellular carcinoma: conclusions of the barcelona 2000 EASL conference. J Hepatol 35:421–430
13. Tateishi R, Shiina S, Teratami T et al (2005) Percutaneous radiofrequency ablation for hepatocellular carcinoma: an analysis of 1000 cases. Cancer 103:1201–1209
14. Tanabe KK, Curley SA, Dodd GD et al (2004) Radiofrequency ablation: the experts weigh in. Cancer 100:641
15. Kagawa T, Koizumi J, Koijima S et al (2010) Transcatheter arterial chemoembolization plus radiofrequency ablation therapy for early stage hepatocellular carcinoma: comparison with surgical resection. Cancer 116:3638–3644
16. Rossi S, Garbagnati F, Lencioni R et al (2000) Percutaneous radiofrequency thermal ablation of non resectable hepatocellular carcinoma after occlusion of tumor blood supply. Radiology 217:119–126
17. Ohmoto K, Yoshioku N, Tomiyama Y et al (2007) Radiofrequency ablation versus percutaneous microwave coagulation therapy for small hepatocellular carcinoma: a retrospective comparative study. Hepatogastroenterology 54:985–989
18. Akahane M, Koga H, Kato N et al (2005) Complications of percutaneous radiofrequency ablation for hepatocellular carcinoma: imaging spectrum and management. Radiographics 25:S57–S68
19. Sato M, Tateishi R, Yasunaga H et al (2012) Mortality and morbidity of hepatectomy, radiofrequency ablation and embolization for hepatocellular carcinoma: a national survey of 54,145 patients. J Gastroenterol 47:1125–1133
20. Howenstein MJ, Sato KT (2010) Complication of radiofrequency ablation of hepatic, pulmonary and renal neoplasms. Semin Interv radiol 27:285–295
21. Frich L, Halvarsen PS, Skulstad H et al (2007) Microbubbles in the pulmonary artery generated during experimental hepatic radiofrequency ablation is correlated with increased pulmonary arterial pressure. J Vasc Interv Radiol 18:437–442
22. Wah TZ, Arellano RS, Gervais DA et al (2005) Image-guided percutaneous radiofrequency ablation and incidence of post-radiofrequency ablation syndrome: prospective survey. Radiology 237:1097–1102
23. Wong SL, Mangu PB, Choti MA et al (2010) American Society of Clinical Oncology 2009 clinical evidence review on radiofrequency ablation of hepatic metastases from colorectal cancer. J Clin Oncol 28:493–508
24. Munireddy S, Katz S, Somasundar P et al (2012) Thermal tumor ablation therapy for colorectal cancer hepatic metastasis. J Gastrointest Oncol 3:69–77
25. Govaert KM, van Kessel CS, Lolkema M et al (2012) Does radiofrequency ablation add to chemotherapy for unresectable liver metastasis? Curr Colorectal Cancer Rep 8:130–137
26. Ruers T, Punt CJ, van Coevorden F, et al (2010) Final results of the EORTC intergroup randomized study 40004 (CLOCC) evaluating the benefit of radiofrequency ablation (RFA) combined with chemotherapy for unresectable colorectal liver metastases (CRLM). J Clin Oncol 28:15 s(suppl; abstract 3526)
27. Weng M, ZhangY Zhou D, et al (2012) Radiofrequency ablation versus resection for colorectal cancer liver metastases: a meta-analysis. PLOS online 7:1–8
28. Donado M, Ribero D, Morris-Stiff G et al (2007) New paradigm in the management of liver-only metastases from colorectal cancer. Gastrointest Cancer Res 1:20–27

29. Shibata T, Yamamoto Y, Yamamoto N et al (2003) Cholangitis and liver abscess after percutaneous ablation therapy for liver tumors: incidence and risk factors. J Vasc Interv Radiol 14:1535–1542
30. Sipperstein AE, Berber E, Ballem N et al (2007) Survival after radiofrequency ablation of colorectal liver metastases: 10 year experience. Ann Surg 246:559–565
31. Abdalla EK, Vauthey JN, Ellis JM et al (2004) Recurrence and outcomes following hepatic resection, radiofrequency ablation and combined resection/ablation for colorectal liver metastases. Ann Surg 239:818–825
32. Bleicher RJ, Allegra DP, Nora DT et al (2003) Radiofrequency ablation in 447 complex unresectable liver tumors: lessons learned. Ann Surg Oncol 10:52–58
33. Hellman P, Ladjevardi S, Kogseid B et al (2002) Radiofrequency tissue ablationusing cooltip for liver metastases of endocrine tumors. World J Surg 26:1052–1056
34. Berber E, Flesher N, Sipperstein AE (2002) Laparoscopic radiofrequency ablation of neuroendocrine liver metastases. World J Surg 26:985–990
35. Massaglia PJ, Berber E, Milas M et al (2007) Laparoscopic radiofrequency ablation of neuroendocrine liver metastases: a 10-years experience evaluating predictors of survival. Surgery 142:10–19
36. Gc Hui, Tunkali K, Tatli S et al (2008) Comparison of percutaneous and surgical approaches to renal tumor ablation: metaanalysis of effectiveness and complication rates. J Vasc Interv Radiol 19:1311
37. Kunkle DA, Uzzo RG (2008) Cryoablation or radiofrequency ablation of the small renal mass: a meta-analysis. Cancer 113:2671
38. Dupuy DE, DiPetrillo T, Gandhi S et al (2006) Radiofrequency ablation followed by conventional radiotherapy for medically inoperable stage I non-small cell lung cancer. Chest 129:738–745
39. Pereira PL, Massala S (2012) Standards of practice: guidelines for thermal ablation of primary and secondary lung tumors. Cardiovasc Interv Radiol 35:247–254
40. De Baere T (2011) Lung tumor radiofrequency ablation: where do we stand? Cardiovasc Interv Radiol 34:241–251
41. De Baere T, Palussiere J, Auperin A et al (2006) Midterm local efficacy and survival after radiofrequency ablation of lung tumors with minimum follow-up of 1 year: prospective evaluation. Radiology 240:587–596
42. Yoshimatsu R, Yamagami T, Terayama K et al (2009) Delayed and recurrent pneumothorax after radiofrequency ablation of lung tumors. Chest 135:1002–1009
43. Sakurai J, Mimura H, Gobara H et al (2010) Pulmonary artery pseudoaneurysm related to radiofrequency ablation of lung tumor. Cardiovasc Interv Radiol 33:413–416
44. Pennathur A, Luketich JD, Abbas G et al (2007) Radiofrequency ablation for the treatment of stage I non-small cell lung cancer in high-risk patients. J Thorac Cardiovasc Surg 134:857–864
45. Kodama H, Yamakado K, Takaki H et al (2012) Lung radiofrequency ablation for the treatment of unresectable recurrent non-small cell lung cancer after surgical intervention. Cardiovasc Interv Radiol 35:563–569
46. Simon CJ, Dupuy DE, DiPetrillo TA et al (2007) Pulmonary radiofrequency ablation: long-term safety and efficacy in 153 patients. Radiology 243:268–275
47. Gillams A, Khan Z, Osborn P et al (2013) Survival after radiofrequency ablation in 122 patients with inoperable colorectal lung metastases. Cardiovasc Interv Radiol 36(3):724–730
48. Davalos RV, Mir LM, Rubinsky B (2005) Tissue ablation with irreversible electroporation. Ann of Biomed Eng 33:223–231
49. Wendler JJ, Porch M, Hühne S et al (2013) Short and mid-term effects of irreversible electroporation on normal renal tissue: an animal model. Cardiovasc Interv Radiol 36(2):512–520
50. Wendler JJ, Pech M, Blaschke S et al (2012) Angiography in the isolated perfused kidney: radiological evaluation of vascular protectionin tissue ablation by irreversible electroporation. Cardiovasc Interv Radiol 35:383–390
51. Sergio A, Cristofori C, Cardin R et al (2008) Transcatheter arterial chemoembolization (TACE) in hepatocellular carcinoma carcinoma (HCC): the role of angiogenesis and invasiveness. Am J Gastroenterol 103(4):914–921
52. Raoul JL, Heresbach D, Bretagne JF et al (1992) Chemoembolization of hepatocellular carcinomas: a study of the biodistribution and pharmacokinetics of doxorubicin. Cancer 70:585–590
53. Nakamura H, Hashimoto T, Oi H et al (1989) Transcatheter oily chemoembolization of hepatocellular carcinoma. Radiology 170:783–786
54. Nakajo M, Kobayashi H, Shimabukuro K et al (1988) Biodistribution and in vivo kinetics of iodine-131 lipiodol infused via the hepatic artery of patients with hepatic cancer. J Nucl Med 29:1066–1077
55. Kan Z, Sato M, Ivancev K et al (1993) Distribution and effect of iodized poppy seed oil in the liver after hepatic artery embolization: experimental study in several animal species. Radiology 186:261–266
56. Malagari K, Pomoni M, Kelekis A et al (2010) Prospective randomized comparison of chemoembolization with doxorubicin-eluting beads and bland embolization with BeadBlock for hepatocellular carcinoma. Cardiovasc Interv Radiol 33(3):541–551
57. Nicolini A, Martinetti L, Crespi S et al (2010) Transarterial chemoembolization with epirubicin-eluting beads versus transarterial embolization

before liver transplantation for hepatocellular carcinoma. J Vasc Interv Radiol 21(3):327–332
58. Lewis AL, Gonzalez MV, Lloyd AW et al (2006) DC bead: in vitro characterization of a drug-delivery device for transarterial chemoembolization. J Vasc Interv Radiol 17:335–342
59. Varela M, Real MI, Burrel M et al (2007) Chemoembolization of hepatocellular carcinoma with drug eluting beads: efficacy and doxorubicin pharmacokinetics. J Hepatol 46(3):474–481
60. Lee KH, Liapi EA, Cornell C et al (2010) Doxorubicin-loaded Quadrasphere microspheres: plasma pharmacokinetics and intratumoral drug concentration in an animal model of liver cancer. Cardiovasc Interv Radiol 33(3):576–582
61. Gupta S, Wright KC, Ensor J et al (2011) Hepatic arterial embolization with doxorubicin-loaded superabsorbent polymer microspheres in a rabbit liver tumor model. Cardiovasc Interv Radiol 34(5):1021–1030
62. Malagari K, Pomoni M, Spyridopoulos TN et al (2011) Safety profile of sequential transcatheter chemoembolization with DC Bead^{TM}: results of 237 hepatocellular carcinoma (HCC) patients. Cardiovasc Interv Radiol 34(4):774–785
63. Brown DB, Cardella JF, Sacks D et al (2006) Quality improvement guidelines for transhepatic arterial chemoembolization, embolization, and chemotherapeutic infusion for hepatic malignancy. J Vasc Interv Radiol 17(2 Pt1):225–232
64. Llovet JM, Real MI, Montana X et al (2002) Arterial embolisation or chemoembolisation versus symptomatic treatment in patients with unresectable hepatocellular carcinoma: a randomised controlled trial. Lancet 359:1734–1739
65. Lo CM, Ngan H, Tso WK et al (2002) Randomized controlled trial of transarterial lipiodol chemoembolization for unresectable hepatocellular carcinoma. Hepatology 35:1164–1171
66. Marelli L, Stigliano R, Triantos C et al (2007) Transarterial therapy for hepatocellular carcinoma: which technique is more effective? a systematic review of cohort and randomized studies. Cardiovasc Interv Radiol 30(1):6–25
67. Malagari K, Pomoni M, Moschouris H et al (2012) Chemoembolization with doxorubicin-eluting beads for unresectable hepatocellular carcinoma: five-year survival analysis. Cardiovasc Interv Radiol 35(5):1119–1128
68. Burrel M, Reig M, Forner A et al (2012) Survival of patients with hepatocellular carcinoma treated by transarterial chemoembolisation (TACE) using drug eluting beads. implications for clinical practice and trial design. J Hepatol 56(6):1330–1335
69. Fiorentini G, Aliberti C, Tilli M et al (2012) Intra-arterialinfusion of irinotecan-loaded drug-eluting beads (DEBIRI) versus intravenoustherapy (FOLFIRI) for hepatic metastases from colorectal cancer: final results of a phase III study. Anticancer Res 32(4):1387–1395
70. Martin RC 2nd, Scoggins CR, Tomalty D et al (2012) Irinotecan drug-eluting beads in the treatment of chemo-naive unresectable colorectal liver metastasis with concomitant systemic fluorouracil and oxaliplatin: results of pharmacokinetics and phase I trial. J Gastrointest Surg 16(8):1531–1538
71. Stuart K (2003) Chemoembolization in the management of liver tumors. Oncologist 8:425–437
72. Burger I, Hong K, Schulick R et al (2005) Transcatheter arterial chemoembolization in unresectable cholangiocarcinoma: initial experience in a single institution. J Vasc Interv Radiol 16:353–361
73. Touzios JG, Kiely JM, Pitt SC et al (2005) Neuroendocrine hepatic metastases: does aggressive management improve survival? Ann Surg 241(5):776–783 (discussion 83–85)
74. Gupta S, Johnson MM, Murthy R et al (2005) Hepatic arterial embolization and chemoembolization for the treatment of patients with metastatic neuroendocrine tumors: Variables affecting response rates and survival. Cancer 104(8):1590–1602
75. Roche A, Girish BV, de Baère T et al (2003) Trans-catheter arterial chemoembolization as first-line treatment for hepatic metastases from endocrine tumors. Eur Radiol 13(1):136–140
76. Stokes KR, Stuart K, Clouse ME (1993) Hepatic arterial chemoembolization for metastatic endocrine tumors. J Vasc Interv Radiol 4(3):341–345
77. Memon K, Lewandowski RJ, Mulcahy MF et al (2012) Radioembolization for neuroendocrine liver metastases: safety, imaging, and long-term outcomes. Int J Radiat Oncol Biol Phys 1 83(3):887–894
78. Salem R, Lewandowski RJ, Mulcahy MF et al (2010) Radioembolization for hepatocellular carcinoma using Yttrium-90 microspheres: a comprehensive report of long-term outcomes. Gastroenterol 138(1):52–64
79. Kennedy AS, Coldwell D, Nutting C et al (2006) Resin 90Y-microsphere brachytherapy for unresectable colorectal liver metastases: modern USA experience. Int J Radiat Oncol Biol Phys 65(2):412–425
80. Kooby DA, Egnatashvili V, Srinivasan S et al (2010) Comparison of yttrium-90 radioembolization and transcatheter arterial chemoembolisation for the treatment of unresectable hepatocellular carcinoma. J Vasc Interv Radiol 21(2):224–230
81. Carr BI, Kondragunta V, Buch SC et al (2010) Therapeutic equivalence in survival for hepatic arterial chemoembolization and yttrium 90 microsphere treatments in unresectable hepatocellular carcinoma: a two-cohort study. Cancer 116(5):1305–1314
82. Lewandowski RJ, Kulik LM, Riaz A et al (2009) A comparative analysis of transarterial downstaging for hepatocellular carcinoma: chemoembolization versus radioembolization. Am J Transpl 9(8):1920–1928

83. Katsanos K, Sabharwal T, Adam A (2010) Stenting of the upper gastrointestinal tract: current status. Cardiovasc Interv Radiol 33:690–705
84. Adam A, Morgan R, Ellul J et al (1996) A new design of the esophageal wallstent endoprosthesis resistant to distal migration. AJR 170:1477–1482
85. Sabharwal T, Hamady MJ, Chui S et al (2003) A randomized prospective comparison of the Flamingo Wallstent and Ultraflex stent for palliation of dysphagia associated with lower third esophageal carcinoma. Gut 52:922–926
86. Sabharwal T, Morale JP, Irani FG et al (2005) Quality improvement guidelines for placement of esophageal stents. Cardiovasc Interv Radiol 28:284–288
87. Farrugia M, Morgan RA, Latham JA et al (1997) Perforation of the esophagus secondary to insertion of covered wallstent endoprostheses. Cardiovasc Interv Radiol 20:428–430
88. Katsanos K, Sabharwal T, Adam A (2011) Stenting of the lower gastrointestinal tract: current status. Cardiovasc Interv Radiol 34:462–473
89. Baerlocher MO, Asch MR, Dixon P et al (2008) Interdisciplinary Canadian guidelines on the use of metal stents in the gastrointestinal tract for oncological indications. Can Assoc Radiol J 59:107–122
90. Adam A, Watkinson A (1996) Interventional radiology-a practical guide. Radcliffe Medical Press, Oxford an.Radcliffe Medical Press, Oxford and New York
91. Lammer J, Hausegger KA, Fluckiger F et al (1996) Common bile duct obstruction due to malignancy: treatment with plastic versus metal stents. Radiology 201:167–172
92. Kaskarelis IS, Papadaki MG, Papageorgiou GN et al (1999) Long-term follow-up in patients with malignant biliary obstruction after percutaneous placement of uncovered wallstent endoprosthesis. Acta Radiol 40:528–533
93. Brountzos EN, Ptochis N, Panagiotou I et al (2006) A survival analysis of patients with malignant biliary strictures treated by percutaneous metallic stenting. Cardiovasc Interv Radiol 30:66–73
94. Krokidis M, Fanelli F, Orgera G et al (2011) Percutaneous palliation of pancreatic head cancer: comparison of ePTFE/FEP-covered versus uncovered nitinol biliary stents. Cardiovasc Interv Radiol 34:352–361
95. Uthappa MC, Kellett MJ (2004) Interventional radiology in malignant urinary tract obstruction. In Adam A, Dondelinger R, Mueller PR (eds): Interventional radiology in cancer. Springer, Berlin
96. Dyer RB, Regan JD, Kavanagh PV et al (2002) Percutaneous nephrostomy with extension of the technique: step by step. Radiographics 22:503–525
97. Silverman SG, Deuson TE, Kane N et al (1998) Percutaneous abdominal biopsy: cost-identification analysis. Radiology 206(2):429–435
98. Smith EH (1991) Complications of percutaneous abdominal fine-needle biopsy. Radiology 178(1):253–258
99. Cham MD, Lane ME, Henschke CI et al (2008) Lung biopsy: special techniques. Semin Respir Crit Care Med 29(4):335–349

Imaging Principles in Pediatric Oncology

5

Georgia Ch. Papaioannou and Kieran J. McHugh

5.1 Introduction

Pediatric oncology presents challenges to imaging due to several differences that the pediatric population possesses in their physiology and pathology. As is widely accepted, children are simply not small-sized adults.

Patient cooperation is often difficult to achieve in younger patients. Technically, pediatric imaging presents further challenges in obtaining high-quality examinations free of motion artifact, ideally with high-spatial resolution despite small-sized viscera. Sedation and application of modern modalities and ultrafast techniques usually overcome these obstacles. It should also be noted that radiologists and others should be aware of the hazards of ionizing radiation (X-rays, fluoroscopy/angiography, CT, and nuclear medicine techniques), considering its long-term effects on a growing child [1].

The median age of cancer diagnosis in children is 6 years, whereas in adults it is 67 years [2]. Among the commonest pediatric cancers are leukemias (usually acute lymphoblastic) and cancers of the brain (most commonly juvenile pilocystic astrocytomas). The most common solid pediatric tumors are gliomas and medulloblastomas. Although cancer is the leading cause of death among children in the US, it is nevertheless rather rare in this age group: only 1–2 children develop cancer each year for every 10,000 children [3].

G. Ch. Papaioannou (✉)
Department of Pediatric Radiology, Mitera Maternity and Children's Hospital, Hygeia Group, 6 Erythrou Stavrou, 151 23, Athens, Greece
e-mail: gpapaio@hotmail.com

K. J. McHugh
Department of Radiology, Great Ormond Street Hospital for Children, Great Ormond Street, London, WC1N 3JH, UK
e-mail: Kieran.McHugh@gosh.nhs.uk

5.2 Pediatric Versus Adult Cancer

Pediatric cancer presents several differences from the adult form. They vary enormously in terms of their histopathology, biology, epidemiology, clinical presentation, responsiveness to treatment, and also with regard to patient outcome [2].

The majority of pediatric cancers are thought to derive from a chromosomal error, which results in an abnormal developmental process and less often from an external insult [4]. For example, the amplification of *Myc*-N proto-oncogene is associated with progressive disease in neuroblastomas and generally poor outcome [5]. Histologically, certain types of pediatric tumors are unique to childhood and carry the suffix "-blastomas" [4]. Blastomas not only originate from primitive tissues with persistent embryonic elements, but they also affect a younger population and are usually malignant [4]. The commoner blastomas, such as neuroblastoma, nephroblastoma (Wilms' tumor), hepatoblastoma, and medulloblastoma represent almost 25 % of the solid pediatric tumors [4].

A. D. Gouliamos et al. (eds.), *Imaging in Clinical Oncology*,
DOI: 10.1007/978-88-470-5385-4_5, © Springer-Verlag Italia 2014

Pediatric malignancies have a natural history and prognosis that can be very different from adult forms of cancer. For example, neuroblastic tumors and more specifically neuroblastomas are classified based on their morphologic histological features and child's age at diagnosis, according to the Shimada classification and the Pediatric Oncology Group (POG), respectively [5]. Adverse prognosis and aggressive biologic behavior in neuroblastomas can be derived from abnormal biochemical measures, such as high serum levels of lactate dehydrogenase and the degree of maturity of tumor-secreted catecholamines [5].

Screening for neuroblastoma, via urinary catecholamine levels, is actually possible but where performed this has lead to overdiagnosis, with the data indicating that screening for neuroblastoma in children less than 1 year old increased the incidence rate of neuroblastoma, but did not lead to any significant reduction in mortality [6]. The incidence increased as favorable tumors, which would have regressed spontaneously, were picked up by the screening process.

Some pediatric malignancies can thus present specific congenital and neonatal forms within the same general tumor family; neuroblastoma represents the commonest malignancy in the first month of life. Although neuroblastoma in a 2 year old tends to be an aggressive cancer with a poor outcome, neuroblastoma in infancy, even metastatic neuroblastoma (MS disease, formerly 4S), can regress spontaneously [5]. In this age group, it is practically indistinguishable from benign pathologies, such as adrenal hemorrhage. They both tend to resolve spontaneously and many are simply observed without histological confirmation; ultrasonographic surveillance and measurements of urine catecholamine levels are advocated instead [5].

5.3 Imaging of Pediatric Cancer

One of the great challenges in pediatric oncology imaging is to exploit the most appropriate of the available imaging modalities that deliver the least radiation burden to the child, while they combine time- and cost-effectiveness. The as low as reasonably achievable (ALARA) Principle and the Image Gently Campaign focus on optimization of the radiation dose. Both are of the highest importance in children bearing in mind that younger tissues are most susceptible to radiation effects (up to 10 times more susceptible to carcinogenesis due to radiation exposure than adults). The cumulative effect of radiation is more severe in children as they carry a longer life expectancy. This is especially relevant to pediatric oncology patients since the childhood cancer survival rates have increased considerably, and so many of these children have a long life ahead of them [3, 7]. There should therefore be reluctance toward the unnecessary use of CT and the scanning parameters (such as kVP, mAs, pitch, table speed, etc.) should be modified to pediatric standards in order to deliver the minimum radiation dose for diagnostic quality imaging. Adult protocols should not be applied to children as the children could undergo six or more times greater radiation exposure [8]. In oncology practice, repeat scans are required in order to monitor tumor response and to detect early relapse. As approximately 70 % of all children with cancer now survive, there must be additional efforts to avoid or reduce the number of CT scans performed in this population. When a CT is required, the amount of radiation applied should be "child-sized" [9]. The website of the Image Gently Campaign [10], originally conceived in 2006 by the Society of Pediatric Radiology, includes educational material for parents, clinicians, radiologists, and technologists [8].

Multimodality imaging in pediatric oncology should be tailored to each child's characteristics, especially in tumors that present variable biological behavior and sites of origin, such as neuroblastoma. Optimal investigation combines ultrasound (US), CT, or MRI with nuclear studies, such as ^{123}I-MIBG ([^{123}I]metaiodobenzylguanidine), ^{18}F-FDG PET ([^{18}F]-fluorodeoxyglucose positron emission tomography), or bone scan as specified by the various international collaborative group trials.

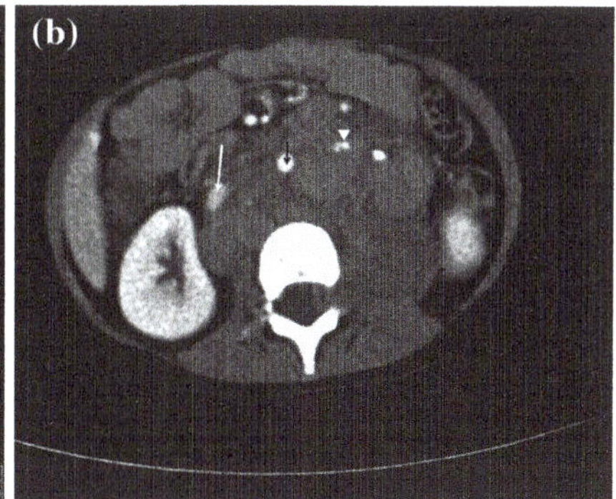

Fig. 5.1 **a** Ultrasound of the abdomen in a 2-year-old with neuroblastoma. The large heterogeneous mass with speckled calcifications (*arrows*) typically develops in the retroperitoneal area encasing the aorta (*arrowhead*), *LI* liver, *V* vertebra. **b** Axial single-phase CT scan of the abdomen. The mass calcifications (*arrowhead*) and the encasement of the aorta (*short arrow*) and the IVC (*long arrow*) are seen again. Additionally, intraspinal extension (*asterisk*) is grossly appreciated and can be further investigated with MRI

Laboratory investigations will often add vital additional information to the initial imaging work-up. For example, a raised serum alpha-fetoprotein usually accompanies a hepatoblastoma, the most common liver tumor less than 4 years of age [5].

Evaluation of suspected pediatric malignancies employs US as the principle initial imaging approach for the majority of different anatomic areas. Superficial lesions, abdominal and pelvic masses, and even intracranial lesions during the first few months of life when the anterior fontanelle is still open should be initially assessed by US (Fig. 5.1), which has the additional potential to evaluate tumor vascularity by Doppler analysis or guide percutaneous biopsy. In mimickers of other malignant tumors, such as proliferating hemangiomas, Doppler analysis may provide typical and specific information. Imaging features of non-CNS pediatric tumors are sometimes nonspecific and diagnosis largely relies on the age of the child and the site of origin of the tumor. Heterogeneity is a feature which usually suggests malignancy. Benign pediatric lesions such as proliferating hemangiomas or fibromatosis of infancy often have a homogenous echotexture. Once US is suggestive of a malignant tumor further detailed investigation is provided by MRI (or CT in case of thoracic lesions) [8]. With modern scanners, the duration of the exam is minimized and usually sedation is not required for CT. CT in children should be only utilized as a single phase post-injection of contrast medium and multiphase scans should be avoided [11]. The superiority of MRI, especially in large abdominal masses, focuses on superb tissue characterization, multiplanar imaging, and lack of ionizing radiation. MRI may overestimate the extent of a mass as it may confuse the margins of a tumor with peritumoral edema or posttreatment fibrosis for residual tumor. Additionally, since the duration of the exam is longer MRI usually requires sedation of children younger than 4–6 years.

Plain radiographs play a crucial role in the initial characterization and the differentiation of aggressive and nonaggressive bone lesions (Fig. 5.2); however, its value is very limited in other pediatric malignancies. Plain film of the chest is, of course, routinely performed during staging of almost all extra-cranial malignancies and during treatment for the evaluation of treatment-related complications.

5.4 Imaging of Specific Pediatric Tumors

Brain tumors in children present several differences which reflect the fact that the skull as well as the brain may be still developing. The distribution of brain tumors in children is strongly

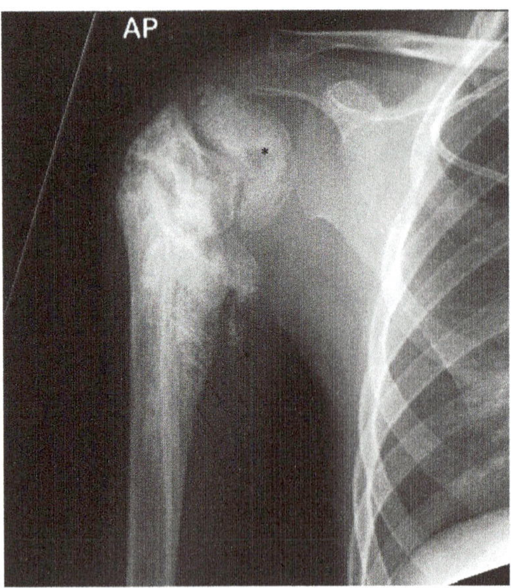

Fig. 5.2 Plain radiography of right humeral osteosarcoma in a 15-year-old boy. A heterogeneous lesion with aggressive imaging features (irregular type of bone destruction and calcification, vertical periosteal reaction—*arrows*, soft-tissue mass with new bone formation—*arrowhead*) is appreciated in the proximal humeral metaphysis. Irregular lytic lesion is also noted in the proximal epiphysis (*asterisk*) indicative of extension of the tumor through the growth plate

affected by age. When the tumor is infratentorial, the differential diagnosis becomes limited, especially by taking into account the patient's gender and the precise anatomical detail from modern MRI techniques, in addition to Diffusion Weighted Imaging (DWI) and Apparent Diffusion Coefficient (ADC) mapping [1]. Brain plasticity in very young children is very important in determining the functional prognosis but also in excluding treatment options, such as radiotherapy. Tumors developing infratentorially that invade the fourth ventricle, such as medulloblastomas or ependymomas, may cause CSF seeding; imaging of the whole neuroaxis is essential to rule out meningeal metastases and should be performed preoperatively to minimize confusion between postoperative leptomeningeal enhancement and tumor seeding [12].

Pediatric renal masses include Wilms' tumor (nephroblastoma) and other entities (such as mesoblastic nephroma, rhabdoid tumor, etc.). Despite advanced imaging renal tumors have similar appearances and accurate diagnosis is made via biopsy or after nephrectomy [13]. Unlike neuroblastoma, Wilms' tumor does not encase adjacent vessels but it often invades the renal vein and inferior vena cava. Wilms' tumor also has certain peculiarities: It may be bilateral (Fig. 5.3) or associated with congenital anomalies or Wilms-predisposition syndromes, such as cryptorchidism, hemihypertrophy, aniridia, Beckwith-Wiedeman syndrome, while chromosomal anomalies are found in certain cases [13]. In renal tumors, the contra-lateral kidney should be scrutinized to rule out focal areas of nephroblastomatosis, which are better depicted with MRI (Fig. 5.3), as these fetal rests predispose to metachronous tumors. In high-risk cases, screening with initial MRI if possible should begin at 6 months of age and be followed by serial ultrasounds every 3 months up to the age of 7 years beyond which the risk for developing Wilms' decreases significantly [13]. Lung metastases should be measured in lung window settings on CT [13]. Within International Society of Pediatric Oncology (SIOP) trials preoperative chemotherapy is applied to induce tumor shrinkage and facilitate surgery, in contrast to the North American approach where immediate nephrectomy at diagnosis is the approach. Preoperative chemotherapy is given everywhere for bilateral tumors which are staged separately, with conservative surgery (hemi-nephrectomy or wedge resections) performed to preserve renal function. The cure rates are over 90 % [13].

In neuroblastomas, MRI is superior to CT in demonstrating in detail intraspinal extension, soft tissue, and bone marrow infiltration. CT is preferred by some surgeons prior to surgery as it provides an excellent multidimensional roadmap of the vessels typically encased by the tumor (Fig. 5.1).

In rhabdomyosarcomas, MRI is overall the most beneficial imaging modality. It can easily be applied in head and neck tumors, paraspinal, limb, or pelvic primary tumors. Regional lymphadenopathy may be assessed by ultrasound and the draining lymph nodal territory must always be evaluated by MRI also.

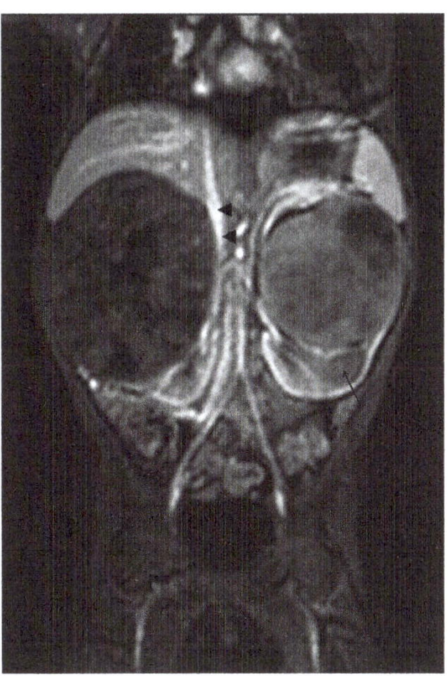

Fig. 5.3 Coronal postgadolinium T1-weighted fat-suppressed image of the abdomen in a 3.5-year-old boy confirms the sonographic findings of bilateral renal tumors (Wilms'). There is additional solid lesion in the lower pole of the left kidney (*arrow*) suggestive of nephroblastomatosis. The IVC appears patent (*arrowheads*)

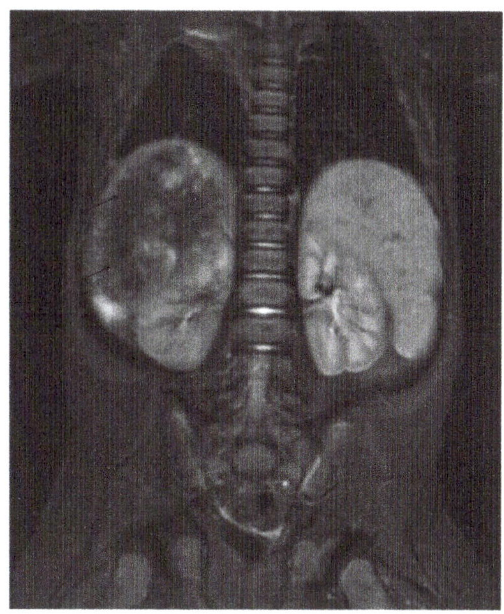

Fig. 5.4 Coronal postgadolinium T1-weighted fat-suppressed image in a 3-year-old reveals a heterogenous lesion in the posterior segments of the liver (*arrows*) in keeping with hepatoblastoma. The precise mapping of the involved hepatic segments is essential for staging

In liver masses, ultrasound is helpful in assessing venous or biliary duct invasion by the mass, while MRI is superb in mapping the exact location of the mass in the varied hepatic anatomical segments (Fig. 5.4). The involvement of liver segments according to the PRETEXT staging system is fundamental to the staging of hepatoblastoma, and reflects its risk prognosis [14].

In bone tumors, plain radiography remains the main imaging modality for the initial evaluation and taken together with the age of the child may provide the correct diagnosis [15]. MRI will provide local intra- and extra-osseous staging in malignant bone tumors (within the bone and across the growth plate, with respect to the joint, the neurovascular bundle, and the adjacent soft-tissues). It will determine the surgical approach with regard to the possibility of limb salvage. Some institutions advocate the role of dynamic MRI in diagnosing local extension and assessing tumor necrosis with chemotherapy more accurately. Diffusion-Weighted MRI and ^{18}FDG-PET CT are complimentary in detecting viable tumor and monitoring response to preoperative neoadjuvant chemotherapy (Fig. 5.5) [16, 17].

5.5 Metastatic Disease

Metastatic disease in pediatric malignancies presents some additional differences. As the skull comprises a high proportion of the skeleton in neonates, it is commonly involved with metastatic disease. As an example, distant metastatic disease in neuroblastoma is encountered at presentation in 60–70 %, the commonest site of distant involvement being the bone marrow, with the base of the skull or calvarium frequently involved by metastatic disease [5]. In this setting, ^{123}I-MIBG nuclear scan is considered essential in the initial diagnostic work-up. PET-CT and Whole-body MRI (WBMRI) are promising modalities to evaluate distant disease in certain pediatric tumors, such as the 10 % of

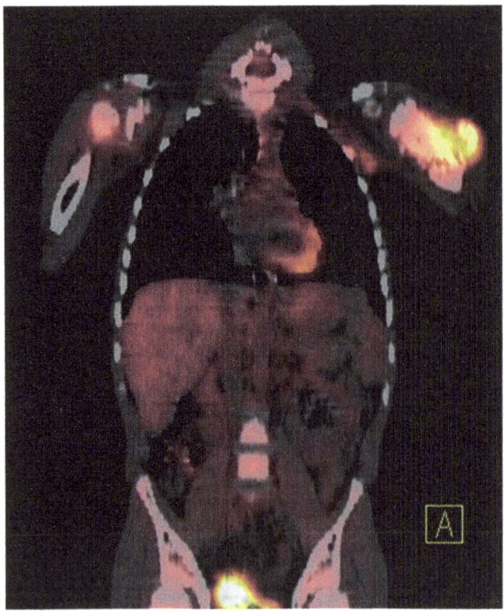

Fig. 5.5 Coronal ^{18}FDG-PET CT image in a 14-year-old boy with left humeral osteosarcoma postadministration of neoadjuvant chemotherapy reveals residual area of avid uptake in the lateral part of the tumor

neuroblastomas which are non-MIBG avid and sarcomas [4].

5.6 Response to Treatment/Tumor Relapse

In many pediatric tumors, the treatment strategy includes initial chemotherapy to reduce tumor size in the hope of allowing complete surgical resection. Some tumors, notably in the head and neck area, however, may remain inoperable after completing chemotherapy and local treatment for these tumors may be done solely with radiotherapy.

The type of imaging surveillance for pediatric malignancies is determined by the relative risk that each tumor exhibits and the need for additional local therapy, as tumor markers alone are not usually sufficient. Imaging is also performed to evaluate response after administration of chemotherapy or to determine the ideal time for surgical intervention. In most tumors, response is determined by tumor size reduction and/or change of its texture [5]. However, in certain cases, residual tumor postoperatively may not worsen a child's prognosis, i.e., intraspinal extension of NBL may be left in situ [5].

During surveillance of abdominal, pelvic, and superficial tumors, US is the key imaging modality as it provides accurate information without any biological burden, although it is operator dependent. It may also confirm invasion of abdominal masses into other adjacent organs by simply demonstrating lack of separate motion between them during inspiration. In immunocompromised children, US is superb with high-resolution techniques in evaluating fungal infiltration of the liver and spleen.

CT or MRI in addition to US is selected according to each institution's availability for monitoring children with high-risk disease. Reformatted CT coronal and sagittal images are very popular with some clinicians for preoperative planning [8]. Obviously, child friendly staff and environment are essential in this group of oncology patients, not only to reduce the need for sedation but also to provide a more pleasant experience to the child with cancer as well as their parents.

Nuclear studies, PET-CT, and WBMRI are promising modalities to evaluate tumor recurrence in certain sarcomas, when bone marrow infiltration or metastases are suspected [1, 5, 7]. WBMRI presents higher sensitivity than bone scintigraphy (early marrow metastases in Ewing sarcoma may be only evident in WBMRI) and almost equal sensitivity and specificity with ^{18}FDG PET-CT [8].

Several new imaging techniques are under investigation for evaluation of response to treatment and tumor recurrence in pediatric oncology. These are based on the assessment of tumoral blood flow in tumors, such as osteosarcoma and neuroblastoma by means of dynamic-enhanced MRI, quantitative contrast-enhanced US, and ^{18}FDG PET-CT [1].

5.7 Summary

Technological advances in diagnostic radiology, such as MRI, have permitted a more accurate assessment of pediatric cancer disease extent and staging, and have aided radiotherapy treatment planning. Repeated MRI has also enhanced tumor surveillance without concomitant irradiation. Those dealing with pediatric oncology patients should be aware of the fundamental differences between cancers in children and in adults, most notably in terms of long-term survival. Consequently, avoidance of ionizing radiation wherever possible should always be at the forefront of the radiology of the malignancies in childhood.

References

1. McCarville MB (2008) New frontiers in pediatric oncologic imaging. Cancer Imaging 8:87–92
2. Weiner MA (2000) Principles and practice of pediatric oncology. In: Bast RC Jr, Kufe DW, Pollock RE et al (eds) Holland-Frei cancer medicine, 5th edn. BC Decker, Hamilton, chapter 137A
3. www.cancer.gov/cancertopics/factsheet/Sites-Types/childhood
4. Papaioannou G, Sebire NJ, McHugh K (2009) Imaging of the unusual pediatric 'blastomas'. Cancer Imaging 9:1–11
5. Papaioannou G, McHugh K (2005) Neuroblastoma in childhood: review and radiological findings. Cancer Imaging 5:116–127
6. Kawada T (2012) Trend in the number of registrations for neuroblastoma in Japan. Jpn J Clin Oncol 42:357–358
7. Goske MJ (2008) The image gently campaign: working together to change practice. AJR 190:273–274
8. States LJ, Meyer JS (2011) Imaging Modalities in Pediatric Oncology. Radiol Clin N Am 49:579–588
9. Voss SD, Reaman GH, Kaste SC, Slovis TL (2009) The ALARA concept in pediatric oncology. Pediatr Radiol 39:1142-1146
10. www.image-gently.org
11. McHugh K, Disini L (2011) Commentary: for the children's sake, avoid non-contrast CT. Cancer Imaging 11:16–18
12. Panigrahy A, Blüml S (2009) Neuroimaging of pediatric brain tumors: from basic to advanced Magnetic Resonance Imaging (MRI). J Child Neurol 24:1343–1365
13. Lowe LH, Isuani BH, Heller RM et al (2000) Pediatric renal masses: Wilms tumor and beyond. Radiographics 20:1585–1603
14. Roebuck D, Aronson D, Clapuyt P et al (2007) 2005 PRETEXT: a revised staging system for primary malignant liver tumours of childhood developed by the SIOPEL group. Pediatr Radiol 37:123–132
15. Miller TT (2008) Bone tumors and tumorlike conditions: analysis with conventional radiography. Radiology 246:662–674
16. Brisse H, Ollivier L, Edeline V et al (2004) Imaging of malignant tumours of the long bones in children: monitoring response to neoadjuvant chemotherapy and preoperative assessment. Pediatr Radiol 34:595–605
17. Hawkins DS, Conrad EU III, Butrynski JE et al (2009) [F-18]-fluorodeoxy-D-glucose positron emission tomography response is associated with outcome for extremity osteosarcoma in children and young adults. Cancer 115:3519–3525

Part II
Bone and soft Tissue Tumors

6 Introduction to Soft Tissue Sarcomas

Ioannis P. Boukovinas

Soft tissue sarcomas (STS) and bone sarcomas comprise a diverse set of separate clinical entities with different degrees of malignancy, biological behavior, and specific therapeutic options. The incidence of STS is relatively low (4–5/100,000/year in Europe) [1], whereas bone sarcomas account for 0.2 % of malignant tumors registered in the EUROCARE database [2].

More than 50 different STS subtypes have been described, showing great variations in clinical course of the disease and chemosensitivity. The choice of treatment is guided by prognostic factors such as tumor stage, histological subtype, location, grade, and patient age and is influenced by the center's experience and philosophy and patient clinical characteristics. Curative-intent treatment strategies almost always include surgery, with (neo)-adjuvant radiation therapy and/or systemic chemotherapy being incorporated in the decisions on multidisciplinary treatment of sarcoma patients. By contrast, less than 10 % of patients with metastatic/advanced soft tissue sarcoma can be cured [3].

During recent years, the development of molecular biology has led to the integration of novel, targeted therapies into the treatment of sarcomas. Due to the ever-increasing number of new molecules, the combination of radiographic imaging and specific molecular techniques is a valuable tool in the decision-making process as to whether their development should be continued. In clinical practice, imaging is used to define criteria for response and progression, allowing for the determining of a suitable treatment strategy that is beneficial for the patient and for the identification of appropriate clinical study primary endpoints. Noninvasive imaging methods, e.g., ultrasonography, computed tomography (CT), magnetic resonance imaging (MRI), and [18F] fluorodeoxyglucose/positron emission tomography (FDG/PET) are analyzed in relation to their impact on the treatment of STS and bone sarcomas.

References

1. Gatta G, van der Zwan JM, Casali PG et al (2011) Rare cancers are not so rare: the rare cancer burden in Europe. Eur J Cancer 47:2493–2511
2. Stiller CA, Craft AW, Corazziari I (2001) Survival of children with bone sarcoma in Europe since 1978: results from the EUROCARE study. Eur J Cancer 37:760–766
3. Clark MA, Fisher C, Judson I et al (2005) Soft-tissue sarcomas in adults. N Engl J Med 353:701–711

I. P. Boukovinas (✉)
Bioclinic Oncology Unit, 86, Mitropoleos street, 54622 Thessaloniki, Greece
e-mail: ibouk@otenet.gr

A. D. Gouliamos et al. (eds.), *Imaging in Clinical Oncology*,
DOI: 10.1007/978-88-470-5385-4_6, © Springer-Verlag Italia 2014

7 Introduction to Bone Sarcomas

Ioannis D. Papanastassiou and Nikolaos S. Demertzis

Sarcomas are malignant tumors of mesenchymal origin, while carcinomas derive from epithelial cells. They comprise approximately 1 % of all malignancies, with soft tissue sarcomas being around 80 % off all sarcomas. Bone sarcomas are seen more often in childhood (except chondrosarcomas) while soft tissue sarcomas predominate in the elderly. Since they have distinct features they will be discussed separately [1].

The most common pathologies are osteosarcoma (OS), chondrosarcoma (CS) and Ewing sarcoma (ES). OS and ES are seen in pediatric patients, especially in the growth spurt. OS have a bimodal distribution, with secondary cases appearing in patients older than 60 years (preexisting Paget's disease, chronic osteomyelitis, implants, previous chemo-radiation etc.). On the other hand chondrosarcomas are only exceptionally seen in the childhood population.

7.1 Histology

OS is characterized by the ability of the tumor cells to produce osteoid or bone. The majority are high grade intramedullary tumors (conventional OS) and are further subcategorized according to the predominant cell population (osteoblastic, chondroblastic or fibroblastic). The remaining OS variants (around 10 %) are: telangiectatic, small cell, surface (peri/parosteal) etc.

ES is named after the famous pathologist James Ewing. They are frequently referred to as Ewing Family of Tumors that also include peripheral primitive neuroectodermal tumors (PNET), Askin's tumor etc., since they share similar characteristics and comprise of characteristic small round blue cells. ES also has a unique chromosomal translocation t(11;22)(q24;q12), that produces the EWS-FLI1 fusion gene that can be detected by cytogenetics (fluorescence in situ hybridization).

CS is comprised of tumor cells capable of producing cartilaginous matrix. Although osteoid may be present, it is reactive and not produced directly by the tumor. The majority are termed conventional CS, while the remainder (less than 10 %) include mesenchymal, dedifferentiated, clear cell etc. Conventional type can appear de novo in the medullary cavity (central type) or from a preexisting osteochondroma (secondary or peripheral type). There are certain diseases that predispose to malignant transformation such as multiple enchondromatosis (Ollier's disease or Mafucci syndrome if coupled with multiple hemangiomas). Unlike OS which are usually high grade, CS are divided into three categories (low- intermediate -high grade), with higher grade tumors being less than 10 % [2].

I. D. Papanastassiou (✉) · N. S. Demertzis
General Oncological Hospital, Kifisias,
Agioi Anargyroi, Athens, Greece
e-mail: ioannis.papanastassiou@gmail.com

A. D. Gouliamos et al. (eds.), *Imaging in Clinical Oncology*,
DOI: 10.1007/978-88-470-5385-4_7, © Springer-Verlag Italia 2014

7.2 Clinical Presentation

Typically the tumor presents as a painful, enlarging lesion. Depending on the location, it may cause stiffness in the adjacent joint, extremity engorgement due to vascular compression, neurological signs, pathological fracture etc. Sometimes onset may be insidious and patients with large tumors may present with subtle symptoms especially in the pelvic region. OS and CS usually lack systemic symptoms, whereas in ES a subset of patients will have constitutional symptoms (fever, malaise, weight loss). Minority will present with metastatic disease (most frequently to the lungs), although most authorities view ES (and OS) as a systemic disease with subclinical metastatic foci upon presentation that should be initially addressed with systematic therapy (chemotherapy).

Laboratory tests are frequently normal. Alkaline phosphatase, LDH and ESR are elevated in up to one/third of the patients. LDH has also prognostic significance in ES.

7.3 Biopsy

Biopsy is a crucial step in the treatment of sarcomas; poorly executed biopsy in non-oncological centers have been shown to be frequently non-diagnostic, change surgical plan and worsen overall prognosis (see Fig. 7.1). Fine needle aspiration (FNA), core biopsy or open biopsies are employed for establishing the diagnosis. The larger the sample, the most likely the test will be diagnostic; in this manner, FNA is not advocated as it yields less diagnostic accuracy. The biopsy tract (either open or percutaneous) should be excised at the time of definitive surgery and therefore should be in line with the anticipated operation. In general, transverse or double incisions should be avoided, technique should be as atraumatic as possible and surgeon should not create dead spaces or insert long retractors (i.e. Homman's) as they may contaminate the field further [3].

7.4 Treatment

Treatment has changed dramatically in the last 4 decades. In the 1970s most of the patients ended up amputated; however, survivorship was limited, around 20 %. The advent of chemotherapy that eradicates systemic disease and subclinical metastasis resulted in a significant rise in survival, which nowadays is estimated to be around 70 %. Furthermore, surgical approach became less aggressive in view of the big retrospective studies from Simon et al. that showed no difference in survival between amputation and limb salvage surgery (LSS). Amputations are exceptionally performed (perhaps in less than 5 %), with relative indications being encasement of

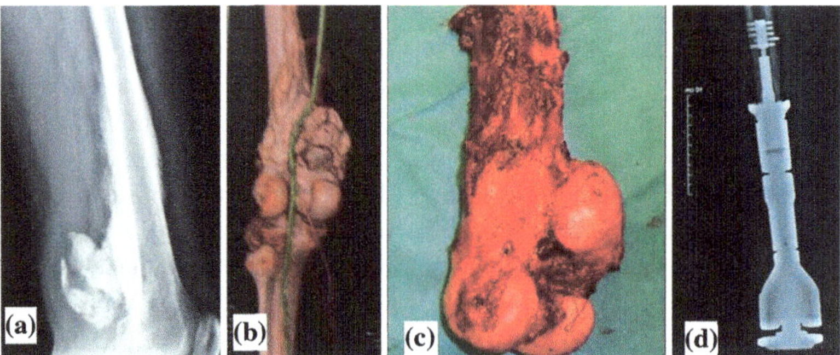

Fig. 7.1 A 35 year old patient with parosteal OS of the distal femur. Plain X-ray (**a**) and CT angiogram (**b**) shows that the tumor arises from the surface of the posterior distal femur abutting the femoral artery. The distal third of the tumor was resected enbloc (**c**) and the bone defect was reconstructed with a distal femoral megaprosthesis (**d**) Compress®, Biomet, Inc., Warsaw

major vessels/nerves, pathological fracture or contaminated wound from previous operations or poor executed biopsy.

7.5 Limb Salvage Surgery

LSS should aim at wide margins after dissection of the tumor from the main vessels has been performed. Reconstruction of the bone defect must be done either by megaprosthetic reconstruction (Fig. 7.1), allograft, combination of allograft- prosthesis (alloprosthesis), implantation of vascularized fibula (Fig. 7.2) [4, 5].

1. OS/ES. Chemotherapy is administered before surgery in most cancer centers (neoadjuvant therapy), although there is no evidence that it increases survival comparing with postoperative (adjuvant) chemotherapy. Neoadjuvant therapy allows for evaluation of tumor necrosis in the surgical specimen and tailoring of the treatment. In OS the most typical drugs administered are cisplatin and adriamycin, along with Methotrexate in younger patients. In ES various regimens are implemented with drug combination of vincristine, cyclophosphamide, etoposide, doxorubicin, dactinomycin, ifosfamide (3–6 drugs). After 3–6 cycles, surgery is performed followed by 3–6 cycles of the same or tailored regimen.
   RT has limited role in OS, basically in inoperable cases or residual tumor after surgery. ES on the other hand, is a radiosensitive tumor, but surgery is preferred over RT, since it allows for evaluation of tumor necrosis and retrospective studies suggest superior local control with surgery, although no head-to-head controlled trials exist. RT is preferred in inoperable cases (or cases where surgery may lead to significant morbidity, such as spino-pelvic region) and certainly in residual disease.
2. *CS* is not a radiosensitive or chemosensitive tumor, (except from some unusual

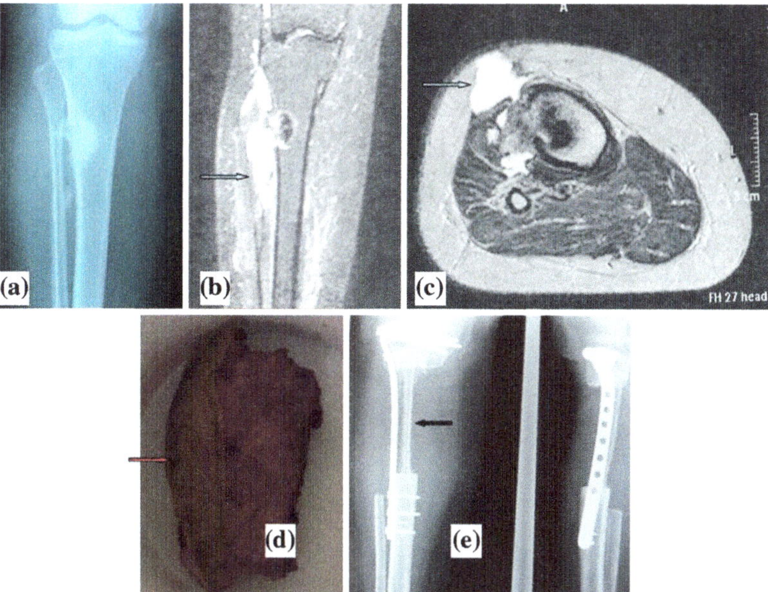

Fig. 7.2 A 45 year old patient with tibial OS. Plain X-ray (**a**) and MRI (**b** Coronal STIR sequence, **c** Axial T1 sequence) depict that the tumor is extracompartmental; *blue arrows* (**b**, **c**) also point a large haematoma contaminating the anterior compartment from a poorly executed biopsy. This necessitated removal of the tibial segment along with the contaminated soft tissue envelope (**d** *red arrow* shows skin incision from previous biopsy), resulting in a foot drop after the operation. Bone defect was reconstructed with transposition of the adjacent vascularized fibula (**e** *black arrow*) along with a long anatomic tibial plate

types such as mesenchymal or dedifferentiated CS), so surgical excision is the mainstay of treatment. Low grade tumors are treated with curettage and cementation, whereas for grade II or III tumors wide excision should be performed. In cases that are deemed inoperable or after incomplete resection, RT may be delivered.

7.6 Recurrent or Metastatic Disease

Local relapse should be dealt with re-excision with negative margins if possible. RT may be also employed to exert local control. Distant metastasis should be treated with metastasectomy (if amenable) and/or systemic chemotherapy.

References

1. NCCN Guidelines (2012) Bone cancer. Version 2. www.nccn.org
2. Fletcher CDM, Unni KK, Mertens F (2002) World Health Organization Classification of tumours: Pathology and Genetics of tumours of soft tissue and bone. IARC Press, Lyon
3. Mankin HJ, Mankin CJ, Simon MA (1996) The hazards of the biopsy, revisited. J Bone Joint Surg Am 78(5):656–663
4. Simon MA, Aschliman MA, Thomas N, Mankin HJ (1986) Limb Salvage treatment versus amputation for osteosarcoma of the distal end of the femur. J Bone Joint Surg Am 68(9):1331–1337
5. Theos C, Koulouvaris P, Kottakis S, Demertzis N (2008) Reconstruction of tibia defects by ipsilateral vascularized fibula transposition. Arch Orthop Trauma Surg 128(2):179–184

8 Introduction to Retroperitoneal Tumors

Dionysis C. Voros and Theodosios C. Theodosopoulos

Retroperitoneal sarcomas (RPS) present specific therapeutic challenges because of their location and frequent close association with several vital structures in the retroperitoneum. This proximity to major vessels, visceral organs, axial skeleton, and neural structures may significantly impair the ability to perform a margin-negative resection, which is the single potentially curative treatment approach in patients who have localized disease. Even in the setting of a complete resection, local recurrence is common.

8.1 Epidemiology

Sarcomas are uncommon malignant tumors arising from mesenchymal stem cells residing in muscle, fat, and connective tissues. Retroperitoneum is the less common site of origin accounting for approximately 10 % of soft tissue sarcomas and less than 1 % of all malignant neoplasms and the overall incidence is 0.3–0.4 % per 100,000 of the population [1].

D. C. Voros · T. C. Theodosopoulos (✉)
Second Department of Surgery, Aretaieion Hospital, Athens Medical School, Athens University, Vas Sofias 76, 11528, Athens, Greece
e-mail: ttheodosopoulos@yahoo.gr

D. C. Voros
e-mail: diovoros@med.uoa.gr

8.2 Clinical Presentation

Most patients who have a RPS present with an abdominal mass, although neurologic symptoms, pain, early satiety, and obstructive gastrointestinal, urinary or vascular symptoms are also seen as presenting symptoms in some patients. Because of the typically silent nature of these tumors until they are large enough to present as an abdominal mass, most retroperitoneal sarcomas are large when diagnosed (>6 cm). Approximately 11 % of patients who have a primary retroperitoneal sarcoma also present with metastatic disease, with lung and liver being the most common site of metastasis. RPS typically present in the sixth decade with a slight male predominance.

8.3 Histological Types

Approximately two-thirds of cases are of high-grade histology, with liposarcomas and leiomyosarcomas representing the most common histologic findings. Retroperitoneal liposarcomas may dedifferentiate to leiomyosarcoma or rhabdomyosarcoma or a less-differentiated liposarcoma and may be associated with worse outcomes, including increased rates of recurrence, increased rates of metastases, and worse survival compared with well-differentiated tumors. Histologically, RPS are predominantly liposarcomas (42–63 %) and leiomyosarcomas

A. D. Gouliamos et al. (eds.), *Imaging in Clinical Oncology*,
DOI: 10.1007/978-88-470-5385-4_8, © Springer-Verlag Italia 2014

(19–23 %). Additional histologic subtypes, such as primitive neuroectodermal tumors (PNET), hemangiopericytoma, and malignant peripheral nerve sheath tumor are less common. Approximately two-thirds of the cases of primary RPS are high grade, whereas the remaining tumors are low grade and mainly lipomatous [2].

Recurrent liposarcomas may also commonly present with dedifferentiation after initial presentation as a well-differentiated liposarcoma and are associated with worse outcomes compared with their differentiated counterparts. Although histologic subclassification may provide prognostic information, patients who have tumors of similar histologic appearance can have quite different clinical courses.

In general, outcomes after therapy for RPS are inferior to those obtained with extremity soft tissue sarcomas, and several factors have been recognized for that fact, including the location of the tumors, inability to obtain negative margins, the size and extent at diagnosis, the multifocality of the lesions or the presence of satellite tumors, and the inability to provide adequate adjuvant therapy because of the proximity to sensitive structures.

Local recurrence-free survival rates of 59 % at 5 years have been reported at high-volume centers. Tumor characteristics that predict a higher risk for local recurrence include higher histologic grade, with patients with high-grade histologic findings having a median survival of 33 months compared with 149 months for low-grade histologic findings, liposarcoma histology, and the completeness of resection. Distant metastases are more likely to occur in patients who have high-grade tumors or a positive resection margin.

References

1. Cormier N, Raphael E, Pollock R (2004) Soft Tissue Sarcomas. CA Cancer J Clin 54:94–109
2. Kotilingam D, Chelouche Lev D, Lazar A (2006) Staging soft tissue sarcoma. Evolution and change. CA Cancer J Clin 56:282–291

9 Conventional Radiology of Bone and Soft Tissue Tumors

Spyros D. Yarmenitis

Under the term "bone tumors," a spectrum of benign and malignant neoplasms as well as non-neoplastic tumorlike lesions is categorized.

The radiographic features of bone tumors have been described in detail since the early 1980s [1–4]. Technical advances of CT and MRI offer strong potentials in diagnosis and staging of bone tumors. However, conventional radiology still plays a primary role in accurately interpreting the characteristics of bone tumors. This is achieved by analyzing the lesions in an organized fashion that may shorten the differential lists and in some occasions to provide a single correct diagnosis.

In contrast to plain film imaging, MRI may overestimate the aggressiveness of some lesions due to its increased sensitivity in depicting marrow and soft tissues edema [5–7].

Systematic diagnostic approach of a detected bone tumor by plain radiography is mainly based on the location of the tumor and the age of the patient. Further radiographic analysis of the lesion includes: margins of lesions, periosteal reaction, radiographic density and patterns of mineralization, size and number of lesions, and the presence of a soft-tissue component.

S. D. Yarmenitis (✉)
Hygeia Hospital, Department of Diagnostic Radiology, 4, Erythrou Stavrou St, 15123, Maroussi, Greece
e-mail: spyros.yarmenitis@hotmail.com

9.1 Patient's Age

Despite existing exceptions, the age predilection of bone tumors (Table 9.1) is the most important clinical information for the evaluation of tumorous lesions of bone.

Over 40 years of age, a malignant lesion is more likely to be metastasis, myeloma, or lymphoma rather than a primary sarcoma. Similarly, in individuals younger than 20 years of age that are not diagnosed as having a primary malignancy, a bone lesion is strongly unlike to be a metastasis (Fig. 9.1). In this age group, Ewing or conventional sarcomas are most possible to occur (Figs. 9.2 and 9.3). However, conventional sarcomas show two age peaks, one in teenagers and the other in over 40 years of age.

9.2 Tumor Location

Bone tumors, according to bone growth rate and/or in regard with their histological origin, often occur at a characteristic location, for example, axial versus appendicular skeleton, long versus flat bone, diaphyseal versus metaphyseal versus epiphyseal, medullary versus cortical (Table 9.2).

Typically Ewing sarcomas arise at red marrow sites, commonly at a diaphyseal location or at flat bones (Fig. 9.2). On the other hand, osteosarcomas tend to arise at sites of rapid bone growth such as the metaphyseal area.

A. D. Gouliamos et al. (eds.), *Imaging in Clinical Oncology*,
DOI: 10.1007/978-88-470-5385-4_9, © Springer-Verlag Italia 2014

Table 9.1 Classification of bone tumor lesions according to age predilection

Age in years	<20	20–40	>40
Malignant	Ewing sarcoma	Osteosarcoma	Metastasis
	Hodgkin disease	Adamantinoma	Myeloma
	Leukemia		Osteosarcoma (Pagetic bones)
	Metastases (rare)		Lymphoma
	Neuroblastoma		Chondrosarcoma
	Osteosarcoma		Malignant fibrous histiocytoma
	Retinoblastoma		
	Rhabdomyosarcoma		
Benign	Aneurysmal bone cyst	Enchondroma	Fibrous dysplasia
	Chondroblastoma	Chondromyxoid fibroma	Paget disease
	Chondromyxoid fibroma	Fibrous dysplasia	
	Enchondroma	Giant cell tumor	
	Fibrous dysplasia		
	Fibrous cortical defect	Osteoblastoma	
	Histiocytosis	Osteoid osteoma	
	Non-ossifying fibroma		
	Osteoblastoma		
	Osteoid osteoma		
	Osteofibrous dysplasia		
	Simple bone cyst		

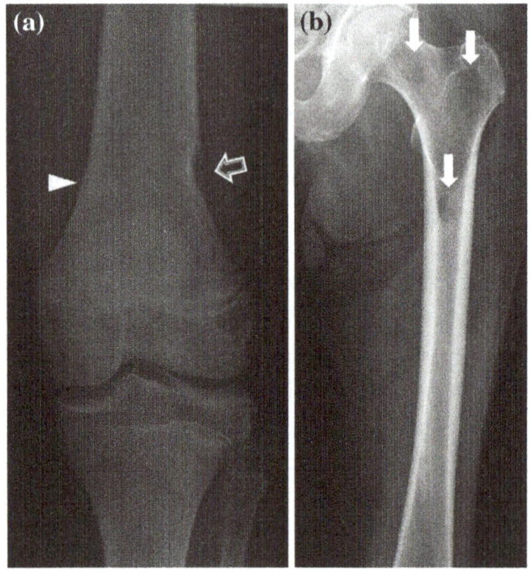

Fig. 9.1 Two cases of osteolytic lesions. According to age predilection and location, the cortical lesion in the left knee of a 16-year-old footballer (**a**) is a fibrous cortical defect (*open arrow*). The lytic lesions (*arrows*) in the left proximal femur of a 68-year-old male (**b**), suffering of lung carcinoma, are osteolytic metastases. In (**a**) a benign periosteal reaction is also seen at the site of a stress fracture (*arrowhead*)

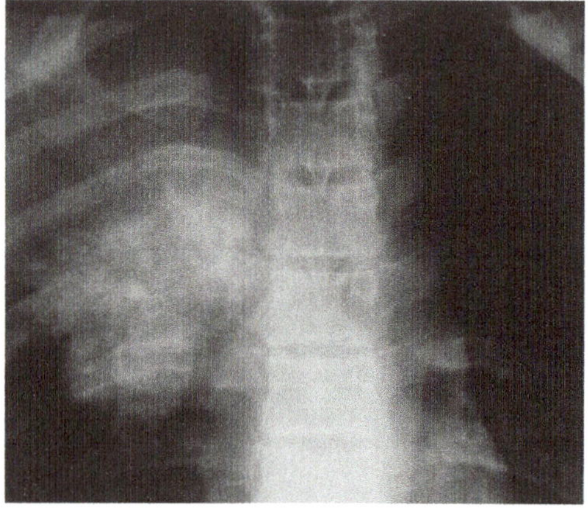

Fig. 9.2 Ewing sarcoma arising from the posterior part of the right 5th rib. Image courtesy of Dr Kosmidou

Both simple bone cysts and non-ossifying fibromas are metaphyseal lesions but the first is a medullary disorder while the second is cortical.

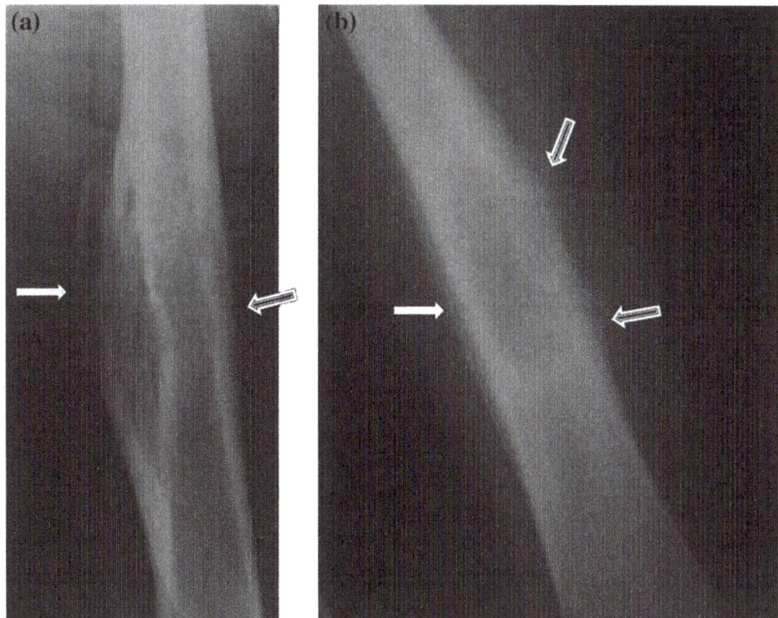

Fig. 9.3 Two cases of diaphyseal lytic type osteosarcomas (**a**) aggressive multilayered periosteal reaction (*arrow*) and spiculated periosteal reaction (*open arrow*). Image courtesy of Dr Ch. Triantopoulou (**b**) Mutilayered periosteal reaction (*arrow*) and destructive periosteal lesion with Codman triangle formation (open arrows). Image courtesy of Dr. Kosmidou

9.3 Margin of Lesions

The margin of a bone lesion and the zone of transition between a lytic lesion and the adjacent bone determine the aggressiveness of a lesion. Sharp margins and narrow sclerotic transition zone are indicative of a non-aggressive lesion (Fig. 9.1a). However aggressiveness should not be confused with malignancy. A very aggressive lesion with ill-defined border and wide transition zone, such as osteomyelitis, is a benign lesion whereas a malignant bone metastasis appears with sharp margins and narrow transition zone (Fig. 9.4).

9.4 Periosteal Reaction

Another feature that may characterize a bone tumor as aggressive or slow growing is the presence and pattern of periosteal reaction.

A non-aggressive or slow growing lesion usually appears with a solid or unilamellated periosteal reaction.

A lesion with an intermediate aggressive process usually shows a multilamellated or "onion-skin" periosteal reaction.

Disruption of anyone of the previous two patterns of periosteal reactions indicates that the tumorous process is very aggressive and has broken through the bone cortex.

A similar pattern of a very aggressive bone tumor is the spiculated or "sunburst" appearance of the periosteal reaction and it is highly indicative of malignancy (Fig. 9.3).

9.5 Radiographic Density and Pattern of Mineralization

Tumor lesions may appear as lytic, sclerotic, or mixed. A mixed appearance is associated with alternating stimulation of the osteoclasts or the osteoblasts by the tumor (Fig. 9.5).

Table 9.2 Characteristic locations of common bone tumors and tumorlike conditions

	Cortical	Medullary
Diaphysis	Adamantinoma	Fibrous dysplasia
	Osteofibrous dysplasia	Ewing sarcoma
	Osteoid osteoma	
	Stress Fracture	
	Chronic osteomyelitis	
	Metastasis	
Metaphysis	Fibrous cortical defect	Fibrosarcoma
	Non-ossifying fibroma	Chondromyxoid fibroma
	Osteochondroma	Aneurysmal bone cyst
	Osteosarcoma	Enchondroma
		Chondrosarcoma
		Simple bone cyst
		Fibrous dysplasia
		Ewing sarcoma
		Osteomyelitis (pyogenic)
Epiphysis	Articular Osteochondroma	Chondroblastoma (child)
		Giant cell tumor (20–40 years)
		Osteomyelitis (Fungal, TB)
		Aneurysmal bone cyst

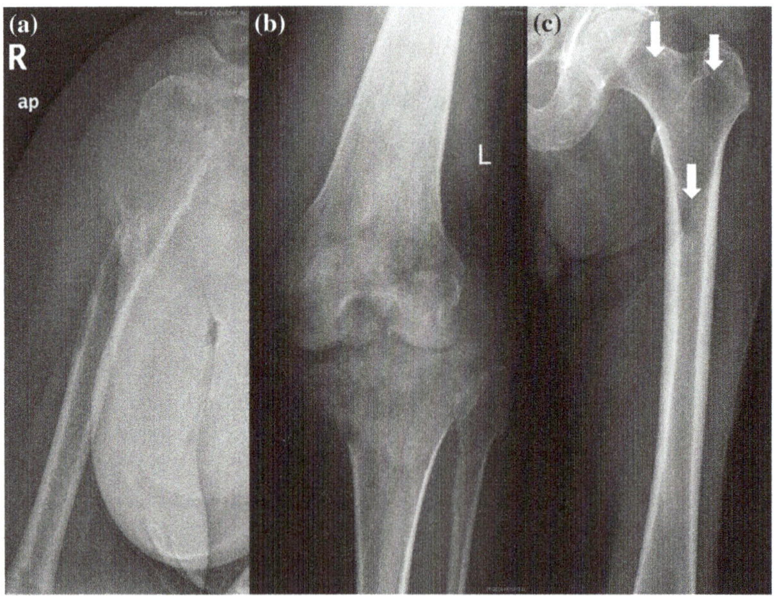

Fig. 9.4 Margin of lesions is indicative of the degree of aggressiveness but not of the malignancy or benignancy. **a** Destructive osteolytic metastatic lesion of right humerus complicated by fracture. **b** Destructive non-neoplastic lesion (tuberculous osteoarthritis) of left knee.**c** Well demarcated non-destructive osteolytic metastases of left proximal femur (*arrows*)

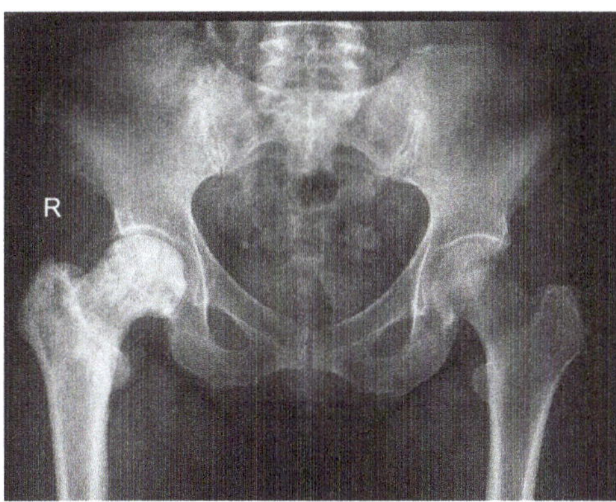

Fig. 9.5 A case of Bone Paget disease in a 70-year-old female Mixed osteolytic and osteoblastic lesions of the right proximal femur with widening of the femoral neck and thickening of the cortical bone

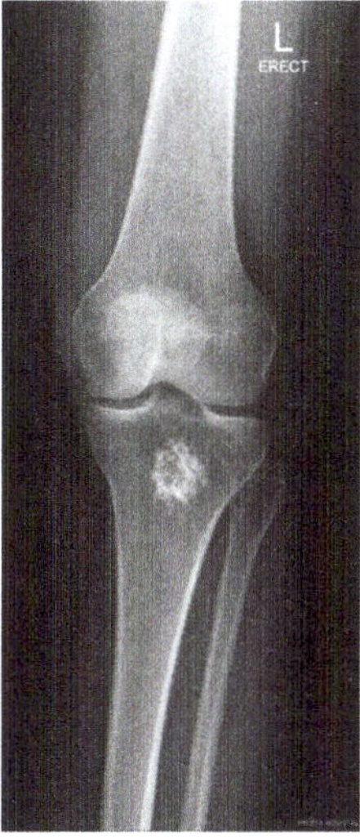

Fig. 9.6 Enchondroma of left tibia: A typical epiphyseal cartilaginous lesion

The type of mineralization (calcification) of the tumor tissue matrix (osteoid, chondral, fibrous, or adipose) also contributes to the radiographic opacity and the specific appearance of the tumors. This may yield adequate information of the type of the underlying tumor tissue matrix and possibly the diagnosis. Calcification of cartilaginous matrix appears as punctuate, flocculent, or ringlike (Fig. 9.6), while bone forming tumors show fluffy, amorphous, cloud-like mineralization. Whenever calcification is faint, CT scan is more sensitive than plain radiographs to assess the mineralization patterns.

9.6 Size and Number

In several processes, the lesion size may be a clue to its diagnosis. A typical example is that of a well-defined cortical lytic lesion with a sclerotic rim. If it is less than 3 cm in length, it is considered as a fibrous cortical defect (Fig. 9.1a). If it is larger than 3 cm, it is termed as non-ossifying fibroma [8].

A 1–2 cm cartilaginous lesion in a long bone is most possible to be an enchondroma (Fig. 9.6). The risk to be a chondrosarcoma increases if it is larger than 4–5 cm [9–11].

Primary bone neoplasms are solitary entities. Metastases, multiple myeloma, and metastatic lymphoma are the most common causes of multiple radiolucent lesions in an adult over 40 years of age (Figs. 9.1b and 9.4c).

Although plain films are often satisfactory to diagnose bone tumors, cross sectional imaging is used for more detailed analysis of the bone neoplasms and in oncologic staging.

CT scan depicts more details in subtle mineralization of lytic lesions, demonstrates occult bone destruction and detects the lucent nidus of an osteoid osteoma.

MRI is considered the standard for staging purposes since, due to its high tissue contrast resolution, it can assess the local extent of the malignant process and the response to treatment [12–14].

However, the concurrent use of conventional radiology is substantial when CT or MR images of bone tumors are interpreted.

References

1. Madewell JE, Ragsdale BD, Sweet DE (1981) Radiologic and pathologic analysis of solitary bone lesions. I. Internal margins. Radiol Clin North Am 19:715–748
2. Ragsdale BD, Madewell JE, Sweet DE (1981) Radiologic and pathologic analysis of solitary bone

lesions. II. Periosteal reactions. Radiol Clin North Am 19:749–783
3. Sweet DE, Madewell JE, Ragsdale BD (1981) Radiologic and pathologic analysis of solitary bone lesions. III. Matrix patterns. Radiol Clin North Am 19:785–814
4. Kricun ME (1983) Radiographic evaluation of solitary bone lesions. Orthop Clin North Am 14:39–64
5. Seeger LL, Dungan DH, Eckardt JJ (1991) Nonspecific findings on MR imaging: the importance of correlative studies and clinical information. Clin Orthop Relat Res 270:306–312
6. Hayes CW, Conway WF, Sundaram M (1992) Misleading aggressive MR imaging appearance of some benign musculoskeletal lesions. Radiographics 12:1119–1136
7. Ma LD, Frassica FJ, Scott WW (1995) Differentiation of benign and malignant musculoskeletal tumors: potential pitfalls with MR imaging. Radiographics 15:349–366
8. Resnick D. (2002) Diagnosis of bone and joint disorders, 4th edn. Philadelphia, PA: Saunders 3757:3922–3924
9. Kendell SD, Collins MS, Adkins MC (2004) Radiographic differ- entiation of enchondroma from low-grade chondrosarcoma in the fibula. Skeletal Radiol 33:458–466
10. Geirnaerdt MJ, Hermans J, Bloem JL et al (1997) Usefulness of radiography in differentiating enchondroma from central grade 1 chondrosarcoma. AJR Am J Roentgenol 169:1097–1104
11. Flemming DJ, Murphey MD (2000) Enchondroma and chondrosarcoma. Semin Musculoskelet Radiol 4:59–71
12. Cerase A, Priolo F. (1998) Skeletal benign bone-forming lesions. Eur J Radiol 27(Suppl 1):S91–S97
13. Pettersson H, Gillespy 3rd T, Hamlin DJ, et al. (1987) Primary musculoskeletal tumors: examination with MR imaging compared with conventional modalities. Radiology 164:237–241
14. Zimmer WD, Berquist TH, McLeod RA et al (1985) Bone tumors: magnetic resonance imaging versus computed tomography. Radiology 155:709–718

US-CT-MRI Findings: Staging-Response-Restaging of Bone and Soft Tissue Tumors

10

Andreas P. Koureas

10.1 Introduction

Primary malignant bone tumors are a rare and diverse group of tumors. Osteosarcoma is the commonest malignant neoplasm among the primary bone tumors (excluding multiple myeloma), accounting for 30 % of all such malignancies.Soft-tissue sarcomas are a rare (1 % adult cancers and 6 % of childhood cancers), heterogeneous group of malignant tumors that can affect any age and gender, and are often highly aggressive. Soft-tissue sarcomas occur in the extremities in about 50 % of cases, with a predilection for the lower extremities (80 %). Malignant fibrous histiocytoma is the commonest histologic subtype, followed by liposarcoma [1]. In the retroperitoneum, the most common tumors are liposarcoma and leiomyosarcoma.

10.2 Staging Bone Tumors

The WHO classification of bone tumors includes ten major categories. Cartilage tumors (chondrosarcoma), osteogenic tumors (osteosarcoma and its subtypes), Fibrogenic tumors (fibrosarcoma), Fibrohistiocytic tumors (malignant fibrous histiocytoma), Ewing's sarcoma, Vascular tumors (angiosarcoma), Muscle tumors (leiomyosarcoma), Hematopoietic tumors (lymphoma, plasma cell myeloma), Lipogenic tumors (liposarcoma), Notochordal tumors (chordoma).

Two staging systems are currently used as far as bone tumours are concerned. The American Joint Commission on Cancer staging system and the Musculoskeletal Tumor Society staging system based on Enneking's work.

The staging of bone tumors is possible with the American Joint Commission on Cancer (AJCC)–International Union against Cancer (UICC) system. These staging systems do not apply to malignant lymphoma and multiple myeloma. The TNM classification consists of T, N and M factors.

The *T* factor represents tumor extent and consists of three stages: T1, tumor greatest diameter less or equal than 8 cm; T2, tumor's greatest diameter more than 8 cm; and T3, skip lesions in the primary bone site. High grade tumors with skip lesions usually have poor outcome.

The *N* factor includes the following two grades: N0, no detectable node metastases; and N1, lymph node metastases. Lymph node metastases are rare in primary bone tumors.

The *M* factor includes metastases to distant organs (lung, liver, brain, lymph node bone marrow, pleura, peritoneum etc.). The commonest site of distant metastases are the lung and the liver.

The M factor is divided into two grades: M0, absence of metastasis; and M1, presence of metastases. M1 is further subdivided in M1a (metastases only in lungs) and M1b (metastases to other distant sites, including lymph nodes).

A. P. Koureas (✉)
Department of Radiology, University of Athens, Medical School, Areteion Hospital, 76 Vas, Sophias Avenue, 11528 Athens, Greece
e-mail: akoureas@yahoo.com

A. D. Gouliamos et al. (eds.), *Imaging in Clinical Oncology*,
DOI: 10.1007/978-88-470-5385-4_10, © Springer-Verlag Italia 2014

The G factor represents the histological grade. Tumors are divided into two grades: low grade G1, and high grade G2.

Accordingly, staging is determined as follows: *IA*, G1 or 2 T1N0M0; *IB*, G1 or 2 T2N0M0; *IIA*, G2 T1N0M0; *IIB*, G2 T2N0M0; *III*, G (any) T(any) skip metastasis; *IVA*, G(any) T(any) N1M0; and IVB, G(any) (any) N(any) M1, [1, 2].

Conventional radiography is often the first examination in patients with primary bone tumors. It plays an important role because it is inexpensive and provides information regarding tumor location, margins, zone of transition, type of periosteal reaction, matrix mineralization, number of lesions and soft-tissue extension. Moreover, radiographs are of vital importance in the differential diagnosis of most primary bone tumors.

Ultrasound has a very limited role in the local staging of primary bone malignancies. Computed tomography (CT) has an important role. CT is the method of choice for imaging—guided biopsies. Also it is very important in assessing distant metastases specially in lung.

Accurate characterization of bone marrow and cortical bone involvement is possible with MR imaging. Muscular involvement and proximity to neurovascular bundles are evaluated effectively with MR imaging.

Magnetic resonance imaging has the most important role in staging and characterizing all primary bone tumors. Every patient should undergo MRI examination prior to biopsy. MR protocols should include T1 weighted spin echo sequences, fat suppressed T2 weighted spin echo sequences in axial, sagittal and coronal planes. Short tau inversion recovery (STIR) sequences are useful in assessing skip lesions but tent to overestimate tumor size. The entire length of the affected bone and the opposite side of the joint must be included in sagittal or coronal planes to exclude skip lesions and transarticular spread of tumor for epiphyseal or metaphyseal lesions which arise close to the joint (Fig. 10.1).

The use of contrast enchantment is controvential. Static gadolinium enhancement does not provide important information for staging and extent assessment because there is sufficient contrast between the tumor and normal bone marrow. Dynamic contrast enhanced MRI can help in differentiating benign from malignant tumors. Malignant tumors tend to enhance more rapidly than benign and to a greater degree. Gadolinium enhancement is preferable in order to identify the cystic and solid components of the lesion for biopsy planning to avoid inadequate specimen [3]. Tumor response to chemotherapy is better assessed with dynamic contrast enhanced MRI especially with the use of subtracted contrast-enhanced T1-weighted images (Fig. 10.2).

Most bone tumors have high signal intensity on (STIR) images. Whole body MRI consists of series of STIR images covering the whole body, in coronal plane. This is a way to scan the whole

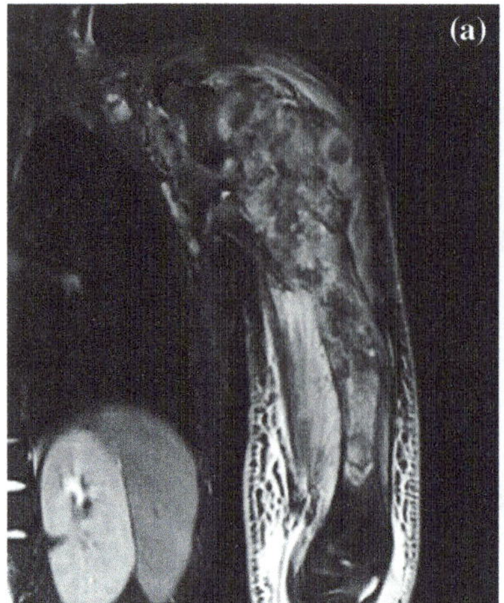

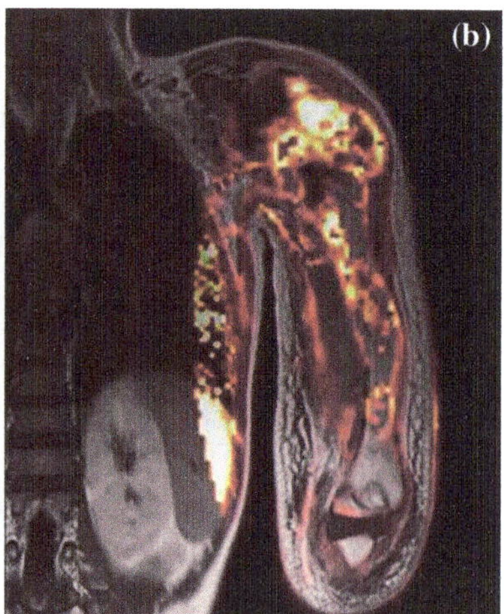

Fig. 10.1 Large humeral osteosarcoma with joint involvement. **a** MRI T2 W image. **b** Contrast enhanced T1 W image. (Courtesy of A. Papadopoulos MD.)

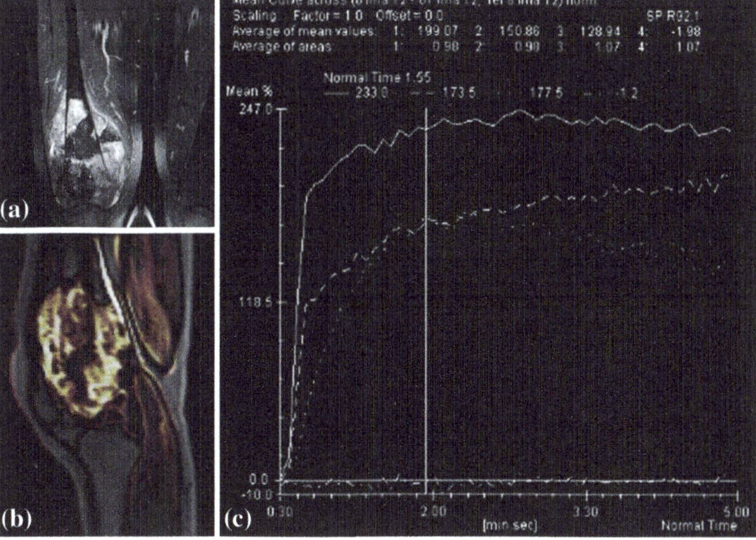

Fig. 10.2 Femoral osteosarcoma non responding to chemotherapy. **a** Coronal MRI T2 W image. **b** Contrast enhanced T1 W image. **c** Enhancing curve

body with MR imaging. It is very useful to screen the skeleton and liver with reasonable sensitivity. Its sensitivity on bone involvement seems to be higher than bone scintigraphy. New techniques such as Diffusion-Weighted (DW) magnetic resonance imaging appear to be very promising in accurately assessing tumors. Whole-body DW imaging can be clinically useful for disease detection, lesion characterization, and assessment of therapy response [4].

10.3 Staging Soft Tissue Tumors

The commonest primary malignant soft tissue tumors are: Malignant fibrous histiocytoma (MFH), liposarcoma, leiomyosarcoma, malignant nerve sheath tumor (MPNST), Synovial sarcoma, fibrosarcoma, rhabdomyosarcoma (commonest soft tissue tumor in children). Despite the advantages in imaging only 25–35 % of primary soft tissue tumors can precisely be characterized with either MRI or CT. The final diagnosis in most cases rests on biopsy [5].

Staging of soft tissue sarcomas is as follows:

Histological grade

Grade 1 (G1): Well differentiated

Grade 2 (G2): Moderately differentiated

Grade 3 (G3): Poorly differentiated

Grade 4 (G4): Undifferentiated

T stage

T1: The sarcoma is 5 cm or less

- T1a: The tumor is superficial
- T1b: The tumor is deep

T2: The sarcoma is greater than 5 cm.

- T2a: The tumor is superficial
- T2b: The tumor is deep

Nodes

N0: The sarcoma has not spread to nearby lymph nodes.

N1: The sarcoma has spread to nearby lymph nodes.

Metastasis

M0: No distant metastases.

M1: The sarcoma has spread to distant organs.

Stage IA: T1, N0, M0, G1:

Stage IB: T2, N0, M0, G1:

Stage IIA: T1, N0, M0, G2 or G3:

Stage IIB: T2, N0, M0, G2:

Stage III: EitherT2, N0, M0, G3 or Any T, N1, M0, any G

Stage IV: Any T, Any N, M1, Any G.

10.4 Staging and Biopsy

Conventional radiography has a limited role in the work up of primary malignant soft tissue tumors. Mainly this is taken to identify calcifications which can help differentiate between

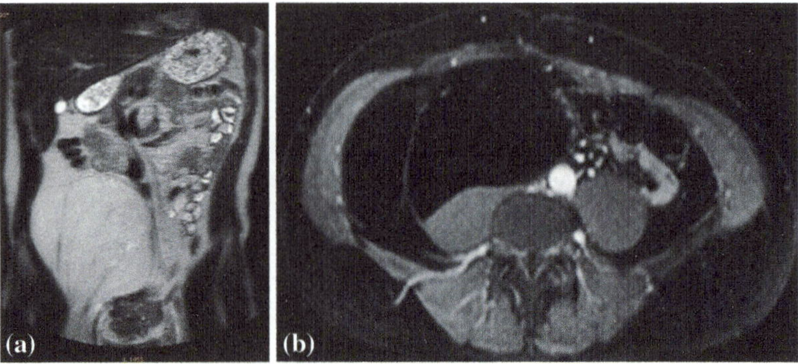

Fig. 10.3 Abdominal liposarcoma extending to the inguinal canal. **a** T1 W image, **b** Contrast enchancent fat suppressed T1 W image showing enhancement of septations within the mass

tumors (phleboliths in hemangiomas, skeletal deformities such as exostosis etc.). Ultrasonography (US) is of the utmost importance in the diagnosis of soft-tissue lesions. This imaging technique aids to distinguish solid masses from cystic lesions. In superficial lesions the relationship with the neurovascular bundles can be accurately delineated. Doppler US demonstrates the extent of internal vascularity of the tumor and also can be used for procedures such biopsy or aspiration of masses under real-time guidance.

MRI is the method of choice for evaluating soft tissue tumors. The technique is similar to that described for bone tumors (Figs. 10.3, 10.4).

The primary goal of treatment is to achieve local control of the disease through a limb- salvage procedure: however, if the lesion is too advanced an amputation or even disarticulation

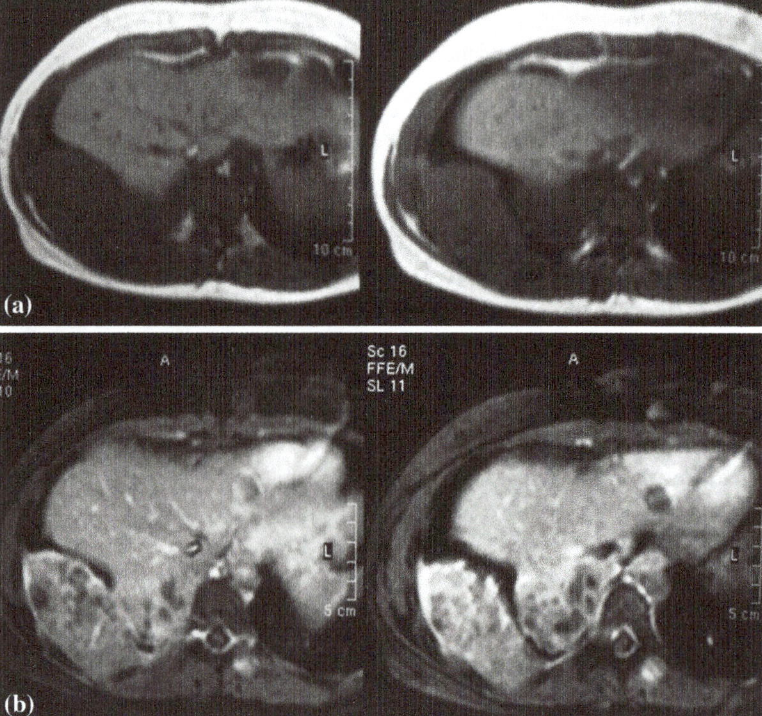

Fig. 10.4 Thoracic cage synovial sarcoma. **a** T1 W image, **b** Axial contrast enhanced T1 W image depicting intense inhomogeneous tumoral enhancement

may be required. The decision depends on many factors such as tumor size, extracompartmental spread, relationship to vessels, nerves and joints. Identification of the compartments is very important in case of imaging guided biopsy. The needle path must be in the same location where the incision for the definitive surgery will be made so that the biopsy track can be resected. Surgeons and radiation oncologists should be consulted regarding the biopsy technique and planned in such a manner as to allow for a complete resection, including the biopsy tract. Also uninvolved compartments, joints and neurovascular bundles must be avoided. In the forearm, the are two compartments volar and dorsal separated by the interosseous membrane. At the thigh, there are three compartments anterior, medial, and posterior. In the calf, there are four compartments, anterior, lateral, superficial posterior and deep posterior. Neurovascular status is determined by the presence of a fat plane which separates the neurovascular bundle from the tumor. If the fat plane between the tumor and the neurovascular structures is obliterated then structures are possibly affected from the tumor and limp—salvage surgery may not be an option (Fig. 10.5).

Bone and lymph node involvement is generally not observed in cases of soft-tissue sarcomas. Nodal metastasis are more frequent in synovial sarcomas, rhabdomyosarcomas, and clear cell sarcoma. The presence of nodal metastasis at presentation upstages the tumor worsening its prognosis. Myxoid liposarcoma has a higher propensity for bone metastases than other sarcomas (Fig. 10.6).

10.5 Response

Chemotherapy is not indicated in most cases of soft tissue sarcomas, as these are relatively chemoresistant. The response rate is <25 %, with more than 75 % of tumors displaying resistance to chemoptherapy. For extremity soft tissue sarcomas the treatment of choice is limb—conserving surgery with adjuvant radiotherapy. The criteria for assessment of tumor response in solid tumors remains a debatable

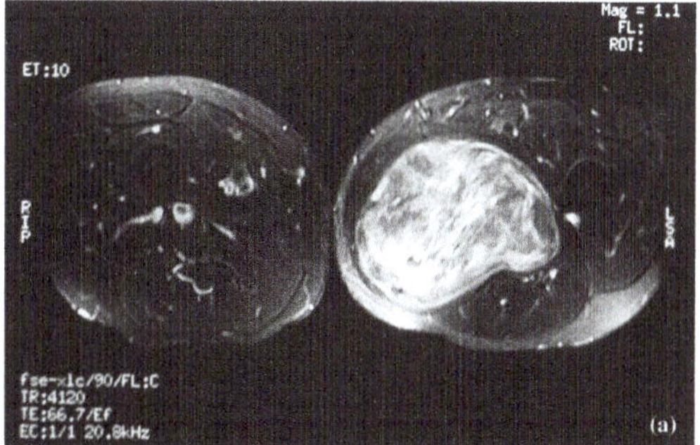

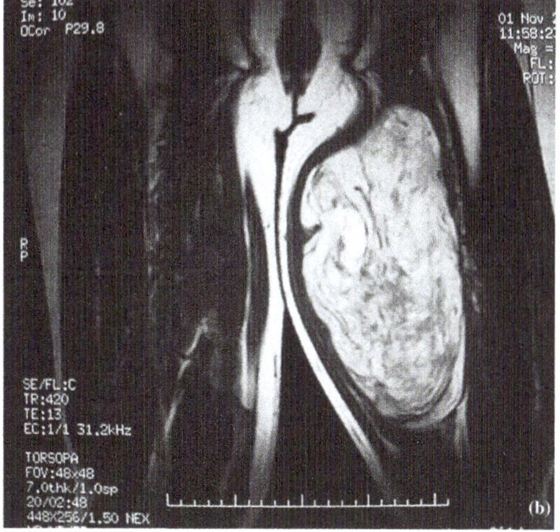

Fig. 10.5 Well - differentiated femoral liposarcoma. **a** T2 W image, **b** T1 W image

topic. The RECIST and adapted Choi criteria were initially used to monitor tumor response. The abovementioned criteria were first described for gastrointestinal stromal tumors (GIST). According to RECIST criteria, tumor response is divided into four categories: Complete response (remission of the disease, no new lesions). Partial response (≥ 30 % decrease in tumor volume, no new lesions), Stable disease (does not meet criteria for complete response, partial response, or progressive disease) and Progressive disease (≥ 20 % increase in the sum of greatest diameters, new lesions). The revised RECIST criteria 1.1 include FDG - PET in the detection of new lesions that define progression [6, 7]. It has been well documented that responding to treatment osteosarcomas may demonstrate tumor necrosis without any decrease in size. To resolve this problem Choi modified RECIST criteria in order to estimate the pathologic response as expressed

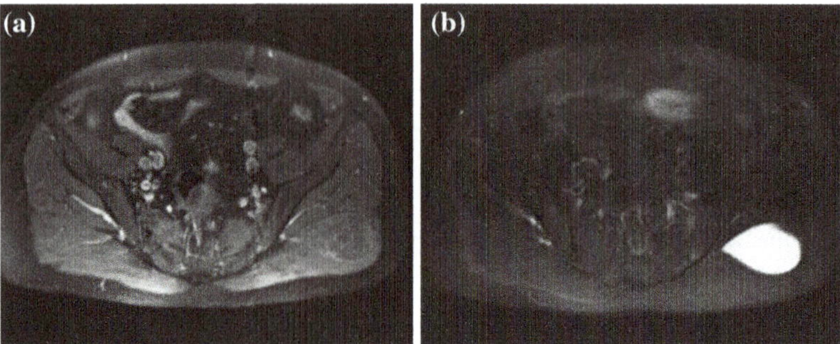

Fig. 10.6 Myxoid liposarcoma. **a** Contrast enhanced T1 W image depicting tumor enhancement. **b** T2 W image, showing very high signal intensity of the tumor

by contrast enhancement. Partial response with the adapted Choi criteria includes ≥10 % decrease in the greatest maximal diameter or ≥15 % decrease of tumor attenuation on CT or contrast-enhanced MR imaging. The diagnosis of progressive disease requires ≥10 % increase in the greatest maximal diameter and absence of criteria for partial response by using tumor attenuation at CT or contrast enhancement at MR imaging or ≥15 % increase in tumor attenuation at CT or contrast enhancement at MR imaging and does not meet the criteria for partial response by using tumor size [8].

10.6 Recurrense

In general the recurrent tumor is characterized by a mass that has the same imaging characteristics as the original tumor. The risk of recurrence depends on tumour grade, surgical margins and additional treatment (radiotherapy, chemotherapy). High Grade Tumours have increased risk of metastases and early local recurrence. Some low grade tumours may dedifferentiate into high grade. Radiologists must be aware of post surgery—radiotherapy changes. Postoperative seromas may have atypical appearance or may co-exist with recurrent tumor in the same patient. Contrast enhanced MRI, Contrast-enhanced and Diffusion-Weighted (DW) magnetic resonance imaging in conjunction with PET may be useful in distinguishing viable tumour from post therapeutic changes. MRI Pitfalls in diagnosing recurrent/residual tumour include: soft tissue infection, hypovascular tumours, muscle flaps and denervated muscle, foreign bodies, mineralized tumours and early postoperative period. Postamputation neuromas must also be differentiated from recurrence.

FDG PET may be useful for the detection of local recurrence and metastasis in soft tissue sarcomas.

Treatment of soft-tissue and bone sarcomas requires a multidisciplinary team that includes radiologists, surgeons and oncologists in order to provide optimal treatment with limb preserving therapies [9, 10].

References

1. Ehara Shigeru (2006) MR imaging in staging of bone tumors. Cancer Imaging 6:158–162
2. Stacy GS, Mahal RS, Peabody TD (2006) Staging of Bone Tumors: A Review with Illustrative Examples. AJR 186:967–976
3. Husband & Reznek's. Imaging in oncology. 3rd Edition. 2010 Informa heallthcare
4. Khoo MM, Tyler PA, Saifuddin A et. al (2011) Diffusion-weighted imaging (DWI) in musculoskeletal MRI:a critical review. Skeletal Radiol 40:665–681
5. Berquist TH, Ehman RL, King BF (1990) Value of MR Imaging in Differentiating Benign from Malignant Soft-Tissue Masses: Study of 95 Lesions. AJR 155:1251–1255
6. Stacchiotti S, Collini P, Messina A et al (2009) High-Grade Soft-Tissue Sarcomas: Tumor Response Assessment—Pilot Study to Assess the Correlation between Radiologic and Pathologic Response by Using RECIST and Choi Criteria. Radiology 251:447–456

7. Nishino M, Jagannathan JP, Ramaiya NH (2010) Revised RECIST Guideline Version 1.1: What Oncologists Want to Know and What Radiologists Need to Know. AJR, 195:281–289
8. Choi H, Charnsangavej C, Faria SC et al (2007) Correlation of computed tomography and positron emission tomography in patients with metastatic gastrointestinal stromal tumor treated at a single institution with imatinib mesylate: proposal of new computed tomography response criteria. J Clin Oncol 25(13):1753–1759
9. Robinson E, Bleakney RR, Ferguson PC (2008) Oncodiagnosis Panel: 2007Multidisciplinary Management of Soft-Tissue Sarcoma. RadioGraphics 28:2069–2086
10. The ESMO/European Sarcoma Network Working Group. Annals of Oncology 23 (Supplement 7): vii92–vii99, 2012 doi:10.1093/annonc/mds253

11 Positron Emission Tomography in Bone and Soft Tissue Tumors

Sofia N. Chatziioannou and Nikoletta K. Pianou

11.1 Introduction

Positron emission tomography /computed tomography with the use of ^{18}F-fluorodeoxyglucose (^{18}F-FDG PET/CT) is an imaging modality that combines both functional and anatomical information. The combination of PET with CT has been established as an imaging modality and is currently widely used in oncology. Bone and soft tissue tumors, as of course the majority of tumors, are characterized of multiple metabolic and molecular alterations, which allow us imaging with positron emitters. These alterations include increased glucolysis, increased amino acid and increased nucleic acid metabolic activity.

There are several radiotracers available for PET imaging, but the most widely used tracer in oncology is ^{18}F-fluorodeoxyglucose (^{18}F-FDG) which is a glucose analogue. Contemporary PET scanners are equipped also with CT (PET/CT scanners) and very recently with MRI (PET/MRI scanners), thus allowing a comprehensive functional and an anatomical assessment of tumors.

^{18}F-FDG follows the pathways of glucose into the cells, meaning that it enters into the cells through membrane glucose transporters (GLOUT 1–GLOUT 7). After its entrance into the cell, it is phosphorylated by an enzyme called hexokinase and converted to FDG-6-phosphate. The difference from glucose is that ^{18}F-FDG is not further metabolized, and it is metabolically trapped into the cell. Taking advantage of the fact that tumors are characterized of increased glucolysis, we can depict images of the tumor. During tumor proliferation, the glucose transporters, especially GLUT 1, are over-expressed, bur other changes as well, like increased hexokinase activity and reduced glucose-6-phosphatase activity, make tumors "visible" to PET.

^{18}F-FDG is injected intravenously to the patient and then the patient remains at rest for about 1 h. Hydration and fasting for at least 6 h prior to the examination are mandatory. Blood glucose levels should also be measured as it is preferred that the glucose level remains <160 mg/dl. Then the patient initially undergoes CT imaging and then PET imaging, usually from the base of the skull to the thighs. In selected patients, the extremities may be in the field of interest. PET images are attenuation corrected with the CT and both images are fused.

S. N. Chatziioannou (✉)
2nd Department of Radiology, Nuclear Medicine Section, National and Kapodistrian University of Athens, "Attikon" University General Hospital, 1, Rimini, Chaidari, 12462 Athens, Greece
e-mail: sofiac@bcm.tmc.edu

N. K. Pianou
Nuclear Medicine Division, PET/CT Department, Biomedical Research Foundation, Academy of Athens, 4, Soranou Ephessiou, 11527 Athens, Greece
e-mail: npianou@bioacademy.gr

A. D. Gouliamos et al. (eds.), *Imaging in Clinical Oncology*,
DOI: 10.1007/978-88-470-5385-4_11, © Springer-Verlag Italia 2014

11.2 Positron Emission Tomography in Sarcomas

Sarcomas are relatively rare and account for about 1 % of all malignancies. They arise from tissue of mesenchymal origin and are very heterogeneous group of malignancies comprising bone sarcomas (BS) and soft tissue sarcomas (STS). However, sarcomas can develop from many types of tissue such as bone, cartilage, muscle, connective tissue, fat, peripheral nerves or vessels, occurring almost anywhere in the body. They usually grow locally, infiltrating surrounding tissues. They occur in both children and elderly. Ewing's sarcoma, which is a malignant primary bone tumor and rhabdomyosarcoma usually occur in children and adolescents, but osteosarcoma may occur in the elderly also. Lungs are the most frequent site for metastases, as sarcomas tend to spread haematogenously, although lymphatic spread is also possible. Extremities, especially lower limbs, are usual sites where sarcomas grow up, but some of them may occur intra-abdominally, like gastrointestinal stromal tumors (GIST), which are the most common sarcomas (mesenchymal tumors) of the gastrointestinal tract.

When the disease is initially diagnosed, there are some parameters which are very important for the management of these tumors, such as the exact location of the tumor, the size and grade of the tumor and the accurate staging. The conventional imaging modalities (CIM) which are used to determine the location and the size of the primary tumor are the magnetic resonance imaging (MRI) and the CT. However, benign soft tissue masses and STS may be difficult to separate with the use of CIM, while sarcomas show very heterogeneous character. Biopsy remains the method of choice for the diagnosis and grading of sarcomas. The biopsy site determines the result which is dependent and directed by anatomical imaging. A problem which often arises when biopsy is performed is that the site of the biopsy taken may not represent the character of the whole mass, therefore, clinically significant high-grade areas of the tumor may be missed. ^{18}F-FDG PET/CT can help improve the localization of the biopsy site, helping for a more accurate staging (Fig. 11.1). However, there are substantial differences in ^{18}F-FDG uptake values between low- and high-grade BS and STS, while ^{18}F-FDG uptake correlates with histological grade in heterogeneous

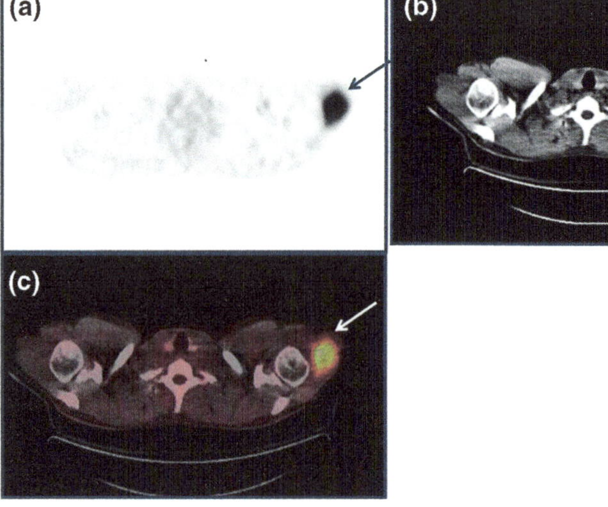

Fig. 11.1 **a–c** Young patient with fever of unknown origin. There is increased ^{18}F-FDG uptake at left humeral soft tissues. Biopsy revealed sarcoma (**a** ^{18}F-FDG PET, *black arrow*; **b** CT, *white arrow*; **c** PET/CT, *white arrow*)

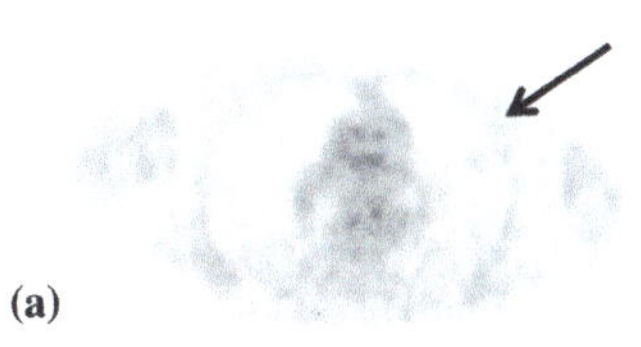

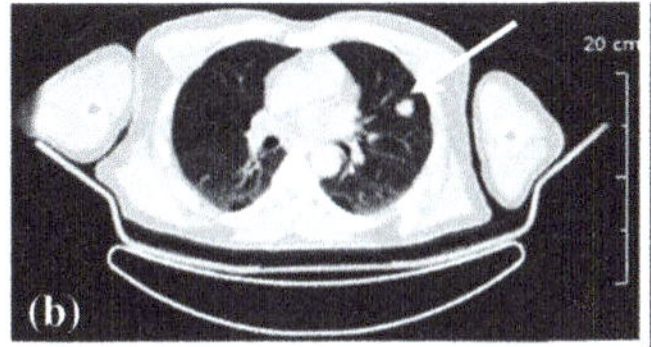

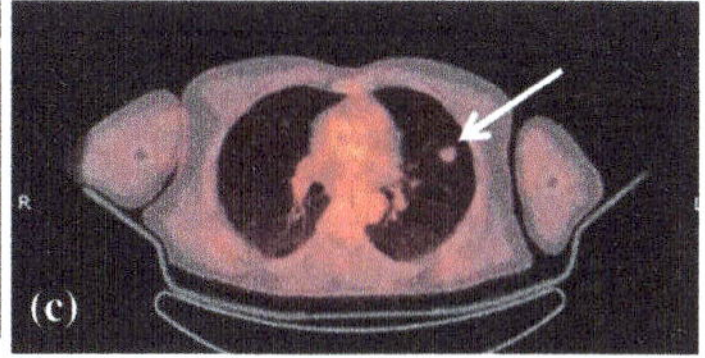

Fig. 11.2 **a–c** Male patient with history of resected low grade synovial sarcoma of the right lower extremity. Lung metastases on CT images showing mildly increased ^{18}F-FDG uptake on PET images (**a** ^{18}F-FDG PET, *black arrow*; **b** CT, *white arrow*; **c** fusion PET/CT, *white arrow*)

sarcomas. High grade sarcomas show more intense ^{18}F-FDG uptake, while low grade sarcomas the opposite, leading sometimes to false negative result (Fig. 11.2). Nevertheless, in clinical practice, the noninvasive assessment of the sites with the highest grade of malignancy is very important for the guidance of biopsy.

A semi-quantitative method which is used to determine the ^{18}F-FDG uptake by the primary tumor is the maximum standardized uptake value (SUV_{max}). SUV_{max} of the primary tumor seems to be a prognostic factor of survival and high SUV_{max} values indicate a poor prognosis. In a recent study of 74 patients with STS, Schwarzbach et al. divided the patients into three groups based on SUV_{max}, those with values <1.59, values >1.59 but <3.6 and ≥ 3.6, with 5-year survival rate 84, 45, and 38 %, respectively [1].

During staging procedure a total body assessment of the metastatic spread of the disease is also important, concerning either the lymph nodes metastases or the distant metastases (Figs. 11.3, 11.4). ^{18}F-FDG PET/CT has high accuracy for staging lymph node metastases and shows high sensitivity and specificity, although lymph node metastases are not very frequent. In a recent study by Fuglo et al. [2] which included 89 sarcoma patients, the ^{18}F-FDG PET/CT revealed a sensitivity of 100 %, a specificity of 90 %, and an accuracy of 91 % for the detection of lymph node metastases. Nevertheless, false negative results may occur if the cancer has low glucose metabolism, if the metastatic lymph nodes are small in size, or a focus may be missed if it is located adjacent to an area of high physiological or pathological ^{18}F-FDG uptake. On the other hand, false positive results may occur due to reactive/inflammatory lymph nodes, as increased glucose metabolism is not specific only to cancer cells but in activated leukocytes and macrophages as well. In situations such as following biopsy, tumor resection or during infection we may have a false positive ^{18}F-FDG uptake in lymph nodes. The tumor itself may also lead to reactive ^{18}F-FDG uptake in the regional lymph nodes due to inflammation. ^{18}F-FDG PET/CT may be used to guide sampling of sites of unexpected nodal metastases.

As for the distant metastases, ^{18}F-FDG PET/CT seems to be a very accurate method of staging (Fig. 11.5). In the study by Fuglo et al. [2], the ^{18}F-FDG PET/CT-detected distant

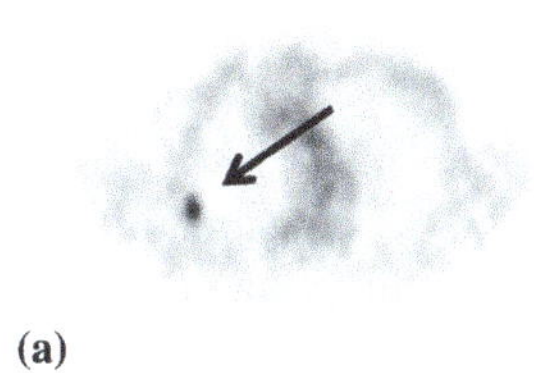

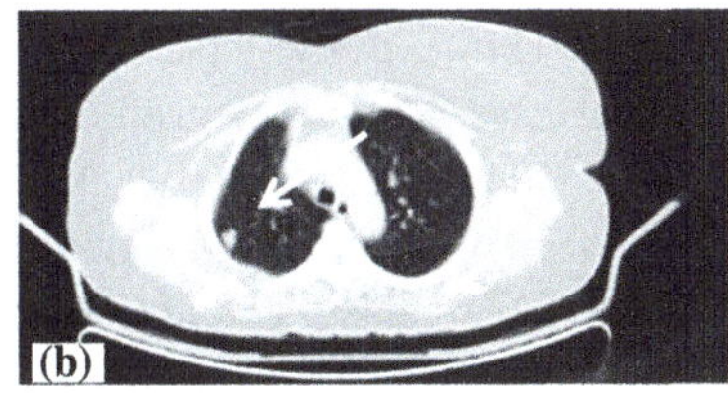

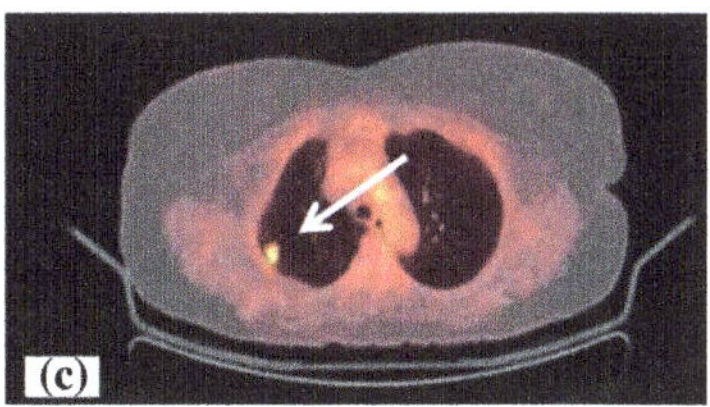

Fig. 11.3 **a–c** Female patient with history of resected uterine leiomyosarcoma. Right pulmonary nodule shows increased ^{18}F-FDG uptake on PET/CT consistent with metastasis (**a** ^{18}F-FDG PET, *black arrow*; **b** CT, *white arrow*; **c** fusion PET/CT, *white arrow*)

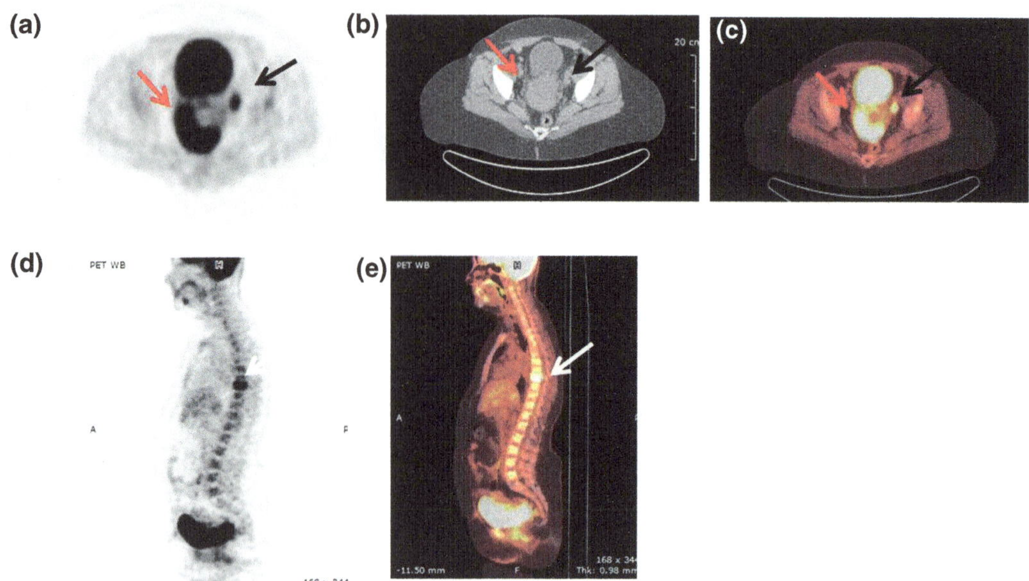

Fig. 11.4 **a–e** Female patient with uterine leiomyosarcoma. ^{18}F-FDG PET/CT performed at initial staging shows increased ^{18}F-FDG uptake at the primary mass (*red arrows*), at left iliac lymph node compatible with metastasis (*black arrows*) and at T8 vertebra compatible with metastasis. (Transverse views: **a** ^{18}F-FDG PET, **b** CT, **c** fusion PET/CT; Sagittal views: **d** ^{18}F-FDG PET, **e** fusion PET/CT)

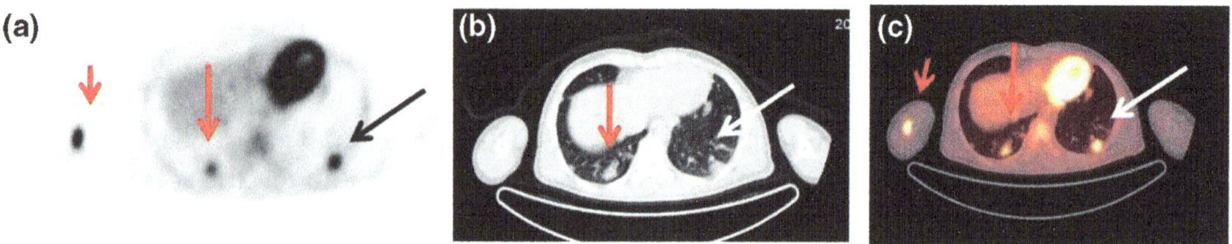

Fig. 11.5 **a–c** Male patient at initial staging of angiosarcoma of the left lung (*black and white arrows*). There is increased ^{18}F-FDG uptake at a right pulmonary nodule consistent with metastasis (*long red arrow*) and at the shaft of the right humerus consistent with bone metastasis (*short red arrow*) (**a** ^{18}F-FDG PET; **b** CT; **c** fusion PET/CT)

metastases with a sensitivity of 95 %, a specificity of 96 %, and an accuracy of 95 %. In this study, the positive predictive value was 87 %, which shows moderate to high ability of 18F-FDG PET/CT to diagnose distant metastases, with not too many false positive results. However, the negative predictive value was high (98 %), which means that ^{18}F-FDG PET/CT may exclude with confidence the presence of distant metastatic disease. In another study by Tateishi et al. [3], which included 117 patients with BS and STS combined PET/CT and CIM helped to avoid surgical resection in 13 % of patients and to alter management in additional 14 % of patients. In the same study the sensitivity, specificity, and accuracy of ^{18}F-FDG PET/CT were found to be 92, 91, and 91 %, respectively. Another advantage of ^{18}F-FDG PET/CT is that the whole body imaging may also reveal incidental findings, such as other malignancies.

In a study of Franzius et al. [4] ^{18}F-FDG PET was compared to bone scintigraphy in the detection of osseous metastases in 38 patients with Ewing sarcoma (ES). The sensitivity, specificity and accuracy of ^{18}F-FDG PET was 100, 96, and 97 %, respectively, on a patient-based analysis. The comparable values for bone scintigraphy were 68, 87, and 82 %. On a lesion-based analysis, the sensitivity of ^{18}F-FDG PET was 88 % and for bone scintigraphy was 69 %. The superiority of ^{18}F-FDG PET over bone scintigraphy for the detection of osseous metastases from ES may be explained by the fact that ^{18}F-FDG PET depicts the increased glucose metabolism of the metastases before bone scintigraphy shows increased osteoblastic activity. Also, ^{18}F-FDG PET has a better spatial resolution than bone scintigraphy. Small metastases adjacent to the growth plates in children, which are areas of normal radiotracer accumulation in a bone scintigraphy, might be missed giving a false negative result. The only exception where bone scintigraphy is superior to ^{18}F-FDG PET is the depiction of metastases to the skull because 18F-FDG normally accumulates in the adjacent cerebral cortex which uses glucose. Bone scintigraphy is more sensitive in that case than ^{18}F-FDG PET. In addition, ^{18}F-FDG PET may detect soft tissue metastases, while bone scintigraphy may not. As for pediatric sarcoma patients, Volker et al. [5] evaluated the impact of ^{18}F-FDG PET in 46 pediatric patients with ES, osteosarcoma and rhabdomyosarcoma at initial staging, compared to other CIM. Authors concluded that ^{18}F-FDG PET and CIM were equally effective in the detection of primary tumors, while ^{18}F-FDG PET was superior to CIM concerning the correct detection of lymph node involvement (sensitivity 95 % vs. 25 %, respectively) and bone manifestations (sensitivity 90 % vs. 57 %, respectively). However, CT was more reliable than ^{18}F-FDG PET in depicting lung metastases (sensitivity 100 % vs. 25 %, respectively).

Local recurrence occurs in approximately 10–15 % of patients with STS, while distant recurrence develops in 35–45 % of patients, even when treated suitably. Surgical resection usually disturbs the normal anatomy of the area and as a result, local recurrence is difficult to be detected (Figs. 11.6, 11.7). In addition,

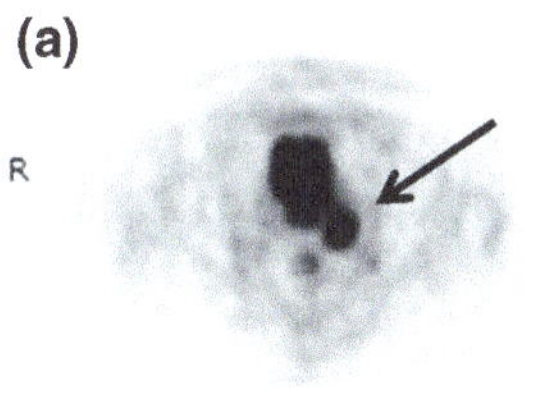

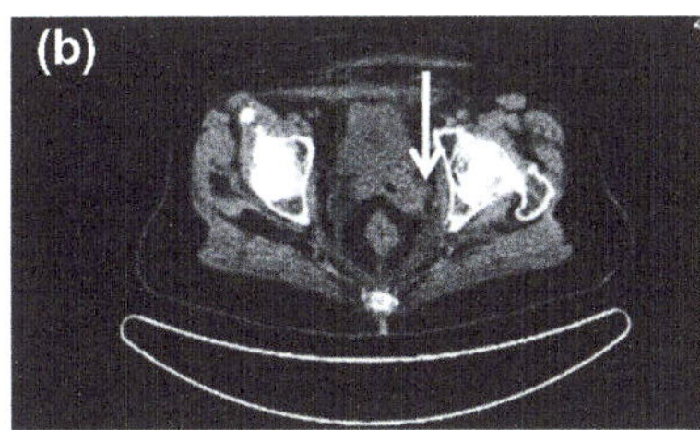

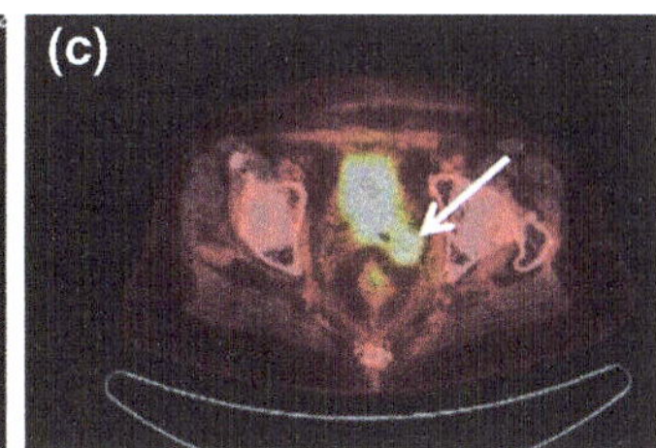

Fig. 11.6 **a–c** Female patient with history of resected uterine leiomyosarcoma. ^{18}F-FDG PET/CT during restaging shows increased ^{18}F-FDG uptake in anatomical position of the uterus, consistent with local recurrence (**a** ^{18}F-FDG PET, *black arrow*; **b** CT, *white arrow*; **c** fusion PET/CT, *white arrow*)

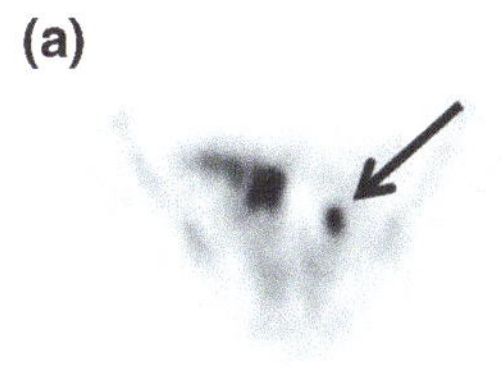

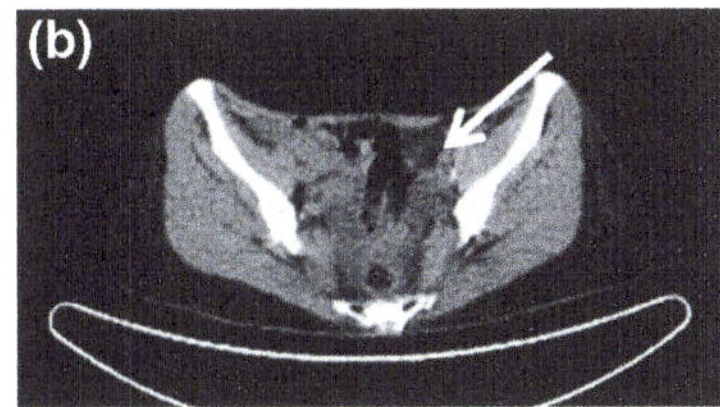

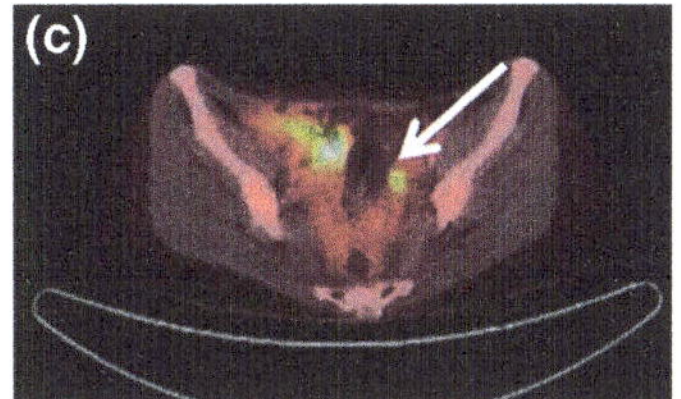

Fig. 11.7 **a–c** Female patient with history of resected uterine leiomyosarcoma. ^{18}F-FDG PET/CT during restaging shows increased ^{18}F-FDG uptake in a left iliac lymph nodes compatible with recurrence (**a** ^{18}F-FDG PET, *black arrow*; **b** CT, *white arrow*; **c** fusion PET/CT, *white arrow*)

radiotherapy may disturb the anatomy of the area, leading to difficulties in detecting local recurrence and ^{18}F-FDG PET/CT may be false positive due to post radiation inflammatory changes. On the other hand, CIM are most prone to errors and CT and MRI, although they are more suitable techniques for visualization of anatomy, usually they cannot differentiate a scar from local recurrence. ^{18}F-FDG PET/CT depicts the increased metabolism associated with abnormal tissues enabling visualization of recurrences. Nevertheless, the study should be performed at least 4–6 months after radiation therapy and the results should be interpreted with caution.

Distant recurrence usually occurs in the lungs. In a study by Franzius et al. [6], ^{18}F-FDG PET was compared to spiral thoracic CT for the detection of pulmonary metastases in 39 patients with ES. There was no patient with a true positive ^{18}F-FDG PET and a false negative CT, and no pulmonary metastasis was detected earlier with ^{18}F-FDG PET than with spiral CT, giving a clear superiority to CT for detecting pulmonary metastases in ES patients. On an examination-based analysis, ^{18}F-FDG PET had a sensitivity of 56 %, a specificity of 91 %, and an accuracy of 82 %, while the same values for CT were 88, 100, and 97 %, respectively. In conclusion, a ^{18}F-FDG PET should not be recommended to exclude lung metastases when the lung CT is negative. However, a positive ^{18}F-FDG PET result can be used to confirm lesions seen on CT as metastatic disease because of its high specificity.

11.3 Positron Emission Tomography in Gastrointestinal Stromal Tumors

As for the monitoring of treatment, ^{18}F-FDG PET/CT seems to have the most important role in GIST therapy [7]. GIST have a common molecular pathogenesis with activating mutations in the gene encoding Kit (a tyrosine kinase and stem cell factor receptor). For that reason, treatment of GIST is currently regarded as the paradigm of molecular-targeted therapy in solid tumors, and targeted therapies by means of the tyrosine kinase inhibitor imatinib mesylate and other similar drugs have been introduced in clinical practice. Conventional cytotoxic chemotherapy and radiotherapy are not effective in this kind of tumors [7].

Most GIST show increased metabolic activity in ^{18}F-FDG PET/CT at initial diagnosis and decreased ^{18}F-FDG uptake during treatment, which is related to a positive treatment result. Treatment with c-Kit inhibitors causes some changes in the tumor structure, such as decreased vascularity, hemorrhage, necrosis, cystic or myxoid degeneration, which may not alter the tumor volume. For that reason the morphologic criteria only, meaning the tumor size, as it is depicted by CT imaging, is not the optimal way to assess treatment response of GIST to drugs, usually underestimating the treatment result. The metabolism of the tumor cell is reflected by the decrease of ^{18}F-FDG uptake, which usually precedes changes in tumor size. There are many studies showing that ^{18}F-FDG PET/CT may identify GIST patient responders to imatinib or other drugs, earlier than CT, while in others ^{18}F-FDG PET/CT is considered as the gold standard technique for the assessment of treatment response in patients with GIST.

Holdsworth et al. [8], studied 63 patients with advanced GIST disease and compared CT bidimensional measurements and ^{18}F-FDG PET/CT SUV_{max} values to determine response to imatinib treatment. The authors concluded that after 1 month of treatment, the SUV_{max} cut off value of 3.4, the reduction of the SUV_{max} value of 40 % compared to the baseline PET and the absence of growth of the tumor are optimal criteria for treatment response.

Unfortunately, 14 % of GIST patients may show primary imatinib resistance, while 50 % of those who responded initially might develop secondary resistance. In these patients, the alteration of therapy with newer tyrosine kinase inhibitors is mandatory [7]. ^{18}F-FDG PET seems to be the most significant independent predictor of progression-free survival (PFS) predicting patient outcome. Demetri et al. [9] studied 97 patients with imatinib-resistant GIST and bulky metastatic disease who were treated with sunitinib. A baseline ^{18}F-FDG PET was performed initially and follow up ^{18}F-FDG PET scans were performed at several points during treatment. In the majority of patients, a partial metabolic response was evident on ^{18}F-FDG PET within 1 week of starting sunitinib. On the contrary, objective responses on CT took much longer to detect. In another study by Fuster et al. [10], 21 patients with locally advanced and/or metastatic GIST refractory to imatinib, treated with doxorubicin (four cycles), followed by imatinib maintenance, were evaluated with CT and ^{18}F-FDG PET at baseline and after completion of therapy. A correlation was found between PET response and PFS. A residual SUV_{max} <5 after treatment correlated with improved PFS while survival curves showed a significant association between PET response and PFS.

11.4 Conclusion

Conclusively, ^{18}F-FDG PET/CT is a useful imaging modality in management of bone and soft tissue tumors. At the initial staging, its role is primarily to indicate the site of biopsy and to detect metastatic disease. During restaging, the differentiation between viable tumor and necrosis is the most important advantage of ^{18}F-FDG PET/CT for the detection of local recurrence, but distant recurrence may be depicted as well. As for the monitoring of therapy, ^{18}F-FDG PET/CT seems to be an important tool to evaluate treatment efficacy primarily in GIST.

References

1. Schwarzbach MHM, Hinz U, Dimitrakopoulou-Strauss A et al (2005) Prognostic significance of preoperative (18-F)fluorodeoxyglucose (FDG) positron emission tomography (PET) imaging in patients with resectable soft tissue sarcomas. Ann Surg 241:286–294
2. Fuglø HM, Jørgensen SM, Loft A et al (2012) The diagnostic and prognostic value of 18F-FDG PET/CT in the initial assessment of high-grade bone and soft tissue sarcoma. A retrospective study of 89 patients. Eur J Nucl Med Mol Imag 39:1416–1424
3. Tateishi U, Yamaguchi U, Seki K et al (2007) Bone and soft-tissue sarcoma: preoperative staging with fluorine 18 fluorodeoxyglucose PET/CT and conventional imaging. Radiology 245(3), 839–847
4. Franzius C, Sciuk J, Daldrup-Link HE et al (2000) FDG-PET for detection of osseous metastases from malignant primary bone tumours: comparison with bone scintigraphy. Eur J Nucl Med 27:1305–1311
5. Völker T, Denecke T, Steffen I et al (2007) Positron emission tomography for staging of pediatric sarcoma patients: results of a prospective multicenter trial. J Clin Oncol 25:5435–5441
6. Franzius C, Daldrup-Link HE, Sciuk J et al (2001) FDG-PET for detection of pulmonary metastases from malignant primary bone tumors: comparison with spiral CT. Ann Oncol 12:479–486
7. Treglia G, Mirk P, Stefanelli A et al (2012) 18F-Fluorodeoxyglucose positron emission tomography in evaluating treatment response to imatinib or other drugs in gastrointestinal stromal tumors: a systematic review. Clin Imag 36:167–175
8. Holdsworth CH, Badawi RD, Manola JB et al (2007) CT and PET: early prognostic indicators of response to imatinib mesylate in patients with gastrointestinal stromal tumor. AJR Am J Roentgenol 189:W324–W330
9. Demetri GD, Heinrich MC, Fletcher JA et al (2009) Molecular target modulation, imaging, and clinical evaluation of gastrointestinal stromal tumor patients treated with sunitinib malate after imatinib failure. Clin Cancer Res 15:5902–5909
10. Fuster D, Ayuso JR, Poveda A et al (2011) Value of FDG-PET for monitoring treatment response in patients with advanced GIST refractory to high-dose imatinib. A multicenter GEIS study. Q J Nucl Med Mol Imag 55:680–687

Clinical Implications of Soft Tissue Sarcomas

12

Ioannis P. Boukovinas

12.1 Diagnosis

The therapeutic strategy depends on disease stage at baseline, tumor grade, and histological subtype. Plain X-rays, CT and MRI scans, angiography, and bone scans are the main diagnostic tools used in the diagnosis and staging of the disease [1]. Depending on tumor location, the preferred methods of diagnostic imaging are:

A. For soft tissue sarcomas (STSs) and bone sarcomas of the extremities and axial joints, MRI scans of the whole compartment with adjacent joints and plain X-rays in two planes
B. For STSs of the trunk, CT and MRI scans; for sarcomas of pelvic bones and surface lesions, MRI scans
C. For flat bone sarcomas, MRI scans and plain X-rays
D. For flat bone sarcomas, MRI scans and plain X-rays

CT of the thorax is usually sufficient for staging purposes, with the exception of some specific histological subtypes, for example, epithelioid sarcoma and clear cell sarcoma, for which regional assessment through CT/MRI is required. Furthermore, an abdominal CT scan should be added for limb myxoid liposarcoma; a brain CT scan is requested for alveolar soft part sarcoma, clear cell sarcoma, and angiosarcoma [2, 3].

It is important to stress the need to perform contrast-enhanced CT for the accurate correlation with neurovascular bundles and inter- and extra-compartmental structures. The exact location of preoperative biopsy can be guided by imaging quality thus avoiding sampling errors, especially in large tumors; additionally, image quality assists the pathologist in tumor identification in 25–40 % of the cases [4], as well as in determining tumor grade.

12.2 Response Assessment

Imaging methods also play a vital role in response assessment in sarcoma, both within the context of phase II/III clinical studies and in everyday clinical practice. Response evaluation criteria in solid tumors (RECIST) is a set of rules used primarily to assess response by CT or MRI. Its latest version (RECIST 1.1) has been adopted worldwide as the precisest, simplest, and most easily reproducible measurement; a series of clinical studies have demonstrated that RECIST 1.1 is linked to patient outcomes. It is based on tumor measurements performed in >6,500 patients [5]. Changes from previous version include:

- A reduction to 5 in the number of target lesions that must be measured, 2 by organ
- A requirement that an increase of at least 5 mm be documented as proof of progression

I. P. Boukovinas (✉)
Bioclinic Oncology Unit, 86, Mitropoleos street, 54622 Thessaloniki, Greece
e-mail: ibouk@otenet.gr

A. D. Gouliamos et al. (eds.), *Imaging in Clinical Oncology*,
DOI: 10.1007/978-88-470-5385-4_12, © Springer-Verlag Italia 2014

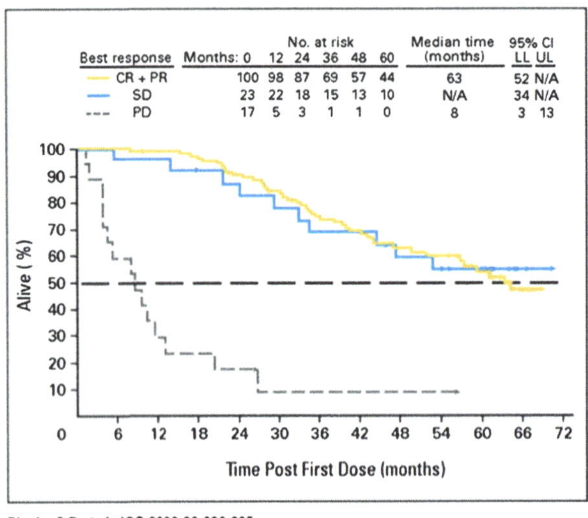

Fig. 12.1 Overall survival according to best response

- A definition for lymph node measurement including the point that the short axis is followed (distinguished from the long axis used for non-nodal masses)

However, a number of implementation issues have arisen with RECIST. For example, lymph nodes with a short axis of at least 15 mm are considered target lesions in clinical studies, but this does not apply in certain settings (e.g., in testicular cancer). Furthermore, there are patterns and locations that cannot be determined precisely, for example, diffuse peritoneal spread, lymphatic spread, and bone metastases. Additionally, results were based on measurements taken by CT that were reproducible with MRI, which makes for a stable assessment, but the latter technique is more difficult to standardize before and after treatment. Most importantly, in this era of targeted therapies, response assessment is based on anatomical change in unidimensional diameter or in the sum of multiple lesions. Today we know that new treatments can improve patient outcome without necessarily shrinking the tumor [6].

The start was made with response assessment in gastrointestinal stromal tumors (GIST), where initial efficacy studies of imatinib showed that patients with stable disease had similarly good outcomes to those who were identified as responders using RECIST criteria (see Fig. 12.1) [7].

RECIST criteria do not consider tumor density in Hounsfield units; response and the degenerative (necrotic) nature of the lesion may lead to initial tumor growth followed by subsequent tumor shrinkage, while RECIST criteria underestimate clinical benefit since response evaluation does not take into account stable disease. Similar difficulties in interpretation have confronted the researchers of the Children's Oncology Group during response assessment to tamoxifen in young patients with recurrent desmoid tumor. Some patients classified as progressive disease by the RECIST criteria on MRI were clinically stable or even improved; this was attributable to an increase in proportion of low signal intensities on T2 W image from including fibrous tissue [8].

GIST have became the paradigm in the development of new response criteria. Initially, Van den Abbeele et al. showed that patients who responded to imatinib by FDG-PET with a decreased standardized uptake value (SUV) to a value <2.5 had longer time to treatment failure (TTF) than those who did not, whereas those who responded by SWOG criteria had the same TTF as those without response [9]. Choi et al. devised new criteria for CT interpretation to discriminate between good and poor responders comparing them with response by FDG-PET, defined as a one-dimensional decrease in tumor size of 10 % or a decrease in tumor density by 15 %; all but one patient fulfilling the above criteria was correctly identified with responders by FDG-PET [10]. The investigators subsequently studied a separate group of patients using the above criteria and found that response was 83 % compared with 45 % by RECIST, that Choi responders had significantly longer time to progression (TTP) than non-responders, and that the RECIST criteria could not separate a group with a longer TTP. Additionally, the Choi responders had equivalent TTP as the RECIST responders, showing that the degree of tumor shrinkage is not directly related to the extent of cell kill. The reproducibility of the Choi criteria remains to be confirmed in prospective multicenter studies and formally adopted in assessing response in GIST.

FDG-PET can be used in GIST to statistically significantly correlate progression free survival (PFS) with early metabolic response. It has been shown that FDG-PET before and after 4 weeks of sunitinib therapy in metastatic GIST is a useful tool for early response to treatment and for the prediction of final outcome [11]. The same was seen with changes in FDG uptake during chemotherapy with imatinib [12, 13]. This finding can be applied especially to the preoperative use of imatinib to avoid major mutilating surgery in resectable GIST, in combination with mutation testing, thus avoiding ineffective treatments and individualizing treatment strategies.

A unique pattern of disease progression was seen in GIST during treatment with imatinib after an initial response, namely, a "nodule within a mass," that is, a nodule growing within a pre-existing tumor, which reflects the emergence of treatment-resistant clones. Such nodules were demonstrable a median of 5 months before documented progression defined by size criteria and should be regarded, at least, as progression. Isolated nodules should be managed with local treatments (radio frequency ablation, embolization, and surgery)[14].

Furthermore, other functional imaging methods could be helpful in assessing response to targeted therapy at an early time point, once again within the setting of GIST. These methods are based on reduced tumor vascularity, impaired microvascular permeability, reduced tissue oxygenation, and the presence of necrosis without change in size. They include contrast-enhanced sonography and dynamic contrast-enhanced magnetic resonance imaging (DCE-MRI). The use of the former method was confirmed in the follow-up of patients with metastatic GIST every 3 months for 3 years showing, in a statistically significant way, that the decrease in tumor contrast uptake at day 7 of treatment with imatinib could predict tumor response, distinguishing good responders from poor responders [15]. Interestingly, contrast-enhanced sonography can be an early predictor of the emergence of resistant tumors, both primary and secondary. The emergence of secondary resistance is seen as revascularization of necrotic areas, redefining therapeutic strategies before the increase in tumor size.

One of the biggest problems with preoperative administration of chemotherapy in STSs and bone sarcomas–and also with isolated limp perfusion and preoperative radiation therapy–is response assessment. In most cases, no difference is seen in imaging after chemotherapy. Thus, an almost complete pathological response cannot be predicted by RECIST criteria.

DCE-MRI can be helpful in such cases, as was shown with response assessment in preoperative administration of chemotherapy in patients with osteosarcoma and Ewing sarcoma [16]. Patients were divided into two groups: those who manifested tumor necrosis exceeding 90 % and those with less than 90 % necrosis. This variable has been found to correlate with clinical outcome. Diffusion scans performed before and during treatment to assess response revealed that changes in mean apparent diffusion coefficient (ADC) are inversely correlated with changes in cellularity after chemotherapy: mean ADC increase was 25 % in poor responders versus 95 % in good responders ($P < 0.003$). Both groups showed no change with traditional imaging methods.

One method that is gaining ground in the assessment of response to preoperative chemotherapy for STSs is 18F-FDG-PET. A necrosis rate of over 90–95 % was initially considered to be a predictor of outcome after preoperative chemotherapy, similarly as in the case of osteosarcoma [17]. However, there are no international consensus guidelines [18, 19]. It has been found that 18F-FDG-PET before, after the initial cycle and after completion of treatment is an important predictor of both response [20–23] and survival. In the study by Herrmann et al. [24], early metabolic response and surgical excision margins were the only predictors of survival. Thus, its use could limit unnecessary treatments and switch from chemotherapy to direct surgery; this risk-adapted therapy could reduce both morbidity and cost. Larger prospective studies should be conducted to verify the 18F-FDG-PET response threshold, which has so far been set arbitrarily in studies.

A peculiar pattern of response has been reported in STS (specifically, in myxoid liposarcoma) with the use of trabectedin. A multicenter retrospective study [25] showed that changes in tumor density on CT scan or in contrast enhancement on MRI (or both) preceded tumor shrinkage. Since trabectedin lacks cumulative toxicity and given that the mean response time is 5 months, treatment should not be discontinued prematurely due to the erroneous understanding that the drug is not active.

A similar pattern of response was seen in chordoma with treatment with imatinib [26].

Intra- and inter-subtype heterogeneity of sarcomas requires new approaches in characterization and treatment. Parallel correlative radiological studies will specify their role in response assessment, both with traditional cytotoxic therapies and with molecular targeted therapies.

12.3 Follow-Up

There are no reliable data to help set the frequency of follow-up for patients with STSs or bone sarcomas. In general, the frequency of follow-up is defined by the risk category for relapse. In general, high-risk patients relapse within the first 2–3 years, while low-risk patients may relapse later. Most relapses are either local or occur in the lungs; their early detection (before they become symptomatic) is important, so that can be treated surgically. MRI is mostly used to detect local relapses while CT is used to detect pulmonary metastases, but this has not been confirmed in randomized, prospective studies. The risk of radiation exposure should also be taken into account in young individuals.

For sarcomas, especially of the extremities, interpreting post-treatment MRI requires experience and often a combination of other methods to positively rule out local relapse. Thus, Vanel et al. [27] found that the presence of low signal intensity on T2-weighted sequences had 96 % sensitivity for exclusion of recurrent or residual tumor. On the other hand, the presence of high signal intensity on T2-weighted sequence is not necessarily indicative of relapse. More specifically, after radiation therapy it may be related with the presence of seroma, hematoma, or post-irradiation inflammation, which may be imaged up to 4 years post-treatment. It is also important to identify marrow changes resulting from radiation therapy or treatment with marrow-stimulating drugs [28].

The generally acceptable follow-up protocol for patients with resected sarcoma at intermediate and high risk for relapse consists of examination every 3 months in the first year, every 4 months in the second year, and 6 months thereafter, by CT of the thorax and local MRI. Low-risk patients could be followed up every 4–6 months for the first 5 years, alternating between X-ray and CT of the thorax, and annually thereafter.

References

1. Panicek DM, Gatsonis C, Rosenthal DI et al (1997) CT and MR imaging in the local staging of primary malignant musculoskeletal neoplasms: Report of the Radiology Diagnostic Oncology Group. Radiology 202:237–246

2. Soft tissue and visceral sarcomas: ESMO Clinical Practice Guidelines for diagnosis, treatment and follow-up (2012). The ESMO/European Sarcoma Network Working Group. Annals of Oncology 23 (Supplement 7): vii92–vii99
3. Bone sarcomas: ESMO Clinical Practice Guidelines for diagnosis, treatment and follow-up (2012). The ESMO/European Sarcoma Network Working Group. Annals of Oncology 23 (Supplement 7): vii100–vii109
4. Crim JR, Seeger LL, Yao L et al (1992) Diagnosis of soft tissue masses with MR imaging: can benign masses be differentiated from malignant ones. Radiology 185:581–586
5. Eisenhauer EA, Therasse P, Bogaerts J et al (2009) New response evaluation criteria in solid tumors: Revised RECIST guideline (version 1.1). Eur J Cancer 45:228–247
6. Michaelis LC, Ratain MJ (2006) Measuring response in a post-RECIST world: from black and white to shades of grey. Nat Rev Cancer 6:409–414
7. Blanke C, Demetri G, von Mehren M et al (2008) Long-Term Results From a Randomized Phase II Trial of Standard- Versus Higher-Dose Imatinib Mesylate for Patients With Unresectable or Metastatic Gastrointestinal Stromal Tumors Expressing KIT. J Clin Oncol 26(4):620–625
8. Dhani N, Tu D, Sargent DJ, Seymour L, et al (2009) Alternate endpoints for screening phase II studies. Clin Cancer Res 15:1873–1882
9. Van den Abbeele AD, Badawi RD (2002) Use of positron emission tomography in oncology and its potential role to assess response to imatinib mesylate therapy in gastrointestinal stromal tumors (GIST). Eur J Cancer 38:S60–S65
10. Choi H, Charnsangavej C, Faria SC et al (2007) Correlation of computed tomography and positron emission tomography in patients with metastatic gastrointestinal stromal tumor treated at a single institution with imatinib mesylate: proposal of new computed tomography response criteria. J Clin Oncol 25:1753–1759
11. Prior J, Montemurro M, Orcurto MV et al (2008) Early Prediction of Response to Sunitinib After Imatinib Failure by 18F-Fluorodeoxyglucose Positron Emission Tomography in Patients With Gastrointestinal Stromal Tumor. J Clin Oncol 27:439–445
12. Stroobants S, Goeminne J, Seegers M et al (2003) 18FDG-Positron emission tomography for the early prediction of response in advanced soft tissue sarcoma treated with imatinib mesylate (Glivec). Eur J Cancer 39:2012–2020
13. Gayed I, Vu T, Iyer R et al (2004) The role of 18F-FDG PET in staging and early prediction of response to therapy of recurrent gastrointestinal stromal tumors. J Nucl Med 45:17–21
14. Desai J, Shankar S, Heinrich MC et al (2007) Clonal evolution of resistance to imatinib in patients with metastatic gastrointestinal stromal tumors. Clin Cancer Res 13:5398–5405
15. Lassau N, Lamuraglia M, Chami L et al (2006) Gastro-intestinal stromal tumours treated with imatinib: monitoring response with contrast enhanced ultrasound. Am J Roentgenol 187:1267–1273
16. Hayashida Y, Yakushiji T, Awai K et al (2006) Monitoring therapeutic responses of primary bone tumors by diffusion-weighted image: Initial results. Eur Radiol 16:2637–2643
17. Eilber F, Rosen G, Eckardt J et al (2001) Treatment-Induced Pathologic Necrosis: A Predictor of Local Recurrence and Survival in Patients Receiving Neoadjuvant Therapy for High-Grade Extremity Soft Tissue Sarcomas. J Clin Oncol 19:3203–3209
18. Collin C, Godbold J, Hajdu S et al (1987) Localized extremity soft tissue sarcoma: an analysis of factors affecting survival. J Clin Oncol 5:601–612
19. Gaynor JJ, Tan CC, Casper ES et al (1992) Refinement of clinicopathologic staging for localized soft tissue sarcoma of the extremity: a study of 423 adults. J Clin Oncol 10:1317–1329
20. Evilevitch V, Weber WA, Tap WD et al (2008) Reduction of glucose metabolic activity is more accurate than change in size at predicting histopathologic response to neoadjuvant therapy in high-grade soft-tissue sarcomas. Clin Cancer Res 14:715–720
21. Benz MR, Czernin J, Allen-Auerbach MS et al (2009) FDG-PET/CT imaging predicts histopathologic treatment responses after the initial cycle of neoadjuvant chemotherapy in high-grade soft-tissue sarcomas. Clin Cancer Res 15:2856–2863
22. Dimitrakopoulou-Strauss A, Strauss LG, Egerer G et al (2010) Impact of dynamic 18F-FDG PET on the early prediction of therapy outcome in patients with high-risk soft-tissue sarcomas after neoadjuvant chemotherapy: a feasibility study. J Nucl Med 51:551–558
23. Tateishi U, Kawai A, Chuman H, et al (2011) PET/CT allows stratification of responders to neoadjuvant chemotherapy for high-grade sarcoma: a prospective study. Clin Nucl Med 36:526–532
24. Herrmann K, Benz M, Czernin J et al (2012) 18-FDG-PET/CT Imaging as an Early Survival Predictor in Patients with Primary High-Grade Soft Tissue Sarcomas Undergoing Neoadjuvant Therapy. Clin Cancer Res 18:2024–2031
25. Grosso F, Jones R, Demetri G et al (2007) Efficacy of trabectedin (ecteinascidin-743) in advanced pretreated myxoid liposarcomas: a retrospective study. Lancet Oncol 8:595–602

26. Casali PG, Messina A, Stacchiotti S et al (2004) Imatinib mesylate in chordoma. Cancer 101:2086–2097
27. Vanel D, Shapeero LG, De Baere T et al (1994) MR imaging in the follow up of malignant and aggressive soft tissue tumors: results of 511 examinations. Radiology 190:263–268
28. Panicek D, Schwartz L (1999) MR imaging of bone marrow in patients with musculoskeletal tumors. Sarcoma 3:37–41

13 Clinical Implications of Bone Sarcomas

Ioannis D. Papanastassiou and Nikolaos S. Demertzis

13.1 Diagnosis

First study should be a plain X-ray of the affected area, followed by CT or MRI. Pulmonary lesions are detected with CT, whereas skeletal foci are detected with bone scan. It is possible that we are currently not staging patients optimally and some metastatic lesions are being misdiagnosed and perhaps other modalities such as total body MRI should be employed. ^{18}F-FDG PET/CT is a useful imaging modality for diagnosis and staging especially in high grade tumors. It is also more sensitive to bone scanning in Ewing sarcomas of the bones. PET is also necessary to distinguish viable residual tumor from necrosis following treatment [1].

13.2 Staging

For bone sarcomas, the most widely used classification systems are the Musculoskeletal Tumor Society system developed by Enneking in the 1980s and the American Joint Cancer Committee (AJCC) system. They have different scope, since AJCC is related to prognosis and includes some parameters (i.e., size) not encountered in Enneking's classification, which on the other hand is related to the surgical approach.

13.3 Surveillance

According to NCCN guidelines, patients should be monitored every 3 months for the first 2 years, every 4 months in the 3rd year, every 6 months for years 4 and 5 and on an annual basis thereafter. Clinical exam, chest imaging (X-ray or CT) and imaging of the primary site (X-ray, MRI or CT), as well as skeleton screening (bone scan or PET) may be performed in regular intervals. Especially for CS, late recurrences (even after 10 years) are more common, so patients should be advised and followed-up accordingly.

Reference

1. Bastiannet E, Groen H, Jager PL, et al (2004) The value of PET/CT scan in the detection grading and response to therapy of soft tissue and bone sarcomas: a systematic review and meta-analysis. Cancer Met Rev 30:83–101

I. D. Papanastassiou (✉) · N. S. Demertzis
General Oncological Hospital Kifisias,
Agioi Anargyroi, Athens, Greece
e-mail: ioannis.papanastassiou@gmail.com

A. D. Gouliamos et al. (eds.), *Imaging in Clinical Oncology*,
DOI: 10.1007/978-88-470-5385-4_13, © Springer-Verlag Italia 2014

14 Clinical Implications of Retroperitoneal Sarcomas

Dionysis C. Voros and Theodosios C. Theodosopoulos

14.1 Diagnosis and Evaluation

RPS account for approximately one-third of all retroperitoneal masses. Differential diagnosis, including lymphoma, testicular neoplasm, germ cell tumor, desmoids, functioning and nonfunctioning adrenal masses, renal tumor, pancreatic tumor, and gastrointestinal stromal tumor, should be considered. If visceral invasion is present, the differential should include tumors of these organs and endoscopy with biopsy, if feasible, to evaluate for intraluminal evidence of involvement (e.g., stomach, duodenum, pancreas, colon), should be performed.

History and physical examination should be focused to narrow the differential diagnosis. Testicular examination for masses or/and testicular ultrasound should be considered.

The initial diagnostic evaluation of patients who are suspected of having RPS should include a contrast enhanced CT of the abdomen and pelvis to evaluate the size and extent of the lesion. MRI of the abdomen has been evaluated as a method of staging and may provide an alternative modality to assess local disease extent.

D. C. Voros (✉) · T. C. Theodosopoulos
Second Department of Surgery, Aretaieion Hospital, Athens Medical School, Athens University, Vas Sofias 76, 11528, Athens, Greece
e-mail: diovoros@med.uoa.gr

T. C. Theodosopoulos
e-mail: ttheodosopoulos@yahoo.gr

Voros et al. (1998) [1] published that in some cases, satellite tumours have been identified in the surrounding sarcoma's fat, which may be quite far from the initial tumour and these may be responsible for local recurrence. Some of these are being seen in the preoperative CT scan and some are being revealed at the pathology report. These satellite tumours are small sarcomatous tumours in the surrounding of the main tumour fat, that could be even some centimetres away from it, and who if they remain could be responsible for local recurrence and so we must always search for them either preoperatively or intraoperatively. The MD Anderson study (2009) [2] defines the multifocality in STS as having more than one noncontiguous tumor and that has been considered a feature of more aggressive disease with worse outcome. They also found that a higher number of tumors (>7), is associated with worse overall survival. In one of our cases, a 64-year-old male presented with four different foci at the time of diagnosis. He complained of non typical mild discomfort and swelling of the left inguinal area. He underwent a CT scan which revealed: (a) left iliac fossa mass 11 × 10, 5 × 9 cm, (b) left inguinal mass 6 × 5, 5 × 2, 5 cm, (c) right iliac fossa mass 4.3 cm, and (d) during the operative exploration a big satellite mass was found (Fig. 14.1).

The performance of biopsy for RPS in the preoperative setting is controversial. Percutaneous biopsy is proposed to perform only when the diagnosis may change the preoperative therapy, such as using neoadjuvant for gastrointestinal

A. D. Gouliamos et al. (eds.), *Imaging in Clinical Oncology*,
DOI: 10.1007/978-88-470-5385-4_14, © Springer-Verlag Italia 2014

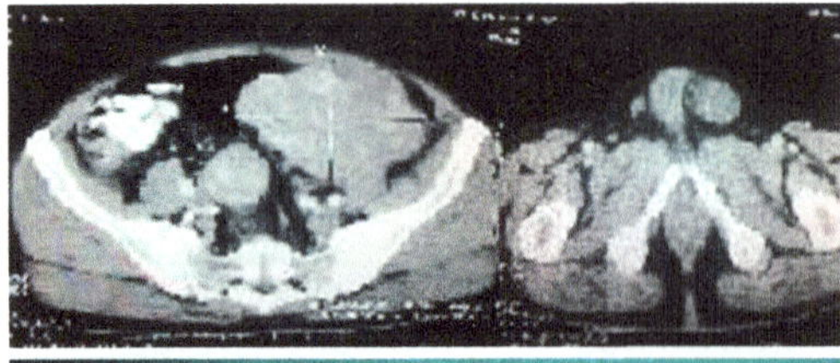

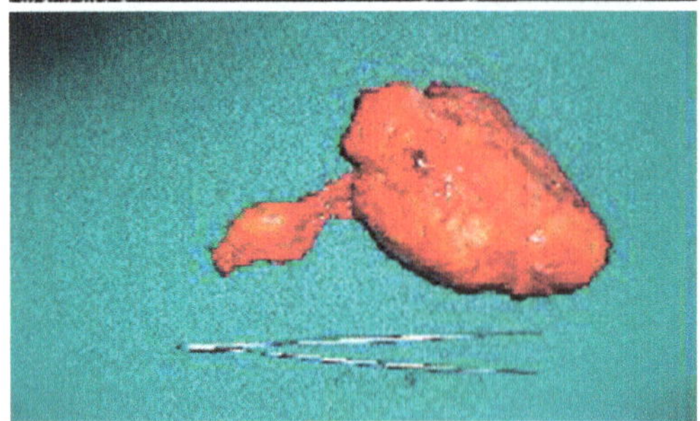

Fig. 14.1 Preoperative imaging and a postoperative specimen of a multifocal disease

stromal tumors or primary chemotherapy for lymphoma. If distant metastases are present and surgical therapy is not being considered for primary management, a biopsy of the primary tumor or a metastatic site may be required for alternative therapy to be administered. In the situation of an incidental finding of a RPS during abdominal surgery, a biopsy should be performed before resection to avoid a potentially morbid and unnecessary resection of a chemotherapy sensitive tumor. CT of the chest is typically performed to evaluate for the presence of lung metastases.

14.2 Management

Disease control for RPS is inferior to those obtained for sarcomas at other locations for a variety of reasons, including the difficulty to obtain wide negative surgical margins, higher rates of unresectability, higher rates of margin-positive resection, and difficulty in delivering adjuvant therapies (e.g., radiotherapy).

Patients who present with a RPS should ideally be evaluated by members of a multidisciplinary sarcoma team and managed at high-volume centers.

14.3 Surgical Therapy

The goal of therapy for most patients is surgical resection with negative margins. The possibility of a margin negative surgical resection depends on several factors, including invasion of adjacent visceral organs, vascular structures, and skeletal structures. Other operative findings that may impair the outcome of the surgical approach include the presence of peritoneal metastases or the presence of distant metastatic disease.

Complete resection rates vary by series but typically range from 54 to 88 %. Disease control outcomes are relatively close to the completeness of resection in surgical series, with inferior outcomes noted after incomplete resection or margin-positive resection [3].

The surgical approach is important to increase the chance of a margin-negative resection and may differ depending on the location and extent of the tumor. In general, a midline incision followed by medial visceral rotation is performed to provide adequate exposure of the tumor bed and surrounding structures. Ideally, dissection then proceeds outside the limits of the pseudocapsule in an effort to increase the likelihood of obtaining a margin-negative resection, although this may frequently require resection of surrounding vasculature or visceral organs. Other incisions that might help the exploration is the thoracoabdominal and abdominoinguinal incision [3] (Fig. 14.2).

Rates of resection of visceral organs at the time of resection of RPS vary significantly by series from approximately 34–75 %. Because disease control outcomes depend significantly

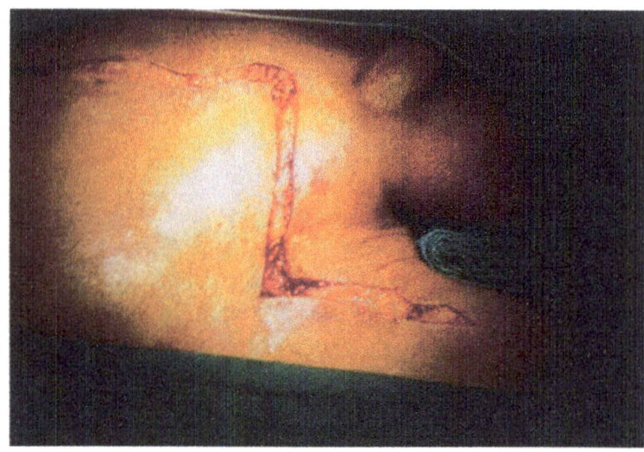

Fig. 14.2 Abdominoinguinal incision

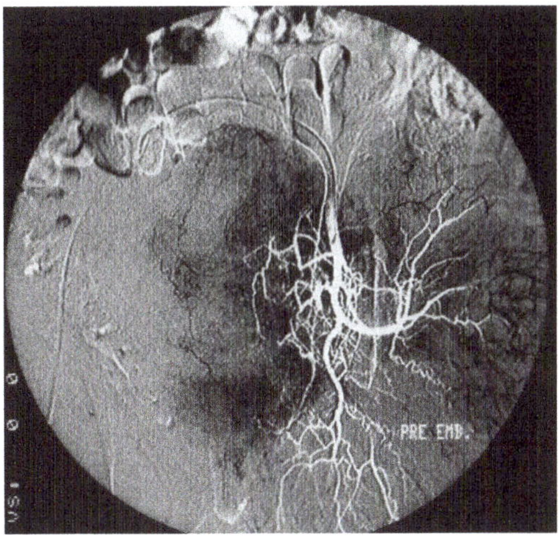

Fig. 14.3 Ischemic embolization of a retroperitoneal tumor

on the adequacy of resection, this approach has also been extended to the setting of vascular involvement highlighting the importance of an aggressive surgical approach. Resection of the tumor and vasculature includes ligation, vessel repair, reimplantation, or bypass grafting in these patients. Morbidity of 36 % and operative mortality of 4 %, compares favorably with other surgical series. Completeness of resection is 60 % and margin-negative resection accomplished in 40 % of patients.

In one pelvic schwannoma of our series, difficult to resect at the initial laparotomy, we performed ischemic embolization and the tumor was completely removed after 1 week (Fig. 14.3). To our knowledge, there are no series in the literature, of ischemic embolization prior to resection for RPS. In the same case, a filter in the IVC was inserted preoperatively to minimize the possibility of pulmonary embolism as the patient already presented with deep vein thrombosis [4] (Fig. 14.4).

14.4 Multimodality Therapy

Because of the high rates of local recurrence after surgical resection of retroperitoneal sarcomas, especially with high-grade tumors or with margin-positive resection, the addition of radiotherapy has been evaluated to improve local control. Unlike extremity sarcomas, radiotherapy dose is often limited by the anatomic constraints of the abdominal compartment, primarily because of the proximity of several radiosensitive structures to the tumor bed, such as bowel, kidney, and neural structures as well as the extended area to be radiated.

In general, radiotherapy may be delivered before surgery, during surgery, or after surgery with a variety of techniques. These techniques include standard external beam radiation delivered before or after surgery, which typically targets the tumor or tumor bed with additional margin for suspected microscopic disease. In addition, such techniques as brachytherapy and intraoperative radiotherapy can be performed in conjunction with surgical resection and may be delivered in combination with external beam radiotherapy as a method to escalate radiation dose locally.

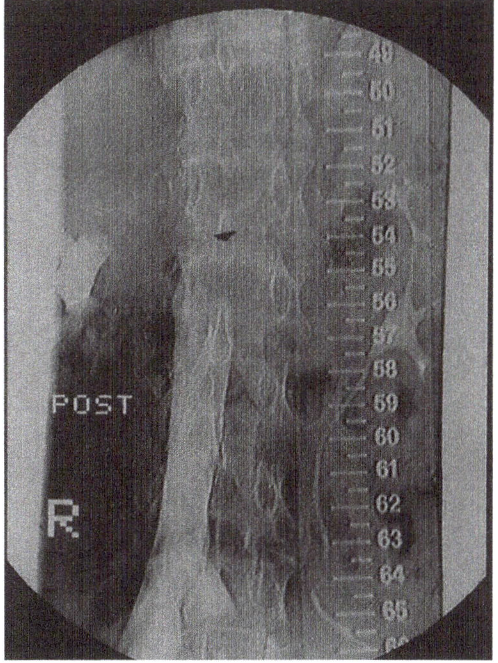

Fig. 14.4 Filter in IVC preoperatively to minimize the possibility of pulmonary embolism

In most centers, radiotherapy is often reserved for patients who have high-grade lesions or in patients in whom a margin-positive resection is anticipated.

The goal of therapy is to allow a margin-negative resection, which would result in better local control and improved survival. Typically, if external radiotherapy is planned, a preoperative approach is preferred in order to decrease the risk for toxicity, to minimize the additional normal tissue that must be irradiated, and to improve the likelihood of a margin-negative resection.

In regard to chemotherapy, there is similar uncertainty regarding the benefit of chemotherapy delivered in the neoadjuvant setting with the intent of improving resectability and the use should be advocated only in the setting of a clinical trial.

The use of adjuvant chemotherapy in the management of sarcomas at any site to reduce the risk for distant disease failure is also controversial. Several prospective trials evaluating adjuvant chemotherapy in patients who have sarcomas have been completed but have not shown consistent evidence of disease-free survival or overall survival benefit. A final option for multimodality treatment of retroperitoneal sarcomas is the combination of radiation and chemotherapy but the efficacy of this approach has not been reported.

14.5 Recurrent Disease

Local recurrence is common for retroperitoneal sarcomas, a situation that presents therapeutic challenges. For lesions that are resectable, surgery remains the preferred treatment modality at the time of local recurrence. The likelihood of obtaining a margin-negative resection is significantly lower at the time of local recurrence and at subsequent recurrences. In general, primary resections result in complete resections in as many as 80 % of patients, whereas complete resection of recurrent disease occurs in 57 % of patients, with lower rates at subsequent recurrences [5].

As in the primary disease setting, complete resection of recurrent disease is associated with improved survival, and this should be the intended goal if surgical therapy is chosen.

If adjuvant therapy was not delivered at the time of the initial resection, this remains an option in the recurrent disease setting. Similar to the primary disease setting, options for additional therapy include neoadjuvant or adjuvant radiotherapy and chemotherapy. In the setting of unresectable local recurrence, palliative radiotherapy or chemotherapy may also be considered to relieve local symptoms or to gain other benefits.

14.6 Follow-Up

In general, patients who have high-grade tumors should undergo frequent clinical and imaging surveillance to be evaluated for recurrent disease.

Surveillance imaging should include CT of the chest, abdomen, and pelvis at intervals of every 3–6 months for the first 2 years for low- and highgrade lesions, followed by biannual evaluations in patients who have high-grade tumors and annual evaluations in patients who have low-grade tumors [6].

References

1. Voros D, Theodorou D, Ventouri K (1998) Retroperitoneal Tumors: Do the satellite tumors mean something? J Surg Oncol 68:30–33
2. Anaya D, Lahat G, Liu J (2009) Multifocality in retroperitoneal sarcoma. Aprognostic factor critical to surgical decision-making. Ann Surg 249:137–142
3. Karakousis C (2010) Refinements of surgical technique in soft tissue sarcomas. J Surg Oncol 101:730–738
4. Theodosopoulos T, Psychogiou V, Yiallourou A (2012) Management of retroperitoneal sarcomas: main prognostic factors for local recurrence and survival. J BUON 17:138–142
5. Gholami S, Jacobs CD, Kapp DS (2009) The value of surgery for retroperitoneal sarcoma. Sarcoma 605840. Epub 8
6. Sogaard AS, Laurberg JM, Sorensen M (2010) Intra-abdominal and retroperitoneal soft-tissue sarcomas–outcome of surgical treatment in primary and recurrent tumors. World J Surg Oncol. 12(8):81

Part III
CNS Tumors

15 Introduction to Brain Tumors

Panagiotis V. Nomikos and Ioannis S. Antoniadis

15.1 Epidemiology

In most cancer registries, brain tumors rank second only to leukemia in incidence for children 0–14 years old with an annual incidence of 3.3–4.8 cases per 100,000 children. More than 23 % of incident childhood cancer arise in the brain and more than 26 % of childhood cancer deaths are attributed to brain cancer. Brain cancer accounts for approximately 1 % of all adult cancers, with an annual age-adjusted incidence of 7.2–9.2 cases per 100,000 adults. More than 2 % of all adult cancer deaths are contributed to brain cancer [1]. Taking into consideration all primary brain and nervous system tumors in adults, the US incidence rate is estimated to be 24.6 per 100,000 persons with approximately one-third of tumors being malignant and the remainder being benign or borderline malignant [2]. The most common intracranial tumor is brain metastasis. They are 10 times more frequent than primary brain tumors and their incidence is increasing during the past decades. More than 75 % of the primary brain tumors are gliomas and meningiomas.

P. V. Nomikos (✉) · I. S. Antoniadis
Department of Neurosurgery and Gamma Knife Radiosurgery, Hygeia Hospital, Erythrou Stavrou 4, 15123 Marousi, Greece
e-mail: pnomikos@hygeia.gr

I. S. Antoniadis
e-mail: iantoniadis@hygeia.gr

15.2 Classification of Primary Brain Tumors

The classification is based on the World Health Organization (WHO) classification of CNS tumors as published in 1979 (Zuelch), followed by revisions in 1993, 2000, and 2007 [3]. Based on morphologic and immunohistochemical features, each tumor entity is classified according to its presumed cell of origin. However, the WHO classification additionally incorporates molecular genetics and immunologic markers in an attempt to construct a cellular classification that is universally applicable and prognostically valid. Based on histological features a grading scheme ranging from WHO grade I (benign) to WHO grade IV (malignant) is established. WHO grade I includes lesions with minimal proliferative potential and the possibility of cure following surgical resection alone. Pilocytic astrocytomas, subependyomas, schwannomas, and most meningiomas are typical examples of WHO grade I tumors. WHO grade II tumors still demonstrate low mitotic activity but also a tendency for recurrence. Diffuse astrocytomas, oligoastrocytomas and ependymomas are classic examples. WHO grade III includes lesions with histologic evidence of malignancy, including nuclear atypia, cellular anaplasia and increased mitotic activity. These lesions have anaplastic histology and infiltrative capacity. Anaplastic astrocytomas and anaplastic ependymomas are typical examples of WHO grade III tumors. The WHO grade IV is reserved for mitotically active, necrosis-

A. D. Gouliamos et al. (eds.), *Imaging in Clinical Oncology*,
DOI: 10.1007/978-88-470-5385-4_15, © Springer-Verlag Italia 2014

prone and rapid preoperative and postoperative progression. These include glioblastoma and the various forms of embryonal tumors.

15.3 Metastatic Neoplasms

These tumors originate from tissues outside the central nervous system (CNS) and spread secondarily to the brain. They occur in up to 40 % of cancer patients. The incidence of brain metastases is increasing over time. Several reasons may contribute, like the prolonged survival of patients due to improved adjuvant therapies, the improvement of neuroradiological techniques with the ability to detect minute lesions and the use of standardized staging protocols to monitor the effect of treatment [4]. The histological type of the primary tumor is associated with the frequency and pattern of CNS dissemination. The most common cancer metastasizing to the brain is lung cancer, accounting for up to 60 % of all brain metastases with breast cancer being the second most common cancer, accounting for up to 30 % of all brain metastasis followed by melanoma (10–15 %). Most tumors spread by hematogenous dissemination within the gray and white matter junction at the watershed areas of the arterial circulation, where the cells are usually trapped. Therefore, 80 % of brain metastases are located in the cerebral hemispheres, 15 % in the cerebellum, and 5 % in the brain stem. A solitary brain metastasis, an absence of systemic metastases, a controlled primary tumors, a high Karnofsky Performance Scale and an age <65 years are factors associated with better prognosis [5, 6].

15.4 Gliomas

Glial tumors (astrocytomas, oligodendrogliomas, mixed gliomas, ependymomas, and choroid plexus tumors) represent more than 40 % of all primary CNS tumors diagnosed. The WHO grading can be used to provide information regarding tumor behavior. Immunohistochemical examination for specific proliferation-associated antigens and differentiation markers as well as molecular markers and can be used to assess diagnosis, proliferation activity, response to adjuvant therapy and prognosis. Immunohistochemistry for antigenes like GFAP and Ki-67 are well established in gliomas. Molecular biomarkers most commonly used to evaluate gliomas include 1p/19q co-deletion, methylation of the O6-methylguanine-DNA methyltransferase gene promoter, alterations of the epidermal growth factor (EGF) receptor pathway, isocitrate dehydrogenase 2 gene mutations and epidermal growth factor, lactophilin and 7 transmembrane domain containing protein 1 on chromosome 1 (ELTD1) [7–9].

The prognosis depends on the grade of tumor, its location, the age of the patient, the percentage of tumor that can be removed surgically and the response to radio- and chemotherapy. WHO grade I is reserved for focal lesions. The pilocytic astrocytoma is the typical WHO grade I lesion. Complete removal of such lesion often means definitive cure for the patient. WHO grade II lesions are diffuse but demonstrate only low proliferation parameters but may recur or change into higher grade tumors. At 5 years after diagnosis 65 % of patients with WHO grade II astrocytomas are alive. The prognosis is significantly worse for grade III anaplastic astrocytomas (30 %) and oligodendrogliomas (40 %) and grade IV glioblastomas (6 %). The age-standarized 10 year relative survival for low grade gliomas is estimated 47 %. The average survival of patients with glioblastoma is less than 12 months and can be extended to 14 months with more recent treatments [10, 11].

In children more than 30 % of CNS tumors are gliomas, with low grade tumors being more often. Most gliomas are pilocytic WHO grade I lesions located in the cerebellum. At 5 years after diagnosis, 98 % of patients are alive. The prognosis of diffuse WHO grade II lesions is worse (48 %). Grade III and IV tumors have the same prognosis as in adults.

15.5 Menigiomas

25 % of CNS tumors are meningiomas, tumors composed by neoplastic meningothelial cells. Women are more commonly affected than men. Meningiomas are sporadic tumors but patients with neurofibromatosis have a significantly increased risk of developing such lesions. The vast majority of them (85 %) are WHO grade I tumors. Atypical WHO grade II meningiomas are uncommon (10 %) and malignant WHO grade III lesions are rare (2–3 %). Since meningiomas are slow growing lesions the prognosis is favorable, even in cases where the lesion can't be completely removed by surgery. Eighty percent of the patients harboring WHO grade I lesions are alive 5 years after diagnosis but the same is true only in 50 % of patients with malignant meningiomas. Menigiomas were the first neoplasm shown to carry a characteristic cytogenetic alteration, monosomy 22. In several studies, loss of expression of protein molecules has been demonstrated and a number of genomic alterations has been associated with progression and atypical histology, including losses of chromosome arms 1p, 6q, 9p, 10, 14q, and 18q, as well as gains/amplifications on 1q, 9q, 12q, 15q, 17q, and 20q [12, 13]. Deletion of the tumor suppressor gene CDKN2 A has also been associated with aggressive and/or anaplastic tumors [14].

References

1. Legler JM, Ries LA, Smith MA et al (1999) Cancer surveillance series [corrected]: brain and other central nervous system cancers: recent trends in incidence and mortality. J Natl Cancer Inst 91(16):1382–1390
2. Kohler BA, Ward E, McCarthy BJ et al (2011) Annualreport to the nation on the status of cancer, 1975–2007, featuring tumors of the brain and other nervous system. J Natl Cancer Inst 103(9): 714–736
3. Louis DN, Ohgaki H, Wiestler OD et al (2007) The 2007 WHO classification of tumours of the central nervous system. Acta Neuropathol 114(2):97–109
4. Gloeckler Ries LA, Reichman ME, Lewis DR et al (2003) Cancer survival and incidence from the Surveillance, Epidemiology, and End Results (SEER) program. Oncologist 8(6):541–552
5. Diener-West M, Dobbins TW, Phillips TL et al (1989) Identification of an optimal subgroup for treatment evaluation of patients with brain metastases using RTOG study 7916. Int J Radiat Oncol Biol Phys 16(3):669–673
6. Lagerwaard FJ, Levendag PC, Nowak PJ et al (1999) Identification of prognostic factors in patients with brain metastases: a review of 1292 patients. Int J Radiat Oncol Biol Phys 43(4):795–803
7. Louis DN (2006) Molecular pathology of malignant gliomas. Annu Rev Pathol 1:97–117
8. Riemenschneider MJ, Jeuken JW, Wesseling P et al (2010) Molecular diagnostics of gliomas: state of the art. Acta Neuropathol 120(5):567–584
9. Towner RA, Jensen RL, Colman H et al (2012) ELTD1, a potential new biomarker for gliomas. Neurosurgery 72:77
10. Stewart LA (2002) Chemotherapy in adult high-grade glioma: a systematic review and meta-analysis of individual patient data from 12 randomised trials. Lancet 359(9311):1011–1018
11. Ohgaki H, Kleihues P (2005) Population-based studies on incidence, survival rates, and genetic alterations in astrocytic and oligodendroglial gliomas. J Neuropathol Exp Neurol 64(6):479–489
12. Lamszus K (2004) Meningioma pathology, genetics, and biology. J Neuropathol Exp Neurol 63(4): 275–286
13. Perry A, Gutmann DH, Reifenberger G (2004) Molecular pathogenesis of meningiomas. J Neurooncol 70(2):183–202
14. Perry A, Banerjee R, Lohse CM et al (2002) A role for chromosome 9p21 deletions in the malignant progression of meningiomas and the prognosis of anaplastic meningiomas. Brain Pathol 12(2): 183–190

16 Conventional Imaging in the Diagnosis of Brain Tumors

Athanasios D. Gouliamos and Nicholas J. Patronas

16.1 Introduction

Computed tomography (CT) and magnetic resonance imaging (MRI) are considered to be the conventional imaging modalities in the investigation of brain abnormalities. MRI having superior spatial and soft tissue contrast resolution has been established as the preferred method. Furthermore, by modifying the imaging parameters of scanning, MR can address a variety of different diagnostic issues. MRI images can be obtained isotropically at 1 mm intervals and can be reconstructed in three dimensions without loss of resolution. Such postcontrast scans are also suitable to measure tumor volume, which is the newest method to evaluate tumor size before and after treatment, replacing the linear measurements.

In the investigation of brain tumors, both CT and MRI are performed before and after administration of contrast media. One needs to be certain, however, that there is no contraindication for the use of iodinated contrast agents in CT or gadolinium-based agents in MRI. Since these agents are eventually excreted by the kidneys, it is imperative to check the renal function, particularly in older patients and in patients with a variety of medical problems that affect the renal function. All commercially available contrast agents have large molecular weight and cannot cross a normal blood–brain barrier (BBB). Thus, leakage of the contrast within a brain lesion indicates disruption of the barrier in that location [1, 2].

In past years, cerebral angiography and spinal angiography were the main diagnostic tools prior to invention of CT, MRI, and PET. Today, the role of these methods is limited and they are usually applied for surgical planning when the road map of the feeding arteries or the draining veins is considered imperative by the surgical team. Additionally, angiography combined with embolization of the tumor vessels prior to surgery, is also performed in certain tumors to minimize excessive blood loss during surgery.

Besides the differences in the cytoarchitecture of the neoplasms as compared to normal tissues, our imaging techniques have allowed us to separate intracranial tumors into two distinct categories. One includes tumors within the brain parenchyma and the other includes a variety of different intracranial tumors outside the brain. Thus, the terms of intraaxial and extraaxial tumors are routinely used to describe the tissue of origin of these tumors. The majority of the extraaxial tumors originate either from the meninges or from the cranial nerves. The majority of the intraaxial tumors are of the glial

A. D. Gouliamos (✉)
Radiology, National and Kapodistrian University of Athens-Aretaieio Hospital, 76, Vas. Sophias Avenue, 115 27 Athens, Greece
e-mail: agouliam@med.uoa.gr

N. J. Patronas
Neuroradiology, National Institute of Health, 9000 Rockville Pike, Bethesda, MD 20892, USA
e-mail: npatronas@cc.nih.gov

A. D. Gouliamos et al. (eds.), *Imaging in Clinical Oncology*,
DOI: 10.1007/978-88-470-5385-4_16, © Springer-Verlag Italia 2014

cells. This simple separation of the intracranial tumors and the identification of their exact location within the intracranial space have proven very valuable in our diagnostic effort and provided clues for the histological characterization in most of these neoplasms.

16.2 Extraaxial Tumors

The imaging features of the meningiomas have been well described in both CT and MRI. The flat surface of dural attachment, the convex medial tumor border compressing the adjacent brain, the dural tail at the margins of the tumor, and the homogeneous enhancement on the postcontrast scans represent the classical features of meningiomas [3, 4]. The presence of psamommatous calcifications within the tumor parenchyma and the focal hyperostosis in the inner table of the skull at the point of tumor insertion also represent diagnostic features, which are best appreciated by CT.

One of the important findings that should be noted in the CT or MRI images is the relationship of the tumor to an adjacent dural sinus or to nearby prominent cortical veins (Fig. 16.1). Invasion of a dural sinus by a meningioma and partial or complete occlusion of its lumen are critical features and very important for surgical planning. The anatomy of a dural sinus and patency of its lumen can be demonstrated by MR or CT venograms. The accelerated growth of a meningioma seen in consecutive CT or MRI examinations within a certain time period represents the most reliable feature of malignant transformation. Other aggressive features include the invasion of the adjacent bone by the tumor associated with extensive bone destruction and extension of the tumor into the scalp. The invagination of the tumor into the brain parenchyma and the participation of the cerebral arteries in the blood supply of the peripheral layers of the tumor also represent ominous features [5].

Tumors that originate from the cranial nerves represent another common extraaxial tumor within the cranial cavity and the spinal canal. Except for the tumors of the first and second cranial nerves, the tumors of the remaining cranial nerves originate from the Schwann cells and are found in the expected location of these nerves.

The tumors of the first cranial nerve, known as olfactory neuroblastomas (previously known as esthesioneuroblastomas), originate from the olfactory neuroepithelium of the neural crest. These tumors typically produce bone destruction of the cribriform plate and although, in some cases, they may be entirely located within the ethmoid sinus, often have prominent intracranial extension. On the postcontrast CT or MRI scans, the tumors enhance heterogeneously. The degree of malignancy of these tumors is variable but the most malignant form often invades the inferior aspect of the frontal lobes and is associated by peritumoral edema in the adjacent brain parenchyma [6].

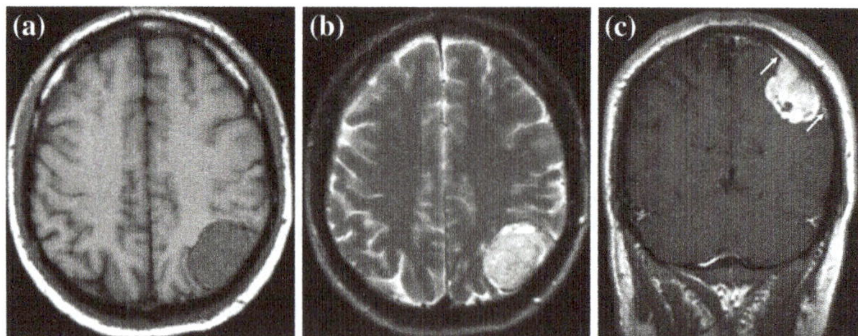

Fig. 16.1 *Left* convexity meningioma: axial T1 (**a**), T2 (**b**) and coronal postcontrast T1-weighted (**c**) images show an extraaxial mass with prominent enhancement. Note dural tail sign in the postcontrast image (*arrows*)

The tumors of the optic nerves and optic chiasm are gliomas. A constant feature found in these tumors is abnormal engorgement of the affected part of the nerve accompanied by increase signal intensity, which is best shown on the flow attenuated inversion recovery (FLAIR) MRI technique. Optic chiasm gliomas often involve one or both optic nerves with or without extension into the orbital compartment. Chiasmatic gliomas may also infiltrate the optic radiation extending at variable distance within the brain parenchyma [7–9]. When first discovered, these tumors may be entirely asymptomatic and their size may remain unchanged for many years. At this stage, the tumor usually do not enhance on the postcontrast scan, which is a feature indicative of the low histologic grade. When visual disturbances develop after years of clinical stability or when abnormal enhancement appears in a previously unenhanced tumor, the question is raised whether the tumor has transformed to a higher grade. Optic gliomas may only involve the intraorbital component of the optic nerve. The MR imaging features of these tumors are identical to those of the intracranial variety. The nerve is enlarged and exhibits high signal intensity. The appearance of intraorbital gliomas may be similar to optic nerve meningiomas, which originate from the sheath of the nerve. The distinction of one tumor from the other can be easily made on the postcontrast CT or MRI scan. In the case of meningioma, the tumor presents as an enhancing mass around the unenhancing and normal in size optic nerve. [10, 11]. The optic glioma, on the other hand, appears as a homogeneous and uniformly enhancing mass incorporating the optic nerve which is not recognized as a separate normal structure within the tumor.

The common finding in schwannomas is that they have a rounded configuration with well circumscribed borders, enhance on the postcontrast scans, and displace but do not invade adjacent structures. These are imaging signs of benign tumors. Schwannomas of intracranial nerves, unlike the schwannomas of peripheral nerves, almost never undergo malignant transformation. Schwannomas of the third, fourth, fifth, and sixth intracranial nerves can be found within the orbit, the cavernous sinus, or the subarachnoid space. The schwannomas of the fifth cranial nerve can also be localized within the Meckel's cave, originating from the Gasserian ganglion. Tumors of ophthalmic division of the fifth cranial nerve can project through the superior orbital fissure into the orbit, whereas tumors from the third division may project through an enlarged foramen ovale into the soft tissues of the nasopharynx [12–14]. The tumors of the seventh nerve, originating from the geniculate ganglion, typically destroy the bony cortex on the anterior aspect the petrous bone and project as a soft tissue extraaxial mass in the middle cranial fossa, compressing the temporal lobe. Schwannomas of the seventh cranial nerve can also occur in any segment of the nerve within the petrous bone. Such tumors are most often encountered in patients with neurofibromatosis.

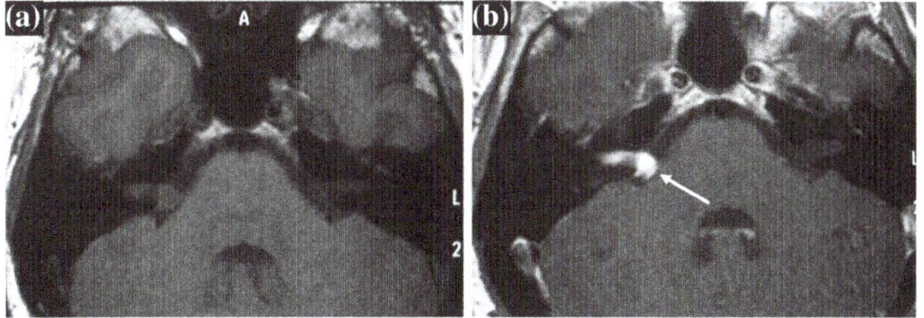

Fig. 16.2 Vestibular schwannoma: axial pre (**a**) and postcontrast (**b**) T1-weighted scans reveal a right internal auditory canal and CPA mass (*white arrow*)

The tumors of the eighth nerve usually originate from the intracanalicular segment of the superior vestibular division. When small in size, they may be entirely confined within the internal auditory canal and they are easily demonstrated on the postcontrast MRI scans where they show intense enhancement (Fig. 16.2). The eighth cranial nerve schwannoma eventually grow outside the internal auditory canal and project into the cerebellopontine (CP) angle cistern. In that location, depending on its size, the tumor often compresses the brain stem or the cerebellar hemisphere [15]. In the CP angle cistern, schwannomas must be distinguished from meningiomas, which are also commonly found in this location. The correct diagnosis of schwannoma can be established by demonstrating the intracanalicular component of the tumor on postcontrast scans. This is a reliable diagnostic sign since meningiomas rarely extend into the auditory canal. Additional diagnostic features include the presence of tumoral calcifications, which are more common in meningiomas or the presence of cystic changes, which are more often encountered in schwannomas. It is of interest to note that both schwannomas and meningiomas can be found in the CP angle in patients with neurofibromatosis 2.

Schwannomas of the ninth, tenth, and eleventh nerves are found with the jugular fossa and the tumors of the twelfth nerve are localized in the hypoglossal canal. Imaging features of chronic bone erosion with enlargement of these canals or even frank bone destruction are best demonstrated by CT scan. The tumors in the jugular fossa often compress and/or occlude the internal jugular vein and depending on their size they may project either superiorly into the cranial cavity or inferiorly into the soft tissues near the base of the skull [16]. The schwannomas of these nerves enhance intensely and homogeneously, with the exception of the cases in which there are cystic components within the tumor parenchyma. Small schwannomas in the jugular fossa may be missed because the enhancement of the tumor is similar to that of the enhancing internal jugular vein and separation of one from the other can be problematic. Another tumor that occurs in the jugular fossa is the paraganglioma, which also enhances intensely on the postcontrast CT and MRI scans. The distinction of schwannomas from paragangiomas can be reliably made by PET scanning with F-18FDOPA having avid uptake in the latter [17].

Besides meningiomas and schwannomas, other tumors or tumor-like lesions are encountered in the cranial cavity, which usually project within the subarachnoid spaces and present as extra axial masses. One of the most common locations for these tumors is the suprasellar cisterns. Pituitary macroadenomas commonly extend above the diaphragm sella and compress

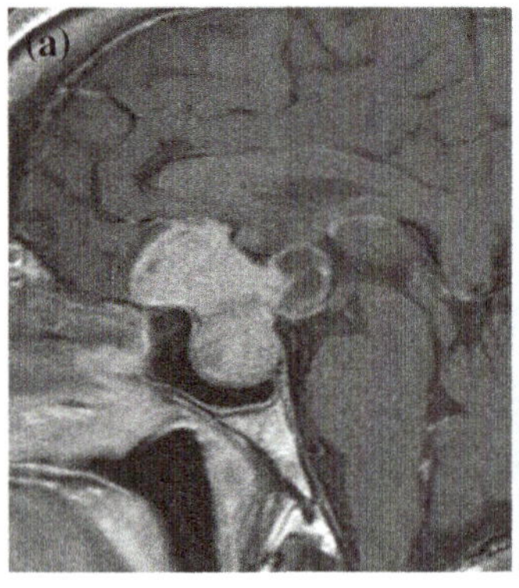

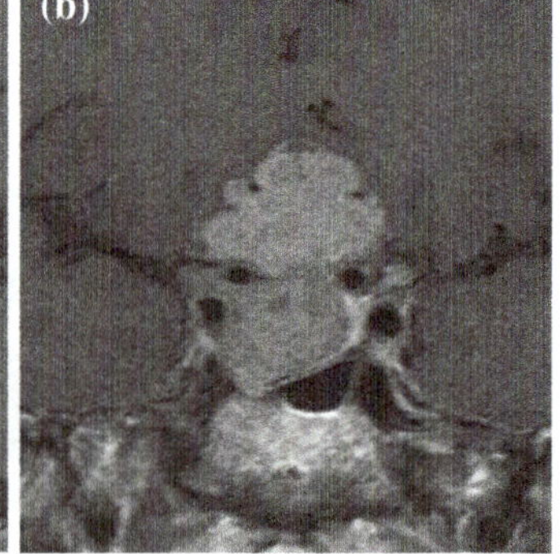

Fig. 16.3 Pituitary macroadenoma presenting as an extraaxial mass: Sagittal (**a**) and coronal (**b**) postcontrast T1-weighted images of the pituitary showing an enhancing mass within the sella turcica extending into the suprasellar cistern and compressing the adjacent brain. A posterior segment of the mass has undergone cystic degeneration. There is invasion of both cavernous sinuses. Note continuity of the intrasellar and supresellar component of the mass

the optic chiasm or the hypothalamus. The anatomic relationship of the adenoma to the pituitary gland is critical for the diagnosis. This is best documented on postcontrast MRI, which will demonstrate a continuity of the suprasellar tumor to the pituitary tissue within the sella [18, 19] (Fig. 16.3). Hemorrhagic elements are sometimes found in the parenchyma of the adenoma, presenting with high signal intensity on precontrast T1-weighted scans due to methemoglobin formation. On other occasions, macroadenomas can undergo cystic degeneration and contain fluid within its cystic component, which is slightly hyperintense with respect to cerebrospinal fluid (CSF) on T1-weighted scans. Pituitary adenomas with suprasellar extension should be differentiated from meningiomas that originate from the diaphragm sella. The diagnosis of meningioma can be easily made by demonstrating a horizontal, relatively hypoenhancing/hypointense diaphragm sella on sagittal postcontrast scans, separating the meningioma above from the normal pituitary gland below.

Another common tumor in the suprasellar cistern is the craniopharyngioma. These tumors are typically connected to the pituitary stalk and can also compress the optic chiasm and the hypothalamus. Besides the visual disturbances, which are one of the most common clinical presentations, these tumors disrupt the communication of the hypothalamus with the pituitary causing pituitary deregulation. In such cases, there is hypopituitarism involving one or more pituitary hormones. They are solid masses but also commonly have cystic components. The cysts often contain oily material and demonstrated high signal intensity on the precontrast T1-weighted scans. A fluid–fluid level is formed within the cyst due to heterogeneous composition of the fluid. Calcifications are commonly encountered in the solid part of the tumor, which always demonstrate increased enhancement on the postcontrast scans. Exceptionally, craniopharyngiomas can be entirely cystic and the features described above are absent.

Rathke's cleft cysts can also present as a suprasellar cystic lesion. A sizable component of the cyst is often located in the pituitary gland. Differentiation of cystic pituitary adenoma from cystic craniopharymgioma or Rathke's cleft cyst is exceedingly difficult by imaging alone [20, 21].

Dermoids are ectodermal inclusion cysts which can present as extraaxial space occupying lesions anywhere in the intracranial cavity but they are most often found in the suprasellar/parasellar regions and in the posterior fossa. Dermoids contain oily material and for this reason cannot be easily distinguished from lipomas, both having high signal intensity on precontrast T1-weighted scans. Lipomas are incidental solid masses that can be found in different intracranial locations and remain unchanged in size and configuration for life. Dermoid cysts, on the other hand, may rupture and droplets of the oily material are disseminated into the subarachnoid space. Chemical meningitis can result from this complication [22].

Epidermoids, similar to dermoids, are also epidermal inclusion cysts with a predilection for the suprasellar cistern or the CP angle cisterns. These thin wall cystic lesions are often multilocular and contain desquamated cells and cellular debris. Unlike dermoids, epidermoid cysts have low or intermediate signal in the precontrast T1-weighted scans. A characteristic imaging feature of epidermoid cysts is the restricted diffusion they exhibit on diffusion weighted images, which is due to increased viscosity of the fluid inside the cysts. Chemical meningitis can also occur in the event of rupture and spilling of the contents of the cyst into the subarachnoid space [23, 24].

16.3 Intraaxial Tumors of Glial Origin

The detection of intracerebral tumors with conventional MR imaging is easy, and the role of CT has diminished since the sensitivity of MRI is by far superior. Intracranial tumors become symptomatic when they have acquired considerable size and demonstrate mass effect, which may be subtle but nearly always present. The signal changes of the tumors on MRI are readily apparent showing high intensity on FLAIR and T2-weighted images and low signal on the T1-weighted techniques. A variety of gliomas have been described by histological examinations and immunohistochemical analysis of excised tumor specimens. Documentation of the different histologic types by imaging often represents a futile exercise and is commonly subject to errors [25, 26].

The conventional thinking in our diagnostic effort is to provide accurate assessment on the degree of aggressiveness of these tumors following the grading system adopted by the World Health Organization [27]. Evaluation of the integrity of the BBB using contrast agents allows the physicians to provide a reasonable assessment of the histologic tumor grade. Thus, the aggressive glioblastoma multiforme (GBM), a grade IV tumor, will demonstrate intense enhancement on the postcontrast scan (Fig. 16.4). Anaplastic astrocytoma (grade III) is a less aggressive tumor as judged by the length of survival when compared to GBM. These tumors usually enhance on the postcontrast scans but the enhancement is less intense and some may not show an obvious disruption of the BBB when first diagnosed (Fig. 16.5). The blood volume in the tumor parenchyma is increased and the FDG uptake has an intermediate value between normal gray and white matter. Infiltrative astrocytomas, oligodendrogliomas and oligoastrocytomas are less aggressive tumors (grade II) but eventually, most if not all, will undergo malignant transformation. These tumors usually have poorly defined margins and are best demonstrated on the FLAIR technique showing increased signal intensity associated with mass effect (Fig. 16.6). There is no disruption of the BBB and the blood volume is either decreased or equal to normal brain on the perfusion scan. Cystic changes are frequently encountered within the tumor parenchyma and calcifications may also be found, the latter being more often in oligodendrogliomas. Subtle tumor growth does occur in these low grade tumors but it takes place over a long period of time and is best demonstrated on the FLAIR technique showing gradual increase in the size of the pathological region. The onset of malignant transformation is herald by BBB disruption accompanied by all other signs described in the GBM and anaplastic astrocytomas. Pilocytic astrocytomas are known to be the least aggressive gliomas (grade I). These tumors are not infiltrative and the peripheral margin of the mass is well demarcated from the adjacent brain. Even though they are of low grade, pilocytic astrocytomas demonstrate increased enhancement on the postcontrast scans (Fig.16.7) and increased capillary density on the perfusion scan. This is due to inherent rich vascularity in the tumor parenchyma and not in the development of new tumor vessels, as is the case of glioblastomas. Another common feature of pilocytic astrocytoma is that they are nearly always associated with a fluid filled cyst, which is eccentrically placed in the periphery of the tumor or within the adjacent normal brain. These features of pilocytic astrocytomas are also encountered in hemangioblastomas, another benign brain tumor.

Gliomatosis cerebri is another type of glioma characterized by its highly infiltrative features. This type of glioma often extends through the corpus callosum into the opposite hemisphere and is readily recognized by FLAIR, exhibiting high signal intensity. The tumor is usually of low grade when first diagnosed and does not enhance on the postcontrast scans. Eventually, there is conversion to a higher grade which is documented by increase in capillary blood volume, scattered foci of enhancement and higher metabolic activity.

Another kind of diffuse infiltrative glioma, most commonly encountered in the pediatric age group, is the glioma that involves the pons. This tumor may also be low grade when first diagnosed. The natural history of these tumors however is that of rapid clinical deterioration within a relatively short period. This is due to

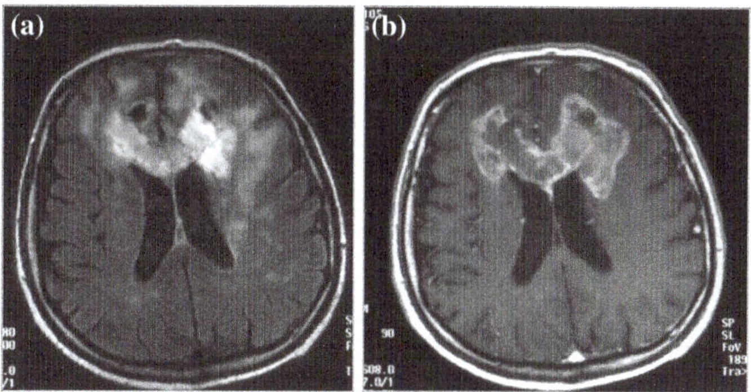

Fig. 16.4 Rapidly growing high grade glioma: Axial FLAIR (**a**) and postcontrast T1-weighted (b) images show classic "butterfly" GBM of the corpus callosum. Central necrosis with an irregular enhancement in the periphery of the tumor

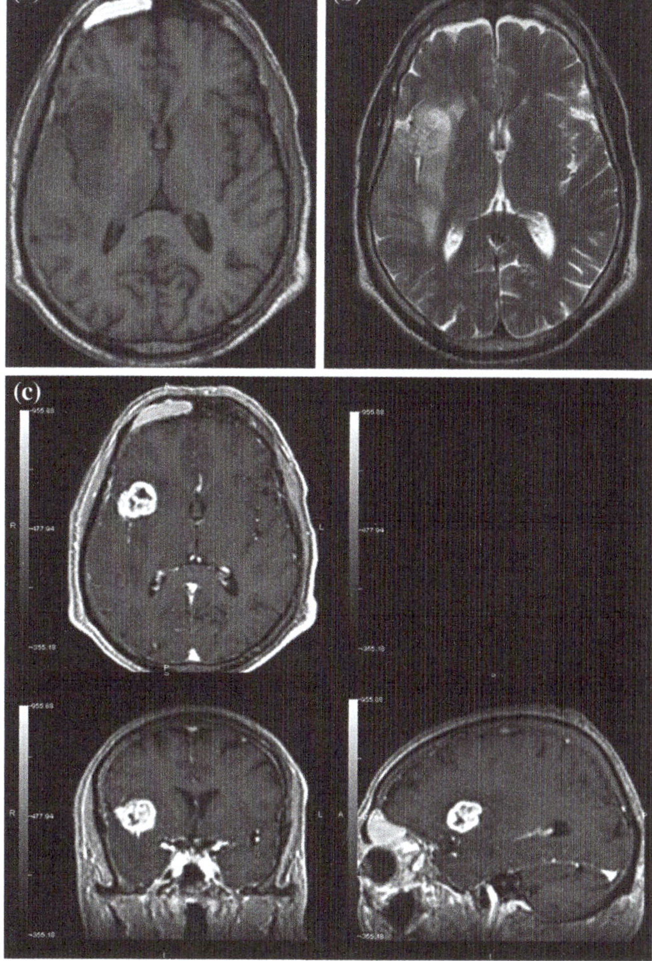

Fig. 16.5 Anaplastic astrocytoma grade III: Axial T1 (**a**), T2 (**b**) and axial coronal and sagittal (**c**) postcontrast T1-weighted images show an infiltrative mass in the right frontal lobe and adjacent insular cortex. There is heterogeneous enhancement in the anterior segment of the mass. As an incidental finding a right frontal mucocele is noted (courtesy of Dr. V. K. Katsaros)

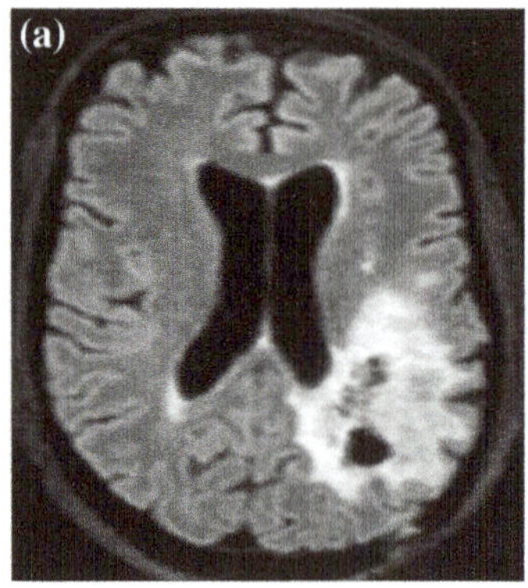

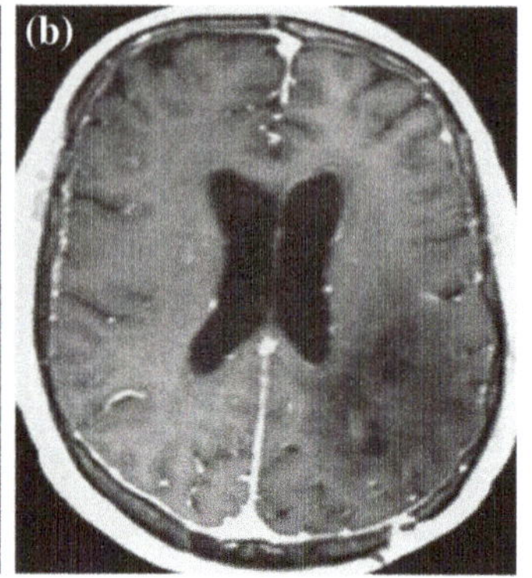

Fig. 16.6 Low grade glioma: Axial FLAIR image of the brain (**a**) shows an infiltrative tumor in the left cerebral hemisphere demonstrating high signal intensity and multiple cysts in its parenchyma. Postcontrast scan image (**b**) reveals no evidence of abnormal enhancement

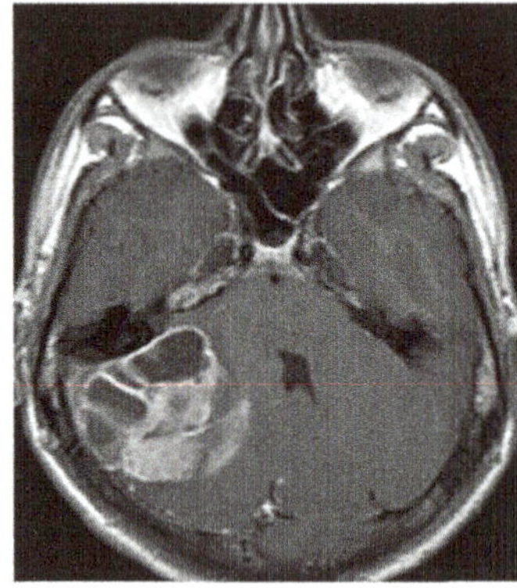

Fig. 16.7 Pilocytic asrtocytoma: axial postcontrast MR image of the brain shows an enhancing mass in the right cerebellar hemisphere. Cystic changes are present in the periphery of the mass. This is a common feature in this type of tumor

the critical location in the brain stem and possible rapid conversion to a higher grade. The MRI scans show engorgement of the pons and abnormal high signal intensity on FLAIR and on T2-weighted scans. These tumors may be only confined in the pons but there is often a variable degree of extension into the medulla or the mid brain. Initially, there is no enhancement on the postcontrast scans but in the course of the disease there is eventual disruption of the BBB. Some of these tumors may develop an exophytic component extending beyond the contour of the pons, encasing the basilar artery without compromising its lumen [28, 29].

Ependymomas represent another type of intraaxial tumors which, as their name implies, originate from the ependymal cells of the ventricular wall. They are often encountered in the pediatric age group and are predominately found in the posterior fossa. A sizable part of these tumors in that location project into the cavity of the fourth ventricle but there is also variable degree of invasion of the cerebellar hemispheres or vermis. The supratentorial ependymomas occur more often in adults. They commonly invade the parenchyma of the cerebral hemispheres and also exhibit a variable degree of extension into the ventricular cavity. On rare occasions, supratentorial ependymomas may be entirely intracerebral with only minimal or no connection to the ependyma of the ventricular wall. These tumors are believed to originate from ependymal rests within the cerebral hemisphere and from the imaging point of view they may be indistinguishable from other gliomas. On the precontrast CT and MRI scans ependymomas often show calcifications and cystic or necrotic areas and enhance heterogeneously on postcontrast scans [30]. The most malignant type of ependymomas has a tendency to metastasize via CSF seeding. A subgroup of tumors in this category, called subependymomas present as a mass which projects within the ventricular cavity. Subendymomas do not usually enhance on the postcontrast scans and generally have a more benign clinical course [31].

16.4 Intraaxial Tumors of Non-glial Origin

Besides the CNS tumors of glial origin, a variety of other neoplasms of primitive bipotential precursors is known to occur within the brain and should be included in the differential diagnosis. Primitive neuroectodermal tumors (PNET) are tumors which originate from primitive neuroectoderal cells and are highly prevalent in the pediatric age group. When PNETs develop in the cerebrum, they are called primary cerebral neuroblastomas, and when localized in the cerebellum they are known as medulloblastomas. The imaging findings of these tumors are similar to those of high grade gliomas presenting with mass effect, abnormal signal changes on T1 and T2 weighted MRI scans and disrupted blood brain barrier. The enhancement of the tumors observed on CT and MRI scans is usually heterogeneous. This is in part due to cystic changes or tissue necrosis although the latter is less pronounced in PNET when compared to glioblastomas. Calcifications can also be encountered within the tumor parenchyma. It is the age of the patient at presentation rather than the morphologic feature on imaging that provides that most valuable clue for the diagnosis of PNET. It should also be noted that medulloblastomas more commonly involve the vermis, but tend to invade the fourth ventricle and the adjacent cerebellar hemispheres early in the course of the disease (Fig. 16.8). Even though these tumors are malignant, the overall prognosis is by far better than that of the malignant glial tumors after surgical resection followed by chemotherapy and/or radiation [32, 33]. It has been known that PNETs have propensity to spread via leptomeningeal seeding throughout the neural axis. Therefore, early detection and proper treatment prior to development of leptomeningeal spread are critical for the best possible outcome. Furthermore, continuous surveillance by postcontrast MRI after completion of the treatments is recommended for several years to rule out recurrence.

Hemangioblastoma is another intraparenchymal brain tumor commonly found in the cerebellum, the brain stem, the spinal cord, and the retina. On rare occasions, these tumors are located within cerebral hemispheres or in the suprasellar cistern. The cells of origin are mesoderm-derived embryologically arrested hemangioblasts located in the wall of small arteries or venules. Hemangioblastomas represent one of the dominant abnormalities in patients with Von Hippel Lindau syndrome but they are also encountered in patients with spontaneous mutation of chromosome three. Hemangioblastomas are benign tumors that can slowly grow in time, and do not metastasize. In the early stage of development, hemangioblastomas appear as small intensely enhancing solid nodules. As the tumor grows in size, edema develops in the surrounding brain parenchyma. The edema is a constant feature of larger tumors and is caused

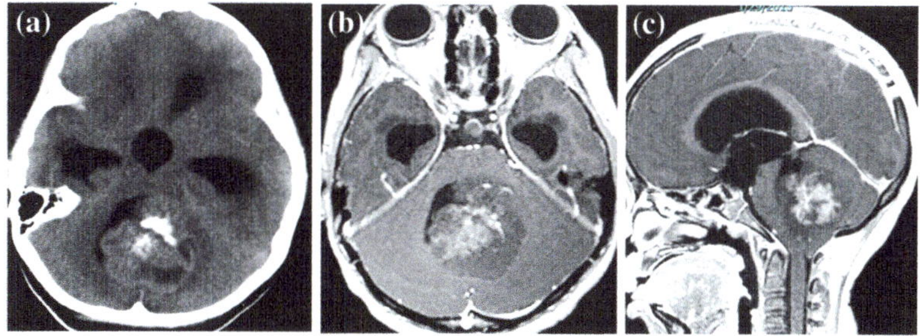

Fig. 16.8 Medulloblastoma: axial precontrast CT of the brain (**a**) shows a large mass originating from the vermis and compressing the forth ventricle. Calcifications and cystic changes are present within the mass. Axial (**b**) and sagittal (**c**) postcontrast MR shows heterogeneous enhancement of the mass. There is also marked hydrocephalus

by extravasation of fluid from the rich vascular bed of the tumor into the interstitial space. Because the amount of fluid in the interstitial space often exceeds the ability of the brain to absorb it, a cyst is formed. Therefore, these cysts represent a byproduct of increased tumor vascularity and there are no tumor cells in their walls. The enhancing tumor nodule is either in direct contact to the outside wall of the cyst or projects within its lumen [34]. This arrangement of the cyst with the nodule is identical to that described in the pilocytic astrocytomas. Often the cyst can reach a large size and is primarily responsible for the patient's symptoms, requiring surgical intervention to drain the fluid and removing the tumor that produced it. Finally, on extremely rare occasions, hemangioblastomas may develop sheaths of tumorous tissues that diffusely infiltrate the leptomeninges in a continuous fashion. The term hemangioblastomatosis has been adopted to describe this unusual manifestation [35].

Tumors that originate from the pineal body are also intraaxial by virtue of origin, although these tumors often grow exophytically and project into the adjacent quadrigeminal or superior vermian cisterns. Several histologic cell types of these tumors have been identified. Germinoma is the most common type comprising about 67 % of pineal body tumors. Other more rare tumors of the pineal body include teratomas, choriocarcinomas, yolk sac tumors , embryonal cell carcinomas, pineocytomas, and pineoblastomas. Excluding the pineocytomas, most of these tumors show strong male predominance. The histologic type in some of these tumors can be suggested by the elevated human chorionic gonadotropin and alpha-fetoprotein levels that are known to occur in choriocarcinomas, yolk sac tumors, and embryonal cell carcinomas. The imaging features on CT or MRI are very similar in all these tumors. The mass of the tumor always enhances and calcifications in the tumor parenchyma are very common [36]. Although physiologic calcifications occur in normal pineal bodies, past experience has revealed that the size of calcification is important and should be considered as a suspicious abnormal finding suggestive of tumor if it is larger than 1.5 cm. CT is the technique of choice for the detection of pineal calcification and for the exact measurements of its size. In pineal body tumors the calcification is often located on the posterior aspect of the tumor, whereas its anterior part is comprised by a non-calcified soft tissue mass encroaching upon the posterior third ventricle. Another constant feature of tumors of the pineal body is the presence of mass effect on the quadrigeminal plate and the obstruction of the aqueduct of Sylvius causing hyprocephalus. Finally, it should be noted that germinomas of the pineal may be, on rare occasions, associated with similar tumors in the suprasellar region. In such cases, it is difficult to determine whether the suprasellar tumor represent spread of the tumor from the pineal or a second primary tumor. Primary germinomas can also be found in the hypothalamic or the suprasellar areas in the absence of tumor in the pineal body (Fig. 16.9).

It is well known that the normal pineal bodies in children under the age of 10 do not calcify. Therefore, the finding of a calcified pineal in this age group has a good chance to be pathologic even when there is no clearly visible mass and the size of calcification is small. Children with normal size but calcified pineal body can clinically present with precautious puberty. If the above-mentioned biochemical markers in the blood or in the CSF are elevated in such children, treatment for pineal body tumor should be considered without need for histology confirmation or other proof.

Other rare intraaxial tumors of mixed or nonglial origin include the following: gangliogliomas, ganglioneuromas, gangiocytomas, and dysembryoplastic neuroepithelial tumors . These are generally benign tumors that are found either incidentally or discovered during the workup for seizure disorder. A mass effect is a constant finding on CT or MR imaging but there are no other specific features that characterize these tumors. They are hypodense on CT, hypointense on T1-weighted, and hyperintense of T2-weighted MRI scans. Cystic changes and calcifications can be found within the mass, which does not usually enhance on the postcontrast

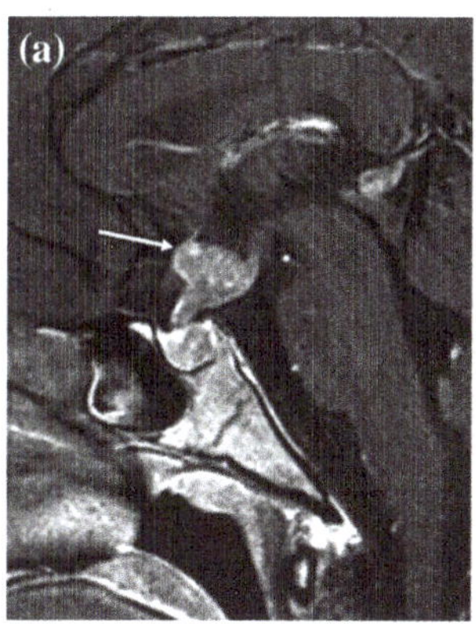

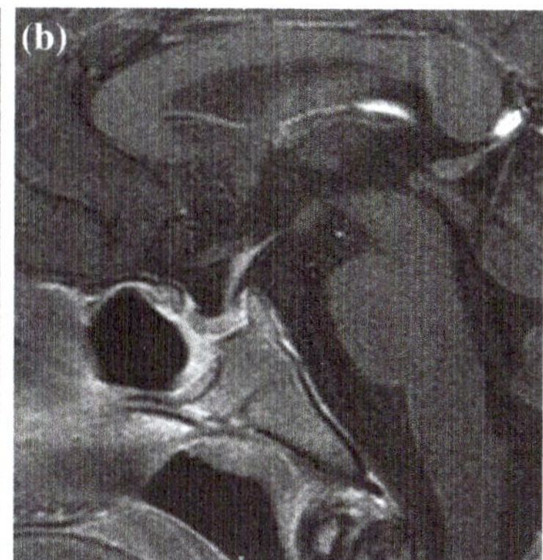

Fig. 16.9 Germinoma in the hypothalamus: On the pretreatment scan (**a**) there is an enhancing tumor in the hypothalamus (*white arrow*) which has also invaded the pituitary stalk and the posterior half of the pituitary gland. On the scan obtained after chemotherapy (**b**), there is complete resolution of the tumor.

scan. These findings are very similar to low grade gliomas from which cannot be distinguished by imaging alone [37]. One interesting abnormality in this group of non-glial lesions is the cerebellar abnormality found in Lhermitte-Dulclos disease, which some consider to be a malformation of brain tissue rather than true tumor. The imaging findings are highly characteristic of this entity on MRI, where there are laminated layers of white and gray matter in parallel arrangement with each other in the center of a cerebellar hemisphere. What is even more interesting in these lesions is the finding of restricted diffusion on MRI and the high metabolic activity on FDG-PET scan [38, 39].

16.4.1 CNS Lymphoma

Primary CNS lymphoma is another tumor of non-glial origin that can be mistaken for a glioma. Conventional CT and MRI studies can often, but not always, provide clues for the diagnosis. Since the treatment of CNS lymphoma and glioma is vastly different, a stereotactic biopsy is routinely done to establish the correct diagnosis. The experience of many years with CT and MRI has established diagnostic criteria suggestive of CNS lymphoma (see Chap. 34).

16.4.2 Metastasis

Metastatic tumors are the most common brain tumors and the diagnostic challenges are relatively small. In many patients, the primary tumor outside the CNS is well known by history. Occasionally, the metastatic brain tumor is the first manifestation of a systemic malignancy. Metastatic tumors are usually round with well-defined borders and may be multiple. Most of these tumors are found at the gray white matter junctions and are entirely surrounded by brain.

Several imaging features seen in different types of metastatic tumors have been described. Frequently, metastatic brain tumors are solid and enhance homogeneously but often they undergo central necrosis and demonstrate a ring-like enhancement on postcontrast scans. The incidence of central necrosis increases with the size of the tumor. It is believed that the necrosis occurs because the rate of tumor growth is not accompanied by a comparable increase of its blood supply. There are certain primary neoplasms that have increased propensity to undergo necrosis when they metastasize to the brain. Such neoplasms include the small cell carcinomas of the lungs and a variety of adenocarcinomas. Hemorrhage can occur within some metastatic brain tumors due to rupture of fragile tumor vessels and often present clinically with sudden deterioration of the neurologic deficit. Among the tumors that tend to bleed, melanoma is the most common. Other highly vascular tumors such as renal cell carcinomas choriocarcinomas and some adenocarcinomas can also become hemorrhagic. The diagnosis of hemorrhage within a metastatic tumor can be easily made on a gradient echo scan showing low signal intensity or on a precontrast T1-weighted scan demonstrating high signal. The hemorrhagic elements may extend throughout the tumor parenchyma and the lesion is indistinguishable from a brain hematoma that has occurred for a variety of different reasons. On other occasions, the hemorrhage is localized in only part of the tumor and in such cases the non-hemorrhagic part of the tumor will enhance and the lesion appears larger on the postcontrast scan. Calcifications within the tumor parenchyma represent a rare phenomenon and are most often encountered in metastatic osteosarcomas.

Metastatic brain tumors are often surrounded by a zone of edema in the adjacent brain parenchyma. This finding occurs in rapidly growing tumors and in tumors that have acquired large size. The presence of edema increases the overall mass effect and is, in part, responsible for the development of symptoms. Although in the majority of cases the diagnosis of brain metastasis can be easily established, on rare occasions a solitary metastatic tumor located on the surface of the brain, loses its round shape and presents with a compressed flat surface against the calvarium, mimicking a meningioma. Another diagnostic problem is encountered when the metastatic tumor is localized in unusual sites such as the pituitary gland, the pituitary stalk, the choroid plexus, or the internal auditory canal. One of the most important issues that need to be addressed in the case of metastatic brain tumors is the accurate documentation of the exact number of lesions. This is a critical issue for the management of these patients, since the selection of surgery, stereotactic radiosurgery, or whole brain radiation is based on this information. The technique of choice for the correct documentation of the number of tumors is the postcontrast 3D gradient echo scan obtained in isotropic one millimeter thin sections. It has been suggested the scanning should be performed with a few minutes delay after the injection so that the maximum concentration of the contrast in the tumor tissue can be achieved. Past experience has shown that tumors as small as one millimeter in diameter can be detected by this method [40].

Metastatic tumors can also occur in the leptomeninges, which is associated with a very poor prognosis. The diagnosis of meningeal carcinomatosis in the brain is best made by using postcontrast FLAIR technique, which is known to have a superior sensitivity compared to conventional postcontrast T1-weighted images.

16.5 Intraventricular Tumors

Primary intraventricular tumors are rare tumors presenting clinically with headaches, visual disturbances, or neurologic symptoms similar to any other neoplastic lesion in the central nervous system. Imaging studies clearly demonstrate the intraventricular location of these tumors. There is often associated hydrocephalus due to partial or complete obstruction of the CSF flow. Intraventricular obstructive hydrocephalus can occur by a variety of non-neoplastic lesions, which may be cystic but need to be distinguished from the true neoplasms. Colloid cysts are located in the vicinity of the foramen Monro and typically demonstrate high density on CT and high signal intensity on T1-weighted MRI scans. Cysticercosis cysts are found in any of the four ventricles. This diagnosis can be suggested if a small, round nodule is found on the interior aspect of the cystic wall representing the scolex. Associated granulomatous calcifications within the brain parenchyma, a cardinal feature of this infectious disease, provide another reliable sign of the diagnosis. Other infectious diseases such as cryptococcosis can also present with intraventricular cysts, abnormal enhancement, engorgement of the choroid plexus, and hyprocephalus [41].

True neoplasms in the ventricles include meningiomas, choroid plexus papillomas, choroid plexus carcinomas, central neurocytomas, and subependymomas and subependymal giant cell astrocytomas, in tuberous sclerosis patients [31, 42, 43] .

The intraventricular meningiomas are solid tumors that often exhibit diffuse or focal calcifications. Invariably, these meningiomas enhance on postcontrast scans but the degree of enhancement is inversely proportional to the amount of calcium deposition within the tumor parenchyma. These tumors are commonly encountered in patients with Neurofibromatosis 2, but they can also be found as an isolated event.

Choroid plexus papillomas and carcinomas are tumors highly prevalent in the pediatric age group and are known to be associated with ventriculomegaly. There is always connection of the tumor to the choroid plexus and the free margin of the tumor projecting within the ventricular cavity is often irregular. Although the prognosis of the papilloma is different from that of carcinoma, differentiation of one from the other cannot be reliably made by imaging and complete surgical excision is recommended in both.

Central neurocytoma is relatively benign intraventricular tumor, which can be of large size when first discovered. On the precontrast CT scan, the tumor is slightly hyperdense with respect to normal brain. Cystic changes and calcifications are nearly always present within the tumor parenchyma which enhances heterogeneously on the postcontrast scans. Unlike the three previous tumors that connect to the choroid plexus, central neurocytoma has its origin in the ventricular wall and sometimes extends within the brain substance. Rare extraventricular neurocytomas have also been described.

Subependymomas also originate from the ventricular wall and usually there in no appreciable involvement of the adjacent brain parenchyma. The majority of these tumors do not enhance on postcontrast scans but when they do, the enhancement is faint and heterogeneous. These tumors are often asymptomatic and are known to have good prognosis after complete surgical excision. Subependymal giant cell astrocytomas are most commonly encountered in patients with tuberous sclerosis and are associated by other stigmata of this entity. A calcification is always present within the tumor and the non-calcified part of the tumor enhances intensely on the postcontrast scan. The tumor is most often found in the vicinity of the interventricular foramina of Monro and in this location can cause hydrocephalus which may be the presenting symptom. The tumor is well circumscribed and often projects within the adjacent brain parenchyma (Fig. 16.10). A complete surgical excision is associated with good prognosis.

In conclusion, the application of our imaging methods has significantly contributed to the diagnosis of brain tumors and influence the management of these abnormalities. Histological characterizations of tumors are not always achieved by our methods and stereotactic biopsies are still widely used for this purpose. Studies of biological behavior and methods assessing the functional status of the microcirculation have provided additional information about the understanding of brain tumors. Such methods are also useful in experimental settings

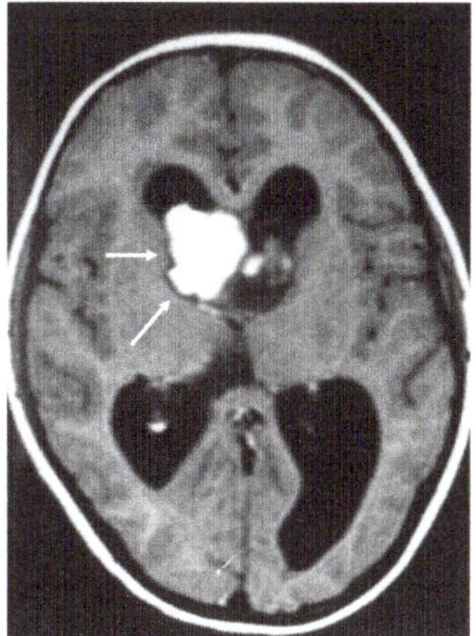

Fig. 16.10 Subependymal giant cell astrocytoma (SGCA): axial postcontrast MR image of the brain shows a right foramen of Monro mass (*arrows*). This tumor is classified as WHO grade I

for the evaluation of new drugs diminishing the cost of these investigations.

References

1. Castillo M, Scatliff JH, Bouldin TW et al (1992) Radiologic-pathologic correlation: intracranial astrocytoma. AJNR Am J Neuroradiol 13(6): 1609–1616
2. Omuro AM, Leite CC, Mokhtari K et al (2006) Pitfalls in the diagnosis of brain tumor. Lancet Neurol 5:937–948
3. Sze G (1993) Diseases of the intracranial meninges: MR imaging features. AJR 160:727–733
4. Elster AD, Challa VR, Gilbert TH et al (1989) Meningiomas: MR and histopathologic features. Radiology 170:857–862
5. Beutow MP, Burton PC, Smirniotopoulos JG (1991) Typical, atypical and misleading features in meningiomas. Radiographics 11:1087–1100
6. Bradley PJ, Jones N, Robertson I (2003) Diagnosis and management of esthesioneuroblastoma. Curr Opin Otolaryngol Head Neck Surg 11(2):112–118
7. Patronas NJ, Dwyer AL, Papathanasiou T et al (1987) Contributions of magnetic resonance imaging in the evaluation of optic glioma. Surg Neurol 28:367–371
8. Astrup J (2003) Natural history and clinical management of optic pathway glioma. Br J Neurosurg 17(4):327–335
9. Tourbah A (2012) Contribution of imaging to the diagnosis of optic neuropathies. Rev Neurol 168(10):702–705
10. Monteiro ML, Goncalves AC, Siqueira SA et al (2012) Optic nerve sheath meningioma in the first decade of life: case report and review of the literature. Case Rep Ophthalmol 3(2):270–276
11. Saeed P, Rootman J, Nugent RA, White VA et al (2003) Optic nerve sheath meningiomas. Ophthalomology 110(10):2019–2039
12. MacNally SP, Rutherford SA, Ramsden RT et al (2008) Trigeminal schwannomas. Br J Neurosurg 22(6):720–738
13. Beges C, Revel MP, Gaston A et al (1992) Trigeminal schwannomas: assessment of MRI and CT. Neuroradiol 34:179–183
14. Celli P, Ferrante L, Acqui M et al (1992) Neurinoma of the third, fourth and sixth nerves: a survey and report of a new fourth nerve case. Surg Neurol 38:216–224
15. Bonneville F, Savatovsky J, Chivas J (2007) Imaging of cerebellopontine angle lesions: an update. Part 2: intra-axial lesions, skull base lesions that may invade the CPA region, and non-enhancing extra-axial lesions. Eur Radiol 17:2908–2920
16. Wan JH, Wu YH, Li ZJ et al (2012) Triple dumbbell shaped jugular foramen schwannomas. J Cranio-Maxillofac Surg 40(4):354–361
17. King KS, Chen CC, Alexopoulos DK et al (2011) Functional imaging of SDHx-related head and neck paragangliomas: comparison of ^{18}F-Fluorodihydroxyphenylalanine, ^{18}F-Fluorodopamine, ^{18}F-Fluoro-2-Deoxy-D-Glucose PET, ^{123}I-Metaiodobenzylguanidine Scintigraphy, and ^{111}In-Pentetreotide Scintigraphy. J Clin Endocrinol Metab 96:2779–2785
18. Boxerman JL, Rogg JM, Donahue JE et al (2010) Preoperative MRI evaluation of pituitary macroadenoma: imaging features predictive of successful transsphenoidal surgery. AJR Am J Roentgenol 195(3):720–726
19. Kaltsas GA, Evanson J, Chrisoulidou A et al (2008) The diagnosis and management of parasellar tumours of the pituitary. Endocr Relat Cancer 15:885–903
20. Donovan JL, Nesbit GM (1996) Distinction of masses involving the sella and suprasellar space: specificity of imaging features. AJR Am J Roentgenol 167:597–603
21. Famini P, Maya MM, Melmed S et al (2011) Pituitary magnetic resonance imaging for sellar and parasellar masses: ten-year experience in 2598 patients. J Clin Endocrinol Metab 96(6):1633–1641
22. Sturiale CL, Mangiola A, Pompucci A et al (2009) Intradural giant dermoid cyst of the petrous apex. J Clin Neurosci 16(11):370–374
23. Rubin G, Scienza R, Pasqualin A et al (1989) Craniocerebral epidermoids and dermoids: a review of 44 cases. Acta Neurochir (Wien) 97(1–2):1–16
24. Konovalov AN, Spallone A, Pitzkhelauri DI (1999) Pineal epidermoid cysts: diagnosis and management. J Neurosurg 91(3):370–374
25. Al-Okaili RN, Krejza J, Wang S et al (2006) Advanced MR imaging techniques in the diagnosis of intraaxial brain tumors in adults. Radiographics 26:S173–S189
26. Upadhyay N, Waldman AD (2011) Conventional MRI evaluation of gliomas. Brit J Radiol 84:S107–S111
27. Kleihues P, Louis DN, Scheithauer BW et al (2002) The WHO classification of the tumors of the nervous system. J Neuropathol Exp Neurol 61:215–225
28. Warren KE (2012) Diffuse intrinsic pontine glioma: poised for progress. Front Oncol 2:205
29. Steffen-Smith EA, Shih JH, Hipp SJ et al (2011) Proton magnetic resonance spectroscopy predicts survival in children with diffuse intrinsic pontine glioma. J Neurooncol 105(2):365–373
30. Spoto GP, Press GA, Hesselink JR et al (1990) Intracranial ependymoma and subependymoma: MR manifefstations. AJNR Am J Neuroradiol 11:83–91
31. Rushing EJ, Cooper PB, Quezado M et al (2007) Subependymoma revisited: clinicopathological evaluation of 83 cases. J Neurooncol 85(3):297–305

32. Vogel H, Fuller GN (2007) Primitive neuroectodermal tumors, embryonal tumors, and other small cell and poorly differentiated malignant neoplasms of the central and peripheral nervous systems. Ann Diagn Pathol 7:387–398
33. Papaioannou G, Sebire NJ, McHugh K (2009) Imaging of unusual pediatric blastomas. Cancer Imaging 9(1):1–11
34. Filling-Katz MR, Choyke PL, Oldfield E et al (1991) Central nervous system involvement in von Hippel Lindau disease. Neurology 41:41–46
35. Courcoutsakis NA, Prassopoulos PK, Patronas NJ (2009) Aggressive leptomeningeal hemangioblastomatosis of the central nervous system in a patient with von Hippel-Lindau disease. AJNR Am J Neuroradiol 30(4):758–760
36. Smith AB, Rushing EJ, Smirniotopoulos JG (2010) From the archives of AFIP. lesions of the pineal region: radiologic-pathologic correlation. Radiographics 30:2001–2020
37. Shin JH, Lee HK, Khang SK et al (2002) Neuronal tumors of the central nervous system: radiographic findings and pathologic correlation. Radiographics 22(5):1177–1189
38. Derrey S, Proust F, Debono B et al (2004) Association between Cowden syndrome and Lhermitte-Dulcos disease: report of two cases and review of the literature. Surg Neurol 61(5):447–454
39. Yako K, Nakazato Y, Hirato J et al (2005) Dysplastic ganglioneurocytoma with increased glucose metabolism: a heterotopia with unique histopathology. Clin Neuropathol 24(6):267–270
40. Patronas NJ, (2011) Brain metastasis. In: Drevelegas A (ed) Imaging of brain tumors with histological correlations, vol 13. Springer, New York, pp 373–400
41. Patronas NJ, Makariou E (1993) MRI of choroid plexus involvement in intracranial cryptococcosis. J Comput Assist Tomogr 17(4):547–550
42. Jelinek J, Smirniotopoulos JG, Parisi JE et al (1990) Lateral ventricular neoplasms of the brain: differential diagnosis based on the clinical, CT and MRI findings. AJR Am J Roentgenol 155(2): 362–372
43. Smith AB, Smirniotopoulos JG, Horkanyne-Szakaly I (2013) From the radiologic pathology archives Intraventricular neoplasms: radiologic-pathologic correlation. Radiographics 33:21–43

17 Diagnostic Issues in Treating Brain Tumors

Nicholas J. Patronas

Our approaches in managing patients with brain neoplasm have been modified in recent years. The recognition that the length of survival or even the possibility of cure depends on the completeness of tumor resection, has led to modification in our operative approaches. Many centers specializing in the treatment of brain tumors have installed MRI scanners within the operating room and perform intraoperative MRI scanning during various stages of the surgical procedure. The intraoperative scans include an isotropic 3D post contrast T1-weighted technique that presents the enhancing part of the tumor in three orthogonal planes. In non-enhancing low grade gliomas, a 3D FLAIR technique can best demonstrate the tumor margins and provides guidance for an appropriate surgical resection. Although tumor cells may have infiltrated the surrounding normal appearing brain parenchyma, the goal of the operation is to remove the visible part of the tumor thus diminishing the tumor burden. During the first 24 hours following surgery, a pre-and postcontrast scan is also obtained for a more accurate documentation of any residual tumor which serves as a baseline for comparison with future studies. This early postoperative scan is important to differentiate residual tumor from enhancing reactive/granulation tissue formation in the wall of the surgical cavity, which is known to develop within a few days after surgery. Furthermore, the early postoperative scan is important to document any complication that may have occurred during or immediately after surgery, such as hemorrhage or ischemic infarction. Either of these two abnormalities will clinically present with deterioration in the neurologic deficits. Hemorrhagic complications can occur in the immediate postoperative period, but also in the course of medical treatment that includes antivascular/antiangiogenic agents. Small ischemic lesions are commonly found near the wall of the surgical cavity and have no clinical significance. Larger ischemic infarctions may occur as a result of endovascular thrombus, arterial spasm, or mechanical occlusion of an arterial branch. An ischemic infarction during the subacute stage will show abnormal enhancement near the surgical bed, which can be mistaken for tumor progression. Such infarctions are best evaluated by a diffusion weighted scan, showing restricted diffusion within minutes after the vascular occlusion (Fig. 17.1). The term pseudoprogression has been adopted to describe such a complication. The phenomenon of pseudoprogression is also encountered in the cases of primary or metastatic brain tumors treated with stereotactic radiosurgery. In the weeks following this type of treatment, there is reactive tissue developing in the tumor area that presents with increase enhancement and a broader zone of edema, producing a false

N. J. Patronas (✉)
Neuroradiology Section, Radiology and Imaging Sciences, National Institute of Health, Bethesda, USA
e-mail: npatronas@cc.nih.gov

A. D. Gouliamos et al. (eds.), *Imaging in Clinical Oncology*,
DOI: 10.1007/978-88-470-5385-4_17,

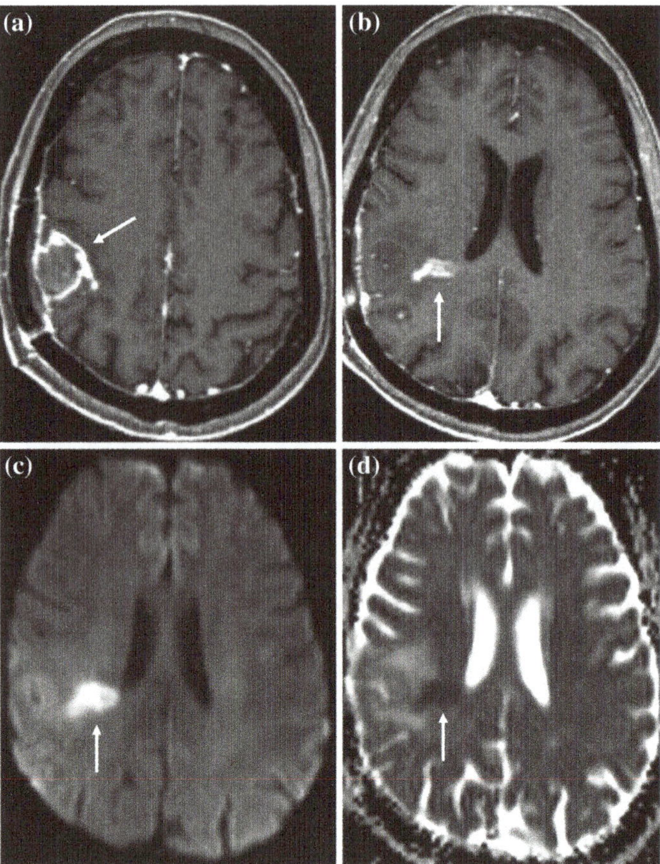

Fig. 17.1 Pseudoprogression: Two axial postcontrast scans of the brain show a postoperative cavity (*arrow*) in the *right* cerebral hemisphere following resection of a glioma (**a**). There is also noted a new area of abnormal enhancement medially to the postoperative cavity (*arrow*) raising the question of recurrent tumor (**b**). Diffusion weighted image (**c**) and ADC map (**d**) shows restricted diffusion in the new enhancing abnormality (*arrows*). This was proven to be an acute ischemic infarction

impression of continuous tumor growth. Past experience in managing these patients has shown that after a variable period of time, which may be up to a few months, there is gradual resolution of the enhancement and only then the beneficial results of radiosurgery become apparent.

On other occasions, tumors that have received focal radiation treatments, with or without chemotherapy, may develop abnormal increase enhancement in the tumor bed followed by breakdown of tissue and cavity formation. This is another treatment-related complication known as radiation necrosis which usually develops within about 2 years after such treatment. Radiation-related necrotic lesions become progressively larger with time exhibiting persistent enhancement within the lesion and increased edema in the adjacent normal brain, both recognized as features of tumor progression. The complication of radiation necrosis may be encountered more frequently in patients who besides radiation therapy also received anti angiogenetic medications. This may be related to the effect both these therapies have in the tumor vessels. The importance of distinguishing true tumor progression from pseudoprogression is obvious since radiation necrosis is compatible with long-term survival whereas tumor progression has a dismal prognosis. Positron emission tomography with FDG has been the method of choice to support

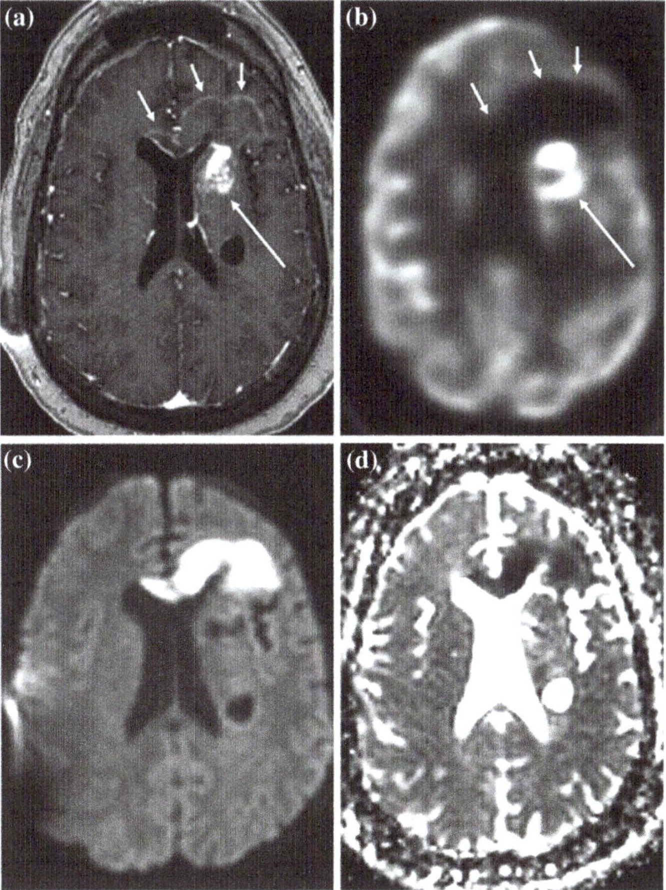

Fig. 17.2 Recurrent glioma associated with radiation necrosis: Axial postcontrast MRI scan of the brain (**a**) shows an abnormal area of increased enhancement in the left basal ganglia (*long white arrow*). This abnormality demonstrates increased metabolic activity on FDG/PET (**b**) indicative of a recurrent high grade tumor (*long white arrow*). A second abnormality is also present in the left frontal lobe which is cavitary and presents with a thin rim of enhancement (*white thin arrows*) in its periphery (**a**). This abnormality extends into the genu of the corpus callosum and shows no metabolic activity on the PET scan (**b**). This second lesion was proven to be radiation necrosis. Diffusion weighted image (**c**) and ADC map (**d**) shows markedly restricted diffusion within the necrotic area

the diagnosis of radiation necrosis, showing decreased metabolic activity in the pathological area [1, 2]. The opposite is true in the case of recurrent or residual tumor. It should be noted however that necrotic areas and persistent viable or recurrent tumor may coexist in different regions of the tumor bed [3]. More recently, diffusion weighted images have also provided a valuable clue to the diagnosis of radiation necrosis. It has been shown that the necrotic areas have increased viscosity and typically demonstrate restricted diffusion. Although a rapidly growing brain tumor can also show restricted diffusion due to increased cellularity, measurements of diffusivity on apparent diffusion coefficient (ADC) maps can separate tissue necrosis from viable tumor with the former showing more severe restriction in diffusion (Fig. 17.2).

Besides DWI, perfusion studies are currently underway in evaluating tissues in the tumor bed that appear to be growing on conventional MRI after treatment. As expected, the early results of such studies indicate that the capillary density and capillary permeability are different in

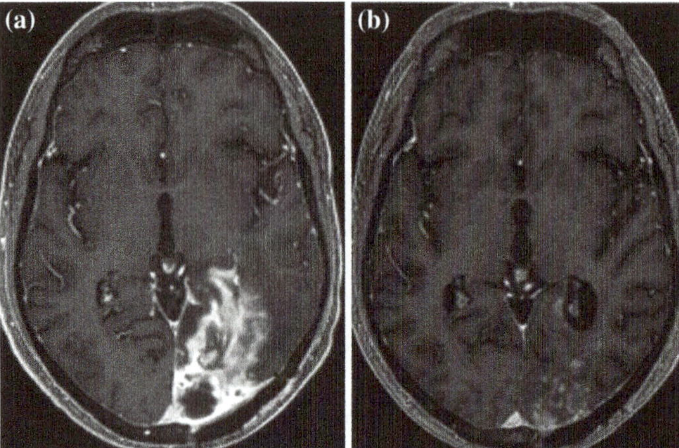

Fig. 17.3 Pseudoresponse: Axial postcontrast MRI scans of the brain. There is a large enhancing glioblastoma in the left occipital lobe prior to treatment (**a**). Patient was subsequently treated with conventional chemotherapy, steroids and an antiangiogenic agent. On follow-up scan 2 months later (**b**) there is marked reduction of the area and degree of enhancement. The apparent improvement is due to partial repair of the blood-brain barrier

recurrent neoplasms as compared to the treatment-related abnormalities.

Another question that is often raised during the posttreatment period is whether resolution or decrease of tumor enhancement is due to successful response to treatment or whether we are dealing with pseudoresponse. The phenomenon of pseudoresponse is most often encountered in patients in whom steroids are included in the treatment regimen. It is well known that steroids repair the BBB and diminish extravasations of both water and injected contrast agents from the endovascular to the interstitial space. This results in decreasing enhancement and edema in and around the tumor area providing a false evidence of good response to chemotherapy. The encouraging imaging findings are accompanied by improvement of the clinical symptoms during the period that follows initiation of such treatments. These beneficiary results are usually short lived as evidenced by the reappearance of the enhancement and deterioration of the clinical symptoms when steroids are not any longer effective in repairing the disruptions of the BBB. It should be noted, however, that the events that take place in the case of primary CNS lymphomas treated only with steroids are different. Lymphomatous cells are actually destroyed by steroids resulting in real reduction of the tumors size. Since steroids do not represent a definitive and completely effective treatment of CNS lymphoma without other chemotherapy drugs, the early good results do not last and in a relatively short period the tumor will reappear.

The phenomenon of pseudoresponse can also be observed in patients treated with antivascular/antiangiogenic agents that are often included in the treatment regimen. These agents are known to constrict tumor vessels which results in decrease extravasations of the contrast. Thus, similar to steroids, antivascular agents provide a false impression of response to treatment (Fig. 17.3). The experience of the last few years has shown that although the patient's symptoms and the quality of life are improved with these treatments the overall survival has not been significantly altered.

The presence of a cavity within a brain tumor is a common finding. Such cavity may be due to previous surgery and partial tumor resection or it may be secondary to spontaneous tumor necrosis. Observations of the behavior of tumor cavities are often useful in determining the behavior of the tumor in time. Increasing size of the cavity

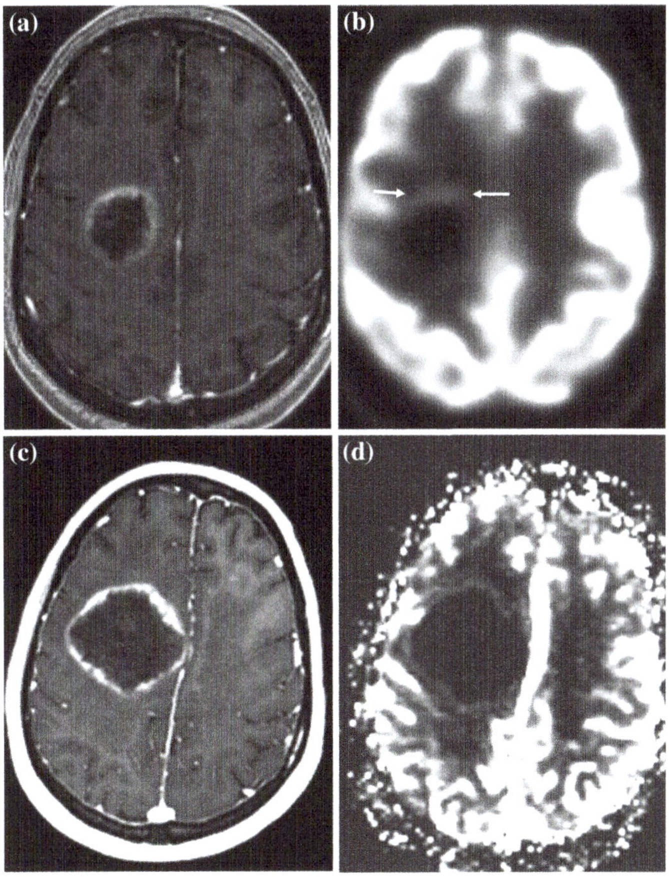

Fig. 17.4 Progressive enlargement of a cavity in brain tumors: a poor prognostic sign. Axial postcontrast scan (**a**) shows a cavitary mass with a rim of peripheral enhancement. Axial FDG/PET at the same level (**b**) shows increased metabolic activity in the anterior wall of the cavity (*arrows*) when compared to the opposite normal white matter. This indicates the presence of viable tumor. A repeat postcontrast scan 3 months later (**c**) shows enlargement of the cavity but the thickness of the enhancing rim is unchanged. A perfusion scan (**d**) shows increased blood volume in the wall of the cavity consistent with viable tumor

with an associated rim of enhancement represents an ominous feature of tumor progression, even when the thickness of the enhancing rim remains thin and stable overtime (Fig. 17.4). The opposite is true when the size of the cavity is decreasing. Another problem that can be encountered in postoperative cavities is the development of a linear enhancement inside the cavity. This may be interpreted as tumor recurrence . Such enhancement when shown to be connected to the leptomeninges and the dura on the surface of the brain is more likely to represent granulation tissue rather that recurrent tumor.

In conclusion we have identified a variety of diagnostic problems that can take place in the course of treatment of brain tumors. Accurate diagnosis of the complications and correct assessment of the effectiveness of the chosen treatment at the earliest possible time are critical for the proper management of these patients.

References

1. Patronas NJ, Di Chiro G, Brooks RA et al (1982) [18F]Fluorodeoxyglucose and positron emission tomography in the evaluation of radiation necrosis of the brain. Radiology 144:885–889
2. Di Chiro G, Oldfield E, Wright DC et al (1987) Cerebral necrosis after radiotherapy and/or intra-arterial chemotherapy for brain tumors: PET and neuropathological studies. AJNR. 8:1083–1091
3. Alexiou GA, Tsiouris S, Kyritsis AP et al (2009) Glioma recurrence versus radiation necrosis: Accuracy of current imaging modalities. J Neurooncol 95:1–11

18 Tumors of the Spinal Cord and Spinal Canal

Athanasios D. Gouliamos and Nicholas J. Patronas

The discussion of the tumors in the spinal canal is simplified by dividing the tumors that occur within the cord and tumors that are located outside the cord but within the thecal sac. Thus, the terms intramedullary and intradural-extramedullary tumors are widely used to describe these abnormalities [1].

Ependymomas are the most common intramedullary tumors in the cord usually originating from ependymal cells of the central canal and the filum terminale. They are most commonly located in the cervical segment of the cord or near the conus extending into the lumbar canal. The intraparenchymal ependymomas are relatively benign tumors classified as grade II. A more aggressive variety can also be encountered and is classified as anaplastic grade III. In their usual presentation, intramedullary ependymomas are well circumscribed round or elongated tumors which enhance on the post contrast scan and are clearly demarcated from the adjacent normal cord. Edema is also found in the cord parenchyma which is proportional to the size and the histologic grade of the tumor. Syrinx can also occur in the normal segment of the cord and is thought to be caused by obstruction of the central canal (Fig. 18.1).

The variety of ependymomas that originate in the conus medullaris and the proximal filum terminale are recognized for their specific histological features and are known as myxopapillary. Myxopapillary ependymomas are usually grade II tumors and present as a multinodular enhancing mass that project from the distal end of the cord into the lumbar canal and incorporating roots of the cauda equina [2–4].

An unusual type of ependymoma has been described in patients with NF2. These tumors are usually small in size and often multiple. They are located in close proximity to the central canal of the cord and enhance intensely on post contrast MRI scans. These tumors are known to be related a subtype of mutation of NF2 patients and have a benign course demonstrating no significant change in size over a period of many years [5–7].

Astrocytomas are the second most common primary tumors of the cord. Four different histologic grades are recognized. Pilocytic, fibrillary, anaplastic, and glioblastomas. The pilocytic are well circumscribed and have good prognosis if successfully removed by surgery. Firbillary are grade II tumors, have a tendency to infiltrate the cord and are not well demarcated from the adjacent cord parenchyma. The anaplastic astrocytomas and the glioblastomas are also infiltrative tumors and have the worse prognosis. Astrocytomas are most commonly found in the cervical cord but occasionally can

A. D. Gouliamos (✉)
Radiology, National and Kapodistrian University of Athens-Aretaieio Hospital, 76, Vas. Sophias Avenue, 11527 Athens, Greece
e-mail: agouliam@med.uoa.gr

N. J. Patronas
Neuroradiology, National Institute of Health, 9000 Rockville Pike, Bethesda, MD 20892, USA
e-mail: npatronas@cc.nih.gov

A. D. Gouliamos et al. (eds.), *Imaging in Clinical Oncology*,
DOI: 10.1007/978-88-470-5385-4_18, © Springer-Verlag Italia 2014

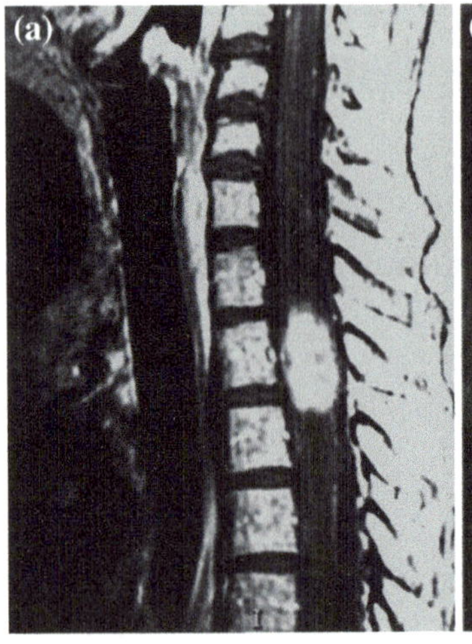

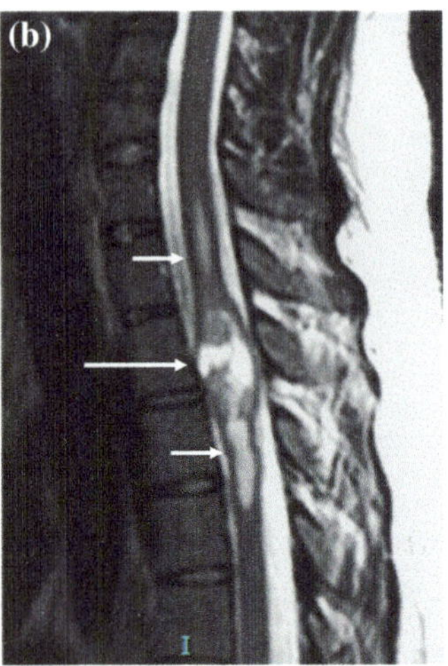

Fig. 18.1 Cord ependymoma. Axial post contrast T1-weighted MRI scan of the spine (**a**) shows an enhancing tumor within the cord parenchyma. The tumor has well defined margins. T2-weighted scan (**b**) demonstrates cystic changes within the tumor (*long horizontal arrow*). There is also evidence of small syrinx both proximately and distally to the tumor (*short arrows*)

infiltrate long segments of the cord in both cervical and thoracic regions. Furthermore, these tumors do not always enhance on post contrast scans and when they do, the enhancement is heterogeneous or it may not extend throughout the entire tumor parenchyma. Therefore, the true margins of the tumor do not always coincide with the area of enhancement. It is for these reasons that complete surgical resection of infiltrative astrocytomas is not often possible. An interesting observation with regards to enhancement is that, unlike the gliomas of the brain, the presence of enhancement in these tumors is not always a sign of high grade malignancy. Another frequent imaging finding of the astrocytomas of the cord is the presence of cavitation within the tumor parenchyma. This is caused by tissue necrosis, which sometimes is rather extensive giving the appearance of syringomyelia. The distinction between these two conditions is rather easy since the necrotic tumor presents with irregular, ragged and nodular inner margins whereas the inner wall of syringomyelia is smooth showing only thin, web-like septations, incompletely subdividing the cavity of the syrinx. Cord astrocytomas with or without tumorous cavitation are occasionally accompanied by benign cysts in the proximal or the distal end of the tumor (Fig. 18.2). A syrinx located within the normal segment of the cord can also be found in some cases. The exact mechanism of syrinx formation is not known, but it may be related to obstruction of the central canal by the tumor or it is caused by disturbance of the bidirectional CSF flow in the subarachnoid space during the two phases of the cardiac cycle [2, 8, 9].

Hemangioblastomas of the cord are also well recognized intramedullary tumors and can be found in patients of the general population, but these tumors represent a common abnormality in patients with Von Hippel Lindau disease . Although hemangioblastomas can originate from vessels within the cord, they often develop from vessels of the leptomeninges on the surface of the cord and later invaginate into its parenchyma. The imaging features of cord hemangioblastomas are similar to those described in the cerebellum. When they are small in size, the tumor is well circumscribed and demonstrates homogeneous enhancement. As they grow bigger, the tumors produce edema in the cord parenchyma. Eventually, the molecules of the extravasated fluid coalesce and form a cavity that increases the overall mass effect and invariably contributes to the patient's symptomatology. Since there are no

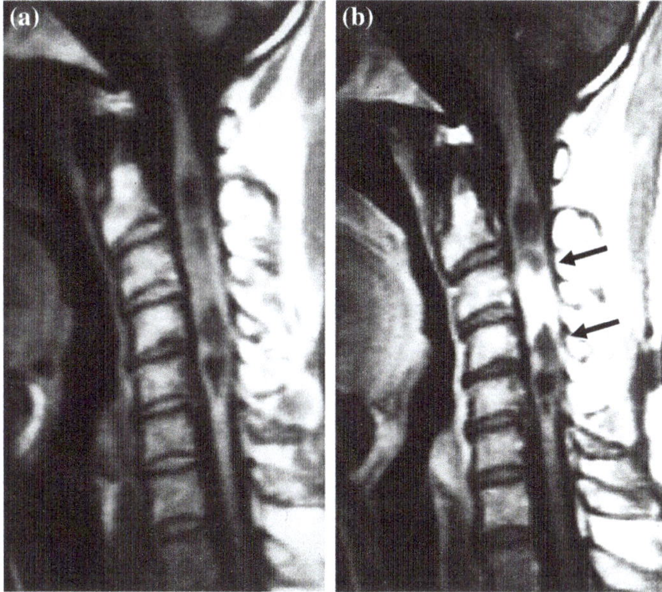

Fig. 18.2 Cord astrocytoma. Sagittal T1-weighted scan of the cervical spine (**a**) shows an expansile mass within the cord at C2-C6 level with cystic areas. Sagittal T1-weighted post contrast image (**b**) shows prominent contrast enhancement of the solid component of the mass with infiltrative margins (*black arrows*)

tumor cells in the wall of the cyst, as in the case of cerebellar hemangioblastomas, during surgery the enhancing nodule is removed while the cavity collapses on its own requiring no excision [10–12].

Hemangioblastomas are often multiple and can also be found in the lumbar canal, originating from leptomeningeal vessels around the cauda equina. The multiplicity of these tumors is not caused by seeding of cells from an existing tumor, as it is the case in meningeal carcinomatosis, but is the result of independent cell mutations in each tumor location. The hemangioblastomas are very vascular tumors and this is a finding that becomes very apparent on post contrast MRI scans demonstrating large draining veins coursing on the ventral and the dorsal aspect of the cord. The prominent vascular pattern can serve as a distinct imaging feature to differentiate hemangioblastomas from schwannomas, neurofibromas or metastatic tumors.

Metastatic tumors within the cord are relatively rare lesions. They are best demonstrated on post contrast MRI scans where they present with mass effect and increased focal enhancement. These imaging features are not unique in metastatic tumors and cannot be used to distinguish metastasis from other intramedullary masses. A clue that an enhancing cord tumor is due to metastasis is provided by finding associated abnormal leptomeningeal enhancement. Unlike intraparenchymal cord metastasis which is a rare phenomenon, meningeal carcinomatosis from primary or metastatic brain tumors is more common complication and is best demonstrated on post contrast T1-weighted technique. The meningeal involvement by metastatic cancer presents with thin linear enhancement on the cord surface or along the roots of the cauda equine. The term "sugar coating" has been used to describe the appearance of this type of tumor metastasis (Fig. 18.3). It should be noted however that this pattern of linear enhancement can also be encountered in cases of leptomeningeal inflammation. The patient's medical history and the analysis of CSF are indispensible in guiding the physicians toward the correct diagnosis. Other rare tumors within the cord parenchyma include oligodendrogliomas with imaging characteristics similar to fibrillary astrocytomas. Neurocytomas, paragangliomas and lymphomas have also been found in the spinal canal and are not easily diagnosed preoperatively. Finally, lipomas are readily identified benign tumors by CT and MRI due to distinct imaging features of fatty tissue [13–19]).

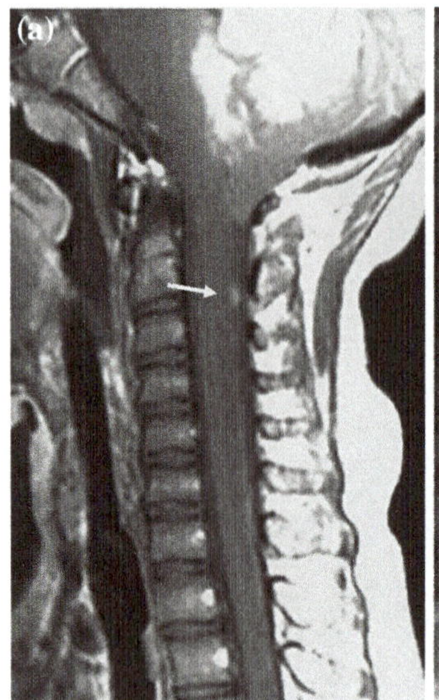

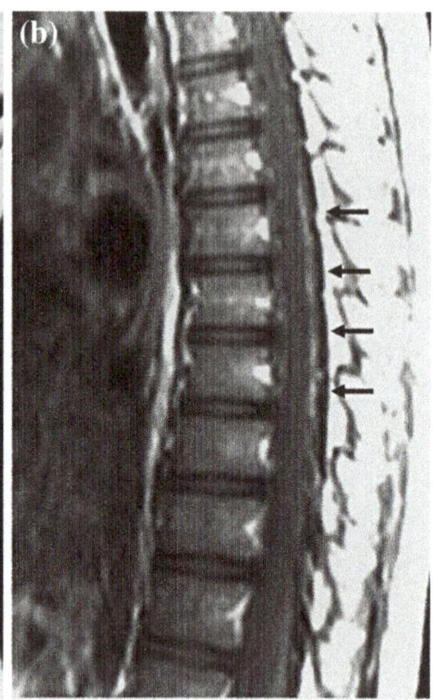

Fig. 18.3 Leptomeningeal metastases in the spinal canal: Sagittal post contrast images of the cervical (**a**) and thoracic (**b**) spine reveal abnormal enhancement in the leptomeninges on the dorsal aspect of the cord (*white arrow in a and black arrow in b*). The enhancing tumor in the posterior fossa (a) was shown to be a medulloblastoma

Neurofibromas and schwannomas are among the most common extramedullary intradural tumors of the spinal canal. It is generally known that these tumors meet the histologic criteria neurofibromas when found in patients with neurofibromatosis 1 and schwannomas when they occur in patients with neurofibromatosis 2. Regardless of the histology, the tumors of the spinal nerves are round masses and enhance homogeneously on post contrast scans. The round contour of the tumor touching the inner dural surface forms an acute angle which is a feature useful in distinguishing neurofibromas and schwannomas from meningiomas. Spinal canal nerve tumors grow slowly and often compress the cord when they are located in the cervical or in the thoracic segment of the spinal canal. Because the cord compression takes place slowly, over a long period of time, symptoms of myelopathy do not usually develop for many years. Large tumors that originate from the roots of the cauda equina cause symptoms from compression of the spinal nerves in the lumbar canal but small neurofibromas and schwannomas can be asymptomatic throughout life.

Another variety of spinal nerve tumors are those found within the neuroforamina of the spinal canal. They are primarily extradural and have a bilobular configuration (dumbbell tumors) with part of the tumor projecting into the paraspinal soft tissues and part into the spinal canal. The intracanalicular component of these spinal nerve tumors can cause compression of the cord and spinal nerves. Both schwannomas and neurofibromas in that location are also slowly growing tumors but often enlarge the neural foramina by chronic and sustained bone erosion.

Spinal canal meningiomas have distinct imaging features, which are identical to those described in the intracranial variety. These tumors enhance after intravenous contrast and the degree of enhancement is inversely proportional to the amount of calcium deposition in their parenchyma. The flat surface of dural attachment and the dural tail are always found in at least one of the imaging planes (Fig. 18.4). Similar to other extramedullary intradural tumors, meningiomas can compress the cord and often require surgical excision [1]. Chronic cord compression,

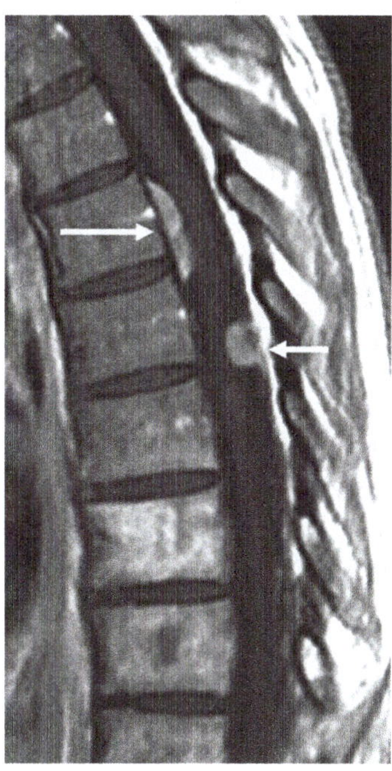

Fig. 18.4 Meningiomas in the spinal canal: Sagittal post contrast T1-weighted scan of the thoracic spine. There are two meningiomas, one ventrally (*long white arrow*) and one dorsally (*short white arrow*) to the cord. Both tumors have a flat surface of dural attachment and enhance homogeneously

regardless of the tumor type, can lead to edema within its parenchyma which can be reversed after surgical resection of the tumor. Chronic cord edema caused by untreated tumors compressing the cord eventually results in myelomalacia, with an irreversible neurologic deficit.

References

1. Abul-Kasim K, Thurnher MM, McKeever P et al (2008) Intradural spinal tumors: current classification and MRI features. Neuroradiology 50:301–314
2. Mechtler LL, Nandigam K (2013) Spinal cord tumors: new views and future directions. Neurol Clin 31(1):241–268
3. Smith JK, Lury K, Castillo M (2006) Imaging of the spinal and spinal cord tumors. Semin Roentgenol 41:274–293
4. Wippold FJ, Smirniotopoulos JG, Moran CJ et al (1995) MR imaging of myxopappillary ependymoma: findings and value to determine extend of tumor and its relation to intraspinal structures. AJR Am J Roentgenol 165(5):1263–1267
5. Patronas N, Courcoutsakis N, Bromley CM et al (2001) Intramedullary and spinal canal tumors in patients with neurofibromatosis 2: MR imaging findings and correlation with genotype. Neuroradiol 128:434–442
6. Plotkin SR, O'Donnell CC, Curry WT et al (2001) Spinal ependymomas in neurofibrosis type 2: a retrospective analysis of 55 patients. J Neurosurg Spine 14:543–547
7. Parry DM, Eldridge R, Kaiser-Kupfer MI et al (1994) Neurofibromatosis 2 (NF2): clinical characteristics of 63 affected individuals and clinical evidence of heterogeneity. Am J Med Genet 52:450–461
8. Koeller KK, Rosenblum RS, Morison AL (2000) Neoplasms in the spinal cord and the filum terminale: radiologic-pathologic correlation. Radiographics 20:1721–1749
9. Smith AB, Soderlund KA, Rushing EJ et al (2012) Radiologic-pathologic correlation of pediatric and adolescent spinal neoplasms: part 1 intramedullary and spinal neoplasms. AJR Am J Roentgenol 198:34–43
10. Wanebo JE, Lonser RR, Glenn GM et al (2003) The natural history of hemangioblastomas of the central nervous system in patients with von Hippel-Lindau disease. J Neurosurg 98:82–94
11. Choyke PL, Glenn GM, Patronas N et al (1995) Von Hippel Lindau disease: genetic clinical and imaging features. Radiology 194:629–642
12. Filling-Katz MR, Choyke PL, Oldfield E et al (1991) Central nervous system involvement in von Hippel Lindau disease. Neurol 41:41–46
13. Fountas KN, Karampelas I, Nikolakakos LG et al (2005) Primary spinal cord oligodendroglioma: case report and review of the literature. Childs Nerv Syst 21:171–175
14. Jallo GI, Freed D, Epstein FJ (2004) Spinal cord gliogliomas: a review of 56 patients. J Neurooncol 68:71–77
15. Faro SH, Turtz AR, Koenigsberg RA et al (2005) Paraganglioma of the cauda equina with associated intramedullary cyst. AJNR Am J Neuroradiol 18:1588–1590
16. Vassiliou V, Papamichael D, Polyviou P et al (2012) Intramedullary spinal cord metastasis in a patient with colon cancer. J Gastointenst Cancer 43:370–372
17. Sung WS, Sung MJ, Chan JH et al (2012) Intramedullary cord metastasis: a 20-year institutional experience with comprehensive literature review. World Neurosurg 2012 [Epub ahead of print]
18. Flanagan EP, O'Neill BP, Porter AB et al (2011) Primary intramedullary spinal cord lymphoma. Neurology 77:784–791
19. Bhatoe HS, Singh P, Chaturvedi A et al (2005) Nondysraphic intramedullary spinal cord lipomas: a review. Neurosurg Focus 18:ECP1

19 Advanced MRI Techniques in Brain Tumors

Stefanos V. Lachanis

Brain tumors are a significant health problem. The annual incidence of primary and secondary central nervous system neoplasms ranges from 10 to 17 per 100,000 persons.

Imaging plays a significant role in intracranial tumor management. Brain tumor treatment without the use of neuroimaging is difficult to imagine in the present era. The role of neuroimaging, particularly magnetic resonance imaging (MRI), can be broadly divided into tumor diagnosis and classification, treatment planning and post-treatment assessment and surveillance. Today, imaging is not limited in providing anatomic details and evaluating tumor complications. In addition to conventional MRI techniques, a variety of advanced MRI techniques are currently in clinical use and are the subject of intense research. These advanced techniques provide functional, hemodynamic, metabolic, cellular and cytoarchitectural information, transforming clinical MR imaging into a comprehensive tool that combines structure with function and physiology. The aims of this article are to provide a summary of established and potential applications of advanced MRI techniques in imaging of brain tumors. The detailed description of the various techniques is beyond the scope of this work.

S. V. Lachanis (✉)
Director MRI Department, 401 General Army Hospital, Athens, Greece
e-mail: steflach61@gmail.com

S. V. Lachanis
Director CT-MRI Department, Iatropolis Medical Center, Athens, Greece

19.1 Perfusion Imaging

The association between angiogenesis and tumor growth and grading is well established. Perfusion methods are indicators of tumor angiogenesis, which is new vessel formation required for tumor growth. There is an increase in vessel diameter, vessel wall thickness, vessel number (microvascular density) and altered vascular permeability in brain tumors. The degree of vascular proliferation is one of the histologic criteria for the determination of the degree of malignancy and grade of gliomas. Perfusion methods have potential applications in diagnosis and staging, determining patient prognosis, predicting which patients respond to a particular treatment and evaluating treatment efficacy.

1. Predicting glioma grade. Conventional MRI with Gd contrast agent provides excellent anatomic imaging of gliomas, but grading is unreliable. Results of many dynamic susceptibility contrast (DSC) perfusion studies suggest that relative cerebral blood volume (rCBV) measurements may improve grading as high-grade gliomas show increased rCBV in comparison with low-grade gliomas. rCBV can be used to predict glioma grade, patient outcome and time to progression, independent of pathologic findings [1]. Longitudinal

A. D. Gouliamos et al. (eds.), *Imaging in Clinical Oncology*,
DOI: 10.1007/978-88-470-5385-4_19, © Springer-Verlag Italia 2014

MR perfusion studies of low-grade gliomas show earlier increase of rCBV in cases of malignant transformation prior to clinical or imaging transformation. rCBV can help identify patients with low-grade gliomas at risk for malignant transformation that might benefit from early aggressive therapy [2]. MR DSC perfusion and spectroscopy can be used to target stereotactic biopsies from the most malignant part of gliomas.

2. Differential diagnosis. Perfusion helps to distinguish high-grade gliomas from lymphomas. Lymphomas have lower rCBV than high-grade gliomas because of the absence of tumor neovascularization. Time signal intensity curves often show an increase above the baseline, following the initial decrease in brain lymphomas. Perfusion may be useful in differentiating high-grade gliomas from solitary metastases. High-grade gliomas tend to have higher rCBV in the peritumoral region than metastases. Perfusion is useful in differentiating tumefactive demyelinating lesions (TDLs) from high-grade gliomas. TDLs show significantly lower rCBV than high-grade gliomas.
3. Post-therapeuting monitoring. The differentiation of radiation-induced necrosis and pseudoprogression after radiotherapy-Temozolamide from recurrent or residual tumor is challenging on conventional MRI. Pathologically often the two entities co-exist. Many studies show that increased rCBV favors tumor recurrence over radiation necrosis but there is a degree of overlap between these two entities. The use of a multiparametric approach that incorporates MR perfusion imaging techniques, diffusion and diffusion tensor imaging (DTI) techniques and spectroscopy adds diagnostic accuracy in differentiating radiation necrosis from recurrent tumor. Advanced neuroimaging methods in pseudoprogression have not yet fully validated but preliminary findings suggest a decrease in rCBV and increase in vascular permeability. A study comparing rCBV before and 1 month after radiotherapy-Temozolomide showed mean increase of 12 % in patients with true progression and decrease of 41 % in patients with pseudoprogression [3].

19.2 MR Spectroscopy

The main metabolites of proton (^{1}H) MR spectrum are choline (Cho), N-acetyl-aspartate (NAA), creatine (Cr), lactate, lipids, and myoinositol. NAA is a neuronal marker and is decreased when tumor cells destroy or displace normal neurons. Cho is a marker of cell membrane turnover and is increased in tumors. Cr is a marker of energy metabolism and, in the clinical setting, is assumed to be stable. Lactate indicates anaerobic glycolysis and is increased in high-grade gliomas and in necrotic-cystic tumors. Lipids are elevated in high-grade tumors, while they are absent in low-grade gliomas. Myoinositol is increased in low-grade gliomas and gliomatosis cerebri. The main clinical applications of MR spectroscopy (MRS) in brain tumors are summarized below [4]:

1. Distinguishing neoplastic from non-neoplastic conditions. MRS can help distinguish tumors from infarcts, cortical dysplasias or encephalitis. The finding of increased Cho makes tumor more likely although there are not clear cut-off values. Acute tumefactive demyelinating plaques may mimic high-grade gliomas. A ratio of Cho/NAA over 2.2 can differentiate high-grade tumors from low-grade tumors and non-neoplastic conditions. The integration of MRS with the other advanced MRI techniques described in this paper may help to improve MRS accuracy.
2. Distinguishing necrotic tumor from abscess. Proton spectra from brain abscess are different from those of high-grade tumors. Abscesses have low Cho, decreased NAA and Cr, and often exhibit compounds such as alanine, acetate, succinate and others. Tumors can exhibit increased Cho in the enhancing rim and peritumoral area.
3. Predicting glioma grade. Whether MRS is useful for grading of gliomas or not still remains controversial. In general, higher Cho/NAA and Cho/Cr ratios suggest a faster

growing neoplasm and a higher tumor grade. Accumulation of lipids or lactate, sometimes associated with Cho decrease, is often seen in hypoxic-necrotic high-grade tumors. Despite many spectroscopic studies indicating high diagnostic accuracy in glioma grading, the possibility that spectroscopy may replace tissue diagnosis and grading is remote.

4. Predicting survival. The ability of MRS to predict survival has been evaluated in both adult and pediatric gliomas. Some studies have indicated that high Cho/NAA ratio and the combined lactate or lipid signal are associated with a higher risk of poor outcome in patients with high-grade gliomas. In patients with gliomatosis cerebri the Cho/Cr ratio has inverse relatioship to survival. Another study showed that increased Cr in low-grade gliomas was predictor of malignant transformation and decreased survival.
5. Tumor recurrence vs radiation necrosis. Increased Cho signal relative to Cho in normal brain is suggestive of recurrence, while significantly reduced Cho levels are indicative of radiation necrosis.
6. Guiding biopsy. MRS can be used to guide biopsy from the most aggressive part of the tumor. Regions with high Cho and Cho/NAA ratio represent good targets for biopsy. In general, regions with increased angiogenesis, vascular permeability and metabolic activity should be sampled.
7. Radiation therapy planning. MRS is valuable to target volumes for radiotherapy. Magnetic resonance spectroscopic imaging (MRSI) may provide complementary and more specific information about the location of active tumor than morphological MRI and can be incorporated in the planning process.

19.3 Diffusion-Weighted Imaging (DWI)

1. DWI and glioma grade. Cellularity, one of the histologic features of glioma grading, has been the target of quantitative assessment with DWI. Several reports have shown that glioma grade correlates inversely with the apparent diffusion coefficient (ADC), likely on the basis of increasing cellularity with grade [5]. However the role of DWI is debated because of the overlap of ADC values between different grades of gliomas. A recent study showed that ADC measurements are better than rCBV values for distinguishing the grade of gliomas, and the combination of minimal ADC and maximal rCBV improves the diagnostic accuracy of glioma grading [6].
2. DWI and non-glial tumors. ADC values have also correlated with cellularity of non-glial tumors. Lymphomas have lower ADC than gliomas. Malignant or atypical meningiomas have lower ADC than grade-1 meningiomas. Pineal cell tumors have lower ADC than germ-cell tumors. Medulloblastomas have lower ADC than pilocytic astrocytomas.
3. DWI and postoperative injury. Immediate postoperative DWI may show areas of restricted diffusion as a result of ischemia and surgical trauma. These areas may enhance on later MRI scans simulating recurrent tumor.

19.4 Functional MRI (fMRI) and Diffusion Tensor Imaging (DTI)

The goal of surgery in brain tumors is to maximize tumor resection and to avoid adjacent eloquent brain structures, because their injury can cause profound neurologic deficits. The eloquent brain can be identified using fMRI for cerebral cortex and DTI for white matter tracts. fMRI can aid planning the surgical approach, assessing surgical risks and maximizing tumor resection [7]. Mapping of the somatotopic motor cortex is the most frequently used presurgical fMRI protocol in patients with perirolandic or central tumors. Paradigms should include finger, toe and tongue movements to localize the motor homunculus in relation to the tumor. Furthermore, fMRI can guide direct electrical cortical stimulation, which is considered the gold standard technique for functional mapping. fMRI helps to identify the foot-leg motor cortex that is, otherwise, difficult to identify

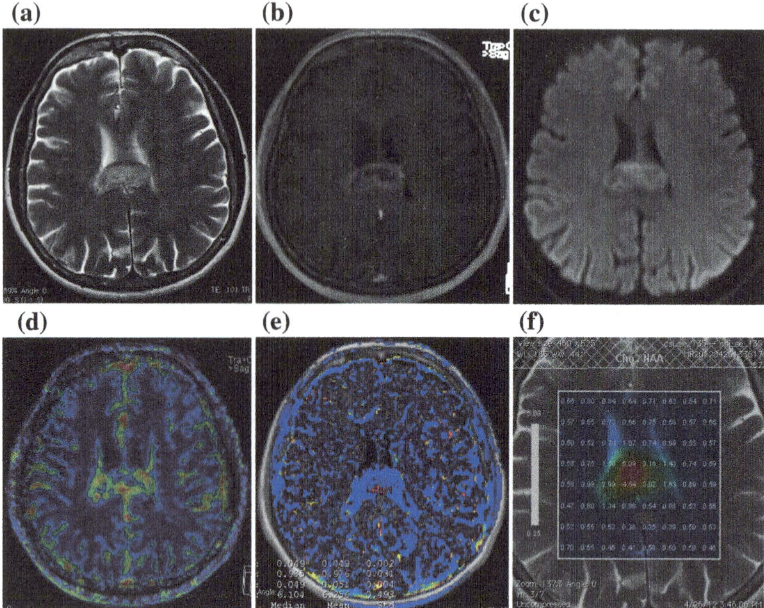

Fig. 19.1 T_2-w shows a mass with moderately increased signal at the posterior body of corpus callosum (**a**), with peripheral enhancing rim (**b**). The lesion shows moderate diffusion restriction on DWI (**c**), increased rCBV with a ratio of 5.2 compared to healthy contralateral (**d**), increased k_{trans} 0.049 s^{-1} on permeability imaging (**e**). Spectroscopic map of Cho/NAA shows maximum value of 5.1(**f**). Biopsy proved glioblastoma multiforme

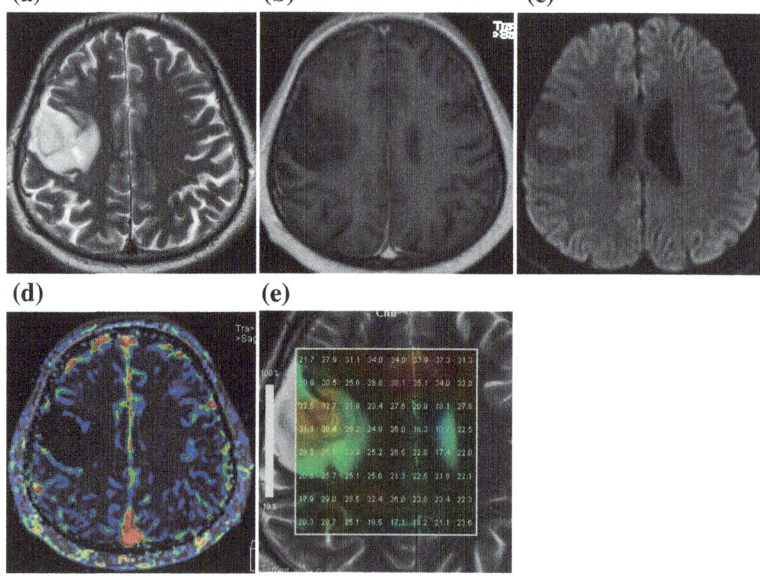

Fig. 19.2 T2-w shows mass with homogeneous increased signal at the posterior right frontal lobe (**a**), with no enhancement (**b**). There is no diffusion restriction on DWI (**c**), and no areas of increased rCBV (**d**). Spectroscopic map of Cho shows moderate increase of Cho (**e**). Biopsy proved Grade two oligoastrocytoma

because of its deep location. The aims of presurgical language fMRI include localizing Broca and Wernicke speech areas in relationship to brain tumors or epileptogenic zones and identifying the language dominant hemisphere. Language fMRI is more complex in comparison to motor fMRI for various reasons (less predictable and complex cortical representation, reorganization, various

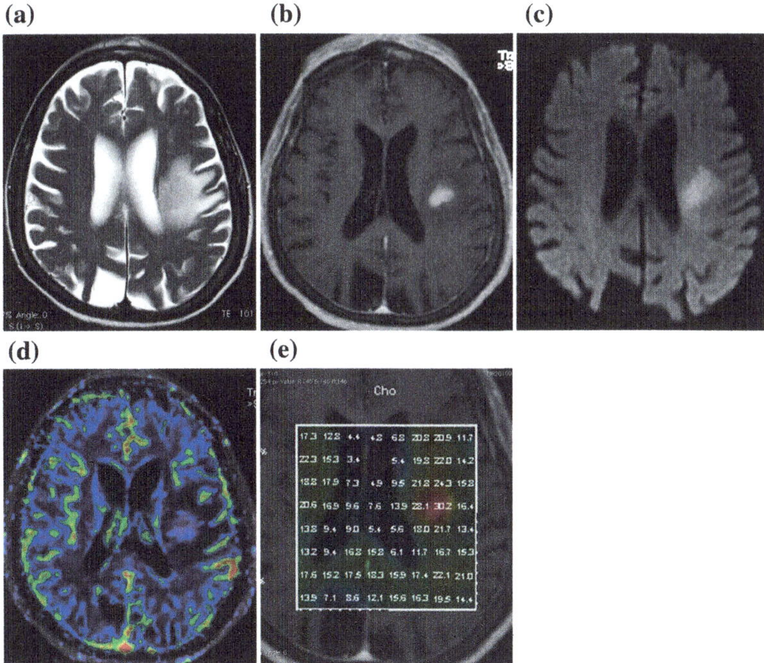

Fig. 19.3 T2-w shows a slightly heterogeneous lesion at the posterior left centrum semiovale (**a**), with homogeneous central enhancement (**b**). There is restricted diffusion on DWI (**c**) with an ADC value of 0.71×10^{-3} mm^2/s, and a moderate increase of rCBV of 2.1 compared to healthy contralateral (**d**). Spectroscopic map of Cho shows moderate increase of Cho. Biopsy proved primary lymphoma of the brain

linguistic components, complex paradigms and methodological issues).

DTI is the only non-invasive method to localize white matter tracts. This is important for brain tumor surgery, where an injury to an eloquent tract may result in serious neurologic deficits. Preoperative DTI tractography can be used to guide the surgical approach and intraoperative stimulation. Several studies have shown that tractography has a role in assessing the deviation, deformation, infiltration or interruption of white matter tracts around brain tumors.

19.5 Integration of Conventional and Advanced MRI Techniques

The integration of advanced MRI techniques with conventional MRI can further improve tumor classification accuracy. A study proposed a diagnostic MRI-based algorithmic approach to differentiate intraaxial brain masses, specifically low-grade from high-grade neoplasms, neoplasms from non-neoplastic disease, and high-grade gliomas and lymphomas from other intraaxial masses. Initial results suggested that intraaxial brain masses could be differentiated with 85–90 % accuracy by using this approach [8]. Another study, integrating preoperative anatomic and physiologic imaging, identified that these data are valuable in characterizing newly diagnosed gliomas and provide information about tumor heterogeneity that may be important assisting the surgeon to obtain representative histology [9]. Examples of multiparametric approach in diagnosis of brain tumors are shown for a glioblastoma multiforme (Fig. 19.1), for a low-grade oligoastrocytoma (Fig. 19.2), and for a primary lymphoma of the brain (Fig. 19.3).

19.6 Summary

MRI is the most valuable imaging modality for imaging of brain tumors but conventional MRI has significant limitations. Neuroimaging of brain tumors today has evolved to more complex studies incorporating perfusion and diffusion MR imaging, and MR spectroscopy. These advanced MRI techniques have become an essential part of the diagnostic armamentarium to diagnose, guide therapy, monitor therapy response, and predict prognosis of patients with brain tumors.

References

1. Law M, Young RJ, Babb JS et al (2008) Gliomas: predicting time to progression or survival with cerebral blood volume measurements at dynamic susceptibility-weighted contrast-enhanced perfusion MRI. Radiology 247:490–498
2. Danchaivijitr N, Waldman AD, Tozer DJ et al (2008) Low-grade gliomas: do changes in rCBV measurements at longitudinal perfusion-weighted MRI predict malignant transformation? Radiology 247:170–178
3. Mangla R, Singh G, Ziegelitz d et al (2010) Changes in relative cerebral blood volume 1 month after radiation-temozolomide therapy can help predict overall survival in patients with glioblastoma. Radiology 250:887–896
4. Horska A, Barker PB (2010) Imaging of brain tumors: MR spectroscopy and metabolic imaging. Neuroimag Clin N Am 20:293–310
5. Cha S (2006) Update on brain tumor imaging: from anatomy to physiology. AJNR 27:475–487
6. Hilario A, Ramos A, Perez-Nunez a et al (2012) The added value of apparent diffusion coefficient to cerebral blood volume in the preoperative grading of diffuse gliomas. AJNR 33:701–707
7. Gupta A, Shah A, Young RJ et al (2010) Imaging of brain tumors: functional magnetic resonance imaging and diffusion tensor imaging Neuroimag Clin N Am 20:379–400
8. Al-Okaili R, Krejza J, Woo JH et al (2007) Intraaxial brain masses: MR imaging-based diagnostic strategy-initial experience. Radiology 243:539–550
9. Chang SM, Nelson S, Vandenberg S et al (2009) Intergration of preoperative anatomic and metabolic physiologic imaging of newly diagnosed glioma. J Neurooncol 92:401–415

20 PET/CT: Is There a Role?

Julia V. Malamitsi

20.1 Introduction

The best anatomic study of brain tumors is acquired by conventional Magnetic Resonance Imaging (MRI). By offering metabolic information, Positron Emission Tomography (PET) has been extensively used in the study of brain tumors. Co-registration of PET with MRI data is nowadays possible, either by software fusion of PET/CT images with MR images or on integrated PET/MR tomographs. This concise review will focus mainly on gliomas, because they represent the majority of primary brain tumors, and on brain metastases from other malignancies, which are more common than primary brain tumors.

20.2 Radiopharmaceuticals

Radiopharmaceuticals used for brain tumor imaging are markers of Glucose metabolism, amino acid transport, proliferation rate, membrane synthesis and hypoxia. Molecular imaging tracers are being developed to select patients for targeted therapies. Besides, somatostatin receptor analogues like [68 Ga]-DOTATOC have been used for cranial meningiomas [1].

Glucose metabolism: 2-[18F] fluoro-2-deoxy-D-glucose (FDG) the most frequently used radiopharmaceutical for PET is taken up by 3–6 % of low grade and 21–47 % of high grade gliomas [2]. FDG is taken up by normal brain tissue, a fact that compromises the detection and delineation of an adjacent brain tumor, and by inflammatory cells. FDG uptake correlates with tumor cell density, grading and malignancy of the tumor.

Amino acid transport: Radiolabelled amino acids being a marker of amino acid transport are increased in malignant transformation, therefore they are taken up by both high and low grade gliomas, and to a minor degree by normal brain tissue. [11C]methionine ([11C]MET), [18F]fluorethyltyrosine([18F] FET) [3] and [18F]fluorodopa ([18F]DOPA) [4] are the most widely used amino acids.

Proliferation Rate: Proliferation markers are taken up by both high and low grade gliomas. [18F]fluorothymidine (FLT), a marker of DNA replication is an index of malignant transformation and therefore of tumor progression and therapy response [5]. FLT is practically not taken up by normal brain tissue, due to low neuronal cell division and intact Blood Brain Barrier (BBB).

Membrane synthesis: [18F]fluorocholine, an index of cell membrane biosynthesis and hence of cell proliferation has been used in distinguishing malignant from benign brain lesions [6].

Hypoxia: [18F]fluoromisonidazole [18F]FMISO shows a high uptake in high grade and not low grade gliomas. Its metabolites are trapped

J. V. Malamitsi (✉)
Medical Physics, Medical School, University of Athens, 75 Mikras Asias, Goudi, 115 27 Athens, Greece
e-mail: j.malamitsi@yahoo.gr

A. D. Gouliamos et al. (eds.), *Imaging in Clinical Oncology*,
DOI: 10.1007/978-88-470-5385-4_20, © Springer-Verlag Italia 2014

exclusively in hypoxic cells. Hypoxia may drive the peripheral growth of glioblastoma. Combined with MRI, images of hypoxia may reveal areas of tumor neoangiogenesis, which are radioresistant and thus help individualize treatment [7].

New tracers: Radiolabelled with PET tracers antisense oligonucleotides, small chains of nucleic acids, have been used to trace specific mRNA in vivo and hence any endogenous gene for imaging and treatment purposes [8]. Antibodies and peptides are eligible ligands for imaging gliomas. 18F-RGD peptides are currently used on a preclinical but also a clinical level for $\alpha v\beta 3$ integrin expression, in order to monitor response to antiangiogenic treatment or to detect early recurrence. [9, 10]. Recently a novel small molecule tracer for apoptosis [18F]-ML-10 has been used to monitor response to radiation therapy of brain metastases [11].

20.3 Role of PET/CT in Primary Brain Tumors

CT and conventional MRI cannot differentiate malignant from benign lesions, especially in cases of anaplastic tumors without contrast enhancement, and recurrence of the tumor from radiation necrosis, given the prolonged period (months or years) of contrast enhancement of the irradiated area. The role of PET/CT in the management of brain tumors is about the following:

20.3.1 Identification of Tumor-Grading-Prognosis

FDG is taken up mainly by high grade tumors and anaplastic areas of low grade tumors [12, 13]. In low grade tumors on repeat FDG scans, newly appearing areas of increased FDG uptake must be interpreted as areas of anaplastic transformation and therefore of higher grading and worse prognosis. The uptake of FDG by inflammatory cells makes differentiation between neoplastic and non neoplastic lesions difficult. In contrast to FDG all amino acid tracers are taken up by both low and high grade gliomas. A comparison between FDG and MET has shown that, by reflecting the biology of gliomas MET PET is more accurate than FDG PET in identifying active tumors [14]. Tumor uptake of FDOPA is similar to that of MET [15]. FET PET detects anaplastic foci and can differentiate histologically grade II from grade III within the same lesion, when dynamic analysis is applied [16]. On a metaanalysis on 462 patients with a newly diagnosed brain lesion, FET PET, used for initial assessment prior to treatment, demonstrated a pooled sensitivity of 0.82 and specificity of 0.76 respectively [17]. Although FDG uptake in brain tumors has prognostic significance, (Fig. 20.1) the most reliable prognostic information is given by FLT PET [18] (Fig. 20.2). Kaplan-Meier curves show that a negative FLT PET scan shows an excellent survival, whereas a positive scan goes along with a fast declining curve. Increased amino acid uptake in remnant glioma tissue goes along with worse survival [19].

20.3.2 Biopsy Guiding

MRI/CT biopsy guidance may be misleading in cases of high grade gliomas and anaplastic astrocytomas when contrast enhancement on gadolinium T1, necessary for stereotactic biopsy, is absent [20], as well as in cases of low grade gliomas with peritumoral edema and contrast enhancement [21]. As brain tumors can be heterogeneous, PET is able to define the most malignant area for a biopsy specimen, and help select anaplastic specimens on previously characterized as low grade gliomas. For stereotactic biopsy, microsurgery and radiotherapy purposes, neuronavigation relies on fusion of MRI/CT with PET, diffusion tensor imaging (DTI), and functional MRI (fMRI) data. FDG is better in selecting site for stereotactic biopsy compared with CT or MRI alone [22], but worse than amino acids especially in low grade gliomas. Although amino acids are useful in biopsy planning and patient selection, they are not adequate to replace histology to assess recurrence or progression.

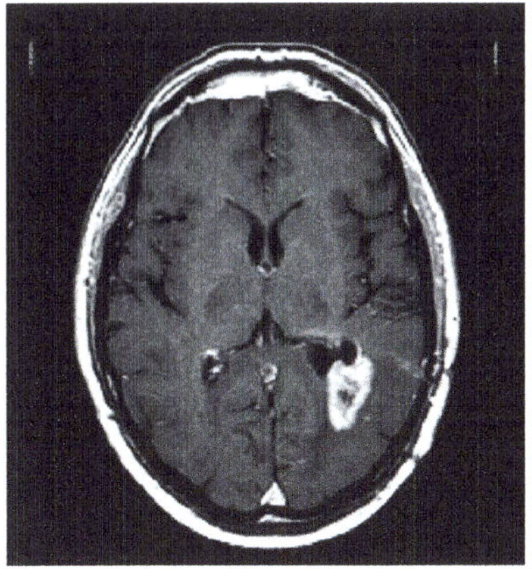
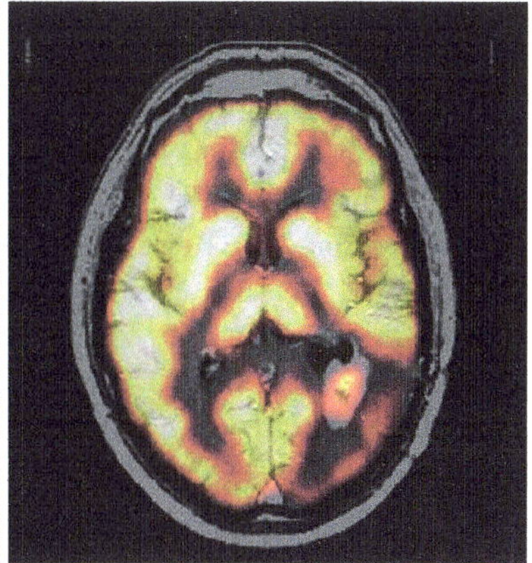

Fig. 20.1 Glioblastoma multiforme in the left parietal lobe post surgery and chemo- radiotherapy. The treated area appears on MRI as contrast enhanced (*left*) and on FDG PET co-registered with MRI as hypermetabolic (*right*), suggestive of recurrence. The patient died 4 months after the PET/CT study. (Courtesy of Dr V. Prassopoulos)

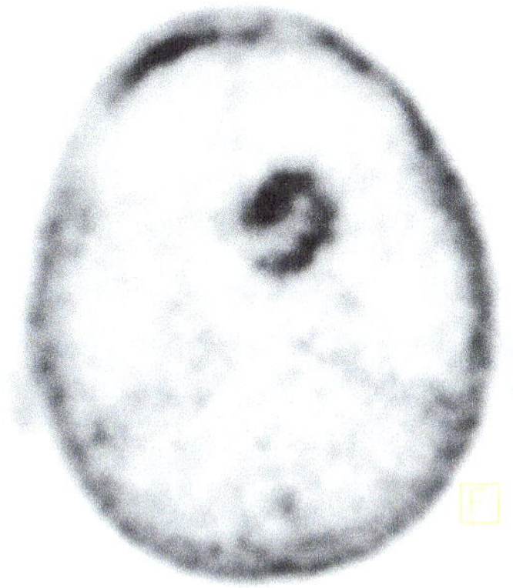
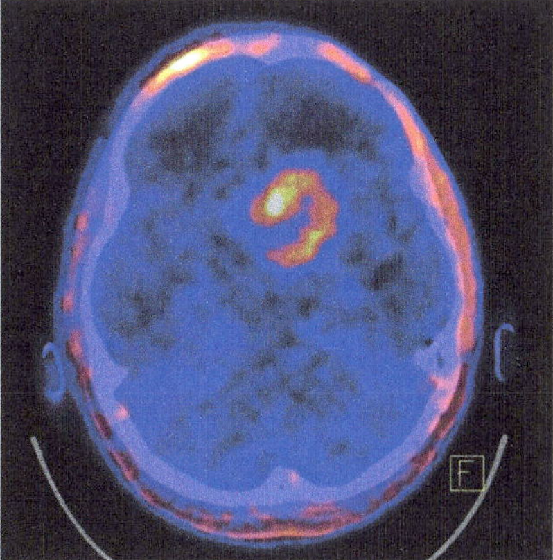

Fig. 20.2 FLT uptake in the left frontal lobe, suggestive of recurrent tumor in the treated area of a glioblastoma. FLT PET (*left*) and FLT PET/CT (*right*) (Courtesy of Dr V. Prassopoulos)

20.3.3 Radiation Therapy Planning

PET data are valuable in all forms of radiotherapy planning i.e. stereotactic radiotherapy, radiosurgery, intensity modulated radiotherapy and brachytherapy because they reveal tumor biology. Biological tumor volume (BTV) based on PET imaging has been proposed for radiotherapy planning since Morphological Gross Tumor Volume (GTV) does not cover adequately the area of the tumor [23]. BTV is promising in sparing normal tissue, reducing toxicity, and better defining the target volume, therefore it has been suggested to identify areas for conformal boost [24]. Treatment planning based on amino acid PET combined with CT/MRI was associated with improved survival than when CT/MRI were used alone [25].

20.3.4 Treatment Monitoring

With multimodality therapy strategies available i.e. surgery, radiotherapy, chemotherapy and novel treatments, early assessment of response is necessary. Whereas with MRI and CT it takes weeks or months to show tumor response to treatment, contrast enhancing lesions on post-treatment MRI cannot be attributed to tumor necrosis or tumor recurrence [26]. Magnetic Resonance Spectroscopy and PET are eligible for this discrimination [27]. Differentiation of recurrence from radiation necrosis with FDG has given a variable sensitivity (40–90 %) and specificity (40–80 %) respectively [2]. Since radiolabelled amino acid tracers are not taken up by inflammatory cells, they are more eligible to discriminate recurrence or progression from adverse radiation effects. FET PET with dynamic data analysis has a sensitivity 100 % and a specificity 93 % in discriminating the two entities [28]. Changes in FLT kinetic parameters early during treatment are a criterion of the efficacy of the applied therapy [29]. Since FLT uptake is BBB breakdown dependent, FLT should only be used to evaluate high proliferating tumors and not for treated low grade gliomas with disrupted BBB.

Effectiveness of new therapeutic agents in gliomas such as antivascular endothelial like growth factor receptor-1 antibody bevacizumab and topoisomerase I inhibitor irinotecan has been evaluated by FLT PET; the metabolic response as assessed by FLT PET was a better predictor of survival than gadolinium contrast MRI response [30]. Besides FET PET and dynamic analysis might help to monitor new treatment modalities like antibody bevacizumab [31]. 18F-Fluciclatide, an 18F-Labeled $\alpha v\beta 3$-Integrin and $\alpha v\beta 5$-Integrin imaging agent has been used to monitor tumor response to antiangiogenic Sunitinib Therapy [32].

20.4 Role of PET/CT in Brain Metastases

PET has been used post chemo/radiotherapy of the whole brain or stereotactic radiosurgery, to discriminate between radiation necrosis and tumor recurrence, since this is not possible on the basis of CT and MRI. FDG PET has been used extensively to differentiate tumor recurrence from radiation necrosis of brain metastases (Fig. 20.3). Dual phase FDG PET differentiates the two entities in a more reliable manner [33].Cerebral metastases are mostly associated with high amino acid uptake, therefore differentiation between recurrence and necrosis is preferable with them. Additionally, due to its low uptake by normal brain, FLT has been used to assess presence of brain metastases [34] (Fig. 20.4).

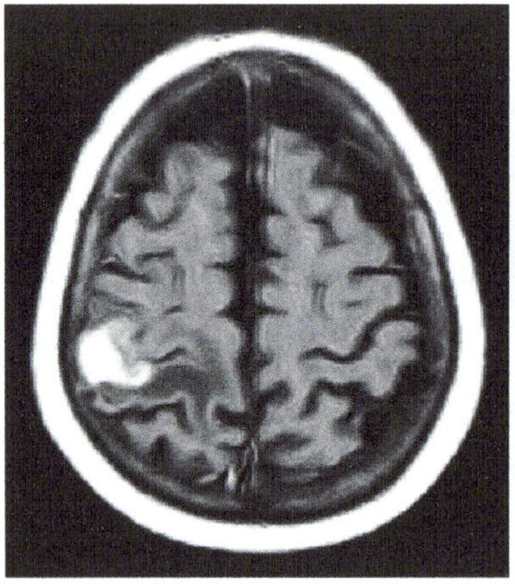

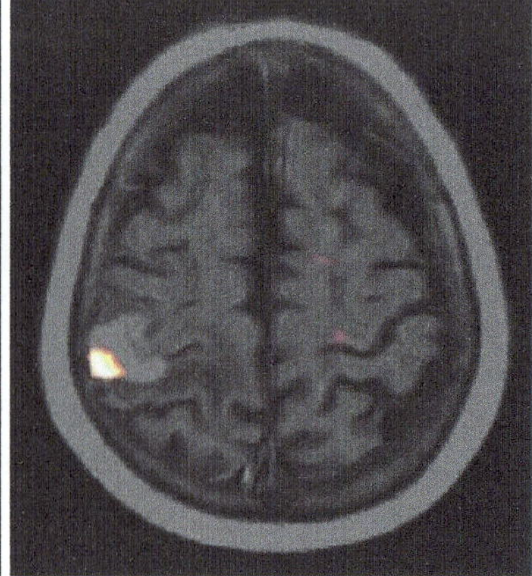

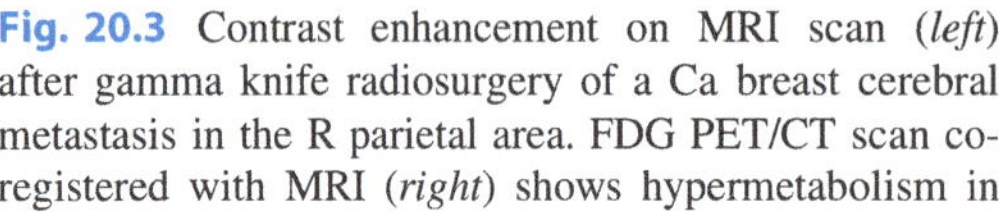

Fig. 20.3 Contrast enhancement on MRI scan (*left*) after gamma knife radiosurgery of a Ca breast cerebral metastasis in the R parietal area. FDG PET/CT scan co-registered with MRI (*right*) shows hypermetabolism in the treated area, suggestive of recurrence. Physiological uptake by normal brain tissue has been suppressed for better distinction of the hypermetabolic lesion (Courtesy of Dr. V. Prassopoulos)

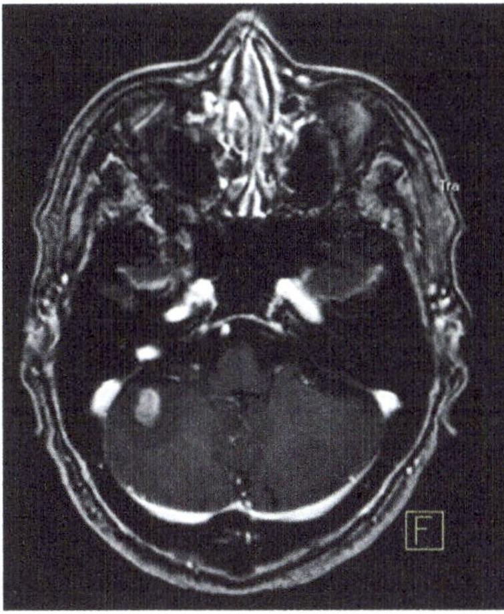

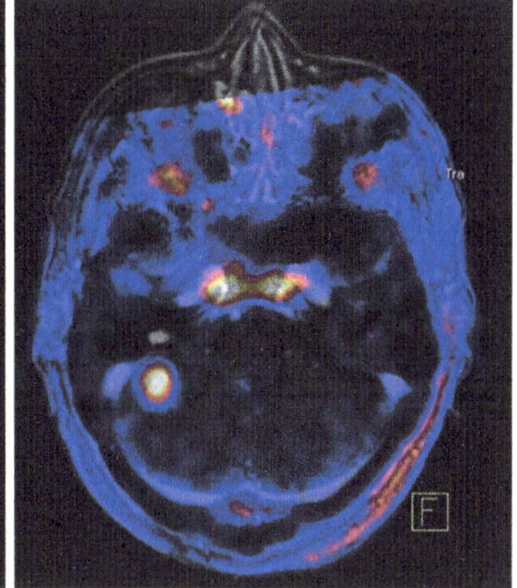

Fig. 20.4 MRI (*left*) shows contrast enhancement of a brain metastasis in the right cerebellum, treated with gamma knife radiosurgery. FLT PET/CT co-registered with MRI shows hypermetabolism in the contrast enhanced area, suggestive of tumor recurrence (Courtesy of Dr V. Prassopoulos)

20.5 Conclusions

Concerning brain tumors FDG PET is useful in grading and prognosis, but not as good as FLT PET, which predicts reliably tumor progression and survival. Amino acids are the preferred PET tracers for stereotactic biopsy guidance, surgical and radiotherapy treatment planning, differentiation between radiation necrosis and recurrence as well as for detection of low grade gliomas. FMISO is promising in detecting radioresistant areas, which need additional treatment.

References

1. Afshar-Oromieh A, Giesel FL, Linhart HG et al (2012) Detection of cranial meningiomas: comparison of 68 Ga-DOTATOC PET/CT and contrast enhanced MRI. Eur J Nucl Med Mol Imaging 39:1409–1415
2. La Fougère C, Suchorska B, Bartenstein P et al (2011) Molecular imaging of gliomas with PET: opportunities and limitations. Neuro-Oncology 13:806–819
3. Heiss P, Mayer S, Herz M et al (1999) Investigation of transport mechanism and uptake kinetics of O-(2-[18F]fluoroethyl)-L-tyrosine in vitro and in vivo. J Nucl Med 40:1367–1373
4. Chen W, Silverman DH, Delaloye S et al (2006) 18F-FDOPA PET imaging of brain tumors: comparison study with 18F-FDG PET and evaluation of diagnostic accuracy. J Nucl Med 47:904–911
5. Chen W, Cloughesy T, Kamdar N et al (2005) Imaging proliferation in brain tumors with 18F-FLT PET: comparison with 18F-FDG. J Nucl Med 46:945–952
6. Kwee SA, Ko JP, Jiang CS et al (2007) Solitary brain lesions enhancing at MR imaging: evaluation with fluorine18 fluorocholine PET. Radiology 244:557–565
7. Swanson KR, Chakraborty G, Wang CH et al (2009) Complementary but distinct roles for MRI and 18F-fluoromisonidazole PET in the assessment of human glioblastomas. J Nucl Med 50:36–44
8. Lendvai G, Estrada S, Bergström M et al (2009) Radiolabelled oligonucleotides for imaging of gene expression with PET. Curr Med Chem 16:4445–4461
9. Battle MR, Goggi JL, Allen L et al (2011) Monitoring tumor response to antiangiogenic sunitinib therapy with 18F-fluciclatide, an 18F-labeled αvbeta3-integrin and αvbeta5-integrin imaging agent. J Nucl Med 52:424–443
10. Iagaru A, Mosci E, Mittra S et al (2012) $\alpha v\beta 3$ integrins as a biomarker of disease recurrence in glioblastoma multiforme: initial clinical results using 18F FPPRGD2 PET/CT. Eur J Nucl Med Mol Imaging 39(2):S244–S245 (abstract)
11. Allen AM, Ben-Ami M, Reshef A et al (2012) Assessment of response of brain metastases to radiotherapy by PET imaging of apoptosis with 18F-ML-10. Eur J Nucl Med Mol Imaging 39:1400–1408
12. Goldman S, Levivier M, Pirotte B et al (1997) Regional methionine and glucose uptake in high-grade gliomas: a comparative study on PET-guided stereotactic biopsy. J Nucl Med 38:1459–1462

13. Yamaguchi S, Kobayashi H, Hirata K et al (2011) Detection of histological anaplasia in gliomas with oligodendroglial components using positron emission tomography with (18)F-FDG and (11)C-methionine: report of two cases. J Neurooncol 101:335–341
14. Pirotte B, Goldman S, Massager N et al (2004) Comparison of 18F-FDG and 11C-methionine for PET-guided stereotactic brain biopsy of gliomas. J Nucl Med 45:1293–1298
15. Becherer A, Karanikas G, Szabó M et al (2003) Brain tumour imaging with PET: a comparison between [18F]fluorodopa and [11C]methionine. Eur J Nucl Med Mol Imaging 30:1561–1567
16. Kunz M, Thon N, Eigenbrod S et al (2011) Hot spots in dynamic (18)FET-PET delineate malignant tumor parts within suspected WHO grade II gliomas. Neuro Oncol 13:307–316
17. Dunet V, Rossier C, Buck A et al (2012) Performance of 18F-fluoro-ethyl-L-tyrosine (18F-FET) PET for the differential diagnosis of primary brain tumor: a systematic review and Metaanalysis. J Nucl Med 53:207–214
18. Chen W, Cloughesy T, Kamdar N et al (2005) Imaging proliferation in brain tumors with 18F-FLT PET: comparison with 18F-FDG. J Nucl Med 46:945–952
19. Nariai T, Tanaka Y, Wakimoto H et al (2005) Usefulness of L-[methyl-11C] methionine-positron emission tomography as a biological monitoring tool in the treatment of glioma. J Neurosurg 103:498–507
20. Barker FG 2nd, Chang SM, Huhn SL et al (1997) Age and the risk of anaplasia in magnetic resonance-nonenhancing supratentorial cerebral tumors. Cancer 80:936–941
21. Law M, Yang S, Wang H et al (2003) Glioma grading: sensitivity, specificity, and predictive values of perfusion MR imaging and proton MR spectroscopic imaging compared with conventional MR imaging. AJNR Am J Neuroradiol 24:1989–1998
22. Pirotte BJ, Lubansu A, Massager N et al (2007) Results of positron emission tomography guidance and reassessment of the utility of and indications for stereotactic biopsy in children with infiltrative brainstem tumors. J Neurosurg 107:392–399
23. Ling CC, Humm J, Larson S et al (2000) Towards multidimensional radiotherapy (MD-CRT): biological imaging and biological conformality. Int J Radiat Oncol Biol Phys 47:551–560
24. Lee IH, Piert M, Gomez-Hassan D et al (2009) Association of 11C-methionine PET uptake with site of failure after concurrent temozolomide and radiation for primary glioblastoma multiforme. Int J Radiat Oncol Biol Phys 73:479–485
25. Grosu AL, Weber WA, Franz M et al (2005) Reirradiation of recurrent high-grade gliomas using amino acid PET (SPECT)/CT/MRI image fusion to determine gross tumor volume for stereotactic fractionated radiotherapy. Int J Radiat Oncol Biol Phys 63:511–519
26. Brandsma D, Stalpers L, Taal W et al (2008) Clinical features, mechanisms, and management of pseudoprogression in malignant gliomas. Lancet Oncol 9:453–461
27. Shah R, Vattoth S, Jacob R et al (2012) Radiation necrosis in the brain: imaging features and differentiation from tumor recurrence. Radiographics 32:1343–1359
28. Rachinger W, Goetz C, Pöpperl G et al (2005) Positron emission tomography with O-(2-[18F]fluoroethyl)-L-tyrosine versus magnetic resonance imaging in the diagnosis of recurrent gliomas. Neurosurgery 57:505–511 (discussion 505–511)
29. Wardak M, Schiepers C, Dahlbom M et al (2011) Discriminant analysis of ^{18}F-fluorothymidine kinetic parameters to predict survival in patients with recurrent high-grade glioma. Clin Cancer Res 17:6553–6562
30. Chen W, Delaloye S, Silverman DH et al (2007) Predicting treatment response of malignant gliomas to bevacizumab and irinotecan by imaging proliferation with [18F] fluorothymidine positron emission tomography: a pilot study. J Clin Oncol 25:4714–4721
31. Galldiks N, Rapp M, Stoffels G et al (2012) Response assessment of bevacizumab in patients with recurrent malignant glioma using [(18)F]Fluoroethyl-L-tyrosine PET in comparison to MRI. Eur J Nucl Med Mol Imaging 2012 [Epub ahead of print]
32. Battle MR, Goggi JL, Allen L et al (2011) Monitoring tumor response to antiangiogenic sunitinib therapy with 18F-fluciclatide, an 18F-labeled αvbeta3-integrin and αV beta5-integrin imaging agent. J Nucl Med 52:424–430
33. Horky LL, Hsiao EM, Weiss SE et al (2011) Dual phase FDG-PET imaging of brain metastases provides superior assessment of recurrence versus post-treatment necrosis. J Neurooncol 103:137–146
34. Dittmann H, Dohmen BM, Paulsen F et al (2003) [18F]FLT PET for diagnosis and staging of thoracic tumours. Eur J Nucl Med Mol Imaging 30:1407–1412

21 Clinical Implications of Brain Tumors

Panagiotis V. Nomikos and Ioannis S. Antoniadis

21.1 Diagnosis

Cerebral metastases are the most common brain tumor in clinical practice since up to 40 % of all patients with a history of cancer will develop metastatic lesions in the brain. Therefore, all cancer patients should undergo an imaging investigation of the brain in regular time intervals which must not exceed, in most cases, 6 months. Additionally, all cancer patients with new neurological symptoms or progressive neurological deficits should promptly perform an imaging of the relevant parts of the central nervous system.

The principal modality for this is MRI. Although CT is cheaper, faster, and easier to perform, it has, in general, a lower screening, diagnostic, and treatment planning value compared to the MRI unless the suspected lesion affects or destroys bone structures- this is the case with most spine metastases- or has prominent calcifications. Iodine contrast enhanced CT of the brain can detect fast growing tumors such as high grade gliomas and metastases but still has the disadvantage of inferior tissue differentiation and anatomical definition compared to MRI, especially in the posterior fossa. Most brain metastases appear in the MRI as well circumscribed, enhancing lesions located at the gray-white matter junction, causing intense edema. More than 70 % of all patients with brain metastases have multiple lesions. Differential diagnoses include astrocytoma (especially high grade glioma), abscess, and non-specific inflammatory reaction.

Distinguishing a high grade primary brain neoplasm from a solitary metastatic lesion is not always an easy task but physiology-based MRI sequences can provide a certain aid. Low apparent diffusion coefficients (ADCs) measured in diffusion-weighted MRI (DWI) are a sign of high tumor cellularity and primary neoplasms infiltrating the surrounding brain parenchyma tend to have lower values in the peritumoral area compared to cerebral metastases. Perfusion MRI (PWI) shows also lower relative cerebral blood volume (rCBV) measurements outside the enhancing portion of the lesion in secondary neoplasms. MRS interrogation in the same areas that shows choline/NAA ratios greater than 1 has an excellent sensitivity for primary brain tumors [1].

Primary brain tumors are most often of glial origin. Low grade gliomas (LGG) are typically solitary lesions, hypointense on T1 weighted MRI images and a diffuse growth pattern on T2 weighted images. Thirty percent of LGGs show contrast enhancement. High grade gliomas (grades III–IV) are complex or ring enhancing lesions and frequently present with a central cyst or necrosis. DWI and MRS have not shown great

P. V. Nomikos (✉) · I. S. Antoniadis
Department of Neurosurgery and Gamma Knife Radiosurgery, Hygeia Hospital, Erythrou Stavrou 4, Marousi 15123, Greece
e-mail: pnomikos@hygeia.gr

I. S. Antoniadis
e-mail: iantoniadis@hygeia.gr

A. D. Gouliamos et al. (eds.), *Imaging in Clinical Oncology*,
DOI: 10.1007/978-88-470-5385-4_21, © Springer-Verlag Italia 2014

clinical value in tumor grading of gliomas, but increased rCBV values in PWI are suggestive of HGG with the exception of tumors with a oligodendrocytic component that present with high rCBV values regardless of tumor grade [2].

Primary CNS lymphoma usually presents as a homogenously enhancing, well circumscribed, lobar or periventricular lesion. Multiple lesions exist in up to 30 % of primary CNS lymphoma patients. Elevated choline, lipid and lactate signals, and reduced NAA signal in MRS are typical for brain lymphoma and can help differentiate it from toxoplasmosis in AIDS patients. Lymphomas also tend to have lower ADC and rTBV values in DWI and PMRI compared to gliomas [1, 3].

Tumor mimicking lesions such as tumeffactive demyelinating lesions (TDL) and brain abscesses can have imaging characteristics that are very similar to HGGs or metastases. Brain abscesses have a distinctive pattern of signals in MRS and TDL rarely shows highly elevated rCBV in PWI.

21.2 Monitoring of the Therapeutic Response of Brain Tumors

MRI is again the imaging modality of choice. Serial imaging controls should be performed in all cases and types of brain malignancy. Cerebral metastases require an imaging follow-up every 3 months for at least 2 years after treatment and the same protocol applies in most HGGs and CNS lymphomas. Follow-up periods of 6 months can be considered if no tumor recurrence has occurred within the first 2 years. LGGs can undergo imaging controls every 6 months for 2 years after an initial postoperative MRI. Yearly controls can be considered after 2 years without tumor recurrence.

Imaging assessment of a brain tumor after surgery or irradiation has always been a challenge for neuroradiologists, neurooncologists, and neurosurgeons. Postoperative changes in the tumor bed and radionecrosis can be mistaken for tumor remnants or recurrence. DWI can be a very useful instrument in differentiating postoperative cellular damage and subsequent contrast enhancement from tumor recurrence, especially in patients receiving adjuvant radio- and chemotherapy [2]. MRS and DWI can also be of some value in recognizing radionecrosis, which exhibits a lower choline signal and higher mean ADC values compared to pure tumor. Finally, PET and SPECT scans have a rather well established efficacy in distinguishing radionecrosis from tumor recurrence.

An important step forward in the accurate assessment of response to therapy in patients with malignant gliomas is the recent introduction of criteria of the response assessment in neuro-oncology (RANO), animprovement of the 1990 established Macdonald criteria [4]. They are based on the product of the maximal cross-sectional diameter of an enhancing lesion but the non-enhancing tumor component is also considered. The RANO criteria take into account new treatment options and changes in imaging procedures. In contrast to the previous criteria measurable (well demarcated) and non-measurable lesions (blurred or cystic) are defined, which are especially important to determine endpoints in clinical studies. If the response rate is the primary endpoint of the study patients with measurable disease are required. If the duration of tumor control is the endpoint of the study, then patients with measurable and non-measurable lesions are eligible. Furthermore, for the first time, tumor size is additionally measured on T2-/FLAIR-weighted images and progress is defined by a significant increase of the T2-/FLAIR lesion.

21.3 Conclusion

The imaging modalities of the central nervous system available to a physician today are many and can provide a considerable amount of information about its anatomy, physiology, and function. Recent advances in computational power and software sophistication have made this information readily available for treatment planning, guidance, and follow-up. In order to improve the quality and diversity of the anatomic imaging, efforts to develop MRI systems with field strength higher than 1,5 Tesla have been made since the late 1980s. High field (3 Tesla) MRI has been available in clinical practice since 2002 and a number of these systems, with a higher spatial resolution and speed, are now operational in many hospitals around the world and tend to become the new standard. These systems provide images of unsurpassed anatomical detail, a feature extremely useful in tumor detection and surgical treatment. Ultra high field (up to 12 Tesla) MRI is currently developed or evaluated in certain neuroscience research facilities mainly in Europe and North America. Technical improvements in electromagnetic source imaging (ESI), i.e., the combination of magnetoencephalography (MEG) and electroencephalography (EEG)-have also made this real-time functional brain mapping technique a valuable complement to the fMRI.

References

1. Al-Okaili RN, Krejza J, Wang S et al (2006) Advanced MR imaging techniques in the diagnosis of intraaxial brain tumors in adults. RadioGraphics 26:S173–S189
2. Cha S (2006) Update on brain tumor imaging: from anatomy to physiology. Am J Neuroradiol 27:475–487
3. Young GS (2007) Advanced MRI of adult brain tumors. Neurol Clin 25:947–973
4. van den Bent MJ, Vogelbaum MA, Wen PY (2009) End point assessment in gliomas: novel treatments limit usefulness of classical Macdonald's Criteria. J Clin Oncol 27(18):2905–2908

Part IV
Lung Cancer

22 Lung Cancer

Paris A. Kosmidis

22.1 Introduction

Lung cancer is the leading cause of cancer incidence and mortality in European countries, accounting for about 21 % of all cancer cases in men. In the United States it is the leading cause of cancer mortality in men and women. Globally, lung cancer incidence is increasing at a rate of 0.5 % per year. In very few countries the incidence is declining due to antismoking policy [1].

Lung cancer is divided into two major groups; Non-Small Cell Lung Cancer (NSCLC) and Small Cell Lung Cancer (SCLC). In this chapter we will deal only with NSCLC.

Patients with advanced disease who receive chemotherapy plus biological agents survive between 12 and 15 months. A small portion of patients, especially with targetable adenocarcinoma, who receive targeted agents, may live longer. Patients with localized non-operable stage treated with chemo-radiotherapy may survive 16–22 months.

On the contrary, lung cancer patients with early operable disease can enjoy long life or even be cured.

Therefore, early diagnosis, accurate staging, response evaluation, and follow-up studies are absolutely mandatory for this group of patients for cure or for better and longer life. Especially, staging is of paramount importance for the decision-making process.

The rapid evolution in imaging techniques and the accumulated experience has introduced new promising standards for early diagnosis, staging, prediction of response, and follow-up for patients with lung cancer.

Reference

1. Brodowitz T, Ciuleanu T, Crawford J et al (2012) Third CECOG concensus on the systemic treatment of non-small cell lung cancer. Ann Oncol 23:1223–1229

P. A. Kosmidis (✉)
2nd Medical Oncology Department, Hygeia Hospital, 4, Er.Stavrou and Vas Sofias Ave, 15123 Marousi, Athens, Greece
e-mail: parkosmi@otenet.gr

A. D. Gouliamos et al. (eds.), *Imaging in Clinical Oncology*,
DOI: 10.1007/978-88-470-5385-4_22, © Springer-Verlag Italia 2014

23 Lung Cancer Screening in High-Risk Patients with Low-Dose Helical CT

Despina I. Savvidou

Most patients with NSCLC are diagnosed at a late stage because of lack of symptoms in early stage disease, resulting in a very low 5-year survival. More than 50 % of patients are diagnosed with metastatic disease [1, 2].

The 5-year survival rate for stage I disease is 60–82 %, while at the same time the 5-year survival rate for stage IV disease is lower than 5 % [1, 2].

Despite the fact that progress in chemotherapy and radiotherapy improved the outcomes for people with lung cancer, the principal hope for curative treatment remains surgical resection. Surgery is very effective when tumors are diagnosed early.

This is why, effective screening methods for early detection of lung cancer are very important, especially for high-risk groups (such as current or former smokers).

Early randomized trials (1970) for lung cancer screening, sponsored by the National Cancer Institute, used chest radiograph with or without sputum cytology (Memorial study, John Hopkins Study, Mayo Lung Project), but no difference was noted in lung cancer incidence or mortality between the control group and the experimental group [2–4].

D. I. Savvidou (✉)
CT and MRI Department, Hygeia Hospital,
Peloponissou 57, 15341, Agia Paraskevi,
Athens, Greece
e-mail: despinasavvidou@yahoo.com

More recently (in 1990s), studies began on Low-Dose Computed Tomography (LDCT) screening for lung cancer [1–4]. The early lung cancer action project and a Mayo clinic study [1], are two of these trials that enrolled a large number of asymptomatic current or former smokers who underwent a baseline LDCT scan and annual LDCT screening. Results of these studies suggest that screening with spiral CT is able to detect lung cancers that are smaller than 2 cm in diameter and of earlier stage (85–93 % at stage I) than those that are depicted with chest radiography and in current clinical practice [1, 2]. However, these trials were observational studies without control groups. As a result, the effects of screening on lung cancer mortality could not be measured. So randomized controlled trials were the best way to show if there is disease-specific mortality benefit using LDCT on lung cancer screening. Screening studies have raised issues regarding false-positive findings, additional interventions, exposure to radiation, and quality of life.

The effect of LDCT screening on mortality is currently the subject of several randomized control trials, underway in the USA and Europe.

The National Lung Screening Trial (NLST) [3–5], launched in September 2002, is a large randomized multicenter study, sponsored by the US National Cancer Institute (NCI). This study was designed to determine whether screening using LDCT compared to chest radiography, can reduce lung cancer-specific mortality in high-risk participants. Total 53,454 participants were

A. D. Gouliamos et al. (eds.), *Imaging in Clinical Oncology*,
DOI: 10.1007/978-88-470-5385-4_23, © Springer-Verlag Italia 2014

randomly assigned to receive either three annual low-dose helical CT scans or posteroanterior chest radiography. The participants were between 55 and 74 years of age, had at least a 30 pack year history of cigarette smoking, and, if former smokers, had quit within the past 15 years. The participants should not have history of lung cancer or other life-threatening cancers in the prior 5 years, no hemoptysis or weight loss to suggest a diagnosis of lung cancer and no chest CT in the prior 18 months. Multidetector scanners with a minimum of four channels were used for the performance of all low-dose CT scans. The average estimated whole-body effective dose of low-dose CT is 1.5 mSV while the dose with diagnostic chest CT is 7–8 mSV. Many of the medical institutions that NLST conducted were recognized for their expertize in radiology and in the diagnosis and treatment of cancer.

Recent data released from the National Lung Screening Trial (NLST) [3–6] demonstrated a statistically significant reduction (20 %) in lung cancer deaths in patients screened with LDCT scans.

Based on these findings, in the May 20, 2012 edition of the Journal of the American Medical Association (JAMA) [6], the American College of Chest Physicians (ACCP), the American Society of Clinical Oncology (ASCO), and several other medical societies recommended annual screening with low-dose computed tomography for smokers and former smokers aged 55–74 years, who have smoked for 30 pack years or more and either continue to smoke or have quit within the past 15 years. At the same time, these societies do not recommend CT screening for individuals who have smoked for less than 30 pack years or are either younger than 55 years or older than 74 years, or individuals who quit smoking before 15 years ago, and for individuals with severe comorbidities that would preclude potentially curative treatment or limit life expectancy. At the same time, it is recommended that individuals should be informed about potential benefits and harms, so they can decide whether to undergo LDCT screening. It is also assumed that the screening will be done at an institute with the resources for managing the findings of screening, similar to those that the NLST was conducted.

Literature supports that LDCT screening can lead to harm [3–6]. In addition to the high-rate of false-positive results (that leads in further evaluation with imaging or invasive diagnostic procedures), other potentially harmful effects of low-dose CT screening are overdiagnosis, radiation exposure, and the effect of screening on quality of life.

All noncalcified nodules, identified in NLST, that were larger than 4 mm in diameter or had suspicious morphology, constituted a positive result, suspicious for lung cancer [5].

The protocol in NLST for the follow-up of these noncalcified solid nodules did not differ substantially from the Fleischner Society guidelines [7] for the management of small pulmonary nodules (Fig. 23.1).

The frequency of invasive evaluation of detected nodules was generally low (Fig. 23.2).

Complications [6] of invasive diagnostic procedures were uncommon, with major complications occurring only rarely (33 per 10,000 individuals screened by LDCT and 10 per 10,000 screened by chest radiograph). The vast majority of severe complications occurred after

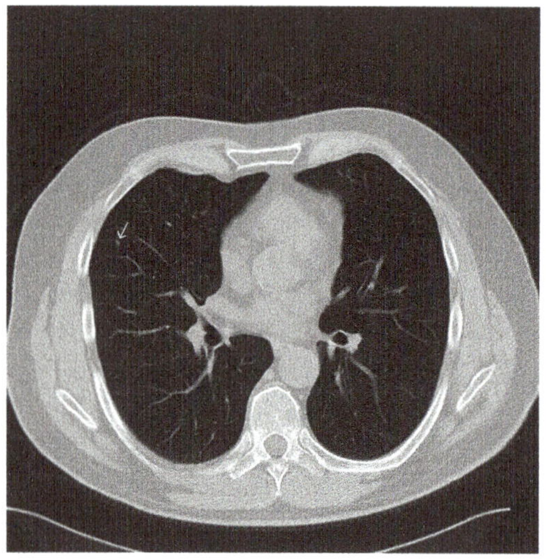

Fig. 23.1 Lung nodule with a diameter of 5 mm (*arrow*) needs follow-up

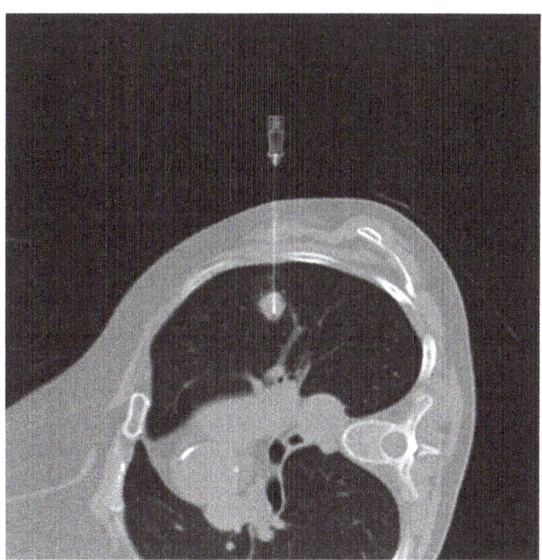

Fig. 23.2 Fine needle aspiration at a 15 mm lung nodule

surgical procedures, particularly among patients with lung cancer. The complications after bronchoscopy or needle biopsy were low.

The false-positive rate, in the NLST study varied between 95 and 98 % on LDCT [3, 5].

Overdiagnosis refers to confirmed slow growing lung cancers identified with screening that a patient dies with and not of. In this category, are included patients who are going to die from another cause.

The estimated effective dose of radiation of LDCT is 1.5 mSV per examination [3, 4, 6]. However, because further investigation is needed when new lesions are detected, the radiation exposure increases in screening studies. It is estimated that participants in NLST received approximately 8 mSV over 3 years (including screening and diagnostic examinations). From such radiation, it is predicted that approximately 1 cancer death may be caused by radiation from imaging per 2,500 persons screened [6]. So, the benefit in NLST in preventing lung cancer deaths is greater than the radiation risk.

The effect of lung cancer screening on quality of life is not determined.

Anxiety from the evaluation of false-positive results may be a disadvantage of lung cancer screening.

The American Association for Thoracic Surgery recommends [8] annual lung cancer screening with low-dose CT for smokers and former smokers, aged 50–79 years with 30 pack year history as well as smokers and former smokers from ages 55 to 79 with a 20 pack year history of smoking and additional comorbidity (such as chronic obstructive pulmonary disorder) that produces a cumulative risk of developing lung cancer of >5 % over the following 5 years.

AATS also recommends guidelines [8], such as those developed by the Fleischner Society, for the management of solid and ground glass nodules identified on LDCT at baseline scan or during an annual LDCT screening examination.

There is a number of ongoing randomized clinical trials in Europe [4, 5], such as the NELSON trial , the Danish Lung Cancer Screening Trial (DLCST) and the Italian Lung Cancer Computer Tomography screening trial (ITALUNG), the Detection and Screening of Early Lung Cancer (DANTE) trial, the LUSI trial in Germany, and the UK Lung Screen (UKLS).

The European studies are expected to address additional questions about low-dose CT screening, such as strageties for the management of nodules observed with screening.

Airway epithelial biomarkers, serum biomarkers, and breath analysis of volatile compounds are new testing techniques that could be a part of a screening algorithm for lung cancer in the future [5].

23.1 Conclusion

Until the NLST, improvement in mortality was questionable when using LDCT scan screening protocols in high-risk patients. With recent information from the NLST, many societies suggest annual screening with low-dose CT in high-risk individuals for lung cancer. However, questions still remain about the harms from false-positive results, overdiagnosis, the costs, and the effect on quality of life. Before public health policy decisions are taken, it must be rigorously analyzed the cost-effectiveness of low-dose CT screening.

References

1. Swensen Stephen J, James R et al (2009) Lung cancer screening with CT: mayo clinic experience 1. Radiology, RSNA
2. Reddy C, Chilla D, Boltax J et al (2011) Lung cancer screening: a review of available data and current guidelines. Hosp Pract 39(4):107–112
3. The National Lung Screening Trial Research Team (2011) Reduced lung-cancer mortality with low-dose computed tomographic screening. N Engl J Med 365:455–457
4. Kramer BS, Berg CD, Aberle DR (2011) Lung cancer screening with low-dose helical CT: results from the National Lung Screening Trial (NLST). J Med Screen 18(3):109–111
5. Nair Arjun, Hansell David M (2011) European and North American lung cancer screening experience and implications for pulmonary nodule management. Eur Radiol 21:2445–2454
6. Bach P, Mirkin Joshua N et al (2012) Benefits and harms of CT screening for lung Cancer. a systematic review. JAMA 307(22):2418–2429
7. MacMahon H, Austin John HM, Gamsu G et al (2005) Guidelines for management of small pulmonary nodules detected on CT scans: a statement from the fleischner society. Radiology 237:395–400
8. Jacobson FL, Austin JH, Field JK et al (2012) Development of the American association for thoracic surgery guidelines for low-dose computed tomography scans to screen for lung cancer in north America: recommendations of the american association for thoracic surgery task force for lung cancer screening and surveillance. J Thorac Cardiovasc Surg

24 CT-MRI in Diagnosis and Staging in Lung Cancer

John A. Papailiou

Non small cell lung cancer stage classification system is correlated with the anatomical extent of the disease based on the characteristics of the primacy tumor, the invasion of the regional lymph nodes, and the presence of distant metastasis. The new TNM staging system (7th edition) is the most widely used staging scheme for non small cell lung carcinoma (NSCLC) and is based on a larger surgical and nonsurgical cohort of patients. CT, MRI imaging are considered useful for precise assessment of tumor extent.

CT is an excellent tool for the detection of lung nodules, and therefore has an important role for lung cancer screening, diagnosis, staging and follow-up. CT is superior to chest X-ray in terms of sensitivity in screening. The detection rate is 1–2.7 % [1], but CT cannot be used as a screening technique, except in a high-risk population [2]. The goal of screening for lung cancer is to identify asymptomatic patients with early stage unrecognized disease and patients at increased risk for developing the disease. Early detection and treatment of preinvasive bronchial lesions as well as accurate diagnosis and staging of primary lung cancer or recognition of synchronous neoplastic lesions have an important impact in treatment and prognosis.

Nodules can be missed by CT but these are either endobronchial, or located close to pulmonary vessels. Missed nodules are also identical in density to those known as ground-glass opacity nodules.

Some morphologic aspects, as spiculated borders, ill-defined contours, presence of air bubbles, eccentric calcifications, are suggestive of a malignancy. Benignity signs of calcification, as total, central, or popcorn-like, are better evaluated on CT. In lesions more than 8 mm in diameter and homogeneous on non-enhanced CT, an increase in attenuation of <15 Hounsfield units has been reported for benignity [3]. Assessing of pulmonary nodules on 3D reconstructions is considered as the most important method for their growth evaluation.

MRI may be identical in details in terms of a tumor location. The MRI technique uses magnetization, and a computer to produce images of body entities, while with MRI there is no exposure to radiation.

MRI is superior to CT in the study of pericardium, heart, and great vessels. Coronal images are useful in the location of tumor in the subcarinal space, aortopulmonary window, and superior vena cava. MRI is limited by poorer spatial resolution, in relation with CT, and by cardiac and respiratory motion artifacts; but these limitations have been diminished with newer MRI.

J. A. Papailiou (✉)
CT Department, Kostantopoulio General Hospital, Agias Olgas, 3–5, Nea Ionia 14233, Athens, Greece
e-mail: johnantpap@ath.forthnet.gr

A. D. Gouliamos et al. (eds.), *Imaging in Clinical Oncology*,
DOI: 10.1007/978-88-470-5385-4_24, © Springer-Verlag Italia 2014

MRI may be used in patients who have had allergic reactions to iodinated contrast media and in patients with renal impairment, because MRI does not use iodinated contrast.

The difference in accuracy between MRI and CT is not significant. The sensitivity of CT is 63 %, and that of MRI is 56 %. In the distinction of T3 and T4 tumors, the specificity of CT is 84 %, and that of MRI is 80 % [4].

There are several limitations to MRI in the lung: the high susceptibility to motion artifacts, the low proton density of lung parenchyma, and the decrease in signal intensity because of air-soft tissue interfaces. The major advantage of MRI is the soft tissue contrast without the use of contrast media. Recent developments including breath-hold acquisitions and gating procedures have increased image quality. The administration of gadolinium that increases the relaxivity is used to enhance tumors and helps to evaluate treated lesions during follow-up. New contrast agents with ultra small iron oxide particles have been proposed to improve the specificity of MRI in detecting invasion of the mediastinum.

The assessment of the staging, i.e., the extent of lung cancer is directly related to the decision for treatment and prognosis. Patients are staged according to the International Staging System. Guidelines have been published providing recommendations on management of patients with non-small cell lung carcinoma. All patients should have a chest radiograph and a contrast-enhanced chest CT that includes the liver and adrenals. MRI is the preferred modality in cases of Pancoast tumors to assess brachial plexus and vascular involvement.

The T staging is relative to the size of primary tumor in long axis or direct extent of the tumor into adjacent entities such as mediastinum or chest wall.

Many changes in staging classification are focused on the T (tumor) staging. These changes are related to the size and location of the primary neoplasm and satellite nodules (Tables 24.1, 24.2).

The new system has five categories in relation to their size, at 2, 3, 5, and 7 cm. Tumors measuring <2 cm are classified as T1a, and those measuring 2–3 cm are classified as T1b. T2 category is subdivided into T2a (>3–5 cm) and T2b (>5–7 cm). Tumors larger than 7 cm are classified as T3. These changes influence treatment.

The new TNM system does not take into account a single tumor which involves two lobes across a fissure. It considers the tumor size and satellite nodules in the same and different lobes. In the new TNM system if additional nodules are

Table 24.1 Primary tumor and its local extent (T status)

	Diameter of the primary pulmonary tumor	Invasion of adjacent structures	Site of nodules
T1	T1a (tumor equal or smaller than 2 cm)		
	T1b (tumor more than 2–3 cm)		
T2	T2a (tumor more than 3–5 cm)	Pleura	
	T2b (tumor more than 5–7 cm)		
T3	Tumor (more than 7 cm)	Thoracic wall, diaphragm, mediastinum, pericardium	In the same lobe
T4		Mediastinum or vertebrae	In the other lobes

Table 24.2 Lymph nodal involvement (N status)

N1	Of the same side peribronchial or of the same side hilar lymph nodes
N2	Of the same side mediastinal or subcarinal nodes
N3	Controlateral scalene or supraclavicular lymph nodes

found in the same lobe, they are classified as T3 in contrast with the previous TNM system where these nodules were classified as T4. Additional nodules outside the primary lobe but in the same lung are now staged from M1 to T4 and patients may be candidate for pneumonectomy. A satellite nodule in the contralateral lung has changed from M1 to M1a to indicate intrathoracic progression, which has a more favorable prognosis in relation to patients with distant metastases (M1b) (Figs. 24.1, 24.2, 24.3, 24.4).

The T status has a significant role to the selection of the therapeutic option, i.e., resection, chemotherapy, or radiotherapy. CT is the principal modality to evaluate tumor size and relationship of the lesion with adjacent organs. The size of the tumor is precisely estimated except in cases of coexisting atelectasis. The location of the tumor within the bronchial tree is determined by bronchoscopy, but CT can be useful in identifying the proximal part of the lesion <2 cm from the carina when transbronchial growth exists. When the lesion is surrounded by lung parenchyma, CT is important to differentiate a tumor that crosses an incomplete fissure from one that involves the fissure. The surgical approach can be modified,

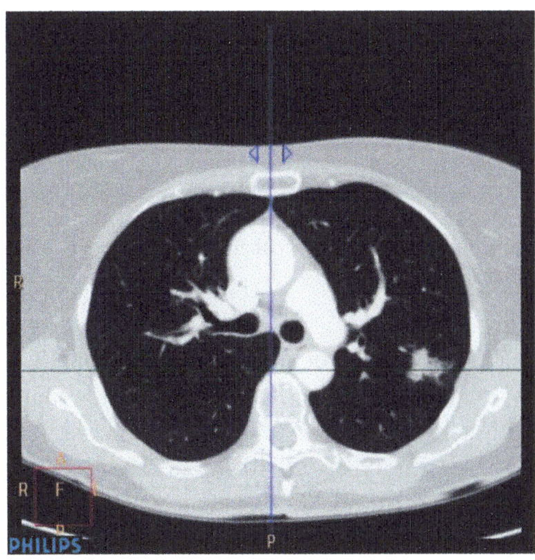

Fig. 24.1 Contrast-enhanced CT image of a 1.9 cm peripheral carcinoma in *left upper* lobe, stage T1a. The spiculated margin is typical of lung cancer

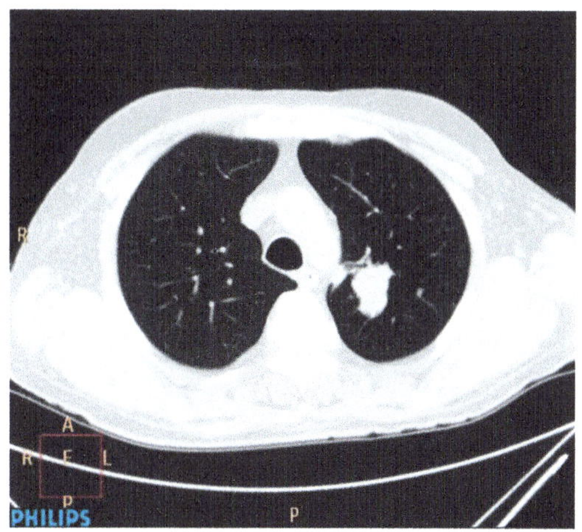

Fig. 24.2 *Left upper* lobe centrally located carcinoma, 3 cm in diameter, stage T1b

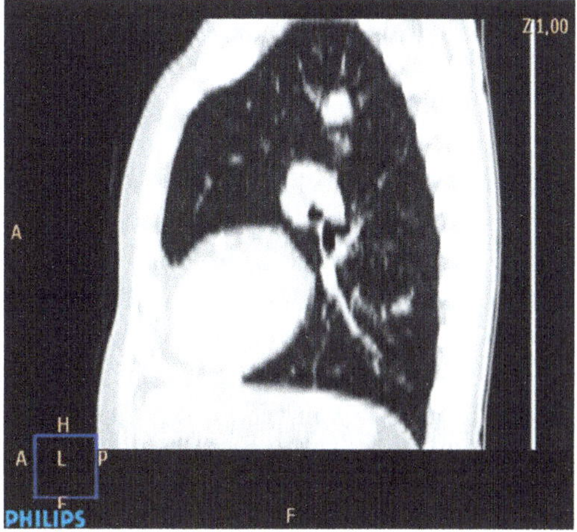

Fig. 24.3 Revisions to T3 designation for non-small cell lung carcinoma. Sagittal multiplanar reformation, CT image, shows as primary tumor a small nodule 1.6 cm in the *left upper* lobe with a satellite 8.0 mm nodule in the left lower lobe. Satellite nodule in the same lung but in different lobe from primary tumor was previously classified as metastatic disease but now is designated as T4

if the pleura is invaded. The situation is difficult with T3 and T4 tumors in which differentiation is not clear if a patient is a candidate for surgery (Fig. 24.3). It is also important to establish the diagnosis of pleural metastases or malignant effusion. On CT, rib destruction is the only reliable sign of chest wall invasion.MR imaging

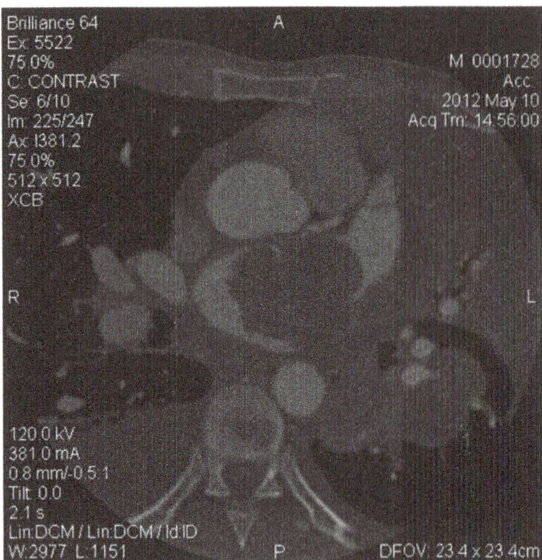

Fig. 24.4 Axial contrast-enhanced CT image shows a *left lower* lobe lung mass (sarcoma), extending into the *left atrium* (T4). Large right malignant pleural effusion in contralateral lung is also seen. It is classified as M1a in the new staging system

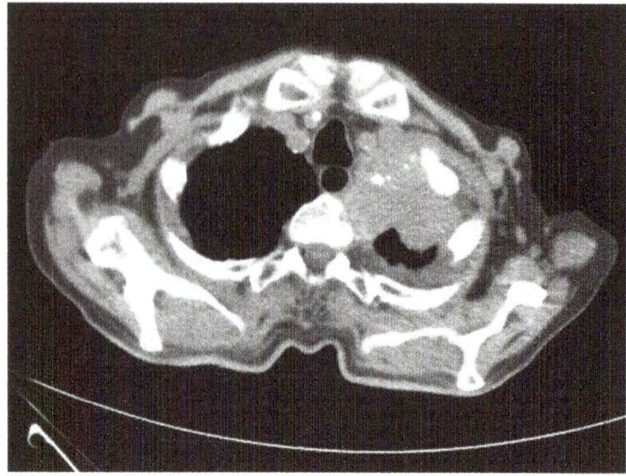

Fig. 24.5 Axial CT image at *left* apex which confirms the left superior sulcus tumor (Pancoast tumor) invading the *left side* of the adjacent thoracic vertebra. Any tumor that invades vertebral body is classified as T4

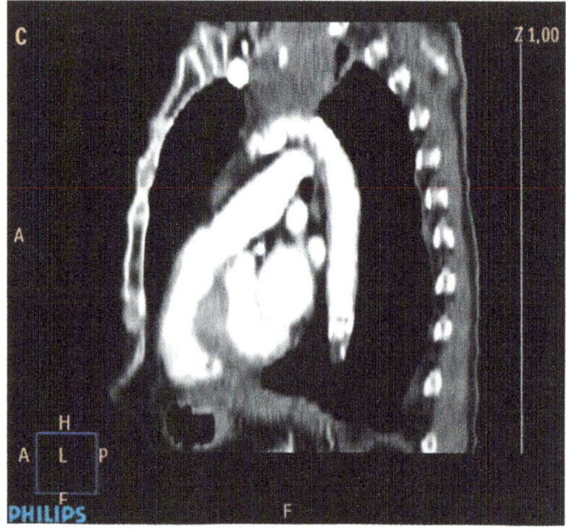

Fig. 24.6 Sagittal contrast-enhanced CT image which confirms at *left* apex, the left superior sulcus tumour (Pancoast tumor) invading aortic arch and the adjacent thoracic wall. Any tumour that invades thoracic wall or heart, is classified as T4

is effective for chest wall invasion assessment. CT or MRI are excellent tools for chest wall invasion, but it is difficult to distinguish by imaging chest wall invasion from cases with fibrous adhesions. With CT and MRI, the diagnosis is easy when mass or bone destruction is present in chest wall (Fig. 24.5). The sensitivity of CT in determining chest wall invasion is 87 %, and the specificity is 59 % [5]. MRI has superior soft-tissue contrast resolution and can be more accurate than CT in chest wall involvement from superior sulcus tumors with respect to involvement of the subclavian vessels (Figs. 24.6, 24.7, 24.8, 24.9), the brachial plexus, and the adjacent vertebra. Axial MRI will demonstrate ingrowth into mediastinum and vertebral canal but sagittal T1 W1 will best demonstrate ingrowths into thoracic and cervical vessels and nerves. Involvement of the brachial plexus and extension into the spinal cord prevent surgical resection. MDCT using coronal and sagittal reformations provides the same information as MRI.

CT features suggesting invasion of mediastinal disease are related to the clarity of fat plane between the mass and mediastinal structures, thickened pleura, or pericardium, lesion >3 cm in contact with the mediastinum and contact with aorta >90°. The use of these criteria, leads to a sensitivity of 27–40 % and an acceptable specificity [6, 7]. Encasement of mediastinal vessels by the tumor is considered as a mediastinal invasion and precludes resection (Fig. 24.10). CT in the assessment of chest wall invasion has a sensitivity of 14 % and specificity

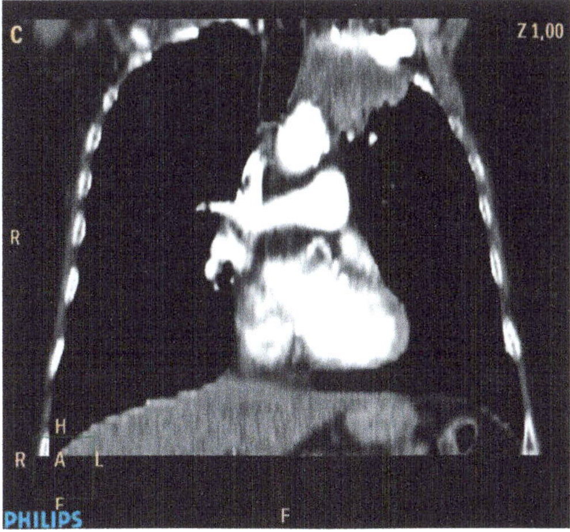

Fig. 24.7 Coronal contrast-enhanced CT image at *left* apex which confirms the left superior sulcus tumor (Pancoast tumor) invading aortic arch and the *left* side of the adjacent thoracic wall. Any tumor that invades thoracic wall or heart is classified as T4

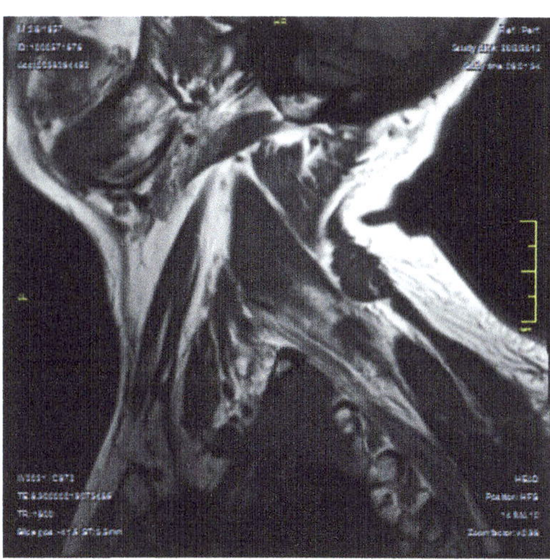

Fig. 24.9 Sagittal contrast enhanced T1-w MR image at lung apex showing a pancoast tumor invading the posterior side of the subclavian artery and the chest wall

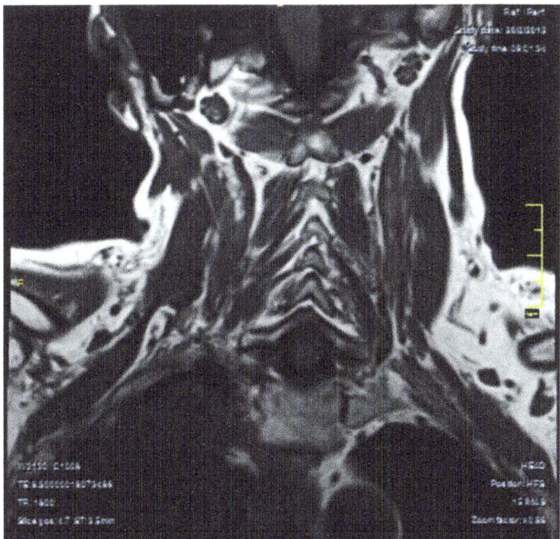

Fig. 24.8 Coronal T1-w MR image showing a large right lung mass (Pancoast tumor), with loss of the adjacent soft tissue plane consistent with local invasion of subclavian artery

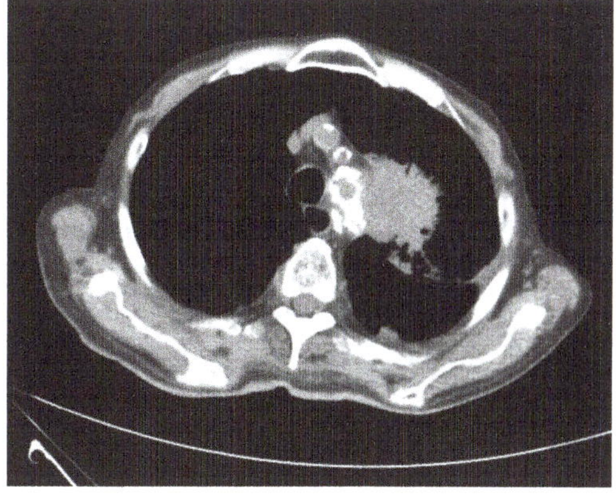

Fig. 24.10 Non small cell lung cancer (NSCLC) using revised TNM system Axial CT image shows a 5 cm tumor (stage T4) extending to the mediastinum and invading the aortic arch without evidence of disease elsewhere. Loss of soft tissue plane between the mass and the tranverse aorta suggests vascular invasion

99 %. In terms of mediastinal invasion CT has sensitivity 50 % and specificity 89 % and in regards for the mediastinal nodal metastases a sensitivity of 61 % and a specificity of 76 % [7]. The multiplanar capabilities and the excellent spatial resolution of MDCT increase the ability to assess mediastinal infiltrations.

When the primary carcinoma has greater than 90° contact to the mediastinal structures, CT could have sensitivity 40 %, specificity 99 %, and positive and negative predictive values 56 and 98 % respectively [6] .

Nodal disease, whether microscopic or gross, bulky >2 cm, or multilevel disease has a markedly negative effect on survival. The combination of advanced T and N status has the worse prognosis with very limited if any survival at 5 years. Accurate mediastinal staging is crucial to the selection of the optimal therapy for patients without distant metastasis. Many different invasive staging tests which should be viewed as complementary to one or another are available. Extend of mediastinal involvement by CT scan is very important for the choice of the appropriate technique.

The CT criterion of nodal (N) metastasis is lymph node enlargement, and is estimated to the short-axis diameter >1 cm. Reactive hyperplasia may be responsible for node enlargement, and metastatic lymph nodes could be normal in size. CT for mediastinal staging has a sensitivity of 57 %, a specificity of 82 %, and positive and negative predictive values of only 56 and 83 %, respectively [8]. It is important to consider that MRI has disadvantages in evaluation of lymph nodes because MRI is insensitive to calcifications and has a poor spatial resolution. A single enlarged node can be a cluster of small nodes on CT. Comparing CT and MRI, the detection rate of nodal metastases was similar [9].

CT has sensitivity and specificity in the detection of mediastinal nodes with ranges of 40–84 % and 52–80 %, respectively [10].

The N classification describes the degree of spread to regional lymph nodes. This staging remained unchanged in the 7th edition (Fig. 24.11). Various techniques are used to identify nodal spread. Lymph node sampling is regarded as the most accurate predictor of nodal status. Mediastinoscopy remains the "gold standard" for staging of the mediastinum, but it is invasive and has limitations in accessing the posterior and inferior mediastinal nodes. The sensitivity for mediastinoscopy is 93 %, and, the specificity 100 %, [11].

The M staging defines the presence of metastases beyond regional lymph nodes. (Table 24.3). In the 7th edition of the lung cancer classification, the pleural, or pericardial dissemination regarding effusions and nodules, are no longer classified as T4, but are now upstaged into a new category (M1a). This category also includes additional nodules that are found in the contralateral lung. Distant metastasis is subclassified as M1b disease.M1a includes malignant pleural effusion and contra lateral lung nodules (Fig. 24.5). M1b refers to extra-thoracic metastases (Table 24.3).

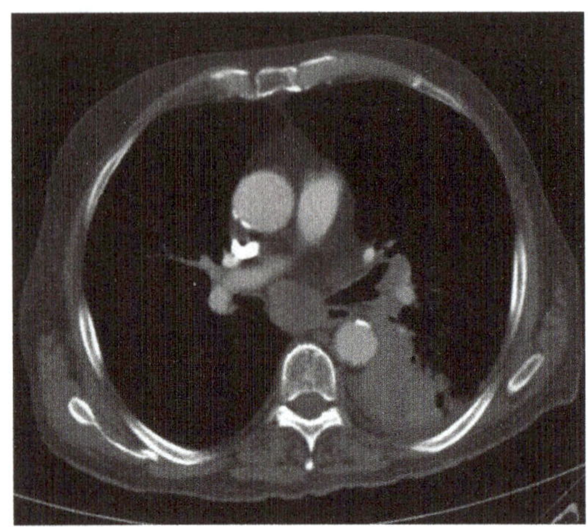

Fig. 24.11 A 7, 5 cm mass in the *left lower* lobe with mediastinal subcarinal lymphadenopathy, N3. As far as size is concerned, the T classification is staged as T3

Table 24.3 Intra and extrathoracic metastases (M status or distant metastases)

M1a	When the spread is local or intrathoracic
M1b	When extrathoracic spread exists

The detection of distant metastases is very important. Metastases occur in about 50 % of patients with NSCLC. These sites include the brain, the liver which can be examined with CT or MRI, and the skeleton, which can be examined with scintigraphy. These sites are imaged as baseline imaging in patients with NSCLC. The probability of metastases is lower for squamous cell cancers and the incidence increases with advancing stage. Adenocarcinoma metastasizes to the brain and adrenals early.

CT scan of thorax usually includes the liver and the adrenal glands. CT scanning has a sensitivity of 85 % in the evaluation of liver metastases [11]. Same results may be obtained with MRI and ultrasonography by experienced imagers. Ultrasonography versus CT is superior in distinguishing metastases from liver cysts.

The adrenals are currently evaluated using extended chest CT examination below the diaphragm.

Adrenal adenomas occur about 1 % in the general population and they should be distinguished from metastases. CT as well as MRI is based on the evaluation of the fat content for assessing benignity. An adrenal mass with an attenuation value of <10 Hounsfield units on a nonenhanced CT is considered benign [12]. Lesions smaller than 1 cm are usually benign. Metastases are usually larger than 3 cm. Adenomas and metastases can also be distinguished by using PET scanning. If all these methods do not demonstrate that the lesion is benign, CT-guided biopsy is necessary.

Pulmonary adenocarcinoma is the most common source of cerebral metastases. MRI is superior to CT, especially in the posterior fossa and the area adjacent to the skull base. The brain is not routinely imaged in asymptomatic patients with NSCLC, because the incidence of silent cerebral metastases is very low ranging from 2 to 4 % [11].

Technetium-99 m (99 m Tc) radionuclide bone scanning is indicated in cases with bone pain or local tenderness. Bone scanning has 95 % sensitivity for the detection of metastases but a high false-positive rate exists because of degenerative disease or trauma. These metastases always require comparison of the bone scans. Spinal metastases may cause spinal cord compression and infiltration. Because only about 5 % of bony metastases detected with radionuclide scans are asymptomatic, routine preoperative bone scanning is not usually a baseline image. Patients with skeletal metastases are thought to be symptomatic or to have abnormal laboratory results. CT or MRI can be recommended in cases of local bone pain.

Pulmonary metastases from a primary NSCLC are not common, but they are present incidentally at autopsy. Differential diagnosis of small lung nodules from granulomas on CT scans may be difficult.

CT is very important imaging technique for needle biopsy and thoracentesis. Needle biopsies are useful if the lung tumor is peripherally located in the lung and not accessible to bronchoscopy (Fig. 24.12). A local anesthetic is given prior to insertion of a thin needle (18 or 23 gauge) through the chest wall into the lung tumor. Cells are suctioned into the syringe and are examined under the microscope. This procedure is accurate when the tissue from the tumor area is correctly sampled. With CT it becomes possible to biopsy lung lesions using cutting needle in selected cases in order to have a small tissue sample. A small risk of pneumothorax, accompanies this procedure.

Lung cancer can very commonly induce pleural effusion. Under CT guidance, with local anesthesia, a needle is inserted into the pleural space from which a small quantity of fluid is taken, to test for cancer cells or a therapeutic drainage in cases of pain or shortness of breath.

Following treatment, a new radiologic evaluation is very important for the prognosis. Imaging techniques in follow-up examinations, include chest X-rays and CT, but no consensus has been established in the use of CT. Extrathoracic imaging with CT is ordered according to clinical symptoms that are suggestive of metastatic disease and a regular follow-up at 3, 6, 12 months, and every year is performed. Changes after pneumonectomy or lobectomy are

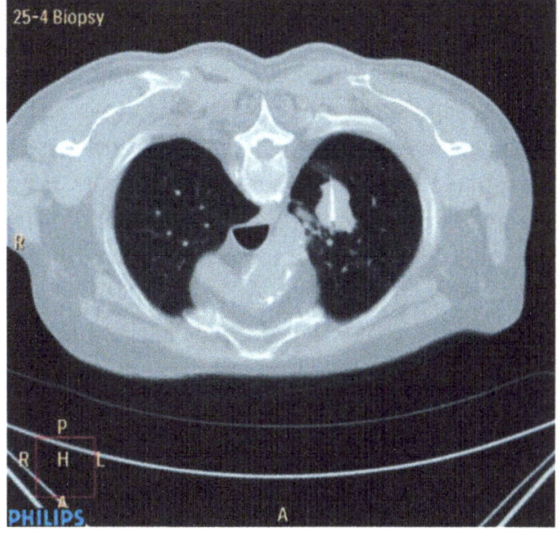

Fig. 24.12 CT-guided biopsy in a carcinoma of the *left upper* posterior lobe. Cutting biopsy needle can be noted posteriorly entering the mass traversing intervening lung

important in interpreting CT images. In patients who are not candidates for surgery, radiotherapy alone or combined with chemotherapy in locally advanced cancers is recommended. After radiation therapy, radiation pneumonitis is seen when ground-glass opacities are visible within the 3 months of treatment. Sometimes pneumonitis appears nodular and simulates metastatic nodules. CT changes are seen within the lung following radiation therapy. The development of fibrosis will usually continue following 3–12 months radiotherapy. Findings of recurrent tumors are nonspecific. For patients treated with chemotherapy, the response is crucial. The method of assessing response to treatment is response evaluation criteria in solid tumors (RECIST). CT is the best method for measuring lung lesions. Recent studies have shown that volumetric CT scanning, which images the tumor at high resolution in order to permit automated calculation of its 3D volume, provides more accurate evaluation of tumor changes, by accounting for its shape and irregularities in its growth. It also permits more precise tumor density measurements for better evaluation of tumor heterogeneity.

In conclusion, CT plays a significant role in the evaluation of lung cancer. CT is an optimal tool for the evaluation of mediastinal metastases and in identifying potential sites of tumor involvement. Additionally, CT is helpful in guiding invasive biopsy procedures. MRI is the noninvasive procedure of choice in the evaluation of superior sulcus tumors and those lesions with suspected vascular, pericardial, or cardiac invasion. MRI is also complementary to CT in the evaluation of chest wall invasion and distant metastases. Many important changes have occurred with the use of new TNM staging system (7th edition) for lung cancer and have been the cornerstone in oncology which allows accurate prognosis and planning of the treatment strategies.

In the multidisciplinary team approach, all medical professionals (pulmonologists, oncologists, thoracic surgeons, pathologists, and radiologists) involved in the clinical management of lung cancer, should become familiar with the updated staging system.

References

1. Henschke CI, McCauley DI, Yankelevitz DF et al (1999) Early lung cancer action project: overall design and findings from baseline screening. Lancet 354:99–105
2. US Preventive Services Task Force (2004) Lung cancer screening: recommendation statement. Ann Intern Med 140:738–739
3. Swensen SJ, Viggiano RW, Midthun DE et al (2000) Lung nodule enhancement at CT: multicenter study. Radiology 214:73–80
4. Hassan I, Gross BH (2011) MD Imaging in lung cancer staging. Med scape reference. Drugs diseases and procedures. Multimedia library. May 27
5. Glazer HS, Duncan-Meyer J, Aronberg DJ et al (1985) Pleural and chest wall invasion in bronchogenic carcinoma: CT evaluation. Radiology 157:191–194
6. Herman SJ, Winton TL, Weisbrod GL et al (1994) Mediastinal invasion by bronchogenic carcinoma: CT signs. Radiology 190:841–846
7. White PG, Adams H, Crane MD et al (1994) Preoperative staging of carcinoma of the bronchus: can computed tomographic scanning reliably identify stage III tumours? Thorax 49:951–957
8. Toloza EM, Harpole L, Detterbeck F et al (2003) Invasive staging of non-small cell lung cancer: a review of the current evidence. Chest 123: 157S–166S
9. Musset D, Grenier P, Carette MF et al (1986) Primary lung cancer staging: prospective comparative study of MR imaging with CT. Radiology 160:607–611
10. Laurent F, Montaudona M, Corneloupb O (2006) CT and MRI of lung cancer. Respiration 73:133–142
11. Coughlin M, Deslauriers J, Beaulieu M et al (1985) Role of mediastinoscopy in pretreatment staging of patients with primary lung cancer. Ann Thorax Surg 40:556–560
12. Boland GW, Lee MJ, Gazelle GS et al (1998) Characterization of adrenal masses using unenhanced CT: an analysis of the CT literature. AJR Am J Roentgenol 171:201–204

25 PET-CT in Lung Cancer

Roxani D. Efthymiadou

An appropriate staging of lung cancer is of great value for patient's management and prognosis. The evaluation includes except the detailed clinical examination, a variety of laboratory tests and imaging methods. PET-CT has much promise as an aid to the noninvasive evaluation of lung cancer. In fact, lung cancer is one of the main and well-established indications of the method [1].

As a product of the advanced technology in imaging, PET-CT combines in one single method the detailed anatomic information provided by CT with the functional data provided by PET. PET-CT has many applications but is widely used in lung cancer because of its superiority, compared to other imaging modalities, in the detection of nodal and metastatic disease. The radiotracer used for PET is 18F-FGD, which is glucose labeled with 18 F, a radionuclide with relatively long half life—of almost 110 min—and small photonic energy of 0,64 MeV. 18F-FDG is the most widely used in oncology radiotracer because cancer cells have increased metabolic activity and exclusively use glucose as a source of energy [2]. After an appropriate preparation, the scan is performed following well predefined instructions. One hour after the 18 F-FDG injection, both a PET and a CT are obtained. The procedure covers the whole body and lasts about 40 min. The amount of radiotracer trapped in cancer sites can be quantified by using methods as the SUV (the Standardized Uptake Value). The PET, CT, and fused PET-CT images are studied by specialists (radiologists and nuclear medicine doctors) in order to combine all the provided data.

18F-FDG PET-CT currently is indicated for the characterization of lung lesions, staging of non-small cell lung carcinoma (NSCLC), detection of distant metastases, diagnosis of recurrent disease, planning radiotherapy, and for treatment monitoring [3].

One of the main indications of PET-CT is the evaluation of the solitary pulmonary nodule (SPN). SPN is opacity in the lung parenchyma that measures up to 3 cm and that has no associated mediastinal adenopathy or atelectasis. CT is considered an excellent tool for the evaluation of the nodule but is characterized by poor specificity (58 %). 18F-FDG PET-CT provides complementary information about the metabolic activity of a nodule that cannot be obtained by radiographic methods. The development of 18F-FDG- PET has taken the evaluation of solitary pulmonary nodules beyond anatomic and predictive analyses to functional and metabolic analyses of disease. PET alone has been described as a better predictor of malignancy than clinical and morphologic criteria combined. A study showed that when an SUV equal to or greater than 2.5 was used for detecting malignancy, the sensitivity, specificity, and accuracy

R. D. Efthymiadou (✉)
CT, MRI and PET-CT Department, Hygeia Hospital, Pittakou 21, Nea Ionia, Attiki 14231, Greece
e-mail: r.efthimiadi@hygeia.gr

A. D. Gouliamos et al. (eds.), *Imaging in Clinical Oncology*,
DOI: 10.1007/978-88-470-5385-4_25, © Springer-Verlag Italia 2014

of PET-CT were 97 %, 82 %, and 92 %, respectively [4]. The negative predictive value of the method is high enough to avoid a biopsy. However, PET-CT may be false negative in small nodules with a diameter less than 8–10 mm. It may also be negative in malignancies with low metabolic activity as focal bronchioalveolar cell carcinoma or carcinoid. A hypermetabolic nodule needs further investigation as increased 18F-FDG is not specific and may represent a malignant as well as an inflammatory lesion [4].

Conventional chest radiography, computed tomography (CT), magnetic resonance imaging, radionuclide scintigraphy, and positron emission tomography (PET) all have been used for NSCLC staging. TNM staging is of great importance for determining the therapeutic strategy [5].

Although CT, until now, has been widely used for the evaluation of tumor size and infiltration of adjacent structures, PET-CT is much more accurate in determination of T staging, as the accuracy of the method is 82 % while the accuracy of CT is 68 %. One of the main advantages of PET-CT is the ability to differentiate the hypermetabolic central neoplasm from the non metabolic postobstructive atelectasis. PET-CT may also reveal subtle areas of invasion which are not occult on CT.

Lymph node status (N staging) is of great importance to determining the resectability of a tumor; PET-CT has been shown to be substantially more sensitive and specific in the detection and characterization of metastases to mediastinal lymph nodes: PET has a sensitivity of 83 % and a specificity of 94 %, while CT has 63 % and 73 % respectively. By combining anatomic and functional data in a one single imaging method, dual-modality PET-CT represents the most efficient and accurate approach to NSCLC staging, with a profound influence on therapeutic management and patient prognosis [6]. Use of PET-CT results in further improved N staging compared with use of CT. The limitations of size-based node characterization system in CT studies are well documented. In CT a lymph node is considered to be abnormal if its short-axis diameter is more than 1 cm. However, a large percentage (44 % according to one study) of small lymph nodes (measured less than 1 cm) is metastatic, whereas an even larger percentage (77 % according to the same study) of enlarged nodes (measured more than 1 cm in the short axis) is proved to be nonmetastatic. PET-CT reveals not only the presence and morphology but also the metabolic activity even of small nodes (< 1 cm) [1]. The method is characterized by 78 % accuracy and 94 % negative predictive value in the detection of mediastinal lymph nodes. Although mediastinoscopy remains the gold standard, PET-CT is the best noninvasive imaging procedure for N staging in NSCLC. The high negative predictive value of PET-CT in the evaluation of mediastinal lymph-node involvement led to the avoidance of invasive methods, such as mediastinoscopy, in most of the PET-CT negative patients.

M status defines the presence or absence of tumor spread to distant lymph nodes or organs. Lung cancer may metastasize to almost every organ of the body but mainly to the brain, the adrenals, the bone, the liver, and the contralateral lung. 30 % of patients with NSCLC have occult distant secondary deposits at the time of presentation of the disease. Detection of distant metastasis (M staging) is another critical step in determining the resectability of the lung tumor. During the past few decades, CT has been used as the method of choice for the detection of metastatic disease in NSCLC. The addition of PET in the evaluation of NSCLC reveals metastatic sites in more patients [7]. PET-CT has high sensitivity in the detection of adrenal metastases . Increased 18F-FDG uptake in an adrenal enlargement can differentiate a metastatic from a benign lesion. PET-CT has also been shown as a sensitive method for the detection of bone and pleural metastases. Although CT may reveal focal thickening at the pleura or the pericardium PET-CT can confirm the diagnosis of malignancy showing increased FDG uptake at the suspicious sites. As a whole body study, PET-CT may reveal distant unexpected metastases not found in conventional staging. Previous studies demonstrated the high accuracy of PET-CT in the detection of unsuspected extrathoracic metastases in up to 17 % of patients. The preoperative use of PET has led to avoid unnecessary thoracotomies in patients considered to be operable on the basis of CT and clinical criteria. Although PET-CT is superior to conventional imaging methods in detection of metastatic disease in the body, MRI of the brain remains the method of choice for detecting metastatic disease.

The ability of PET-CT to detect both intra- and extrathoracic metastatic sites in one single examination with a better accuracy than conventional procedures has a potential impact on patient's management. The PET in Lung Cancer Staging (PLUS) trial and the American College of Surgeons Oncology group trial confirmed that PET-CT—when added to the standard work-up of patients with NSCLC—led to upstage up to 25 % of them and to improve selection of patients who can benefit from curative surgical resection.

PET-CT is an excellent tool for radiotherapy planning . PET-CT—guided planning devices will further refine three-dimensional conformal radiotherapy. PET-CT can demonstrate more accurately the sites of active tumor, which may probably have an impact on radiation therapy volume delineation in NSCLC. PET-CT provides safe delivery of high dose of radiation to the neoplasmatic site protecting the normal tissues, as it can differentiate tumor from nontumor lesions such as atelectasis, consolidation, or scar tissue. According to a study of 26 patients with stages I through III of NSCLC, Bradley et al. 24 found changes in radiation therapy planning in over 40 % of patients after integrated PET-CT in comparison with CT-guided treatment [8].

Although PET-CT is the best noninvasive imaging method for the evaluation of NSCLC, numerous pitfalls exist. The most frequently observed false-positive findings are due to brown fat, foci of infection, benign tumors like adenomas, post-therapeutic thymic hyperplasia, attenuation-related artifacts, recent trauma, surgery, or radiotherapy, but also to sites with physiologically increased 18F-FDG uptake as the brain, the myocardium, the vasculature, the bowel, and the collecting urinary system [5]. False-negative findings can be found in tumors with low metabolic activity as the bronchioalveolar cell carcinoma and the carcinoid, in cases of hyperglycemia but also in very small pulmonary nodules (with a short-axis diameter less than 8 mm).

Many studies have established the role of 18-FDG PET-CT in lung cancer restaging, concerning the detection of residual or recurrent tumor and the response to first line therapy. With the use of FDG PET-CT, residual or recurrent disease should, when possible, be differentiated from therapy-related changes in the lungs. 18F-FDG PET-CT has prognostic value and

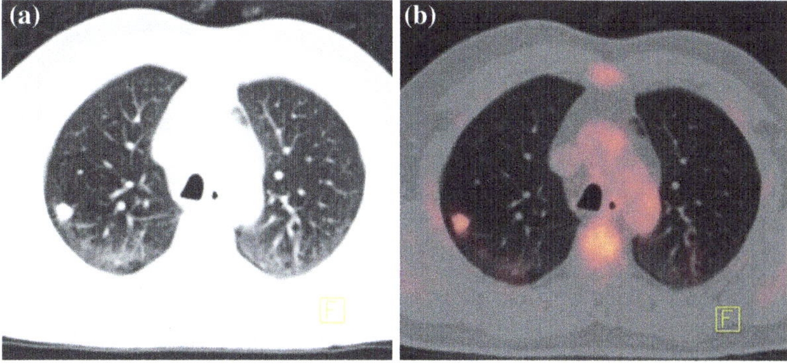

Fig. 25.1 Hypermetabolic SPN at the right lung on CT (**a**) and PET-CT images (**b**), proved- on biopsy-to represent primary lung cancer

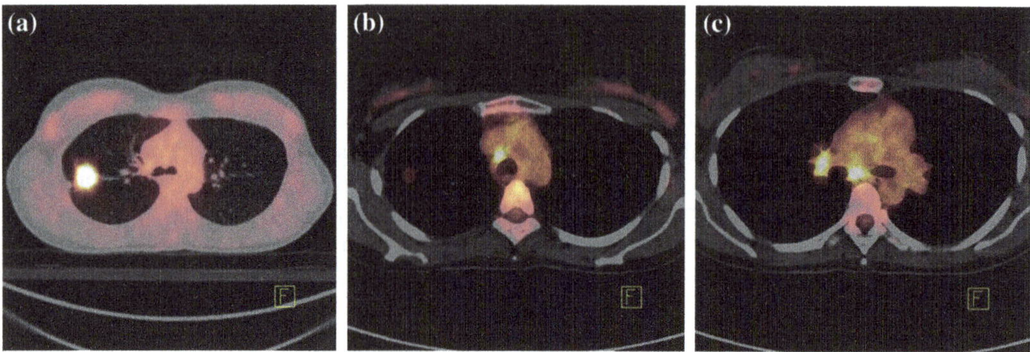

Fig. 25.2 Fused PET-CT images: primary tumor at the right lung (**a**) with hypermetabolic lymph nodes at the mediastinum (**b, c**)

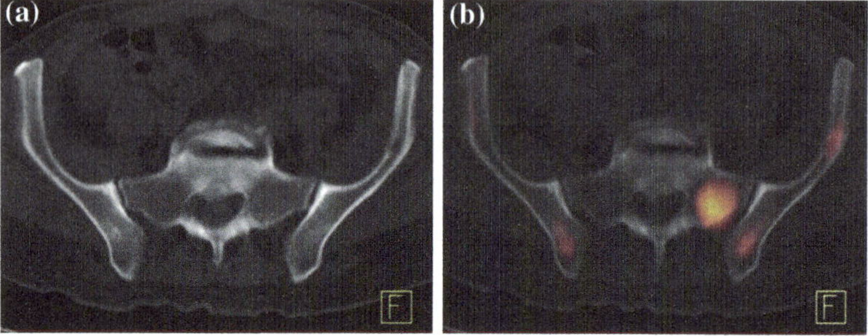

Fig. 25.3 Hypermetabolic metastasis at the iliac bones and the sacrum (**b**) which are not obvious or have subtle appearance on CT images (**a**) in NSCLC restaging

correlates strongly with rates of survival of patients with treated NSCLC meaning that patients with positive 18F-FDG PET-CT results have a significantly worse prognosis than patients with negative results [6, 9]. It was found that a reduction in metabolic activity correlated closely with the final outcome of the therapy. An early metabolic response (drop in SUV more than 50 %) predicted better survival while as poor response predicted progression of the disease.

Despite its high cost, PET-CT—when properly used—has proved to be a cost-effective method in the evaluation of lung cancer [10]. In about 35 % of cases first staged with CT, the stage of the disease has changed—in most cases the disease is upstaged—after subsequent PET-CT, with resultant changes in patient's management.

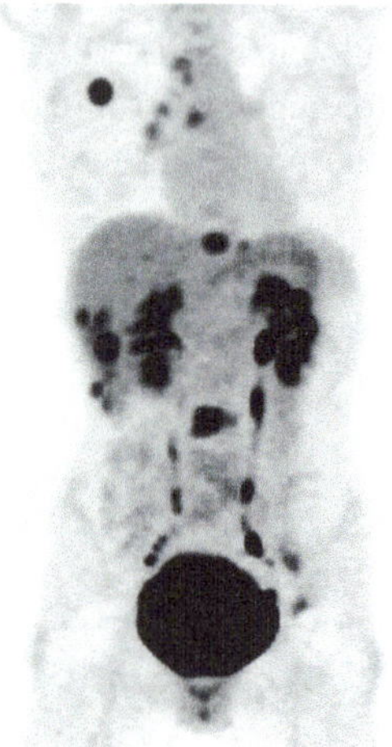

Fig. 25.4 Whole-body PET image: widespread metastatic NCSLC

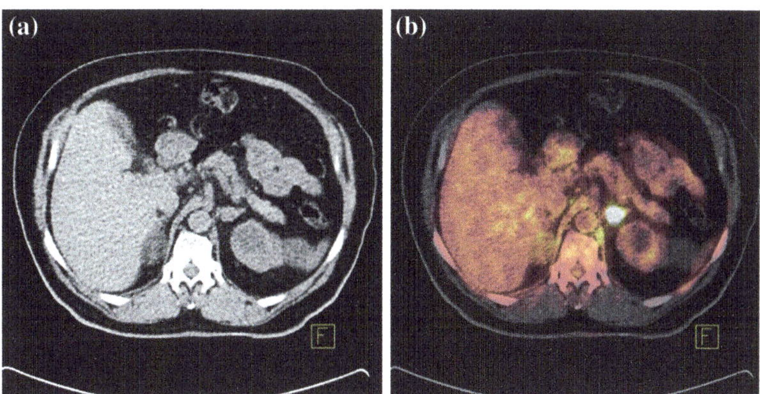

Fig. 25.5 Secondary deposit at the left adrenal on CT (**a**) and PET-CT images (**b**) in a NSCLC patient

According to NCCN practice guidelines PET-CT is recommended in NSCLC for:

(a) diagnosis in patients with one or two pulmonary nodules,
(b) initial staging except if multiple distant metastases exist,
(c) restaging stage III or IV after 2 to 3 months after treatment or before surgery,
(d) restaging in patients with symptoms suggestive of recurrence, and
(e) radiation therapy.

Small cell lung cancer accounts for 15 % of all lung cancers and is characterized by rapid growth and early spread to regional lymph nodes and to distant sites. The role of PET-CT in the evaluation of SCLC is still under study [3, 11]. SCLC is 18F-FDG avid at the primary site and at metastatic sites. PET-CT may be used in staging patients with SCLC in order to select potential candidates for the addition of thoracic radiation therapy to chemotherapy. PET-CT may also lead to upstaging or downstaging of patients and to alteration of radiation fields due to the detection of additional sites of nodal involvement.

By combining anatomic and functional data in a single imaging method, dual-modality PET-CT represents the most efficient and accurate approach to NSCLC staging, with a profound influence on therapeutic strategy and patient prognosis. It also represents a useful and promising method for SCLC management. (Figs. 25.1, 25.2, 25.3, 25.4, 25.5)

References

1. Bunyaviroch T and Coleman R (2006) PET Evaluation of Lung Cancer. J Nucl Med Vol. 47 No. 3
2. Fanti S, Franchi R, Batista G et al (2005) PET and PET-CT. State of the art and future prospects. Radiol Med 110:1–15
3. Ambrosini V, Nicolini S, Caroli P et al (2012) PET/CT imaging in different types of lung cancer: an overview. Eur J Radiol 81(5):988–1001
4. Vahid R, Dabbagh K (2007) Positron emission tomography (PET) in the management of lung cancer. Review. Pneumon 20(1):43–48
5. UyBico SJ', Wu C, Suh R et al (2010) Lung Cancer Staging Essentials: The New TNM Staging System and Potential Imaging Pitfalls. RadioGraphics 30:1163–1181
6. Kligerman S, Digumarthy S (2009) Staging of Non–Small Cell Lung Cancer Using Integrated PET/CT. AJR 193(5):1203–1211
7. Czernin J Schelbert H (2004) PET/CT imaging: facts, opinions, hopes, and questions J Nucl Med 45(*supl*): 1S.
8. Bradley J, Thorstad WL, Mutic S et al (2007) Impact of FDG-PET on radiation therapy volume delineation in non-small-cell lung cancer. Int J Radiat Oncol Biol Phys 59:4–5
9. Hanin FX, Lonneux M, Cornet J et al (2008) Prognostic value of FDG uptake in early stage non-small cell lung cancer. Eur J Cardiothorac Surg 33:819–823
10. Saif MW, Tzannou I, Makrilia N et al (2010) Role and cost effectiveness of PET/CT in management of patients with cancer. Yale J Biol Med. 83:53–65
11. Fischer BM, Mortensen J, Langer SW et al (2006) PET/CT imaging in response evaluation of patients with small cell lung cancer. Lung Cancer. 54:41–49

26 EBUS Staging and Lung Cancer

Nikolaos I. Papanikolaou, Charalampos A. Papagoras, Georgios N. Chrisocherakis and Emmanuil K. Zachariadis

Endobronchial ultrasound is a major advance in the field of diagnostic bronchoscopic procedures.

The technique was first applied in late 1990s and nowadays is widely recognized as a valuable tool for staging and restaging of lung cancer thus diminishing dramatically the need of surgical approach. Radial and Linear EBUS are the two different types of this sophisticated procedure.

26.1 Radial EBUS

The technique is based on the use of small catheters with incorporated on their tip a rotating ultrasound source (20 MHz), which provides a radial scanning image (4.5 cm depth) of parabronchial structures (Fig. 26.1). The catheter is able to pass through the working channel of the bronchoscope and reach the bronchial tree. A fluid interface between the probe and the bronchial wall is obtained by covering the tip of the catheter with a disposable balloon filled with sterile solution.

N. I. Papanikolaou · C. A. Papagoras ·
G. N. Chrisocherakis · E. K. Zachariadis (✉)
Respiratory Clinic, Euroclinic of Athens,
Athanasiadou 7-9, 11521 Athens, Greece
e-mail: rrapti@euroclinic.gr

N. I. Papanikolaou
e-mail: nkpapanikolau@gmail.com

26.2 Indications

Evaluation of the bronchial structure and its main layers.

In practice, we can differentiate between tumor infiltration and compression of the bronchial wall.

We can also determine a cancerous endobronchial lesion as in situ or invasive (the latter erodes the cartilaginous layer) (Fig. 26.2). The procedure is accepted as a necessary step to assess the option of endobronchial treatment (Fig. (26.3). EBUS combined with autofluorescence increases further the diagnostic yield for early tumors (Fig. 26.4).

Diagnosis of peripheral lung lesions

The diagnostic accuracy for lesions bigger than 2 cm combined with the bronchus sign on chest CT is more than 60 %. The use of guide sheath and special curettes offers better localization of the lesion especially under fluoroscopic guidance or in combination with electromagnetic navigation. For nodules less than 2 cm, the diagnostic accuracy is near 45 %[1].

Radial EBUS is considered a safer approach than CT-guided FNA for peripheral lesions especially in emphysematic patients with high risk of pneumothorax.

Evaluation of tumoral margins

EBUS can reliably localize the cancerous borders and their distance from main carina (T2-T3).

A. D. Gouliamos et al. (eds.), *Imaging in Clinical Oncology*,
DOI: 10.1007/978-88-470-5385-4_26, © Springer-Verlag Italia 2014

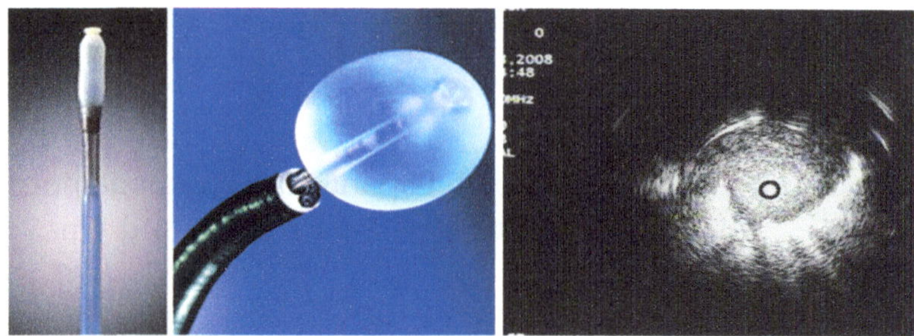

Fig. 26.1 Radial EBUS mini probe. Hypoechoic lesion (15 mm) of the left upper lobe (AdenoCa)

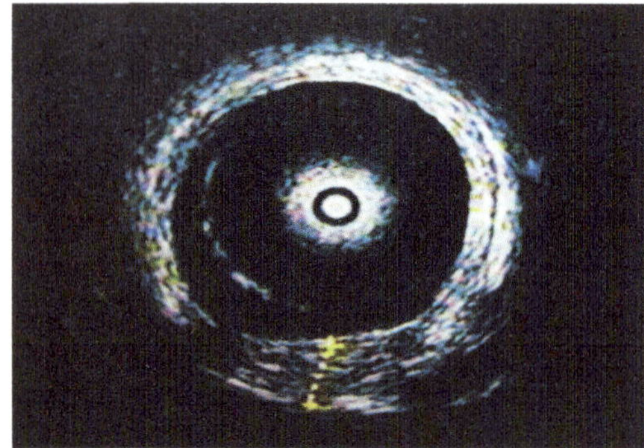

Fig. 26.2 Radial EBUS shows in situ lesion which does not erode the cartilage layer

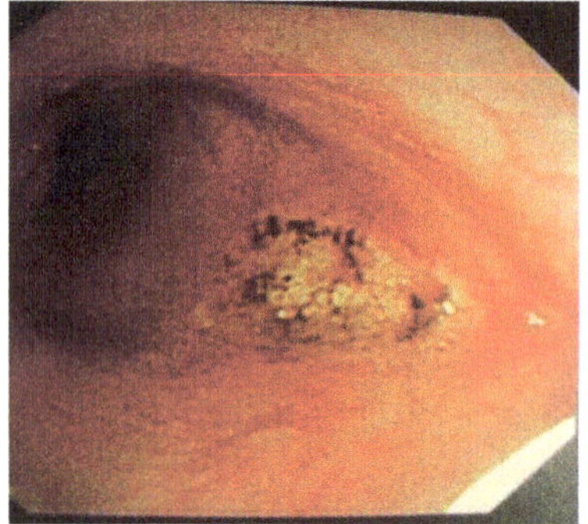

Fig. 26.3 Endobronchial laser resection of carcinoma in situ (subglotic area)

26.3 Linear EBUS (Endobronchial Ultrasound Bronchoscope)

The advent of EBUS bronchoscope in 2004 has greatly expanded the diagnostic field of bronchoscopy. Since that time, mediastinal masses were approached by blind TBNA method (diagnostic accuracy 45–70 % depending of the size and location of the lesion and mainly by the experience of the bronchoscopist).

The EBUS device incorporates on its tip an ultrasound transducer (7 MHz) which provides a real-time vision of biopsy procedure (EBUS TBNA) even in lymph nodes smaller than 1 cm (Fig. 26.5). Penetration depth is 5 cm.

It also combines a Doppler mode which permits the visualization of great vessels and their relation with the mass (Fig. 26.6) offering:

- Protection from vascular trauma or hemorrhagic (non diagnostic) biopsy specimen.
- Staging information based on great vessels involvement.

In a systematic review published in Eur J Cancer 2009, [2] EBUS-TBNA from CT-enlarged lymph nodes has been showed to have remarkable levels of sensitivity (90 %) and specificity (100 %).

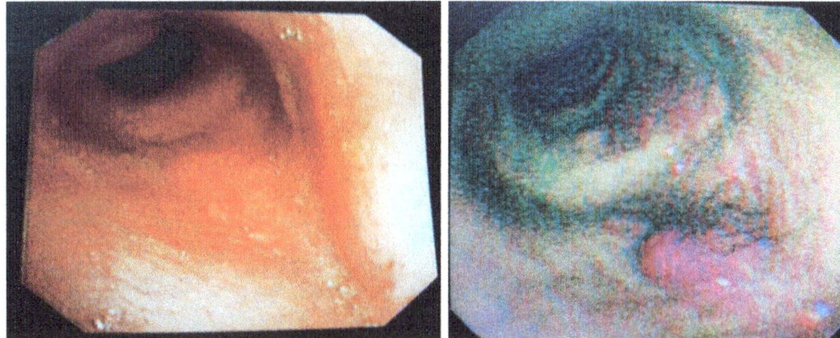

Fig. 26.4 Normal mucosa in subglottic trachea. Autofluorescence identifies a suspected lesion (carcinoma in situ)

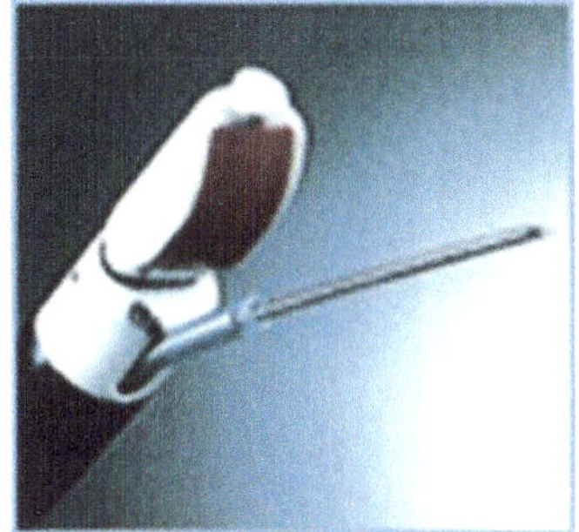

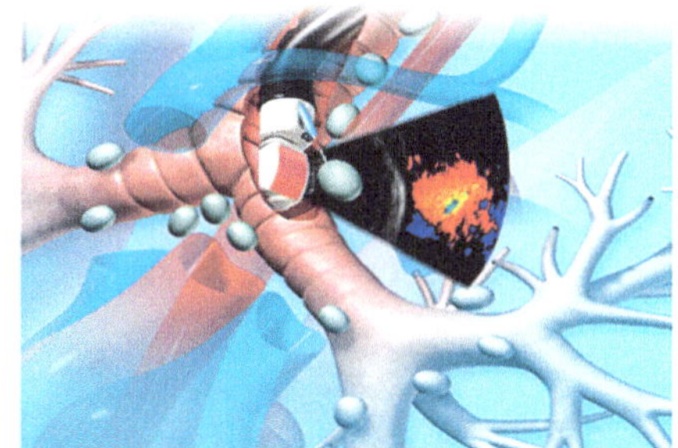

Fig. 26.5 Tip of linear EBUS bronchoscope (courtesy of Olympus)

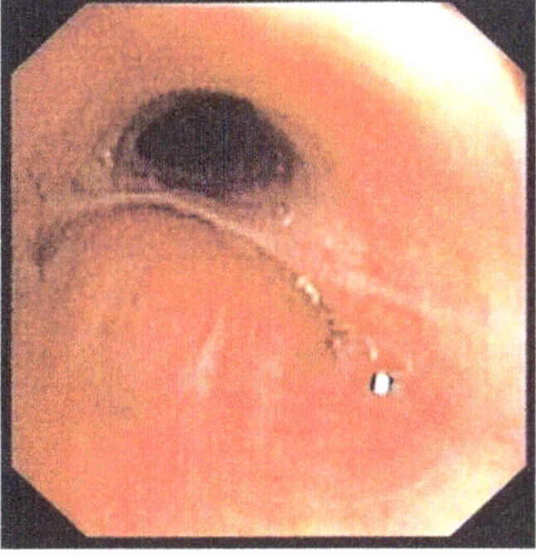

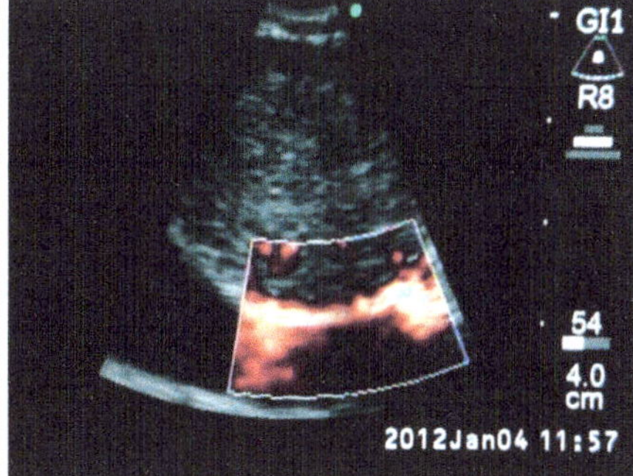

Fig. 26.6 Doppler mode reveals the contact of the mass with pulmonary artery. No signs of vascular invasion are noted

Emerging studies underline the fact that although the needle is 21G, 72 % of the EBUS samples are suitable for molecular analysis [3]. The latter depends of the reliable localization of the lesion (Fig. 26.7), the accurate preparation of the smear and the cell block procedure.

Three or more needle passes are necessary in order to achieve adequate tissue.

Rapid on site evaluation (ROSE) by an expert cytologist increases further the diagnostic accuracy.

Several publications confirm the importance of EBUS staging in mediastinal disease.

Lymph nodal stations of the anterior mediastinum [2, 4, 5] are feasible for diagnosis.

If combined with endoscopic ultrasound (EUS), practically the whole mediastinum can be reached (ad exception of stations 5, 6). Nevertheless, EBUS bronchoscope is feasible for nodal biopsy through esophagus (Fig. 26.8).

As a general rule, every pathological lymph nodal enlargement on CT or PET of lung cancer patients must be approached firstly by EBUS–EUS. In case of negative results, mediastinoscopy must be performed.

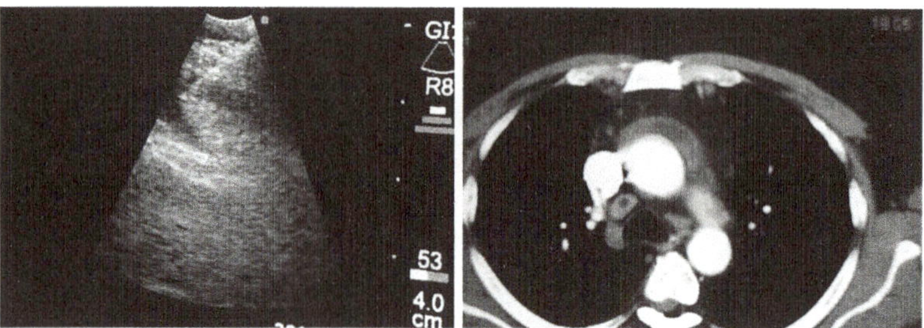

Fig. 26.7 Paratracheal lymph node (4R) with central necrosis. EBUS TBNA permits biopsy from peripheral nodal zone avoiding necrotic material (increased bioptic reliability)

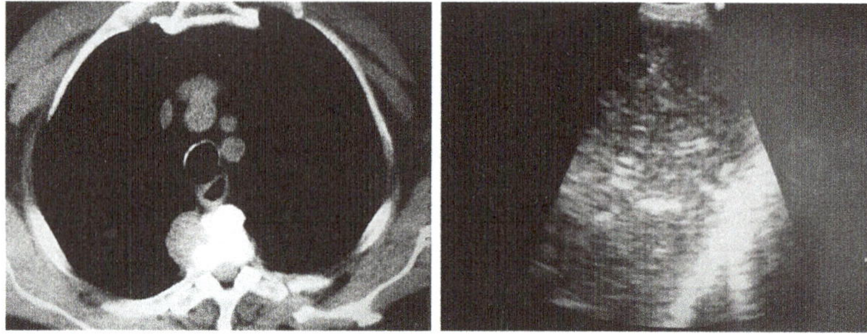

Fig. 26.8 Peripheral mass of the right lung, distant 2 cm from esophagus. EBUS bronchoscope localized the lesion through esophagus

In case of normal mediastinal findings on CT, EBUS investigation revealed N1-2 disease in 15 % of patients [6]. and in 8-10% of negative PET CT scan. Regardless the relatively low percentage of cases, generally is recommended to proceed to EBUS bronchoscopy in high risk lesions for nodal involvement. These are:

- centrally located tumors,
- peripheral T2a
- T2(5–7 cm)–T3 (>7 cm)
- N1 disease
- Tumors with low FDG uptake on PET CT

In conclusion, EBUS, EUS, and mediastinoscopy are complementary procedures in mediastinal staging.

Advantages of EBUS

- The procedure is performed in outpatient basis under mild sedation.
- Biopsy from lymph nodes not accessible with mediastinoscopy is feasible (posterior carinal, hilar, and paraesophageal stations).
- In case of restaging after diagnostic and therapeutic procedures (thoracotomy, radiotherapy, etc.), mediastinoscopy might have technical limitations. EBUS bronchoscopy can be applied several times without complications.

Disadvantages

- EBUS-TBNA negative predictive value (85 %) is the major disadvantage. Consequently, in suspicious lesions, mediastinoscopy (NPP 92 %) must be performed in all the cases of negative EBUS biopsies.
- The accuracy depends of the learning curve of the bronchoscopist. EBUS requires intensified training (at least 50 sessions) and long practical experience in interpreting sonographic images.
- The cost of the equipment is high, thus it is not widely available.
- Most contraindications do not differ from standard bronchoscopy. Special attention must be paid in case of respiratory failure and bleeding disorders.

26.4 Conclusions

- Radial and linear EBUS are widely accepted as very important tools concerning the routine bronchoscopy practice. The procedure is minimally invasive, safe and highly sensitive (90–94 %) and specific (100 %) for mediastinal staging. Nevertheless, its contribution in early lung cancer diagnosis, peripheral tumor approach and restaging after adjuvant treatment is increasingly recognized.
- In the new era of personalized treatment, EBUS TBNA bioptic marerial is suitable for molecular studies.
- EBUS helps in minimizing the need for invasive surgical procedures improving significantly the quality of life of lung cancer patients.

References

1. Eberhardt R, Ernst A, Herth JF (2009) Ultrasound-guided transbronchial biopsy of solitary pulmonary nodules less than 20 mm. Eur Respir J 34(6):1284–1287
2. Gu P, Zhao YZ, Jiang LY et al (2009) Endobronchial ultrasound-guided transbronchial needle aspiration for staging of lung cancer: a systematic review and meta-analysis. Eur J Cancer 45:1389–1396
3. Navani N, Brown JM, Nankivell M et al (2012) Suitability of Endobronchial Ultrasound-guided Transbronchial Needle Aspiration Specimens for Subtyping and Genotyping of Non–Small Cell Lung CancerA Multicenter Study of 774 Patients Am. J Respir Crit Care Med 185(12):1316–1322
4. Vilmann P, Puri R (2007) The complete ''medical'' mediastinoscopy (EUS-FNA + EBUS-TBNA). Department of Surgical Gastroenterology, Gentofte University Hospital, Copenhagen, Denmark. pevi@-geh.regio. Minerva Med 98(4):331–338
5. Chin R Jr, Ward R, Keyes JW et al (1995) Mediastinal staging of non-small-cell lung cancer with positron emission tomography. Am J Respir Crit Care Med 152(6 Pt 1):2090–6
6. Felix J, Herth MD, Ralf Eberhardt MD et al (2005) EBUS guided biopsy for the diagnosis of mediastinal lymph nodes in a radiologically normal mediastinum CHEST. 128 (4_MeetingAbstracts):211S–211S

Clinical Implications of Lung Cancer 27

Paris A. Kosmidis

For several years, efforts have been undertaken to increase the number of operable patients by making the diagnosis earlier in pre-symptomatic stage, in an effort to eliminate mortality.

The National Lung Screening Trial (NLST) was the most successful and promising trial for lung cancer screening and early diagnosis. They concluded that annual low-dose spiral CT screening of high risk participants was associated with a 20 % mortality reduction. The eligibility criteria for this study were current or former smokers (aged 55–74 years) with a smoking history of at least 30 pack-years and with no history of lung cancer [1].

Lung cancer is generally first imaged and often, first detected by chest radiography. This is the preferred initial imaging modality because of its availability, low-cost, low radiation dose, and high sensitivity. The radiological diagnosis is confirmed by CT scan. Following diagnosis, staging is by all means, the cornerstone in the decision-making process [2].

Computed tomography (CT) and occasionally magnetic resonance imaging (MRI) of the chest and upper abdomen are used to stage a known or suspected lung cancer. It is generally agreed that all patients with abnormal mediastinal lymph nodes at CT need further imaging with FDG-PET and probably lymph node biopsy. Therapy should not be planned based only on positive CT findings. Roughly 40 % of all nodes which are supposed to be malignant by CT are benign and 20 % of all nodes which are looked benign by CT are malignant. CT has a sensitivity and specificity of 51 and 86 % respectively, which are considered moderate. The role of MRI in the detection and staging of bronchogenic cancer has been limited and tends to be used only to answer very specific questions such as chest wall invasion, superior sulcus tumors, involvement of cardiac chambers, or pericardium. CT is superior for adrenals while MRI is more accurate in brain metastasis [3, 4].

Today, the most accurate staging is done by integrated PET/CT because it combines morphologic and metabolic information. Especially for lymph nodes PET/CT can accurately distinguish N_1, N_2, N_3 disease. PET/CT will detect non visible otherwise distant metastases in 10–15 % and mediastinal lymph node metastases in 10 % of NSCLC patients. PE/CT has a sensitivity of 74 % and a specificity of 85 % in the assessment of mediastinal lymph nodes. The sensitivity is poor for small lymph nodes (20 % false negatives) and poor specificity for large nodes (20 % false positive) [5, 6].

Tissue biopsy is necessary to confirm the diagnosis. Especially in small lymph nodes of mediastinum without FDG uptake with a centrally located tumor or hilar lymph nodes with increased FDG uptake. In these cases, mediastinal lymph nodes are found positive for malignancy in 6–30 % [3].

P. A. Kosmidis (✉)
Hygeia Hospital, Athens, Greece
e-mail: parkosmi@otenet.gr

A. D. Gouliamos et al. (eds.), *Imaging in Clinical Oncology*,
DOI: 10.1007/978-88-470-5385-4_27, © Springer-Verlag Italia 2014

The biopsy is done with either Endoscopic ultrasound-guided fine-needle aspiration (EUS–FNA) or Endobronchial ultrasound transbronchial needle aspiration (EBUS–TBNA) or both [3, 7, 8].

In patients with normal biopsies with the above two methods one may proceed with surgical mediastinoscopy only in those with abnormal mediastinum [3].

PET/CT is not useful in neuroendocrine lesions and generally in tumors with low FDG uptake. Inflammatory lymphadenitis may give false positive results. This is the reason why in positive results, tissue biopsy is necessary [6]. With the more extensive use of PET/CT, staging has become more accurate and treatment more tailored. Many operations have been cancelled and in localized disease chemoradiotherapy has been selected. In addition to staging PET scan has prognostic and predictive value. The higher the FDG uptake as it is expressed by SUV, the more aggressive the tumor. A reduction of SUV by >30 % (20–35 %) following one cycle of Cisplatin-based chemotherapy is correlated with better response and survival with sensitivity and specificity 95 and 76 % respectively [9]. The repeat PET/CT must be done 3 weeks following chemotherapy. The difference in SUV appears earlier in patients who are treated with EGFR-TKI's and respond. There are very preliminary studies with (F) FLT-PET on this matter. PET/CT is also useful for radiotherapy planning. It better discriminate between tumor and peritumural atelectasis or necrosis. It helps radiotherapy to be more accurate and to eliminate toxicity [9]. Also PET/CT will evaluate the response following chemoradiotherapy. When SUV was decreased by more than 50 % following treatment in comparison to the SUV prior to chemoradiotherapy, this may be considered a good indication for response. The repeat PET/CT must be done at least 3 months following the end of radiation.

The radiological follow-up of patients after treatment is not defined and is a matter of debate. Purpose of the follow-up is the early detection of relapse or metachronous primary tumors. In locally advanced NSCLC following radiochemotherapy, CXR every 4–6 months for the first 5 years and then annually is a preferred option. CT may replace CXR in high risk patients [10]. It seems that intensive follow-up does not have any impact on overall survival. In patients with early disease and surgery, CT scan with sections of the liver and adrenal glands and fiberoptic bronchoscopy every 6 months for the first 3 years and then annually has been proposed [11]. Although, there is no agreement, this schedule may improve survival by detecting recurrences or second primaries at an asymptomatic stage. Regarding brain metastasis, although there is no consensus, MRI could be done in suspicious or symptomatic patients [12].

In summary, the co-operation of Radiologist and Oncologist, the explosion of imaging techniques along with the experience have lead to better screening, diagnosis, staging, and follow-up of patient with lung cancer.

References

1. The National Lung Screening Trial Research Team (2011) Reduced lung cancer mortality with low-dose computed tomographic screening. N Engl J Med 365:395–409
2. Swensen SJ, Viggiano RW, Midthum DE et al (2000) Lung nodule enhancement at CT: multicentre study. Radiology 214:73–80
3. Tournoy KG, Keller SM, Annerma JT (2012) Mediastinal staging of lung cancer: novel concepts. Lancet Oncol 13:221–229
4. Gould MK, Kuschner WG, Rydzak CE et al (2003) Test performance of positron emission tomography and computed tomography for mediastinal staging in patients with non-small cell lung cancer, a meta-analysis. Ann Intern Med 139:879–892
5. Reed CE, Harpole DH, Posther KE et al (2003) Results of the American College of Surgeons Oncology Group ZOO50 trial: the utility of positron emission tomography in staging potentially operable non-small cell lung cancer. J Thorac Cardiovasc Surg 126:1943–1951
6. Van Tinteron H, Hoekstra OS, Smit EF et al (2002) Effectiveness of positron emission tomography in the preoperative assessment of patients with suspected non-small cell lung cancer: the PLUS multicentre randomised trial. Lancet 359:1388–1392
7. Gu P, Zhao YZ, Juang LY et al (2009) Endobronchial ultrasound-guided Transbronchial needle aspiration for staging of lung cancer: a

systematic review and meta-analysis. Eur J Cancer 45:1389–1396
8. Navani N, Brown JM, Nankivell M et al (2012) Suitability of endobronchial ultrasound-guided Transbronchial needle aspiration specimens for subtyping and genotyping of non-small cell lung cancer. A multicentre study of 774 patients. Am J Resp Crit Care Med 185:1316–1322
9. Skoura E, Datseris IE, Platis I et al (2012) Role of Positron Emission Tomography in the early prediction of response to chemotherapy in patients with non-small cell lung cancer. Clin Lung Cancer 13:181–187
10. Benamore R, Shepherd FA, Leighl N et al (2007) Does intensive follow-up alter outcome in patients with advanced lung cancer. J Thorac Oncol 2(4):273–281
11. Westeel V, Choma D, Clement F et al (2000) Relevance of an intensive postoperative follow-up after surgery for non-small cell lung cancer. Ann Thorac Surg 70:1185–1190
12. Schmidt-Hansen M, Baldwin D, Hasler E et al (2012) What is the most effective follow-up model for lung cancer patients? a systematic review. J Thorac Oncol 7(5):821–824

Part V
Head and Neck Cancer

28 Introduction to Head and Neck Cancer

Amanda K. Psyrri

28.1 Epidemiology

Worldwide, an estimated 6,44,000 new cases of head and neck squamous cell cancers (HNSCC) are diagnosed per year [1]. More than 90 % of these cancers are of squamous histology, which are frequently related to tobacco and alcohol use. Growing evidence over the past two decades suggests that human papillomavirus (HPV) 16 infection is implicated in the etiology of a subset of oropharyngeal squamous cell cancers in individuals who have little or no history of alcohol or tobacco use [2, 3].

28.2 Management According to Stage

Early stage tumors (TNM stages I and II) are managed with single modality therapy, surgery alone or radiation alone. In addition to surgery, radiotherapy is one of the pillars for treatment in HNSCC. Radiotherapy is applied as a single modality or as component of multimodality treatment. The choice of therapy largely depends on the stage of the disease: at early stages either surgery or radiotherapy can be sufficient, but in more advanced stages a combination of therapies yields better treatment results. Radiotherapy is also an essential component of organ preservation strategies. Imaging plays an important role in radiotherapy treatment planning. Optimal application of radiotherapy in head and neck cancers is often challenged by several tumor-related factors: total tumor burden, delineation of tumor borders, potential damage to healthy tissues around the tumor, tumor heterogeneity such as hypoxia and cell proliferation [4]. Advances in radiation therapy such as three-dimensional conformal radiation (3D-CRT) , intensity-modulated radiation therapy (IMRT), image-guided radiotherapy (IGRT), stereotactic body radiation (SBRT) and proton therapy aim to selectively deliver radiation to tumor tissues and spare the surrounding healthy tissues. Precise three-dimensional delineation of target volumes is the hallmark of high accuracy radiotherapy. Contrast-enhanced computed tomography (CECT) is the current standard for delineating tumors of the head and neck for radiotherapy. Modern imaging techniques may increase the therapeutic ratio and are currently being utilized.

28.3 Locally Advanced Disease

Patients with HNSCC often present locally advanced disease associated with significant local or regional spread of disease. Locally advanced HNSCC requires a multidisciplinary approach and is often curable with combined modality treatment including surgery, radiotherapy (RT), and chemotherapy. Treatment

A. K. Psyrri (✉)
Internal Medicine-Section of Medical Oncology, Attikon University Hospital, Rimini 1, Athens 12461, Greece
e-mail: dpsyrri@med.uoa.gr

A. D. Gouliamos et al. (eds.), *Imaging in Clinical Oncology*,
DOI: 10.1007/978-88-470-5385-4_28, © Springer-Verlag Italia 2014

selection for patients with locally advanced disease usually relies on organ-sparing/preserving approaches, taking into consideration the potential side effects, quality of life and patients' performance status and preferences. Historically, surgery followed by radiotherapy was the cornerstone in the management of locally advanced OSCC. However, these approaches often produced suboptimal control of locoregional disease and significant long-term functional impairment.

Concurrent chemoradiotherapy has been established as the optimal combination of chemotherapy and radiotherapy in locally advanced disease by randomized trials and metaanalyses [5–7]. Assessment of tumor response routinely includes clinical examination and radiographic imaging. These methods and criteria for tumor response assessment, however, after chemoradiotherapy have several limitations. Established Response Criteria guidelines, such as RECIST, use tumor measurements obtained by computed tomography (CT) or magnetic resonance imaging (MRI). CT or MRI assessments are based on anatomy and reflect changes in tumor volume. RECIST criteria were mainly developed for the evaluation of response in metastatic solid tumors treated with palliative systemic therapies. Complete response (CR) is defined as complete disappearance of all lesions, including lymph nodes. Subcentimeter lymph nodes can be a residual finding after shrinkage of pathologic lymph nodes after chemoradiotherapy. In this setting, defining CR using RECIST can be challenging [8].

28.4 Imaging

Positron emission tomography (PET) provides measurement of metabolic activity within a target lesion. A variety of PET tracers have been developed to assess metabolic differences between normal and cancer cells and tumor hypoxia. Therefore, they may be useful in selecting tumors for hypoxia modifiers or dose escalation. FDG PET can be useful in detecting recurrence even when disease is undetectable by conventional radiologic imaging. Combined functional and anatomical imaging offers advantages in response assessment.

References

1. Al-Sarraf M (2002) Treatment of locally advanced head and neck cancer: historical and critical review. Cancer Control 9:387–399
2. Weinberger PM, Yu Z, Haffty BG et al (2006) Molecular classification identifies a subset of human papillomavirus–associated oropharyngeal cancers with favorable prognosis. J Clin Oncol 24:736–747
3. Ang KK, Harris J, Wheeler R et al (2010) Human papillomavirus and survival of patients with oropharyngeal cancer. N Engl J Med 363:24–35
4. Arens AI, Troost EG, Schinagl D et al (2011) FDG-PET/CT in radiation treatment planning of head and neck squamous cell carcinoma. Q J Nucl Med Mol Imaging 55:521–528
5. Adelstein DJ, Li Y, Adams GL et al (2003) An intergroup phase III comparison of standard radiation therapy and two schedules of concurrent chemoradiotherapy in patients with unresectable squamous cell head and neck cancer. J Clin Oncol 21:92–98
6. El-Sayed S, Nelson N (1996) Adjuvant and adjunctive chemotherapy in the management of squamous cell carcinoma of the head and neck region. A meta-analysis of prospective and randomized trials. J Clin Oncol 14:838–847
7. Munro AJ (1995) An overview of randomised controlled trials of adjuvant chemotherapy in head and neck cancer. Br J Cancer 71:83–91
8. Passero VA, Branstetter BF, Shuai Y et al (2010) Response assessment by combined PET-CT scan versus CT scan alone using RECIST in patients with locally advanced head and neck cancer treated with chemoradiotherapy. Ann Oncol 21:2278–2283

US Findings in Head and Neck Cancer 29

Angelos A. Kalovidouris

29.1 Introduction

Ultrasound (US) is the initial imaging modality for evaluating superficial neck masses. In most cases, US aids in achieving an exact diagnosis or at least in determining the relation of the lesion to one or more neck organs, as well as its size, structure, margins, and vascularity. US is the preferred modality of guiding needle aspiration of all types of superficial lesions on the neck. Several technical improvements in the last years have contributed to improve image quality.

Compound imaging reduces artifacts and speckle noise and improves contrast resolution. Color and power Doppler are used to assess the degree of vascularity of neck organs. Lately, US-elastography is a new method for qualitative and quantitative estimation of tissue elasticity. US is considered as the modality of choice for evaluating thyroid and parathyroid neoplasms. It is used routinely for evaluating salivary gland tumors and cervical nodes.

A brief review of the main applications of US in the study of the neck cancer is presented emphasizing mainly in the cancer of the superficial organs of the neck, especially of the thyroid, parathyroid glands, salivary glands, and cervical lymph nodes.

A. A. Kalovidouris (✉)
Department of Radiology, Areteion University Hospital, University of Athens Medical School, 76, Vas. Sophias Avenue, 11526 Athens, Greece
e-mail: akalovidouris@windowslive.com

29.2 Ultrasonography in Thyroid Neoplasms

Nodules in the thyroid gland are common. The vast majority are benign. The likelihood that a nodule is cancerous is influenced by a variety of risk factors. As regards age malignancy is more common in patients younger than 20 and older than 60 years of age. The primary role of imaging in thyroid cancer is to differentiate between benign and malignant nodules. The most common tests used are US and US-guided FNA (USGFNA) Imaging also has a role in preoperatively staging and follow-up of patients treated for thyroid cancer.

The overall incidence of thyroid cancer in impalpable nodules is approximately 10 % regardless of the number of nodules present at sonography [1].

Several sonographic features present within a thyroid nodule are related to an increased risk of thyroid cancer.

29.3 Sonographic Features of Thyroid Neoplasms

Many US features of thyroid nodules such as size, shape, margins, echo structure, echogenicity, nodular growth, calcifications, vascularity, and elasticity are closely related to malignancy. Although these US findings have high sensitivity no single sonographic feature can reliably

A. D. Gouliamos et al. (eds.), *Imaging in Clinical Oncology*,
DOI: 10.1007/978-88-470-5385-4_29, © Springer-Verlag Italia 2014

distinguish benign from malignant thyroid nodule. However, when taken more than one US features, specificity improves. The sensitivity of US in the diagnosis cancer is 69–98 % and it has a specificity of 50–92 % and a diagnostic accuracy of 80–99 %.

The following 10 US features of a thyroid nodule may differentiate a benign from a malignant nodule:

1. Nodule size

Size was used as a criterion in the decision for thyroid nodule biopsy. Nodule size has not been found to be significantly indicative of malignancy. Thyroid cancers, smaller than 1 cm in size, have been shown to act clinically similar to larger cancers, and therefore these lesions should be followed with periodic US examination with the possibility for further evaluation with USGFNA, if growth or suspicious features are observed on sequential scans.

2. Nodule shape

Prognostic significance has been implicated with nodule shape. Nodules with irregular or more spherical shape found to have a higher incidence of malignancy than oval shape nodules. These features have fairly low sensitivity and cannot be considered pathognomonic of malignancy.

3. Echo structure

Considering composition nodules are classified as cystic, solid, or mixed. Malignancy has been more closely related to solid compared with cystic or mixed nodules. Purely cystic or mixed nodules as are those with microcystic, spongiform appearance are unlikely to be malignant [2].

4. Echogenicity

Most thyroid carcinomas are hypoechoic relative to surrounding thyroid parenchyma. Hypoechogenicity is a sensitive sign but is not specific. On the other hand, the combination of hypoechogenicity with another characteristic that has high specificity creates a useful pattern for triaging nodules to FNA. Over 30–55 % of benign nodules are also hypoechoic. An echogenic appearance is commonly associated with benign nodule. Follicular neoplasms, both benign and malignant, and rarely papillary cancers may have an echogenic appearance.

5. Margins

An irregular, speculated, or ill-defined margin has been associated with increased risk of malignancy. Well-defined, smooth margins are suggestive of benign lesion. Hypoechoic circumferential halo is often associated with benign lesions, believed to represent a capsule and flattened thyroid tissue. An incomplete or absent halo may be displayed in neoplasms and its presence or absence has been found to be suggestive but not diagnostic. Ill-defined margins are seen in both benign and malignant lesions.

6. Calcifications

Calcifications have been found in papillary, medullary, and anaplastic thyroid carcinomas as either psammoma bodies or as amorphous granular deposits. Of all the sonographic features associated with thyroid malignancy, microcalcifications are the most specific. Microcalcifications are defined as punctuate echogenic foci without acoustic shadowing or associated comet-tail artifact. The positive predictive value of a finding of microcalcifications in thyroid nodule ranges from 24 to 70 % [3].

7. Vascularity

Almost all solid nodules display some flow on color Doppler with current generation ultrasound equipment. In general, a peripheral flow pattern tends to be a feature of benign nodules, and malignant nodules tend to have internal vascularity but there is considerable overlap. A cystic nodule without any internal flow is unlikely to be malignant. Although marked internal vascularity was more often present in malignant than benign nodules, more than half of nodules with internal hypervascularity were benign. Papillary cancers were hypovascular, but none were entirely avascular. A cystic nodule without any internal flow is unlikely to be a papillary carcinoma.

8. US-Elastography

Elastography is a rapidly evolving imaging technique for the US measurement of tissue stiffness. Soft tissues deform more while hard tissues deform less. The rationale behind

US-elastography is that a cancerous nodule is harder and deforms less than the surrounding tissue. US-elastography scores were based on four classes of tissue stiffness (a. class 1 for soft nodules, b. class 2 and 3 for nodules with an intermediate degree of stiffness, and c. class 4 for anelastic lesions). Several studies have documented the application of US-elastography to thyroid nodules with sensitivity and specificity ranging from 80 to 97 % with an accuracy of approximately 80 % [4]. Although the use of US-elastography in combination with other US modalities has not been established and lacks standardized measurements for widespread use, it improves clinical outcomes and may help in differentiating benign from malignant lesions as well as in the selection of nodules for further evaluation by needle biopsy.

9. Nodule growth

Nodule growth is not pathognomonic of malignancy. While benign nodules may decrease in size, they often increase in size. The rate of thyroid nodule growth cannot distinguish alone between benign and malignant nodules. Although there is no general agreement on the definition of nodule growth, some suggest a 15 % increase in nodule volume, while others recommend measuring a change in the mean nodule diameter. American Thyroid Association (ATA) recommends a reasonable definition of growth as 20 % increase in nodule diameter with a minimum increase of at least 2 mm, in two or more dimensions.

10. Multiplicity of nodules

Patients with multiple thyroid nodules have the same danger of malignancy as those with solitary nodules. In patients with multiple nodules, the cancer rate per nodule decreases but the decrease is approximately proportional to the number of nodules, so that the overall rate of cancer per patient is the same as in patients with a solitary nodule. Although thyroid cancer found in patients with multiple nodules is often located in the dominant or larger nodule, in one-third of cases the cancer is in a nondominant nodule.

29.4 Malignant Thyroid Neoplasms: Histological Classification: The Main US Findings

Thyroid cancer can arise from different cell types and histological classification and is an important determinant of prognosis. There are four main types of thyroid cancers: tumors, arising from thyroid cells, ranging from papillary and follicular to anaplastic carcinomas, medullary cancer arising from parafollicular cells, primary thyroid lymphoma, and rare tumors arising from the stromal cells of the gland, such as sarcoma.

29.4.1 Papillary Carcinoma

Papillary cancer is the most common thyroid malignancy accounting for 75–80 % of thyroid cancer. Papillary carcinoma appears as a hypoechoic nodule with irregular margins, microcalcifications, and hypervascularity. The most specific sonographic finding of papillary cancer includes a solid hypoechoic lesion with microcalcifications and ill-defined margins. Although this finding has high specificity (85–95 %), sensitivity is only 25–59 % [1]. Most papillary cancers are solid (87 %) and hypoechoic (86 %) (Fig. 29.1). Some evidence of intrinsic vascularity is generally seen, though the distribution

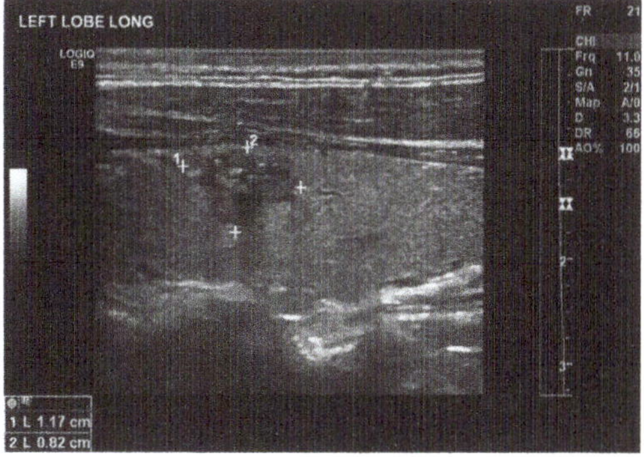

Fig. 29.1 Papillary carcinoma appearing as a solid nodule, hypoechoic with irregular shape, and calcifications

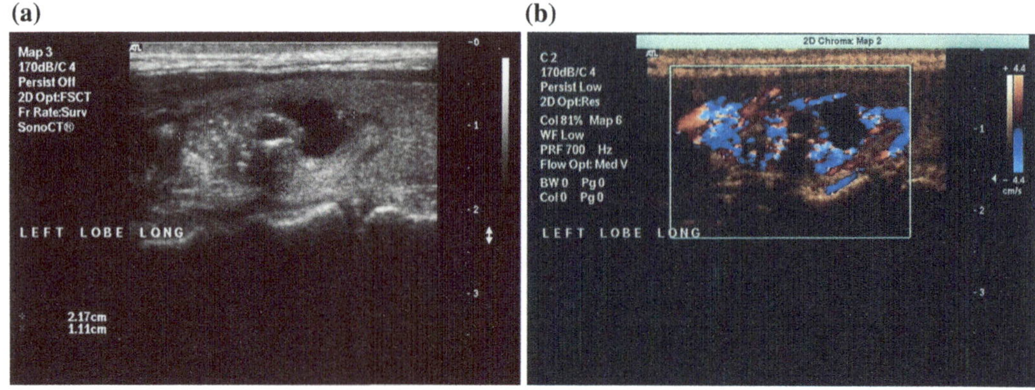

Fig. 29.2 Papillary carcinoma. (**a**) Solid inhomogeneous nodule with cystic changes and calcifications in the solid part of the nodule. (**b**) Color Doppler demonstrates internal vascularity

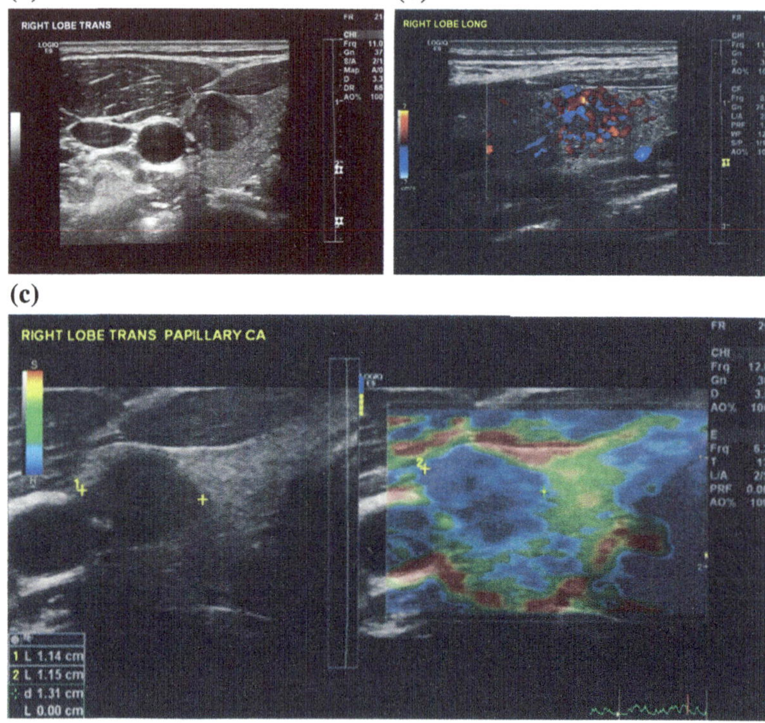

Fig. 29.3 Papillary carcinoma. (**a**) Inhomogeneous solid nodule. (**b**) CDI chaotic internal vascularity. (**c**) Elastography demonstrating high elasticity index

of vascularity has not been found to be a reliable feature [5] (Figs. 29.2 and 29.3).

29.4.2 Follicular neoplasms

Follicular carcinomas account for about 10 % of all thyroid cancers. Differentiation of follicular adenoma from a follicular carcinoma is based on the presence of capsular or vascular invasion on histologic examination and this cannot be made by sonography or by FNAC. On sonography, follicular adenomas and follicular carcinomas are usually solitary encapsulated tumors often with a well-defined peripheral hypoechoic halo representing the fibrous capsule. Two histologic patterns of growth of follicular carcinomas can be observed. The minimally invasive type is encapsulated, in contrast to widely invasive type, which extends beyond the tumor capsule into blood vessels and adjacent parenchyma. Echogenicity of follicular neoplasms is variable and can be echogenic, isoechoic, or hypoechoic (Fig. 29.4). Cystic components and calcifications are rare, and surrounding halo is often seen. In contrast to papillary carcinomas, follicular carcinomas metastasize hematogenously to bones, brain, and liver rather than by way of lymphatics.

29.4.3 Medullary Carcinoma

Medullary thyroid cancer is a neuroendocrine tumor arising from the parafollicular cells located in the upper two-thirds of thyroid gland and accounts for 2–10 % of all thyroid cancers. Although medullary cancer is associated with MEN 2A, 80 % occur sporadically. Patients who have sporadic medullary carcinoma typically present with a painless palpable nodule in the fifth or the sixth decade of life, but the disease is often metastatic to cervical lymph node at presentation. Medullary carcinoma appears solid and hypoechoic on US with irregular contours and often has calcifications with disorganized hypervascularity. The value of serum calcitonin screening measurement in patients who have thyroid nodules is dubious, because levels are often falsely elevated and FNA is highly accurate. On sonography, medullary carcinomas are typically solid hypoechoic, and often have coarse central calcifications (Figs. 29.5 and 29.6).

29.4.4 Anaplastic Carcinoma

Anaplastic carcinoma of the thyroid is a rare tumor of the thyroid, but extremely aggressive, represented the terminal stage in the dedifferentiation of a follicular or papillary carcinoma. Anaplastic carcinoma accounts for 1.6–12 % of all malignant tumors of the thyroid gland. Patients are usually elderly with a history of goiter and present with a rapidly growing neck mass. The tumor characteristically invades locally and involves adjacent muscles and blood vessels. Distant metastases most commonly involve the lungs, bones, brain, and liver. On sonography, anaplastic carcinomas are generally large, fixed, hard, and heterogeneous in appearance. Internal calcifications and cystic or necrotic areas may be seen. Adjacent enlarge lymph nodes are common. Invasion of nearby structures, such as the carotid sheath, trachea and muscles, and the overall extent of tumor are often better assessed on CT or MRI imaging.

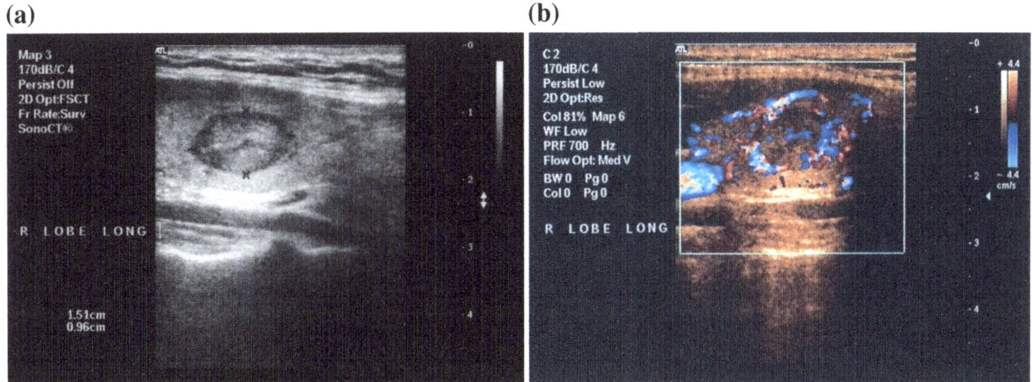

Fig. 29.4 Follicular carcinoma. (**a**) Solid mass with hyperechoic and hypoechoic components. (**b**) Color Doppler demonstrates marked increased vascularity

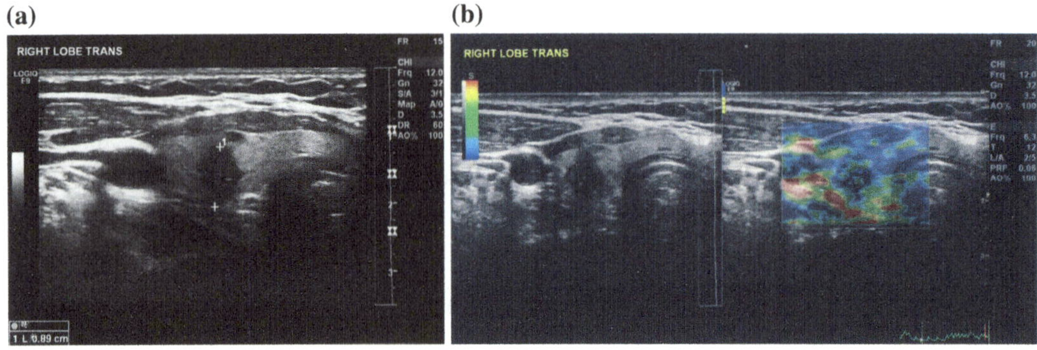

Fig. 29.5 Medullary carcinoma. (**a**) A solid nodule of 8.9 mm, hypoechoic with irregular shape and microcalcifications. (**b**) Elastography demonstrating high elasticity index

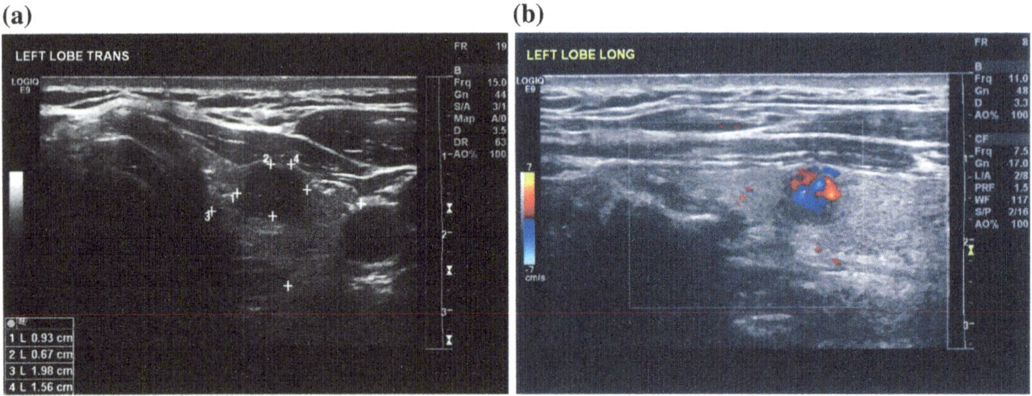

Fig. 29.6 Medullary carcinoma. (**a**) Gray-scale image of 9.3 mm hypoechoic mass in thyroid with microcalcifications. (**b**) Color Doppler demonstrates marked internal vascularity

29.4.5 Lymphoma

Primary lymphoma of the thyroid is uncommon accounting for 2 % of extra nodal lymphomas and less than 5 % of all malignant thyroid tumors. Patients present with a rapidly enlarging painless neck mass. Primary lymphoma may occur in preexisting case of Hashimoto thyroiditis. On US thyroid lymphoma is characteristically very hypoechoic with a pseudocystic pattern and tuberous contours.

29.5 USGFNA of Thyroid Nodules: Current Selection Criteria

Clearly no single sonographic feature predicts malignancy. Several groups have tried to develop multivariable predictors of malignancy using variable sonographic features as variables margin, shape, hypoechogenicity, internal architecture, and calcification (Tables 29.1, 29.2 and 29.3).

The ATA guidelines, revised in 2009, divide the thyroid nodules into four categories. On the basis of their composition. nodules are characterized as:

a. Entirely solid,
b. Mixed cystic-solid,
c. Spongiform, or
d. Purely cystic.

The American Association of Clinical Endocrinologists (AACE), in collaboration with the Associazione Medici Endocrinologi (AME), and the European Thyroid Association (ETA), published revised guidelines for the diagnosis and management of thyroid nodules in 2010.

Table 29.1 ATA thyroid needle biopsy guidelines (2009)

a. All solid hypoechoic nodules >1 cm in diameter
b.Isoechoic or hyperechoic nodules >1–1.5 cm in size
c. Mixed cystic-solid nodules that exceed 1.5–2 cm, if they have irregular margins, microcalcifications, or infiltration of the nearby tissue
d. Mixed cystic-solid nodules without suspicious US features if they are >2 cm in diameter
e. Nodules exhibiting a spongiform echotecture only if they are >2 cm in diameter
f. Purely cystic nodules do not require biopsy

Table 29.2 AACE/AME/ETA thyroid nodule biopsy guidelines (2010)

a. Nodules of any size with marked hypoechogenicity, irregular or microlobulated margins, taller than wide configuration, microcalcifications, or "chaotic arrangement of intranodular vascular images" or "chaotic intranodular vascular spots"
b. Independent of dimensions if US suggests the presence of metastatic lymph nodes or if extracapsular growth is noted in the nodule
c. The solid component of all complex cystic nodules because of the risk of cystic papillary carcinoma. *Note* Nodules that are "hot on scintigraphy" do not require biopsy

Table 29.3 KSTR thyroid nodule guidelines (2011)

a. Nodules considered probably benign and <1 cm in diameter: no follow-up US is needed
b. Nodules >1 cm and probably benign: follow-up US study at 2 years and at 3–5 years
c. "Selective use of biopsy" for those nodules thought to be probably benign but exceed 2 cm in diameter
d. All nodules reflecting any feature suspicious for malignancy: US may be used to guide percutaneous biopsies (USGFNA)
e. Nodules smaller than 5 mm: selective USGFNA based on the risk factors of the patient and the experience of the radiologist performing the procedure
f. All nodules >5 mm with a suspicious feature, "if feasible": US may also be used to guide percutaneous biopsies (USGFNA)
g. Any suspicious nodule with benign initial cytological findings: repeated USGFNA
h. Nodules considered indeterminate, with neither benign nor suspicious features: follow- up US if the nodule is <1 cm and biopsy for all such nodules >1 cm in diameter
i. Any nodule showing growth should undergo USGFNA. Growth is defined as a 20 % increase in diameter or a 50 % increase in volume [9]

The Korean Society of Thyroid Radiology (KSTR) published guidelines for the management of thyroid nodules in 2011, using a different approach. Thyroid nodules have been divided into three categories:

a. *Probably benign*. Spongiform nodules, completely cystic, or predominantly cystic nodules;
b. *Suspicious for malignancy* . Nodules with taller than wide shape, irregular margins, marked hypoechoic echotecture, macrocalcifications, extracapsular extension, or a spiculated margin; and
c. *Indeterminate*. Nodules that cannot be classified in category a (probably benign) or b

(suspicious for malignancy). In this case follow-up US is recommended.

29.6 The Role of US for Preoperative Staging (Mapping) of Patients with Thyroid Carcinoma

In patients with known or suspected thyroid carcinoma US examination should include assessment of extension of thyroid carcinoma to thyroid capsule or infiltration of beyond the thyroid capsule to adjacent soft tissues or vascular bed. US also provides an objective means of documenting lymph mode size, location, and characteristics suggestive of nodal metastases. Sonography has been established as the most sensitive imaging test to diagnose those nodal metastases. Lymph node metastases are noted in up to 60 % of patients on histologic review in centers performing ipsilateral and central neck dissections in all patients. US evaluation identified nonpalpable lateral compartment infiltrated lymph nodes in 14 % of patients undergoing initial surgery. Even when lymph nodes were palpable, sonographic assessment of the extent of lymph node involvement altered 40 % of the operative procedures by changing the extent of resection [6].

29.7 Metastatic Lymph Nodes

Various sonographic features have been described to aid in the differentiation of metastatic lymph nodes from normal nodes, including increased lymph node size, rounded shape, absence or deformation of echogenic hilus, hyperechogenicity, cystic changes, presence of calcifications, and increased vascularity (Fig. 29.7). Cervical lymph node size is unreliable as the sole criterion of metastatic thyroid carcinoma, because hyperplastic nodes may be large and metastatic nodes may be normal in size [7].

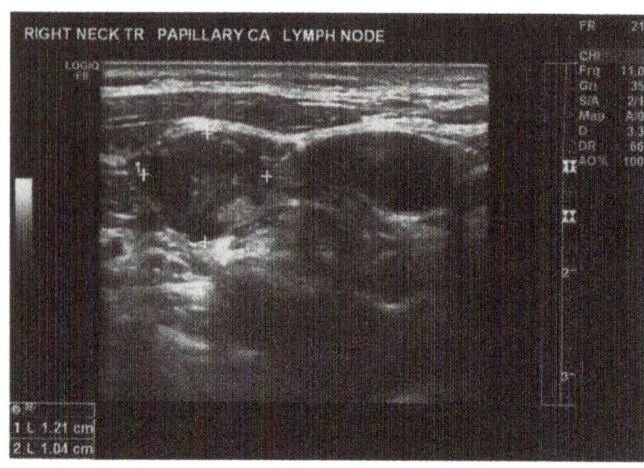

Fig. 29.7 Infiltrated lymph node. A rounded shape lymph node with heterogeneously disorganized consistency and microcalcifications lateral to internal jugular vein

29.8 Evaluation of the Post Thyroidectomy Bed

The primary goal of follow-up in patients who have operated for thyroid carcinoma is the early discovery of recurrence, either in cervical lymph nodes. The combination of a detectable stimulated serum thyroglobulin level with neck sonography identifies 95 % of patients who have metastatic lymph nodes and has a negative predictive value of 99 % [7, 8].

The American thyroid association guidelines support the use of only stimulated thyroglobulin and cervical ultrasound rather than the use of radioiodine scanning for surveillance in low-risk patients who have DTC.

Thyroid cancer recurrence is usually 2–10 years after operation. It is usually seen on the side of primary lesion (43–80 %), on the opposite side in 30.2 % and on both sides in 26 %.

Following thyroidectomy and remnant ablation, only a minimal of echogenic tissue, like reflecting tissue and scar tissue is noted in the thyroidectomy bed. Recurrent thyroid cancer in the bed typically appears as a solid or mixed cystic and solid soft-tissue mass, often with marked vascularity (Fig. 29.8). If large masses or posterior positioned masses are noted in the central compartment of the neck CT or MRI may be necessary to evaluate for invasive disease into

(a) (b)

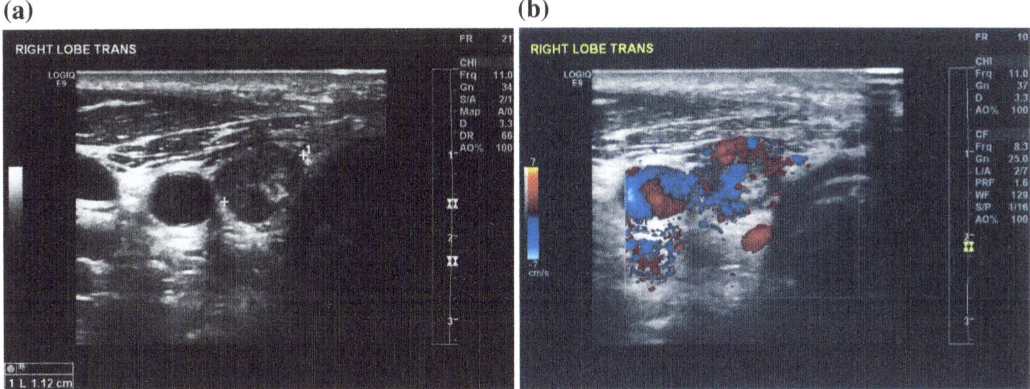

Fig. 29.8 Recurrence of medullary carcinoma. (**a**) Solid inhomogeneous mass of 11 mm, appearing 1 year after thyroidectomy in the thyroid bed. (**b**) Color Doppler demonstrates increased vascularity

the trachea, esophagus, retropharyngeal space, or skull base, because sonography is limited in evaluating these masses. Following thyroidectomy, metastatic disease to the paratracheal lymph nodes can be detected by identifying enlarged cystic calcified or vascular paratracheal lymph nodes.

Sonography has been established as the most sensitive imaging modality to access the neck for metastatic thyroid carcinoma. The sensitivity of US to local recurrence of thyroid cancer is 83–93 %, its specificity is 90–92 %, and its diagnostic accuracy is 90–91 %.

Lymph node metastases may vary from subtle alterations in echogenicity or vascular patterns to more obvious findings of calcifications and cystic changes within an affected node. If US findings are not diagnostic enough USGFNA should be performed on the suspicious node. Sonographic surveillance and USGFNA offer to the ability to document early thyroid cancer recurrence in the neck [8].

29.9 Parathyroid Cancer: US Findings

Parathyroid carcinoma is an unusual cause of hyperparathyroidism representing less than 2 % of all cases. The diagnosis is made during pathomorphological examination especially in the setting of primary hyperparathyroidism and

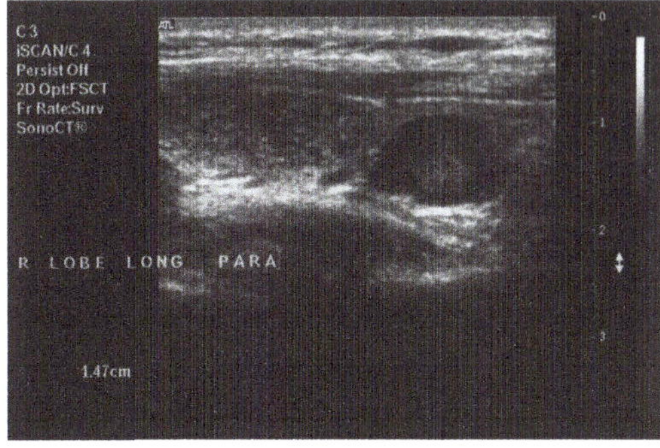

Fig. 29.9 Parathyroid carcinoma: An oval shape mass inhomogeneous 14.7 mm in size with irregular margins and absence of echogenic capsule

recurrent nerve paralysis. Patients usually have typical symptoms associated with hypercalcaemia and high levels of blood PTH. Grossly parathyroid carcinomas tend to be large and exhibit a roundish or oval shape, irregular indistinct margins, and absence of an echogenic capsule (Fig. 29.9). Parathyroid carcinomas have no characteristic imaging features and may not be distinguishable from adenomas or other soft-tissue masses. The metastatic lymph nodes of the neck can serve as an additional sign of parathyroid carcinoma in the absence of malignancies in the other organs of the neck and mediastinum. Regional cervical and mediastinal lymph node metastasis may occur in up to one-third of patients, and distal metastases in approximately 25 % of patients. The US is not efficient for tumors less than 10 mm in size. It is also of little value for retrotracheal, retroesophangeal, mediastinal, and other locations of parathyroid lesions. Scintigraphy (99mTc-sestamibi) CT or MRI is preferable on such cases.

29.10 Malignant Tumors of the Salivary Glands: US Findings

There are many types of malignant epithelial tumors, which may account for 20 % of the salivary tumors. Malignant tumors may grow rapidly and may be fixed to the skin of the underlining soft tissues, or bones. They may be painful or tender to palpation can be associated with lymph node metastases and cause facial nerve paralysis or paresis. The most frequent are mucoepidermoid cancer (5–10 % of all salivary gland tumors) adenocystic carcinoma and acini cell tumors. US may be used to determine whether a superficial lesion is intrinsic or extrinsic to the parotid gland or to the submandibular gland and to follow such a mass. US may also be used to guide percutaneous biopsies of the major salivary gland masses that cannot be done by palpation alone and may help to improve the diagnostic yield of those procedures by ensuring that the sampling is from the mass and not adjacent normal gland. Malignant tumors often show irregular borders, attenuated posterior echoes, heterogeneous internal echoes, or a irregular and polygonal shape (Fig. 29.10). There are no consistent criteria to differentiate between malignant and benign lesions. Malignant tumors may also be homogeneous, well defined, cystic, and even lobulated similar to pleomorphic adenomas. US, however, is fundamentally limited by the bony confines of the mandible and mastoid. MRI or CT is necessary to show the extent of disease, particularly to demonstrate perineural spread of tumor tissue.

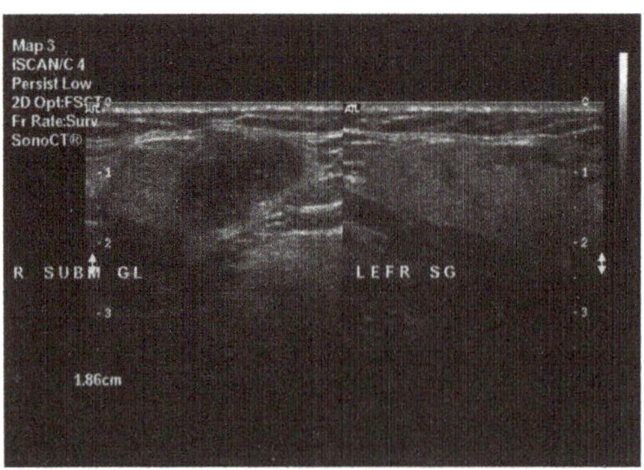

Fig. 29.10 Carcinoma of submandibular gland. Double picture of the right and left submandibular gland. An inhomogeneous hypoechoic solid mass is seen in the right submandibular gland. Normal left submandibular gland on the left half of the picture

References

1. Nam-Goong I, Kim H, Gong G et al (2004) Ultrasonography-guided fine-needle aspiration of thyroid incideltaloma: correlation with pathological findings. Clin Emdocrinol 60:21–28
2. Moon WJ, Jung SL, Lee JH et al (2008) Bening and malignant thyroid nodules: US differentiation-multicenter retrospective study. Radiology 247:762–770
3. Frates MC, Benson CB, Charboneau JW et al (2005) Management of thyroid nodules detected at us society of radiologist's in ultrasound, consensus conference statement. Radiology 237:794–800
4. Asteria C, Giovanardi A, Pizzocaro A et al (2008) US-elastography in the differential diagnosis of bening and malignant thyroid nodules. Thyroid 18:523–531
5. Chan BK, Desser TS, Mc Dougal IR et al (2003) Common and uncommon sonographic features of papillary thyroid carcinoma. J Ultrasound Med 22:1083–1090
6. Gharib H, Papini E, Valcavi R et al (2006) AACE/AME Task force on thyroid nodules. American association of clinical endocrinologists and associazone medici endocrinology medical guidelines for clinical practice for the diagnosis and management of thyroid nodules. Endocrinol Pract. 12:63–102
7. Leboulleux S, Girard E, Rose M et al (2007) Ultrasound criteria of malignancy for cervical lymph nodes in patients follow-up for differentiated thyroid cancer. J Clin Endocr Metab 92(9): 3590–3594
8. Frasoldati A, Pesent M, Gallo M (2003) Diagnosis of neck recurrences in patients with differentiated thyroid carcinoma. Cancer 97:90–96
9. Levine RA (2012) Current guidelines for the management of thyroid nodules: poster 9128/2012 Endocrinol Pract 18(4):596–599
10. Papini E, Guglielmi R, Bianchini A (2002) Risk of malignancy in nonpalpable thyroid nodules: predictive value of ultrasound and color-doppler features. J Clin Endocrinol Metab 87:1941–1946

CT and MR Findings in Head and Neck Cancer

30

Elias C. Primetis and Apostolos V. Dalakidis

30.1 Introduction

Accurate assessment and staging in head and neck cancer is crucial for patients' management and planning the appropriate treatment. In such setting, the main goals of imaging are to define the extent and size of primary tumor, to assess nodal involvement, to evaluate for possible perineural tumor spread, and to differentiate between recurrent/residual tumor and post-treatment changes. Both Computed Tomography (CT) and Magnetic Resonance Imaging (MRI) are particularly well-suited for the evaluation of deep and submucosal spaces of head and neck region; however, each one is bounded by its own limitations.

30.2 Indications

The introduction of CT in the 1970s and the following advent of MRI have enriched our diagnostic armamentarium and increased diagnostic accuracy and confidence. MRI has the following advantages:

E. C. Primetis (✉) · A. V. Dalakidis
Department of Radiology, University of Athens Medical School, Aretaieion Hospital, 76, Vas. Sophias Avenue, 11528, Athens, Greece
e-mail: elprimetis@yahoo.gr

A. V. Dalakidis
e-mail: tolisroma@gmail.com

- Superior soft tissue contrast resolution, which results in better definition of tumor extent;
- Lack of iodine-based contrast agents (gadolinium-based contrast agents instead); and
- High sensitivity in the detection of perineural or intracranial disease.

The disadvantages of MRI include lower patient tolerance, contraindication in case of pacemakers, or certain other implanted metallic devices and artifacts related to multiple causes, including motion-related artifacts. Additionally, MRI is not reliable for detecting small tumor deposits in normal-sized lymph nodes.

The advantages of CT are the following:

- It is a fast and readily available imaging modality;
- It is well tolerated; and
- It is more suitable to depict bony structures and calcifications.

On the other hand, CT has inferior contrast resolution and requires iodinated contrast media and ionizing radiation.

MRI is considered the modality of choice for the evaluation of nasopharyngeal (Fig. 30.1), sinonasal (Fig. 30.2) and parotid tumors because of better contrast resolution, ability to detect perineural spread and less prominent motion artifacts in the above anatomic regions. It is the appropriate modality to delineate any intraorbital or intracranial extent of malignant tumors. It is also the initial study of choice for tumors confined to the tongue and possibly for other locations of the oral cavity, since it is superior in the detection of tumor spread in the bone/bone

A. D. Gouliamos et al. (eds.), *Imaging in Clinical Oncology*,
DOI: 10.1007/978-88-470-5385-4_30, © Springer-Verlag Italia 2014

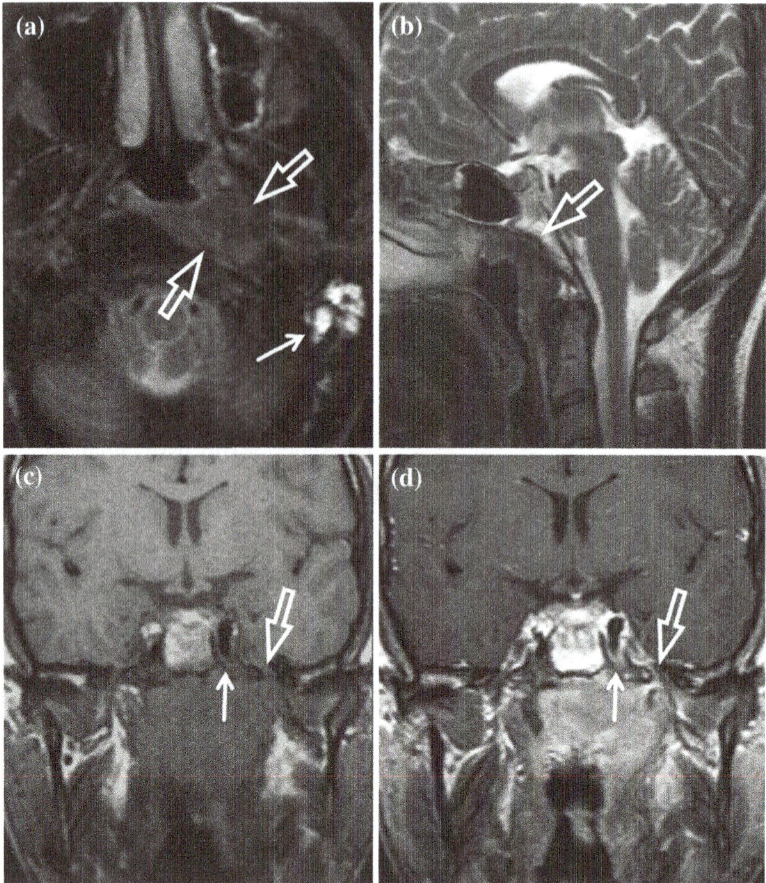

Fig. 30.1 Nasopharyngeal Carcinoma: MRI: (**a**) Axial T2 W: Mass centered in the *left* lateral pharyngeal recess (*open arrows*). Retained secretions in the *left* mastoid air-cells (small arrow), due to eustachian tube dysfunction. (**b**) Sagittal T2 W: Invasion of anterior clivus by the tumor (*open arrow*). (**c**) Coronal T1 W. (**d**) Coronal T1 W post contrast shows contrast enhancement of the mass. Proximity of the mass to internal carotid artery (*small arrows* c, d), to foramen ovale and mandibular nerve (V3) (*open arrows* c, d) is well depicted

marrow and it is not influenced by the presence of dental amalgams.

On the other hand, tumors of the oropharynx (Fig. 30.3), larynx (Fig. 30.4), and hypopharynx are initially assessed with CT, which is less affected by breathing and swallowing artifacts. Patients with difficulty in handling their oral secretions because of prior head and neck surgery, especially after tracheotomy or partial glossectomy, cannot tolerate lying still for the time required for MR scanning. In such cases, the rapid imaging of multislice helical CT is more suitable to yield studies unmarred by motion artifacts. CT is also the modality of choice to evaluate for obstructing salivary ductal calculi (sialoliths) or for the detection of fractures, since calcifications and bone structures are better depicted [1, 2]. Some authors rely heavily on CT for initial evaluation, preoperative planning, biopsy targeting, and postoperative follow-up. They reserve MRI in case perineural, cartilaginous, or bony invasion is suspected after CT imaging or for tumors which tend to spread via these routes, such as adenoid cystic carcinoma (Fig. 30.5).

The evaluation of nodal status is a controversial topic since there is no clear advantage of CT over MRI. In the last few years, the advent of

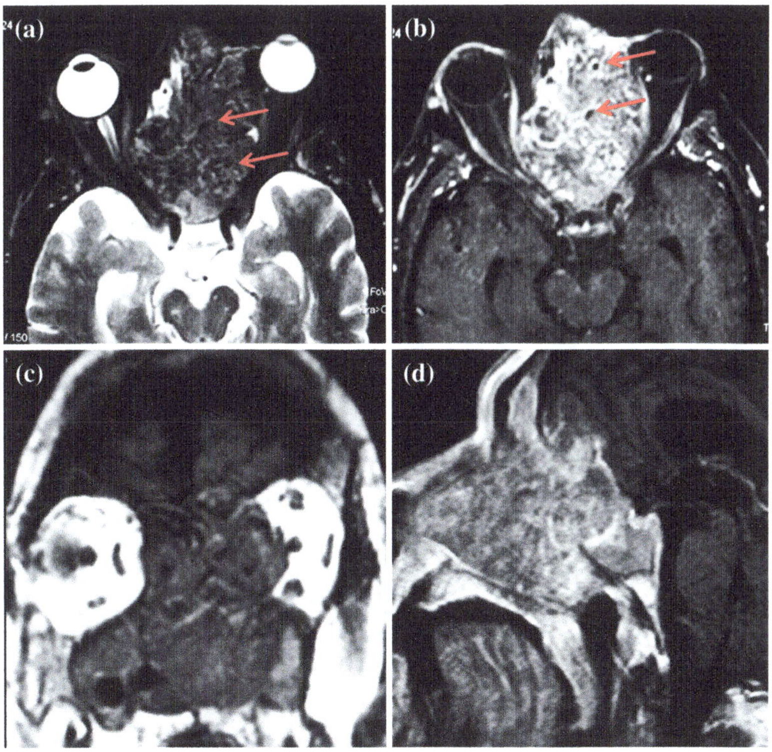

Fig. 30.2 Ethmoid cells giant adenocarcinoma: MRI: Axial T2 W (**a**) and Post Contrast-Fat Suppression-T1 W (**b**): A large mass occupying nasal cavity. T2 signal of the mass is intermediate to low due to high cellular component as well as small extracellular space and water content. Small intra-tumoral signal voids (*red arrows*) correspond to high flow vessels and calcifications. The mass enhances avidly with contrast medium due to increased vascularity. Coronal T1 W (**c**) shows invasion of the left orbit. Sagittal T1 W post contrast (**d**) shows invasion of the anterior cranial fossa

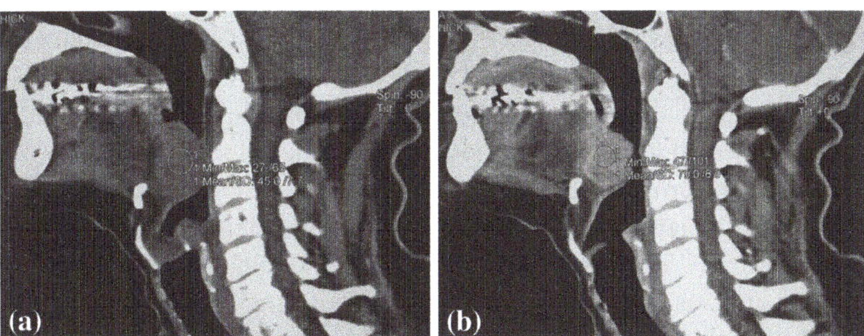

Fig. 30.3 Oropharyngeal (lingual tonsil) carcinoma: CT: Non-enhanced (**a**) and enhanced (**b**) sagittal reconstructions. Enhancing mass of the lingual tonsil invading the base of the tongue, occupying epiglottic vallecula and displacing epiglottis posteriorly

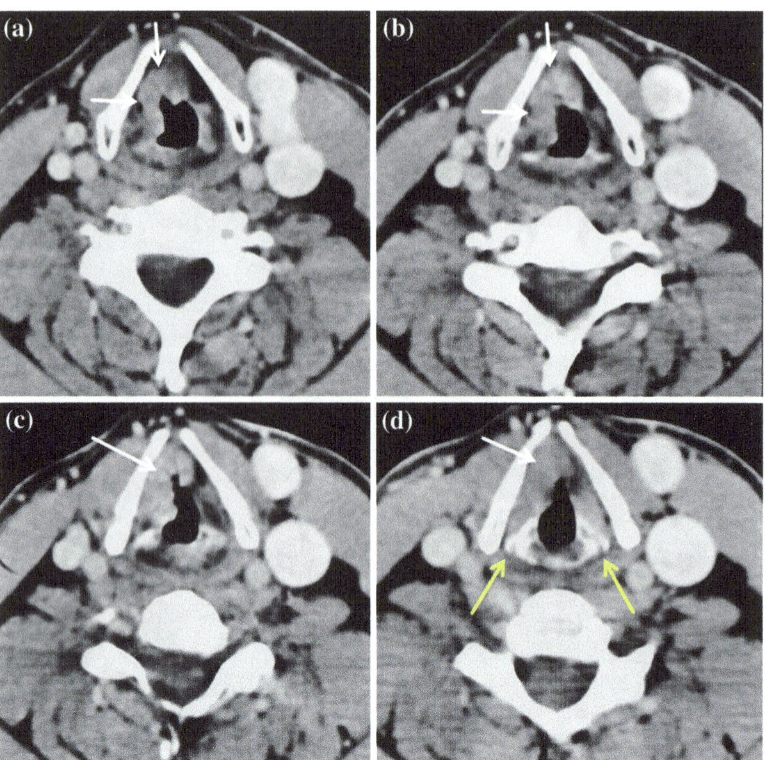

Fig. 30.4 Transglottic Laryngeal carcinoma (supraglottic and glottic): Consecutive axial post contrast CT slices (**a–d**). Moderately enhancing soft tissue density lesion infiltrating the right false vocal cord, paraglottic space, laryngeal ventricle, and right true vocal cord (*white arrows* **a–d**). Cricoarytenoid joints (*yellow arrows* **d**)

new MR techniques (diffusion imaging, USPIO) seems to favor MRI in assessing nodal disease.

30.3 Imaging Findings

Clinical and demographic data should be taken into account when interpreting imaging studies. The patient's age is an important discriminatory factor in the differential diagnosis. In the pediatric age group, a variety of benign entities (congenital or inflammatory) comprises the majority (>90 %) of lesions. In the same age group, the majority of malignant lesions are lymphomas (e.g. Burkitt lymphoma if rapid growth is noted) and rhabdomyosarcomas. On the other hand, a head/neck mass-lesion (excluding thyroid lesions) in adults, most probably (>90 %) corresponds to malignancy. In younger adults (20–40 years), the most frequent malignancy is lymphoma; whereas in adults older than 40 years, the most common neck mass is a nodal metastasis from squamous cell carcinoma [3].

In the past, neck findings were classified according to the cervical triangles. This classification has limited value, since it cannot localize and describe the deep head and neck lesions. Therefore, it is important to adapt a new classification system based on the deep spaces of the neck. The majority of radiologists have adapted the following spatial approach. The deep anatomic structures are subdivided by the superficial, middle, and deep layers of the deep cervical fascia into the following suprahyoid (above the hyoid bone) spaces: superficial pharyngeal mucosal, parapharyngeal, carotid, parotid, masticator, retropharyngeal, and pre-paravertebral (Fig. 30.6). The infrahyoid (below hyoid bone) neck spaces (site of important structures such as

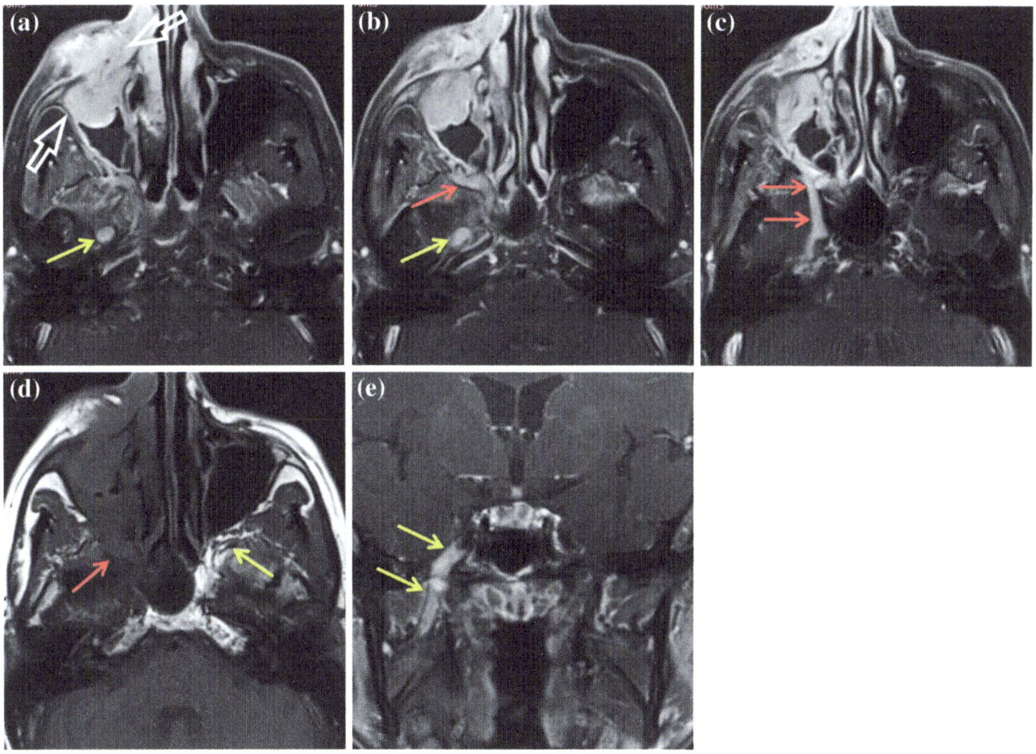

Fig. 30.5 Adenoid cystic carcinoma with perineural spread: MRI: Consecutive axial T1 W fat-suppressed post contrast images (**a–c**). Axial T1 W (**d**). Coronal T1 W fat-suppressed post contrast (**e**). Large enhancing mass invading the anterior wall of the right maxillary sinus (*open arrows* **a**). Effacement of fat in the *right* pterygopalatine fossa (*red arrow* **d**) compared to the normal *left* one (*yellow arrow* **d**). Abnormal enhancement of the *right* pterygopalatine fossa (*red arrow* **b**), along the route of V2 (*red arrows* c), and V3 nerve (*yellow arrows* **a**, **b**, and **e**) due to perineural tumor invasion

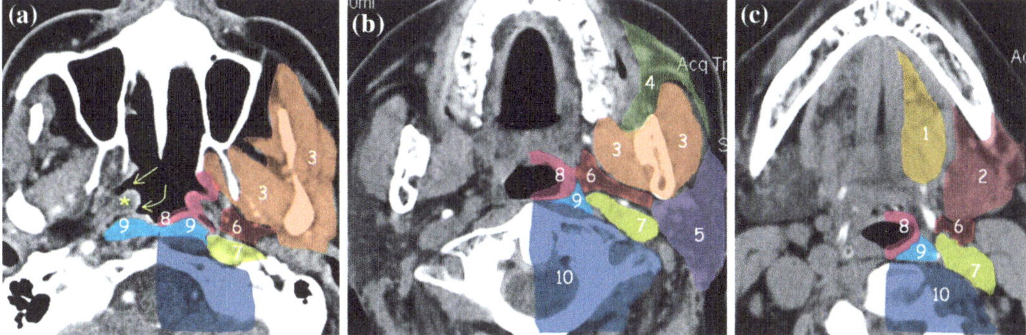

Fig. 30.6 Axial CT slices at the level of: (**a**) Maxillary sinuses, (**b**) Maxilla, (**c**) Mandible. Anatomic spaces: *1 Sublingual space, 2 Submandibular space, 3 Masticator space, 4 Buccal space, 5 Parotid space, 6 Prestyloid parapharyngeal space, 7 Carotid space (poststyloid parapharyngeal), 8 Pharyngeal mucosal space 9 Retropharyngeal space 10 Pre*paravertebral space. Torus Tubarius: [Asterisk]. Pharyngeal ostium of the auditory (eustachian) tube: [*Straight arrow*]. Lateral pharyngeal recess (fossa of Rosenmuller): (*Curved arrow*)

the thyroid gland and the larynx) include the visceral (site of the thyroid), posterior cervical, anterior cervical, carotid, parapharyngeal, and pre-paravertebral spaces.

The initial step when evaluating a neck lesion is to determine the space from which the lesion originates, since only a limited number of structures are located within each space. Specific lesions are found within these separate anatomic spaces, markedly limiting the differential diagnosis. As an example, the principal structures within the parotid space are the parotid gland and parotid lymph nodes. Consequently, if a parotid space mass is identified, the diagnosis is primarily limited to either a parotid tumor or nodal disease.

Soft tissue neck masses have few specific imaging characteristics, but many hints may drive the radiologist toward either a benign or a malignant process [4]. The imaging features suggestive of malignancy are:

- Large volume;
- Extra-compartmental extension (extension outside a neck space);
- Ill-defined margins;
- Broad interface with underlying fascia;
- Inhomogeneous MR signal intensity;
- High-signal intensity on T2-weighted MR;
- Invasion of bone or neurovascular structures;
- Intra-tumoral hemorrhage;
- Intra-tumoral necrosis; and
- Marked, primarily peripheral enhancement.

It is important to evaluate the lymph node status . In cross-sectional imaging, the assessment of a node mainly relies on its size and the presence of central necrosis. Evaluation of the shape is more difficult: a metastatic node is usually round (a ratio of the longitudinal-to-transverse diameter of less than 2). It has been suggested that a short-axis diameter of >10 mm in a lymph node should be considered abnormal. Heterogeneous nodal enhancement on CT or MR imaging is a specific feature of malignancy, particularly for/in squamous cell carcinoma. Pathologically, tumor cells initially involve the marginal sinus of the nodal cortex. Subsequently, they invade the medullary portion of lymph nodes, blocking the lymphatic flow, which results in medullary necrosis. In patients with squamous cell carcinoma, nodes with central necrosis are considered as metastatic, regardless of their size.

In case of laryngeal carcinoma, endoscopy plays an important role in diagnosis. The role of imaging in such case is to evaluate tumor extent and to contribute to treatment planning and patient follow-up. When interpreting imaging studies of laryngeal carcinoma we should be attentive to the following issues: (1) tumor volume; (2) presence of and/or degree of cartilaginous invasion; (3) invasion by the tumor into supraglottic, glottic, and subglottic compartments; (4) pre-epiglottic, paraglottic, and soft tissue dissemination; and (5) extent of nodal disease. It is important to note that cartilaginous invasion is a key factor in planning treatment strategy. CT findings indicative of such involvement are: sclerosis, erosion or lysis of cartilage, irregular cartilage margin, extra-laryngeal tumor beyond the cartilage, and expansion of cartilage. Whereas sclerosis is the most sensitive (83 %) criterion, it often histopathologically corresponds to reactive inflammation, particularly in the thyroid cartilage (specificity, 40 %) [5]. MR imaging findings suggestive of cartilaginous invasion are:

1. High-signal intensity within the cartilage on fat-suppressed FSE T2-weighted images,
2. Low signal intensity on T1-weighted images in the involved hyaline cartilage or in an ossified cartilage with fat marrow, and
3. Cartilaginous enhancement on fat-suppressed T1-weighted images.

These MR findings can also be found in cases of cartilage inflammation and edema with no histologically proven tumor invasion. Nevertheless, if these findings are absent, cartilage invasion is less likely [6].

30.4 Results

The vast majority of head and neck cancers are squamous cell carcinomas. Early stage cancer confined to the mucosa is usually undetectable on cross-sectional imaging. Endoscopy is frequently able to detect these tumors. Cross-sectional imaging is useful in accurate staging, since clinical staging often results in downstaging in case of laryngeal tumors, extension to the deep soft tissues and laryngeal cartilage invasion is better assessed by cross-sectional imaging, with CT and MRI being able to assess areas hidden from the clinician. Cross-sectional imaging will result in upstaging the primary tumor in approximately 25 % of patients. In the hypopharynx, the initial clinical tumor stage was upgraded after cross-sectional imaging in up to 90 % of patients.

In many head and neck regions (such as sinuses, nasopharynx, skull base, oral cavity and hypopharynx-larynx), CT and MR imaging have complementary roles. CT is more accurate and sensitive in assessing the margins of osseous anatomic structure and cavities and may demonstrate early skull base erosion. MRI offers higher soft tissue contrast and multiplanar capabilities. Whereas CT may detect cortical erosion of the skull base, MR imaging is probably more sensitive in assessing skull base invasion. It is particularly well suited to study bone marrow, because it can differentiate fat from other tissues.

Sensitivity of MRI (89 %) is higher than that of CT (64 %) in the detection of tumoral cartilage invasion (e.g. laryngeal cartilages). Higher sensitivity comes at a cost of decreased specificity (79 %). The specificity of CT is higher than that of MRI in all reported studies. The overall accuracy of MRI is higher than that of CT by an increment of 2–10 %; however, these differences were not found statistically significant. In a meta-analysis of the major studies, the accuracy of MRI (83.6 %) was calculated higher than that of CT (80.8 %). Many authors therefore recommend MR as the primary imaging modality for cartilage assessment in patients with laryngeal carcinomas. [5].

Lymph node status is an important prognostic factor. CT, MRI, US, and especially US-guided FNA cytology proved to be more reliable than clinical palpation for detection of metastatic lymph nodes in a recent meta-analysis. In cross-sectional imaging lymph node evaluation mainly relies on size criteria. The following size criteria have been proposed as optimal: a minimum axial diameter of 11 mm for jugulodigastric node and a corresponding 10 mm diameter for the remainder of nodes. These criteria had a sensitivity of 89 % and a specificity of 73 % per neck dissection specimen, and a sensitivity of 41.7 % and specificity of 99.3 % per node [7]. Lymph node size clearly is of limited diagnostic value. Other morphologic features include the shape and the number of lymph nodes. A metastatic node tends to be round, whereas a normal node is often oval, oblong, or kidney shaped. It has been reported that metastatic nodes had a ratio of the longitudinal-to-transverse diameter of less than 2 (sensitivity, 97 %; specificity, 97 %; accuracy, 97 %) [8]; however, it was found that lymph node shape did not increase the accuracy of the minimal axial diameter criterion. Newer MRI techniques (Diffusion MRI) and the development of tissue specific contrast agents (USPIO) offer new options in the diagnostic work-up of potentially metastatic lymph nodes. Another important parameter in assessing lymph node status is the presence of central necrosis. As mentioned earlier, central necrosis is highly indicative of nodal involvement. Some authors have reported that CT is more sensitive than MR imaging for the evaluation of nodal necrosis. MR imaging findings that indicate central necrosis show a heterogeneous signal on a T2-weighted image and ring enhancement on a gadolinium-enhanced image. Both fatty replacement and nodal abscess may mimic central necrosis. Thus, the use of fat-suppression and non-contrast T1-weighted images is essential to differentiate these conditions.

30.5 Conclusions

The assessment of head and neck malignancies requires a multidisciplinary team approach. Nowadays, medical imaging with CT and MRI plays substantial role in the management of head and neck cancer. Pretreatment diagnostic work-up with both modalities has predictive value for patient outcome. Based on pretreatment imaging, individualized replanning during radiotherapy may improve tumor control rates and spare normal tissues from unnecessary irradiation. Post-treatment CT or MRI is of great value when recurrent disease is suspected, to confirm its presence, to define its extent and differentiate between post-treatment inflammatory/fibrotic changes and tumor recurrence.

References

1. Rumboldt Z, Gordon L, Gordon L et al (2006) Imaging in head and neck cancer. Curr Treat Options Oncol 7:23–34
2. Alberico RA, Husain SH, Sirotkin I (2004) Imaging in head and neck oncology. Surg Oncol Clin N Am 13:13–35
3. Harnsberger HR et al (2004) Diagnostic Imaging. Head and neck, Amirsys, Salt Lake City
4. Razek AA, Huang BY (2011) Soft tissue tumors of the head and neck: imaging-based review of the WHO classification. Radiographics 31:1923–1954
5. Yousem DM, Tufano RP (2002) Laryngeal imaging. Magn Reson Imaging Clin N Am 10:451–465
6. Som PM, Curtin HD (2011) Head and neck imaging. Mosby Elsevier, St. Louis
7. Anzai Y, Brunberg JA, Lufkin RB (1997) Imaging of nodal metastases in the head and neck. J Magn Reson Imaging 7:774–783
8. Steinkamp HJ, Cornehl M, Hosten N et al (1995) Cervical lymphadenopathy: ratio of long- to short-axis diameter as a predictor of malignancy. Br J Radiol 68:266–270

PET-CT Findings in Head and Neck Cancer

31

Fani J. Vlachou

Multimodality imaging is not only the present, but also the future of diagnostic imaging. PET/CT is a hybrid device, which has the capability to provide a combination of anatomical and functional imaging due to the high spatial resolution of CT and the molecular imaging of PET.

PET/CT uses 18F-FDG, a radiolabeled glucose analogue which accumulates in tumor cells that have increased glucose metabolism, and seems to contribute to a great extent in the management of head and neck squamous cell carcinoma (HNSCC) patients including staging, restaging, treatment planning and surveillance of these patients [1].

The American Joint Committee on Cancer recommends the TNM staging for squamous cell carcinomas, which represent the 90–95 % of head and neck cancers [1].

In T staging, MRI is considered the gold standard, although recent studies have shown PET/CT's capacity to detect a primary lesion with high precision (94–98 %), to generate total sensitivity and specificity results ranging from 93 to 100 % and 90 to 100 %, respectively [2]. Regarding HNSCC at an early stage, it is hard to say whether the PET component of PET/CT imaging adds any valuable information to the primary cancer as opposed to a contrast-enhanced CT scan. Moreover, an extended meta-analysis carried out showed that a higher primary site SUV is related to lower percentages of disease-free survival, overall survival and local control [3]. FDG-PET/CT can identify primary tumors whose total volumes are at least 1 ml, nevertheless the sensitivity lowers as the size becomes smaller [4].

During evaluation of regional lymph nodes metastases, which plays a significant role in defining the progression of the disease and therefore the suitable treatment, PET/CT outclasses conventional imaging modalities which regard the size of the lymph nodes as pathologic criterion. Its capacity to detect lymph node metastases in unexpected areas, like the axilla, infraclavicular regions and the upper mediastinum is another benefit. In head and neck cancer, the presence of metastasis to cervical lymph nodes is regarded as a crucial matter. The most significant HNSCC parameter related to diagnosis is the existence and the amount of pathologic nodes. Patients diagnosed with nodal disease and extranodal spread decreases their likelihood to survive by 50 %. It is well known that some lymph nodes smaller than 1 cm can possibly represent metastases and these "small lymph nodes" are usually "missed" when using CT or MRI. In situations like these, FDG PET/CT is more accurate as it can detect small size lymph nodes larger than 6 mm that have increased radiopharmaceutical up-take. For smaller lymph nodes or for micro metastases FDG PET/CT's precision is restricted by the limited spatial resolution of PET/CT systems, which provides false negative results.

F. J. Vlachou (✉)
Department of Nuclear Medicine, Hygeia Hospital, Kifissias Ave. and 4 Erythou Stavrou Str. Maroussi, 15123, Athens, Greece
e-mail: fanivlachou@yahoo.com

A. D. Gouliamos et al. (eds.), *Imaging in Clinical Oncology*,
DOI: 10.1007/978-88-470-5385-4_31, © Springer-Verlag Italia 2014

Another problem in using FDG PET/CT for N staging is the false positive lymph nodes attributed to increased radiopharmaceutical uptake in inflammatory lymph nodes. The metabolic activity observed in lymph nodes is measured by standardized uptake values (SUV). Benign and malignant diseases are defined with cutoff values, however they are not applicable in head and neck malignant diseases. Rodrigues et al. conducted a study in which SUV values could help in discrimination of a benign lymph node inflammation from metastatic involvement in cases where they surpass 6.5 for a whole body protocol of PET/CT and 11 for and neck contrast-enhanced study of PET/CT. Lymph nodes false-positive findings can provide critical evidence concerning staging and treatment and are connected to HNSCC inflammation. A study by Kovács et al. was conducted to compare PET/CT contribution in neck dissection with directed lymph node biopsy in terms of accurate staging. The results demonstrated PET/CT prevalence in excluding any vain neck dissections in patients with false-positive findings [4].

However, various studies have demonstrated the sensitivity of FDG PET/CT in the evaluation of nodal metastatic disease is higher than that of CT (96 versus 78 %) [1] and slightly higher than that of MRI (93 %). Another remarkable benefit of FDG PET/CT is its ability to alter N staging in 10 % of HNC patients [2]. According to Schöder et al. documented PET/CT's sensitivity (87 to 90 %) and specificity (80 to 93 %) of the cervical lymph node diagnosis compared with MRI and CT sensitivity (61 to 97 %) and specificity (21 to 100 %) [4].

To sum up, in the evaluation of HNSCC patients for cervical nodal metastases, FDG PET/CT is considered better than the conventional imaging modalities (CT, MRI), but the guided fine needle aspiration biopsy remains the gold standard (Figs. 31.1, 31.2, 31.3 and 31.4) [2].

In order to exclude or to confirm the presence of distant metastases, especially in patients with advanced HNSCC, FDG PET/CT is considered the modality of choice, because in one examination not only are we able to visualize the whole body and have the opportunity to identify foci of increased metabolic activity that may represent distant metastasis (most common in the lungs, liver or skeleton), but we can also detect a possible second primary tumor. It is worth mentioning that numerous studies have shown that the use of FDG PET/CT has significantly changed the stage of the disease (overstaging or understaging) in about 30 % of HNC patients [5].

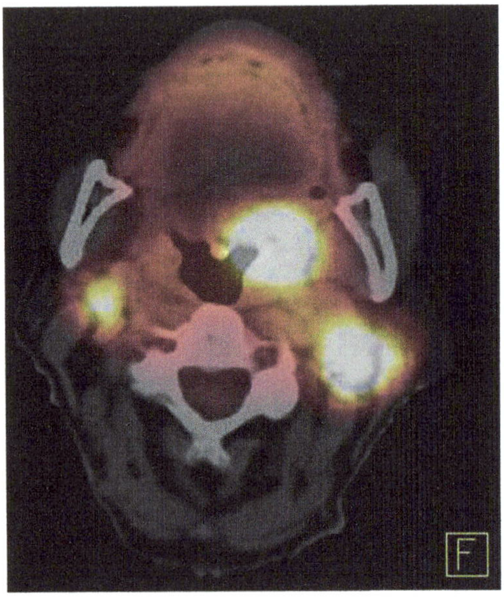

Fig. 31.1 Squamous cell carcinoma of the left oropharynx. Hypermetabolic lymph nodes in the left and right lateral neck

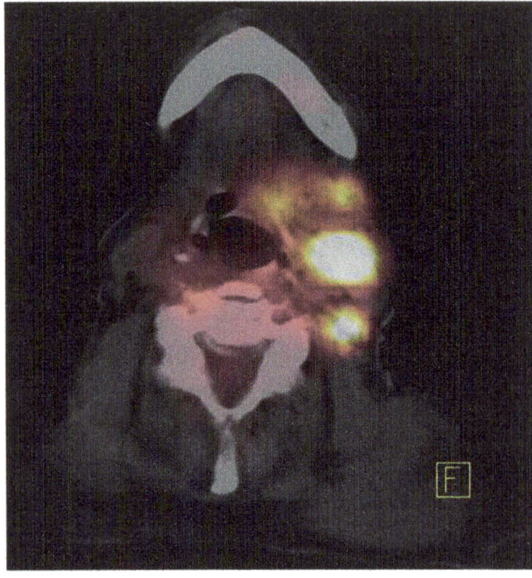

Fig. 31.2 Multiple hypermetabolic lymph nodes in the left lateral neck

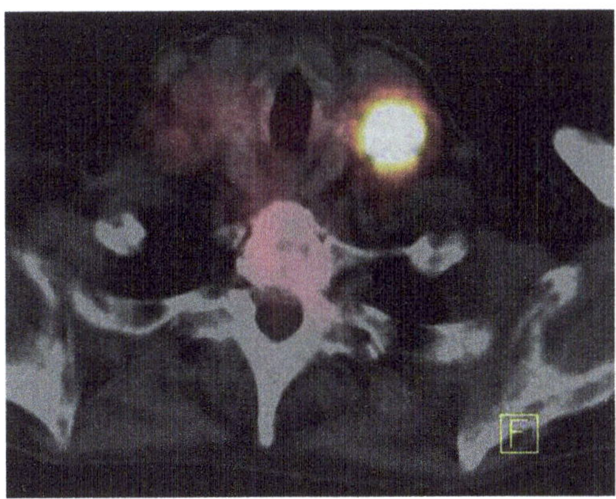

Fig. 31.3 Hypermetabolic lymph node in the left supraclavicular region

Various studies approve of the use of PET/CT in metabolic imaging during the pretreatment assessment of patients diagnosed with advanced stage (III/IV) HNSCC. The optimized accuracy in stage detection as well as distant disease diagnosis in appreciable amount of patients constitute its main advantages, but are not applicable to those who are diagnosed with an early stage HNSCC and those unlikely to be found with distant disease.

Lonneux et al. monitored a group of 233 HNSCC patients who had never undergone PET/CT before. Their aim was to discover any differences in staging and treatment with the aid of PET imaging compared with same work routine by using anatomic imaging. The results showed that 86.3 % of patients were not affected at all or were affected negligibly by PET, however management changes were considered necessary in 13.7 %. These adjustments entailed different surgical and radiation plans due to alterations in TNM staging and diagnosis of distant disease that resulted in implementing a different therapy. In 100 (43 %) out of 233 patients, TNM staging pre-PET and post-PET imaging were found inconsonant. The following assessments included only 60 out of these 100 patients, in which PET showed precise aggravated severity of the disease in 30, precise decreasing severity in 17 and provided false results in 13 patients. PET detected all distant metastases and second primaries.

Connell et al. conducted a study during which therapy was changed to a great extent in 11 % of patients due to PET/CT imaging. In addition to this, Krabbe et al. tested the accuracy of PET/CT in diagnosis by examining the chest for second primary and distant metastatic disease. Results showed that PET sensitivity was 100 % and that of chest CT was 92 %, regarding intrapulmonary disease in both cases. As for specificity, PET was considered superior (93 %) as opposed to that of CT (63 %).

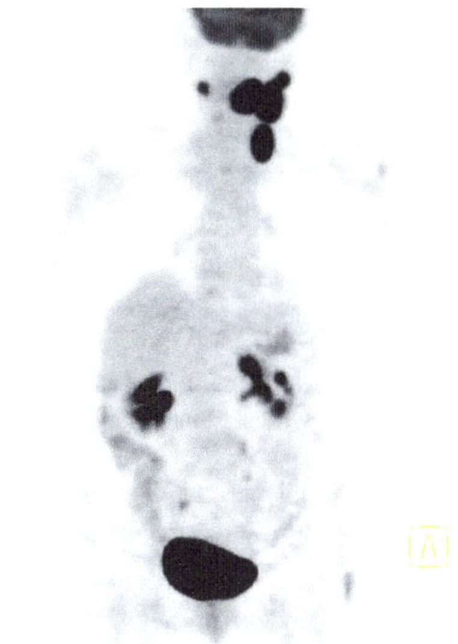

Fig. 31.4 MIP: multiple hypermetabolic lesions in the oropharynx, left and right neck and left supraclavicular

Roh et al. examined the mediastinum and lungs in order to assess sensitivity and specificity for both PET and CT. In the former case, PET values were 80 and 85 % respectively, whereas in the latter case CT values were 53 and 73 % correspondingly. Gourin et al. evaluated patients diagnosed with recurrent advanced-stage HNSCC in which PET/CT had a 95 % NPV for distant metastasis or second primary lung cancer. The SUV values led to elevated PPV of this study. Thus, leaving out distant metastasis, it was possible to make out a treatment plan for patients highly likely to suffer from a distant disease [3].

PET/CT imaging for lesions smaller than 10 mm produce low sensitivity values. Moreover, the case of an elevated SUV during PET or PET/CT imaging entails high metabolic activity of inflammatory tissue resulting in reduced NPV for low-volume disease and a gradually deteriorating PPV for metabolic imaging. Research for positive or negative findings entails high expenditure and delay related to the treatments of HNSCC patients. What is more, PET/CT demonstrates poor results in the diagnostic field during the early stage of disease. Taking into consideration these studies, it is widely accepted that PET/CT should be included in pretreatment evaluation concerning patients with advanced stage (III/IV) and recurrent HNSCC who are highly possible to be found with regional and distant metastasis and second primary disease, whereas its contribution in the early stage (I/II) HNSCC's is minor (Figs. 31.5, 31.6, 31.7 and 31.8) [3].

Apart from the situations where the primary tumor is known, there are patients with cervical enlarged lymph nodes of metastatic squamous cell carcinomas of unknown primary tumor, whose evaluation made by physical examination, panendoscopy with blind biopsy, CT or MRI is negative. In about 25 % of these patients, FDG PET/CT can identify the primary tumor with an overall sensitivity and specificity of 88 and 75 % [6]. Patients diagnosed with nodal metastasis along with an unknown HNSCC primary site constitute a small proportion (3 to 5 %).

On the detection of the primary site it is feasible to implement targeted therapy and eliminate the distress. PET/CT could ideally be used to find an unknown primary HNSCC. Meta-analyses conducted by Dong et al. and Rusthoven et al. concerned this matter. PET/CT detected an additional 31.5 % of primary tumors after physical examination and CT or magnetic resonance. Panendoscopy with directed biopsies and tonsillectomy were not included. Also, there was an additional 15.9 % of regional metastasis as well as 11.2 % of distant metastasis traced by PET imaging. As far as the tonsil and the base of the tongue are concerned, the false-positive values were high (nearly 40 and 20 % correspondingly), whereas false-negative values were less (13 and 17 % correspondingly).

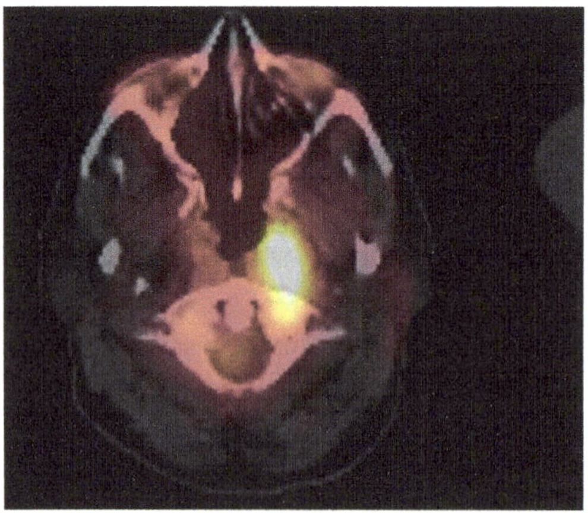

Fig. 31.5 Squamous cell carcinoma of the left rhinopharynx

However, the existence of cancer cannot be supported by a positive PET/CT result, whilst the deficiency of PET/CT localization should not discourage the surgeon to run a panendoscopy test along with tonsillectomy and directed biopsies. Therefore, a PET/CT evaluation for the unknown primary HNSCC, performed before panendoscopy and directed biopsies, offers a direction to the surgeon and enables him to detect additional regional and distant metastasis. A PET/CT evaluation performed after directed biopsies and tonsillectomy is demanding due to the inflammation following the surgery resulting in possible risk of PET/CT imaging in directing the surgeon to primary site [3].

During the early stage of HSNCC, especially those of the oral cavity, the status of the neck nodes plays a significant role in treatment and prognosis plan. Treatment is intensified in case of nodal metastasis and the recommended assessment of the cN0 neck includes pathologic examination of the diagnostic neck dissection specimen or sentinel lymph node(s). As for the disease recognition in the cN0 neck, PET/CT generated results in relation to sensitivities (25 to 83 %), specificities (58 to 100 %) and negative predictive values (88 to 98 %). It is commonly accepted that PET/CT imaging results should not define management decisions concerning the cN0 neck. The presence of occult metastasis smaller than 10 mm on a highly frequent basis is the main flaw of PET/CT imaging. PET/CT provides low sensitivity for metastatic foci less than 5 mm. In cases where PET/CT demonstrates positive findings for small metastases, this may be attributed to the surrounding desmoplastic inflammatory reaction as the cancer itself. Less than 50 % of nodal metastasis

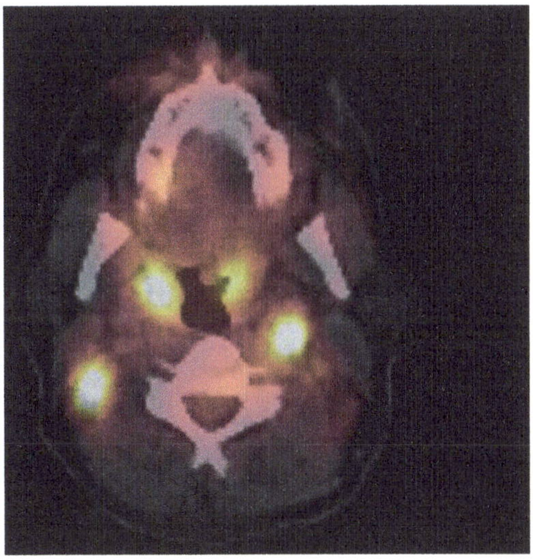

Fig. 31.6 Hypermetabolic lymph nodes in the neck

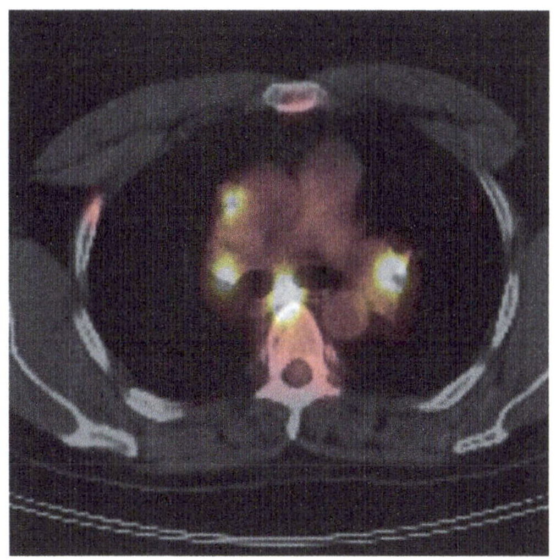

Fig. 31.7 Hypermetabolic lymph nodes in the mediastinum

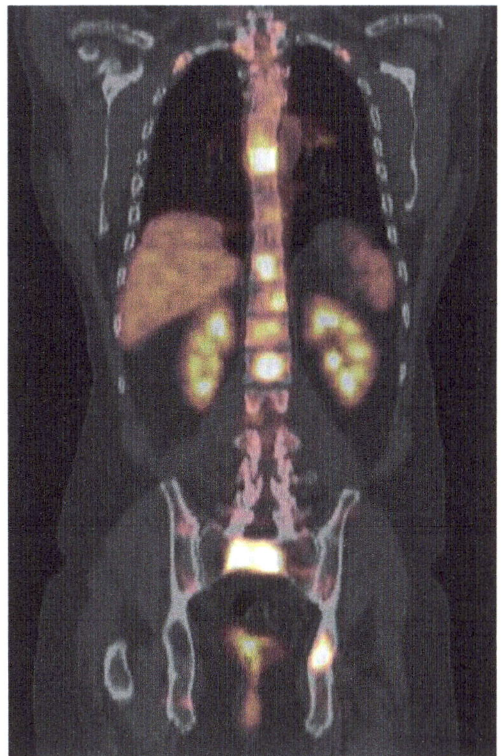

Fig. 31.8 Hypermetabolic lesions in the skeleton

smaller than 6 mm and only 60 % that is 6–10 mm in size are detected by PET/CT scanning. Kyzas et al. conducted a meta-analysis demonstrating the total sensitivity for PET of the cN0 neck was 50 %. Additionally, PET/CT can prove to be helpful with selected primary tumor images as they could be indicative of nodal metastasis just as the depth of tumor invasion is. However, pathologic examination still remains the decisive means in cN0 neck staging and has not been displaced by PET/CT imaging [3].

Radiotherapy is one of the therapeutic methods concerning head and neck cancer patients. The use of PET/CT in the radiation therapy planning is very helpful for more accurate selection and delineation of target volumes, including in the field of radiation not only the primary lesion, but also the lymph nodes metastases.

Retrospective studies have shown that the integration of PET/CT into IMRT planning leads to the reduction of GTV size which entails higher radiation dose in a smaller volume and better protection of the nearby normal tissues. In these studies the results were very encouraging considering that 91 % of patients treated with IMRT based on FDG PET/CT had 2-year overall survival and 80 % of them had event-free survival rates [2].

The development of new radiation technologies, such as Intensity-Modulated Radiation Therapy (IMRT), enables radiotherapists to "sculpt" areas of lower and higher radiation dose in HNSCC patients resulting in reduction of radiotherapy side effects such as dysphagia, osteonecrosis, xerostomia etc.

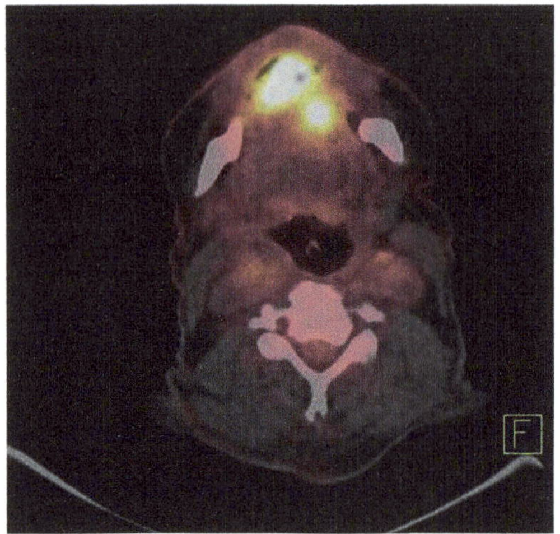

Fig. 31.9 Squamous cell carcinoma of the oral tongue

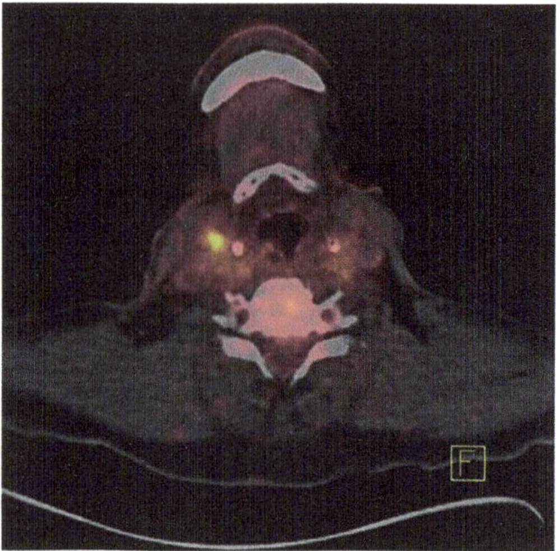

Fig. 31.10 Hypermetabolic lymph node in the right neck at the level of arytenoid cartilage

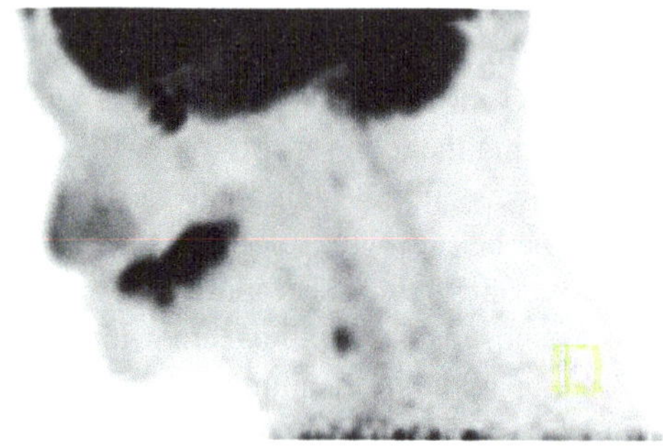

Fig. 31.11 MIP: Hypermetabolic lesions in the tongue and right neck

Functional FDG-PET/CT images are very useful in defining target volumes in order to determine the areas that will receive the highest dose of radiation. Additionally, they prove to be helpful in protecting normal tissues.

Gross Tumor Volume (GTV) is indicated by images and physical examination. GTV areas are usually three dimensional varying from 0.5 to 1.5 cm in order to define the PTV (Planning Target Volume). Therefore, any changes concerning GTV have a direct impact on the PTV and the radiation dose.

The sufficient radiation of gross disease is crucial in order to avoid locoregional and distant spread as well as recurrence of the disease. This is the reason why the adequate coverage of gross tumor volume plays an important role in radiation treatment of HNSCC patients.

Many published studies comparing the delineation of GTV by CT or PET/CT usage conclude that PET/CT delineated volumes are usually smaller than CT ones. It is estimated that PET/CT changed the radiation planning in about 55 % of HNSCC patients [7].

The presence of hypoxia in squamous cell carcinomas of the head and neck is a major negative prognostic factor not only for tumors' progression, but also for response to therapy including radiation treatment. In order to identify hypoxic tumor subvolumes, new hypoxia specific PET tracers based on 18F-labeled 2-nitroimidazole compounds such as 18F-FMISO, 18F-FAZA, 18F-EF1, 18F-EF3 and 18F-EF5 may potentially be useful for the selection and monitoring patients for hypoxia-directed therapies [8].

As it is well known, in clinical practice the modality of choice for monitoring treatment response is Computed Tomography (CT) and the guidelines universally accepted criteria are those of the World Health Organization (WHO) which have been modified by the Response Evaluation Criteria In Solid Tumor (RECIST) [9].

However, in head and neck cancer patients the post-therapy identification of residual tumor uses conventional anatomical imaging modalities that is not satisfying because it takes only morphological changes into account while PET/CT imaging, apart from morphological changes, can additionally evaluate metabolism and differentiate the fibrotic or necrotic post-therapy tissues from viable residual tumor.

Metabolic activity in cancers, such as HSNCC is decreased before any decrease in tumor volume occurs. Regarding primary site or metastatic nodes, PET/CT outclasses CT and MRI combined in recurrent disease detection. Sensitivities of PET/CT in identification of a residual/recurrent disease at the primary site vary from 82 to 100 %. Average sensitivity of nodal detection after chemoradiation was 74 %, however PET/CT negative predictive value surpassed 90 %. Surveillance with the aid of PET/CT during from 6 weeks to 4 months following the end of therapy plays a crucial role in sensitivity (90.9 %) and specificity (93.3 %) concerning residual disease, distant metastases or possible second neoplasm. Although there is no protocol, PET/CT is best implemented 8–10 weeks after chemoradiation has ended and according to a meta-analysis of studies the highest sensitivity is achieved 10 weeks following therapy [4].

PET/CT is considered to have affected post-treatment restaging and oncologic surveillance to a great extent for HNSCC patients. There is a debate concerning the utility of PET/CT scanning for this reason and especially for HNSCC patients diagnosed with an N+ neck and are given radiotherapy and chemoradiation treatment. The number of neck dissections after chemoradiation for advanced disease has been reduced due to the use PET/CT scanning into post-treatment surveillance algorithms. Isles et al. carried out a meta-analysis which was published in 2008 and included 27 articles on post treatment assessment of the primary site referring to values of sensitivity (94 %), specificity (82 %), PPV (75 %) and NPV (95 %), resulting from PET/CT.

In cases where PET was conducted at least 10 weeks following the treatment, sensitivity results were improved greatly. Extensive studies in relation to the identification of the neck disease assessed by PET/CT during post-treatment led to sensitivities of 71 to 100 %, specificities of 87–97 %, PPVSs of 38–71 % and NPVs of 97–100 %. Also, it was observed that during the post-treatment PET/CT had a significantly

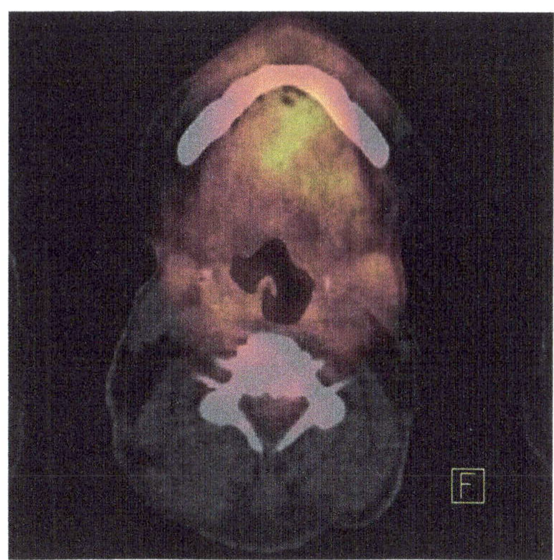

Fig. 31.12 Slightly increased metabolic activity in the tongue (post therapy improvement)

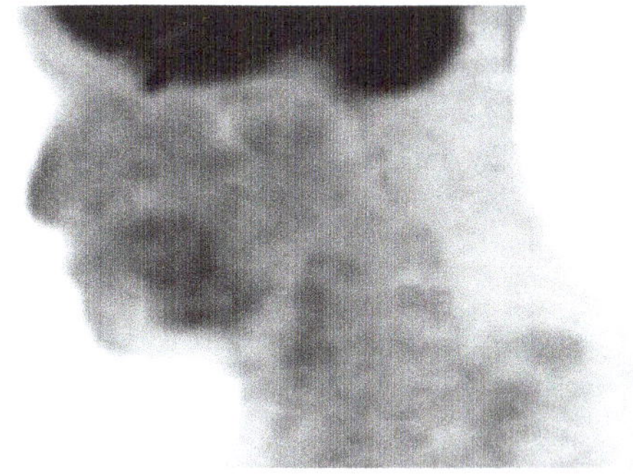

Fig. 31.13 MIP post treatment: improvement

positive effect on 37 % of patients. However, the low PPV seems to be the greatest flaw of post treatment PET/CT and it is attributed to inflammatory tissue at the primary site or inside the lymph nodes. If PET/CT negative findings occur for 12 weeks or more following the most recent directed treatment concerning cancer, there is low probability of detecting a viable neck cancer.

PET/CT scanning in post-treatment is performed best when the background normal tissue inflammation has been restrained in order to detect easily residual disease as well as when the inflammation of a treated primary tumor and lymph nodes has also been constrained. The first scan during post-treatment is performed by most centers upon completion of 12 or more weeks leading to the decrease of false-positive scans and

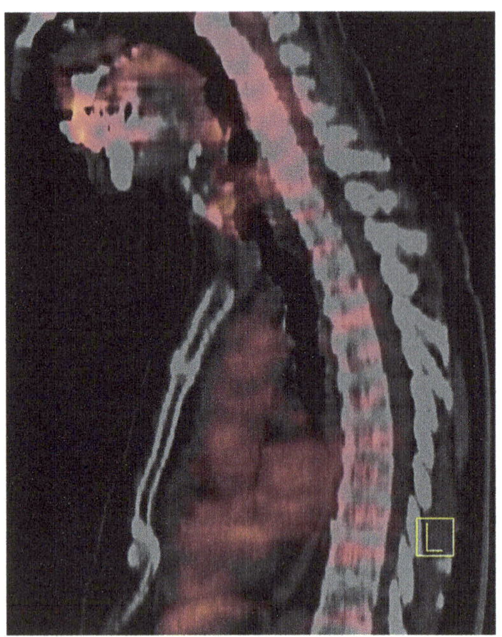

Fig. 31.14 PET/CT (05/2011) squamous cell carcinoma of the larynx, post treatment findings: slightly increased metabolic activity in the larynx (SUV = 3.2)

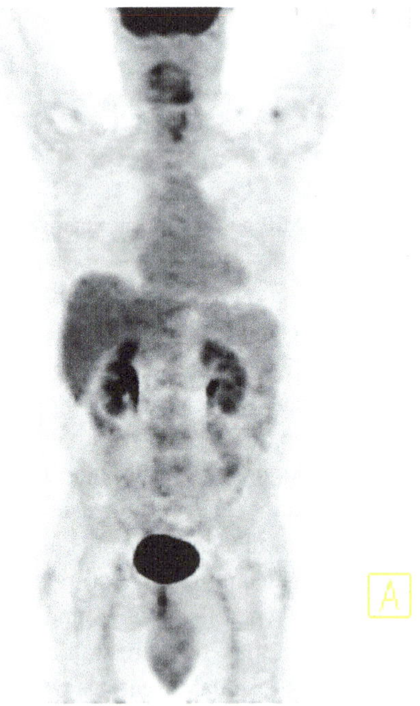

Fig. 31.15 PET/CT (05/2011) MIP post treatment

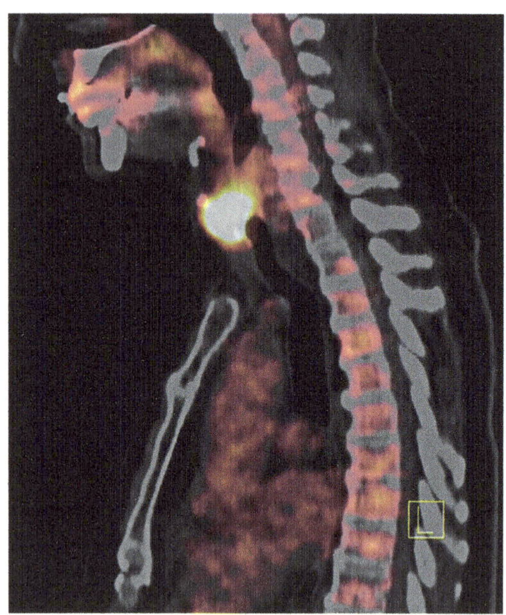

Fig. 31.16 PET/CT (06/2012) Recurrence in the larynx

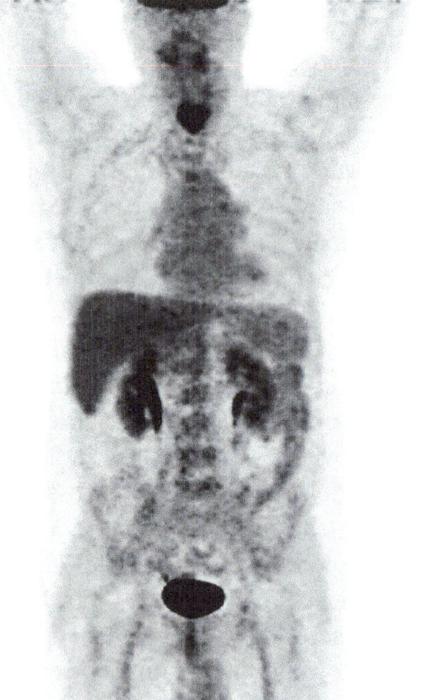

Fig. 31.17 PET/CT (06/2012) MIP: Hypermetabolic lesion in the larynx

to the prevention of any harmful survival impact in case of a salvage surgery. Additional scanning following the negative findings of PET/CT scanning 12 weeks after a last-cancer directed treatment has not been extensively tested. Post-

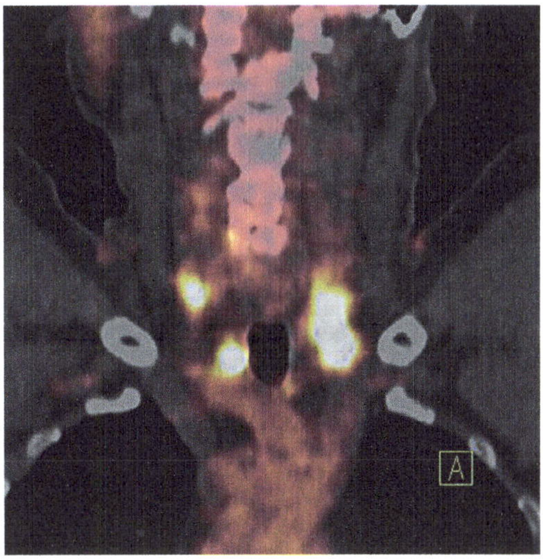

Fig. 31.18 Differentiated thyroid carcinoma, thyroidectomy. I131 whole body scan: negative, increased serum Tg levels. PET/CT: Hypermetabolic lesions in the thyroid bed, multiple metabolic lymph nodes in the posterior neck triangles

treatment scans were performed at 3, 6, 9 and 12 months by Krabbe et al. and resolved that the greatest clinical profit was achieved by conducting 1 post-treatment study at 3 or 6 months. According to Lee et al., the first study should be conducted in less than 6 months after treatment and concluded that a positive follow-up study after a negative post-treatment PET study was highly impossible. There was no useful information provided, but the team supported the idea of conducting a second surveillance study, considering that one year would be sufficient to excel diagnostic capacities [3].

The majority of authors agree that the optimal timing to practice PET/CT in HNC patients is at 2–3 months after the chemoradiation treatment in order to reduce the false positive results that arise due to treatment induced inflammation changes. In the case that the post-therapy PET/CT is performed on the right time, it generates a high negative predictive value, the method is implemented with higher precision and the false positive results are reduced about 30 % [10].

A more detailed evaluation of the therapy using PET/CT could be accomplished, if a baseline PET/CT study in initial staging was conducted enabling us to compare the studies during

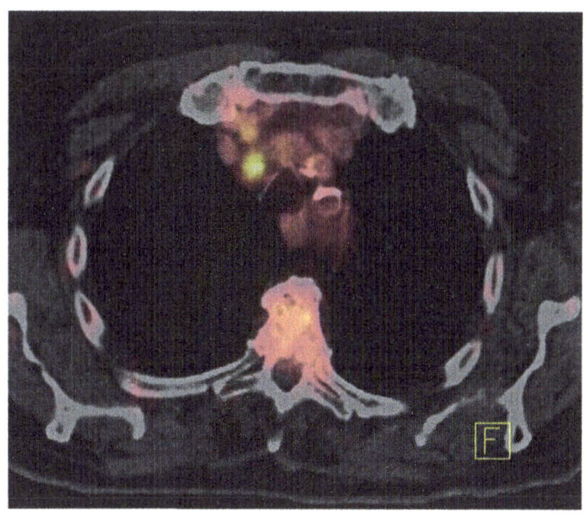

Fig. 31.19 Medullary thyroid carcinoma, thyroidectomy. Increased serum calcitonin levels. PET/CT: Hypermetabolic lymph nodes in the mediastinum

and after the completion of therapy as well as to evaluate the morphological and metabolic changes that have occurred in order to assess the effectiveness of the therapeutic methods (Figs. 31.9, 31.10, 31.11, 31.12 and 31.13).

Over 80 % of the patients with early-stage HNC radiation and surgery are usually curative. However, in patients with advanced stage HNC the overall survival is less than 50 % due to high rates of recurrence [9]. PET/CT demonstrates great sensitivity results varying from 93 to 100 %, whereas specificity results range from 63 to 94 % for the detection of recurrence. Due to the fact that most of the recurrences occur in the first year after the therapy, surveillance PET/CT can be done after a regular six-month interval for the first 18 months and then on a yearly basis, depending on clinical suspicion of recurrent disease (Figs. 31.14, 31.15, 31.16 and 31.17) [10].

Some authors consider that if negative PET/CT scans occur 14 months after therapy, then the surveillance of the patients may stop, but anytime a patient is treated for HNC and has clinical evidence of recurrent disease, PET/CT must be implemented [1].

As far as thyroid carcinoma is concerned, the role of FDG PET/CT is well established regarding the differentiated thyroid carcinoma (DTC-papillary and follicular) as well as the medullary and anaplastic thyroid cancer. DTC patients are treated by thyroidectomy followed by I-131 therapy. The follow-up of these patients includes measurement of serum thyroglobulin levels (Tg) and whole body I-131 scan. FDG PET/CT is useful in the detection of recurrence and metastatic disease in patients with increased serum Tg whose whole-body I-131 scan is negative, having a high accuracy of 93 %, sensitivity 95 %, specificity 91 % and NPV 95 % (Fig. 31.18) [2].

The follow-up of medullary thyroid carcinoma (MTC) treated patients includes evaluation of serum calcitonin levels and ultrasound, CT or MRI imaging. Moreover, FDG PET/CT proves to be helpful in the identification of metastatic disease in patients diagnosed with treated MTC who have increased serum calcitonin levels without any morphological findings (Fig. 31.19).

In patients with anaplastic thyroid cancer, FDG PET/CT may be useful for the delineation of disease and detection of distant metastases [1].

All in all, 18-FDG PET/CT contributes greatly in administration of head and neck cancer patients. In the initial staging, PET/CT excels conventional imaging modalities in the detection of lymph nodes metastases, distant metastases and of unknown primary tumor and second primary tumor as well as in monitoring patients' response to the treatment and in longstanding surveillance, having high accuracy and sensitivity in identifying recurrence and metastatic disease.

In radiotherapy, PET/CT may be helpful by providing more accurate delineation of targets volumes. The use of new hypoxia PET/CT radiotracer will contribute in the near future, not only in radiotherapy by increasing the radiation dose in the hypoxic volumes of the tumors, but also in chemotherapy by using therapeutic methods that increase the oxygen into the tumors (erythropoietin, blood transfusion, hyperbaric oxygenation) or by using hypoxia-activated drugs such as tirapazamine [8].

A new hybrid imaging technique recently introduced in clinical practice is PET/MRI. Even though the published studies referring to the use of PET/MRI in oncology are limited, this new diagnostic tool seems to have a potential value in oncologic imaging.

Especially regarding squamous cell HNC, the reported sensitivity of PET/MRI in the detection of primary tumor is 100 %, the sensitivity, specificity and accuracy for the N staging is 85, 92 and 89 %, while in the evaluation of treatment response the reported sensitivity and specificity of PET/MRI is up to 93 % [11].

References

1. Agarwal V, Branstetter IV BF, Johnson JT (2008) Indications for PET/CT in the head and neck. Otolaryngol Clin N Am 41:23–49
2. Grosu AL, Weber WA (2010) PET for radiation treatment planning of brain tumors. Radiother Oncol 96:325–327
3. Funk GF (2012) Head and neck surgeon's perspective on best practices for the use of PET/CT scans for the diagnosis and treatment of head and neck cancers, clinical challenges in otolaryngology. Arch Otoralyngol Head Neck Surg 138(8):748–751
4. Lauren VZ, Wiggins RH (2012) A head and neck radiologist's perspective on best practices for the usage of PET/CT scans for the diagnosis and treatment of head and neck cancers, clinical challenges in otolaryngology. Arch Otoralyngol Head Neck Surg 138(8):754–758
5. Ha PK, Hdeib A, Goldenberg D et al (2006) The role of positron emission tomography and computed tomography fusion in the management of early-stage and advanced-stage primary head and neck squamous cell carcinoma. Arch Otolaryngol Head Neck Surg 132(1):12–16
6. Rusthoven KE, Koshy M, Paulino AC et al (2004) The role of fluorodeoxyglucose positron emission tomography in cervical lymph node metastases from an unknown primary tumor. Cancer 101(11):2641–2649
7. Ahn PH, Garg MH (2008) Positron emission tomography/computed tomography for target delineation in head and neck cancers. In: Seminars in Nuclear Medicine, Department of radiation oncology, pp 141–147
8. Souvatzoglou M, Grosu AL, Roper B, Krause BJ, Beck R, Reischl G, Picchio M, Machulla HJ, Wester HJ, Piert M (2007) Tumor hypoxia imaging with FAZA PET in head and neck cancer patients: a pilot study. Eur J Nucl Med Mol Imaging 34:1566–1575
9. Kostakoglu L, Valk PE (2006) Assessment of treatment response by FDG-PET, Positron Emission Tomography, Springer, 405:387–389
10. Quon A, Fischbein NJ, Ross McDougal I, Le Q-T, Loo BW, Pinto H, Kaplan MJ (2007) Clinical role of F-FDG PET/CT in the management of squamous cell carcinoma of the head and neck and thyroid carcinoma. J Nucl Med 48:58S–67S
11. Buchbender C, Heusner TA, Lauestein TC, Bockisch A, Antoch G (2012) Oncologic PET/MRI, Part1: tumors of the brain, head and neck, chest, abdomen and pelvis. J Nucl Med 53:1–11

32 Clinical Implications of Head and Neck Cancer

Amanda K. Psyrri

The survival of tobacco-associated HNSCC has not substantially changed over the past 30 years. Novel agents and strategies are being tested in several clinical trials. Quantitative imaging using computed tomography, magnetic resonance imaging and positron emission tomography modalities will play a pivotal role in the design of clinical trials addressing molecularly targeted therapies. The clinical investigation of molecularly targeted therapies introduces new complexities in the assessment of response. The Quantitative Imaging Network [1] addresses the necessity for imaging technologies which can accurately and reproducibly measure not only change in tumor size but changes in relevant metabolic parameters, modulation of relevant signaling pathways, drug delivery to tumor and differentiation of apoptotic cell death from other changes in tumor volume. Quantitative imaging has potential applications from phase 0 through phase 3 oncology trials. In HNSCC, PET/CT for example can be used for staging, follow-up and surveillance. In staging, the diagnostic problem is distinguishing reactive lymph nodes from metastatic disease. Quantitation has not been particularly helpful in this setting since the tracer uptake in tiny nodes is markedly underestimated due to the partial volume effect. Modifications such as partial volume correction may be useful in improving the accuracy of assessment of nodes for metastatic disease. The current approach is to evaluate the most likely distribution of nodal metastases and to dismiss as false positives mild uptake signals in sites that are less likely to be involved. This process is currently done using observer experience. More objective evaluation of nodal status could combine partial volume correction with probabilities of nodal involvement for different anatomic sites.

New imaging modalities are also utilized in management of thyroid cancer. Thyroid cancer is now the 5th most commonly diagnosed cancer in women in the United States [2]. However, fewer than 2000 people die per year of their disease and mortality rates have not changed for the past several decades. The most common type of thyroid cancer, differentiated thyroid cancer (DTC), is derived from the follicular cells of the thyroid, and it includes papillary and follicular thyroid cancers [3]. While the majority of patients are cured or have indolent disease, a small percentage develops metastases refractory to radioactive iodine or TSH suppressive therapy. Medullary thyroid cancer (MTC) accounts for approximately 2–3 % of thyroid cancers and is derived from the neuroendocrine "C" cells of the thyroid gland. The only curative treatment for medullary thyroid carcinoma is complete surgical resection.

A. K. Psyrri (✉)
Internal Medicine-Section of Medical Oncology, Attikon University Hospital, Rimini 1, 12461 Athens, Greece
e-mail: dpsyrri@med.uoa.gr

A. D. Gouliamos et al. (eds.), *Imaging in Clinical Oncology*,
DOI: 10.1007/978-88-470-5385-4_32, © Springer-Verlag Italia 2014

Therapy with tyrosine kinase inhibitors (TKIs) has extensively been studied in thyroid cancer. The identification of BRAF (in papillary and anaplastic thyroid cancers) and RET (in MTC) mutations, as well as the discovery that angiogenesis plays a significant role in tumorigenesis in DTC and MTC has led to several clinical trials of multikinase inhibitors over the past decade. Sorafenib, sunitinib, and pazopanib are TKIs which have shown favorable results in phase II trials in DTC [4–6]. A phase III, randomized study of vandetanib versus placebo in MTC has reported favorable results [7]. Vandetanib was recently approved by the Food and Drug Administration for symptomatic or progressive MTC. Vandetanib is therefore the first drug to be approved for this disease.

To conclude, imaging modalities play essential role in diagnosis, staging and management of patients with head and neck cancers. The aim of this section is to summarize how application of these modalities in the management of head and neck cancers will revolutionize the outcome of these diseases.

References

1. Kurland BF, Gerstner ER, Mountz JM et al (2012) Promise and pitfalls of quantitative imaging in oncology clinical trials. Magn Reson Imaging 30:1301–1312
2. 2010 ACSCFaFACS
3. Cabanillas ME, Hu MI, Durand JB, Busaidy NL (2011) Challenges associated with tyrosine kinase inhibitor therapy for metastatic thyroid cancer. J Thyroid Res 985780
4. Bible KC, Suman VJ, Molina JR et al (2010) Efficacy of pazopanib in progressive, radioiodine-refractory, metastatic differentiated thyroid cancers: results of a phase 2 consortium study. Lancet Oncol 11:962–972
5. Carr LL, Mankoff DA, Goulart BH et al (2010) Phase II study of daily sunitinib in FDG-PET-positive, iodine-refractory differentiated thyroid cancer and metastatic medullary carcinoma of the thyroid with functional imaging correlation. Clin Cancer Res 16:5260–5268
6. Kloos RT, Ringel MD, Knopp MV et al (2009) Phase II trial of sorafenib in metastatic thyroid cancer. J Clin Oncol 27:1675–1684
7. Wells SA Jr, Gosnell JE, Gagel RF et al (2010) Vandetanib for the treatment of patients with locally advanced or metastatic hereditary medullary thyroid cancer. J Clin Oncol 28:767–772

Part VI
Lymphomas

Introduction to Lymphomas

33

Theodoros P. Vassilakopoulos and George J. Pissakas

Lymphoproliferative neoplasms are mainly divided into two major categories: Hodgkin lymphoma (HL) with an annual incidence of ~3/100,000 and non-Hodgkin lymphomas (NHL), which are approximately 8-fold more common. NHL constitutes a heterogenous group of disorders: 85 % are of B cell and 15 % of T-cell origin. Lymphomas are classified according to the 2008 World Health Organization classification scheme (Table 33.1). Among NHL, diffuse large B-cell lymphomas (DLBCL) are the most common subtype (31 % of the total), followed by follicular lymphomas (~25 %), extranodal marginal (MALT) lymphomas (8 %), mantle cell lymphoma (6 %) and primary mediastinal large B-cell lymphoma (PMLBCL) (2–3 %). Altogether, the common "nodal" T-cell lymphomas (peripheral T-cell NOS, angioimmunoblastic and anaplastic large cell lymphoma) comprise ~8 % of the total cases of NHL. It should be noted that small lymphocytic lymphoma and B-chronic lymphocytic leukemia (B-CLL) are reported to account for ~10 % of NHL cases. However, this figure is based on histologic data, whereas many cases of B-CLL are diagnosed by blood flow-cytometry without a lymph node and frequently without bone marrow biopsy. Thus, B-CLL is a separate entity with an annual incidence of 4–5/100,000 [1].

In contrast to solid tumors, which are generally staged based on TNM classification schemes, lymphoma staging is based on the Ann Arbor system (see next chapter, Table 34.1). The Ann Arbor staging system was primarily developed for HL and reflects the tendency of this disease to affect lymph nodes in an anatomically contiguous manner [2, 3]. Its use was extended to NHL as well, although its performance may be inferior in this setting. Specific NHL subtypes cannot be practically staged by the Ann Arbor system. Thus, specific staging systems have been reported for gastric MALT lymphomas, Burkitt lymphoma, primary CNS diffuse large B-cell lymphomas, cutaneous T-cell lymphomas, etc.

Before the introduction of computed tomography (CT), "pathological" staging was routinely used in order to assess disease extent in a more accurate way, especially in patients with "seemingly" localized or limited HL, who could be treated with radiotherapy alone. Pathological staging included staging laparotomy with splenectomy, nodal sampling, liver, and bone marrow biopsy. The introduction of CT in the everyday practice facilitated the evaluation of abdominal disease and pathological staging was gradually substituted by clinical staging. However, there were still normal-sized nodes on CT, which were involved by the disease. Bipedal

T. P. Vassilakopoulos (✉)
Department of Haematology, National and Kapodistrian University of Athens, Laikon General Hospital, 17 Ag. Thoma Str, Goudi, Athens, Greece
e-mail: theopvass@hotmail.com

G. J. Pissakas
Head of Radiation Oncology Department, Alexandra General Hospital, Athens, Greece

A. D. Gouliamos et al. (eds.), *Imaging in Clinical Oncology*,
DOI: 10.1007/978-88-470-5385-4_33, © Springer-Verlag Italia 2014

Table 33.1 The 2008 World Health Organization (WHO) classification of lymphoid neoplasms in immunocompetent patients

Precursor Lymphoid Neoplasms
B-cell lymphoblastic leukemia/lymphoma (either NOS or 7 subtypes with recurrent cytogenetic abnormalities)
T-cell lymphoblastic leukemia/lymphoma
Mature B-Cell Neoplasms
Chronic lymphocytic leukemia / Small lymphocytic lymphoma
B-cell prolymphocytic leukemia
Lymphoplasmacytic lymphoma / Waldenstrom's macroglobulinemia
Heavy chain diseases
Including: Gamma, Mu, Alpha heavy chain disease
Hairy cell leukemia
Splenic B-cell lymphoma/leukemia, unclassifiable
Including: splenic diffuse red pulp small B-cell lymphoma, hairy cell leukaemia variant
Splenic marginal zone lymphoma
Extranodal marginal zone lymphoma of Mucosa-Associated Lymphoid Tissue (MALT lymphoma)
Nodal marginal zone lymphoma
Follicular lymphoma
Including variants: pediatric, primary intestinal, other extranodal, intrafollicular neoplasia (in situ)
Follicle center cell lymphoma, primary cutaneous
Mantle cell lymphoma
Diffuse large B-cell lymphoma (DLBCL), NOS
T-cell/histiocyte rich large B-cell lymphoma
Primary DLBCL of the CNS
Primary cutaneous DLBCL, leg type
EBV positive DLBCL of the elderly
Primary mediastinal (thymic) large B-cell lymphoma
Intravascular large B-cell lymphoma
DLBCL associated with chronic inflammation
Lymphomatoid granulomatosis
Large B-cell lymphoma arising in HHV8-associated multicentric Castleman disease
ALK positive large B-cell lymphoma
Plasmablastic lymphoma
Primary effusion lymphoma
Burkitt lymphoma
B-cell lymphoma, unclassifiable, with features intermediate between DLBCL and Burkitt lymphoma
B-cell lymphoma, unclassifiable, with features intermediate between DLBCL and classical Hodgkin lymphoma
Plasma cell neoplasms

(continued)

Table 33.1 (continued)

Including: Monoclonal gammopathy of unknown significance (MGUS), Plasma cell myeloma, Solitary plasmacytoma of bone, Extraosseous plasmacytoma, and Monoclonal immunoglobulin deposition diseases [Primary amyloidosis, monoclonal light and heavy chain deposition diseases, osteosclerotic myeloma (POEMS syndrome)]
Mature T- and NK-Cell Neoplasms
T-cell prolymphocytic leukemia
T-cell large granular lymphocytic leukemia
Chronic lymphoproliferative disorders of NK cells
Aggressive NK-cell leukemia
Adult T-cell leukemia/lymphoma
Extranodal NK/T-cell lymphoma, nasal type
Enteropathy-associated T-cell lymphoma
Hepatosplenic T-cell lymphoma
Subcutaneous panniculitis-like T-cell lymphoma
Mycosis fungoides
Including variants: folliculotropic, pagetoid reticulosis, granulomatous slack skin
Sezary syndrome
Primary cutaneous CD30 positive T-cell lymphoproliferative disorders
Including: Primary cutaneous anaplastic large cell lymphoma, Lymphomatoid papulosis
Primary cutaneous peripheral T-cell lymphomas, rare subtypes
Including: Primary cutaneous $\gamma\delta$ T-cell lymphoma, Primary cutaneous CD8 positive, aggressive, epidermotropic, cytotoxic T-cell lymphoma, and Primary cutaneous CD4 positive, small/medium T-cell lymphoma
Peripheral T-cell lymphoma, NOS
Angioimmunoblastic T-cell lymphoma
Anaplastic large cell lymphoma, ALK positive
Anaplastic large cell lymphoma, ALK negative
EBV-positive T-cell lymphoproliferative disorders of childhood
Including: Systemic EBV positive T-cell lymphoproliferative disease of childhood, and Hydroa vacciniforme-like lymphoma
Hodgkin Lymphoma
Nodular lymphocyte predominant Hodgkin lymphoma
Classical Hodgkin lymphoma
Subtypes: Nodular sclerosis, lymphocyte rich, mixed cellularity, lymphocyte depleted

NOS=Not Otherwise Specified

lymphangiography could provide a qualitative means to identify infradiaphragmatic disease at that time. Despite false negatives by CT scanning, technical difficulties and the more common use of systemic chemotherapy led to the abandonment of lymphangiography.

CT remained the gold standard for staging of malignant lymphomas for many years. MRI and ultrasonography (US) could be used for further evaluation of certain CT findings and bone scanning was used for the evaluation of osseous disease in patients with relevant symptoms.

However, CT cannot reliably assess the significance of residual masses after the end of therapy, which are very common in HL, PMLBCL, and DLBCL and may occur in almost every disease subtype. Gallium scanning has been traditionally used for the evaluation of the presence of viable lymphoma in residual masses, although its accuracy was relatively limited. The introduction of positron emission tomography (PET-scan and PET/CT-scan) during the recent years provided a much more reliable tool for response assessment and evaluation of residual masses as well as a very sensitive means for accurate baseline staging [4, 5].

In everyday practice, "clinical staging" according to the Ann Arbor system is based on clinical examination, chest X-rays, whole-body CTs (except of brain) and bone marrow biopsy. Specific studies, including MRI, ultrasonography US, brain imaging (CT and/or MRI), bone scanning, upper and lower GI endoscopy, etc., are performed in the appropriate clinical setting. Recently, positron emission tomography combined with CT (PET/CT) has been introduced for staging and evaluation of response to therapy in various lymphoma subtypes, mainly HL and aggressive B-cell lymphomas [6–8].

This chapter aims to review the contribution of each of these methods in lymphoma imaging, acknowledge their limitations and summarize recent clinical results related to the application of novel imaging methods, mainly PET/CT.

References

1. Swerdlow SH, Campo E, Harris NL, Jaffe ES, Pileri SA, Stein H et al (eds) (2008) WHO classification of tumors of haematopoietic and lymphoid tissues, 4th edn. International Agency for Research on Cancer, Lyon
2. Carbone PP, Kaplan HS, Musshoff K, Smithers DW, Tubiana M (1971) Report of the committee on Hodgkin's disease staging classification. Cancer Res 31:1860–1861
3. Lister TA, Crowther D, Sutcliffe SB, Glatstein E, Canellos GP, Young RC et al (1989) Report of a committee convened to discuss the evaluation and staging of patients with Hodgkin's disease: cotswolds meeting. J Clin Oncol 7:1630–1636
4. Juweid ME, Stroobants S, Hoekstra OS et al (2007) Use of positron emission tomography for response assessment of lymphoma: consensus of the imaging subcommittee of international harmonization project in lymphoma. J Clin Oncol 25:571–578
5. Cheson BD, Pfistner B, Juweid ME et al (2007) Revised response criteria for malignant lymphoma. J Clin Oncol 25:579–586
6. Connors JM (2011) Positron emission tomography in the management of Hodgkin lymphoma. Hematology, Am Soc Hematol Educ Programm Book pp 317–322
7. Seam P, Juweid ME, Cheson BD (2007) The role of FDG-PET scans in patients with lymphoma. Blood 110:3507–3516
8. Tsukamoto N, Kojima M, Hasegawa M et al (2007) The usefulness of 18F-fluorodeoxyglucose positron emission tomography (18F-FDG-PET) and a comparison of 18F-FDG-PET with 67Gallium scintigraphy in the evaluation of lymphoma. Relation to histologic subtypes based on the World Health Organization classification. Cancer 110:652–659

34 Lymphomas: The Role of CT and MRI in Staging and Restaging

Vassilis C. Koutoulidis

34.1 Introduction

Lymphoma is a heterogeneous group of more than 30 distinct types, differing widely in epidemiology and clinical behavior. There is, furthermore, a great variety in both prognosis and optimal treatment among the various lymphoma types [1]. Lymphoma is a tissue-based diagnosis and excisional lymph node biopsy -which allows morphologic, immunohistochemical, and even genetic assessment- remains the standard of care in most cases for accurate histopathologic classification at initial presentation [1–3]. Once the pathologic diagnosis is established, the next step is clinical staging, which is mandatory for prognostication and appropriate treatment planning [2]. Clinical staging of lymphoma is based on physical examination, imaging and bone marrow biopsy. Additional procedures such as lumbar puncture and endoscopy play a role in staging a few specific subtypes. In practically all cases, imaging –anatomic cross sectional imaging (CT and/or MRI) and/or functional imaging (PET or PET/CT)—plays a central role in staging. Staging is usually based on the Ann Arbor classification (Table 34.1) which takes into account the number and location of involved sites and the type of lesions (nodal and extranodal) [4, 5]. Clinical prognostic models developed for common lymphoma types, including Hodgkin Lymphoma (HL) and Diffuse Large B cell Lymphoma (DLBCL), incorporate the Ann Arbor stage -usually in the form of presence or absence of advanced (i.e. III/IV) stage disease- in their scoring systems [1]. In addition to being an important prognostic determinant, initial staging affects the overall therapeutic strategy. Moreover, correct knowledge of the distribution of disease before treatment is necessary to accurately restage at the end of therapy and document or exclude a complete remission.

34.2 CT in Lymphoma Staging

CT is a widely used, although imperfect, imaging modality for pretreatment staging of lymphoma. Advantages of CT include its widespread availability, easiness to perform and relatively low cost. Moreover, its impact on prognosis determination and treatment planning has been repeatedly documented in multiple large-sample studies. On the other hand CT, as opposed to PET, provides only structural information. It, therefore, fails to detect pathologic changes in normal-sized structures, such as presence of disease in normal-sized nodes or diffuse involvement of a normal-sized spleen. It also cannot easily diagnose lesions that have poor contrast with surrounding tissue, which can be the case with lymphomatous deposits in parenchymal organs like the liver or spleen [2].

V. C. Koutoulidis (✉)
Department of Radiology, University of Athens Medical School, Areteion Hospital, 76, Vas. Sophias Avenue, 11528, Athens, Greece
e-mail: vkoutoulidis@med.uoa.gr

A. D. Gouliamos et al. (eds.), *Imaging in Clinical Oncology*,
DOI: 10.1007/978-88-470-5385-4_34, © Springer-Verlag Italia 2014

Table 34.1 Ann Arbor staging classification

Stage I	Involvement of a single lymphatic site (i.e., nodal region, Waldeyer's ring, thymus, spleen) (I); or localized involvement of a single extralymphatic organ or site in the absence of any lymph node involvement (IE)
Stage II	Involvement of two or more lymph node regions on the same side of the diaphragm (II); or localized involvement of a single extralymphatic organ or site in association with regional lymph node involvement with or without involvement of other lymph node regions on the same side of the diaphragm (IIE)
Stage III	Involvement of lymph node regions on both sides of the diaphragm (III), which also may be accompanied by extralymphatic extension in association with adjacent lymph node involvement (IIIE) or by involvement of the spleen (IIIS) or both (IIIE, S). Splenic involvement is designated by the letter S
Stage IV	Diffuse or disseminated involvement of one or more extralymphatic organs, with or without associated lymph node involvement; or isolated extralymphatic organ involvement in the absence of adjacent regional lymph node involvement, but in conjunction with disease in distant site(s). Stage IV includes any involvement of the liver or bone marrow, lungs (other than by direct extension from another site), or cerebrospinal fluid

From Ref. [5]

In a typical Multidetector CT (MDCT) protocol for lymphoma staging, contiguous thin-collimation slices are acquired in the neck, thorax, abdomen and pelvis. Intravenous administration of iodinated contrast is necessary to increase extranodal (e.g. liver and spleen) lesion conspicuity (Fig. 34.1). Acquiring images during a single phase of contrast enhancement (roughly approximating the so-called portal-vein phase) is sufficient. The use of i.v. contrast does not allow differentiation between benign and malignant lymph nodes but it can be helpful in distinguishing nodes from vessels, especially in the neck, mesentery and pelvis. Oral contrast material administration is recommended to optimize delineation of stomach and bowel.

Nodal disease. When staging lymphoma with CT, size criteria are used to diagnose pathologic lymph nodes [2, 5–7]. Morphologic features and contrast enhancement patterns are not useful for differentiating involved from uninvolved nodes. Affected nodes are homogeneous, soft-tissue density structures with variable (usually mild to moderate) contrast enhancement (Fig. 34.2). Imaging findings of necrosis are uncommon, even in markedly enlarged nodes and, when present, are often associated with aggressive disease [7]. Calcifications are very rare prior to treatment, although they may be seen following therapy (especially radiotherapy) [6]. While different measurement techniques (long axis, short axis or ratio) have been used in various

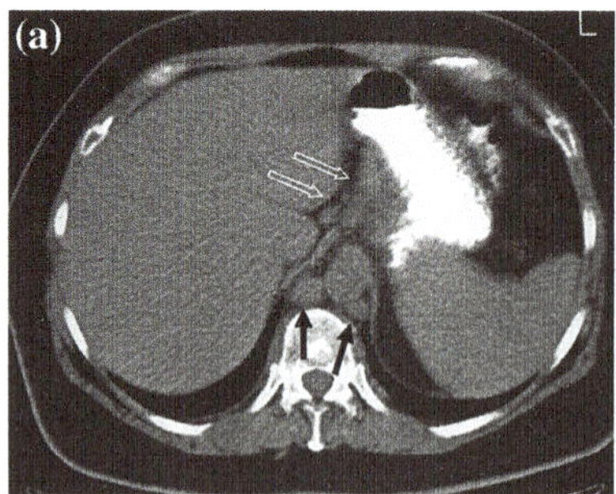

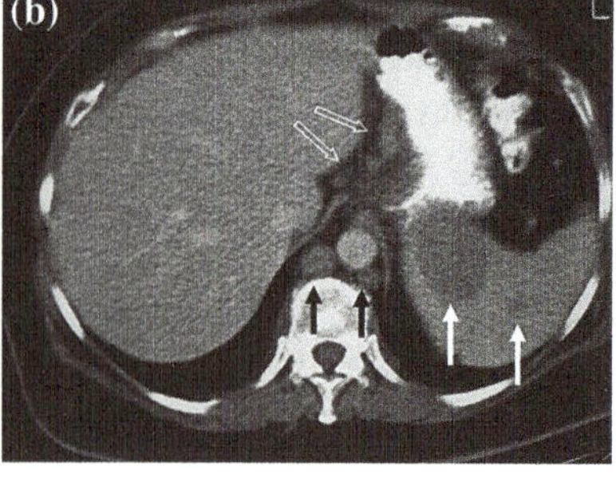

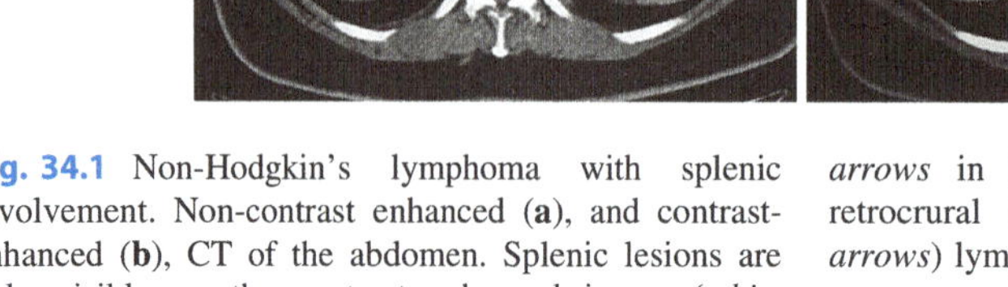

Fig. 34.1 Non-Hodgkin's lymphoma with splenic involvement. Non-contrast enhanced (**a**), and contrast-enhanced (**b**), CT of the abdomen. Splenic lesions are only visible on the contrast enhanced image (*white arrows* in **b**). Note also the presence of enlarged retrocrural (*black arrows*) and gastrohepatic (*open arrows*) lymph nodes

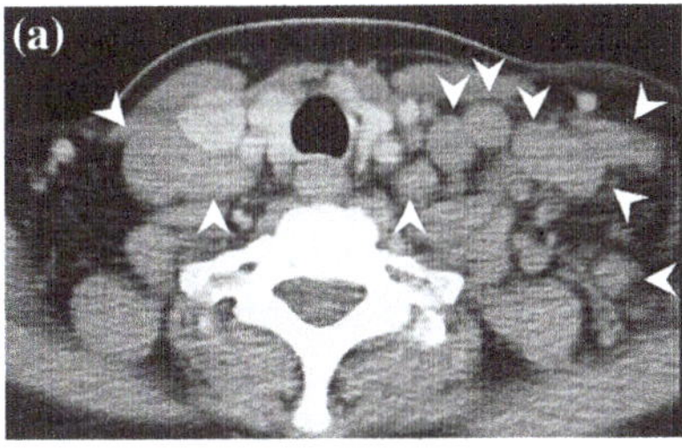

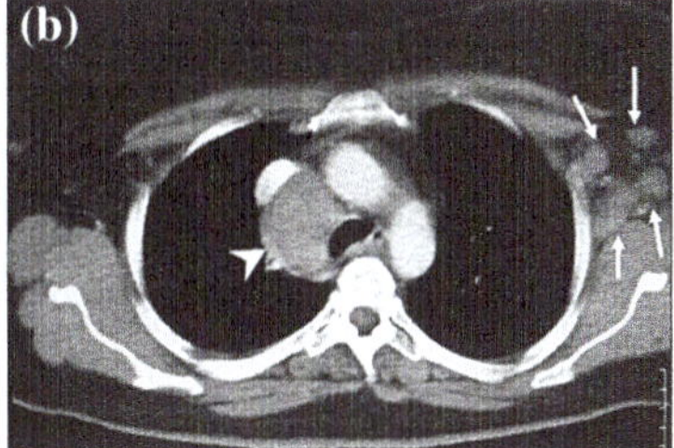

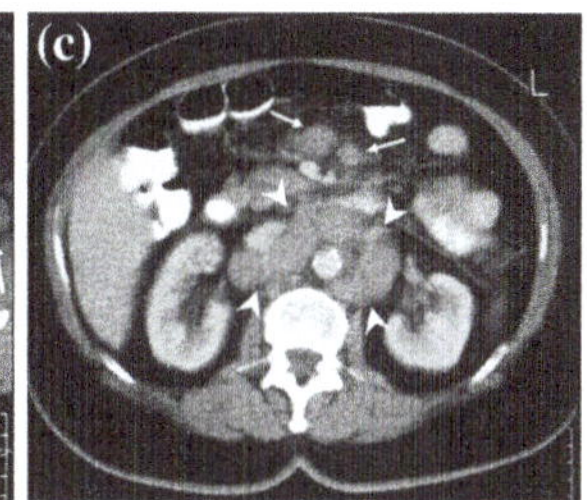

Fig. 34.2 CT of the neck (**a**), chest (**b**), and abdomen (**c**), in a patient with stage III Non-Hodgkin's lymphoma. Multiple enlarged cervical (*arrowheads* in **a**), paratracheal (*arrowhead* in **b**), left axillary (*white arrows* in **b**), retroperitoneal (*arrowheads* in **c**) and mesenteric (*white arrows* in **c**) lymph nodes are seen. All enlarged nodes exhibit homogeneous soft-tissue density, without calcifications or necrosis

studies, short axis diameter is considered by many as the most reliable parameter of nodal size. Furthermore, short axis diameter measurement is less dependent on the spatial orientation of the lymph node relative to the plane of scanning and is easily obtained and reproduced in sequential scans [8]. Different upper limits of normal short-axis diameter at CT have been proposed, depending on location. In most nodal stations a short-axis diameter exceeding 10 mm is considered abnormal. Different values have been proposed for retropharyngeal nodes (8 mm), retrocrural nodes (6 mm), gastrohepatic ligament and porta hepatis nodes (8 mm), internal iliac (7 mm) and obturator nodes (8 mm) [9]. It must be emphasized that applying a higher cut-off for the normal lymph node diameter increases specificity at the expense of sensitivity and vice versa. Therefore, professional judgment and common sense should be used by the radiologist in applying these recommendations in everyday practice (as opposed to clinical trials, where absolute standardization is mandatory). Furthermore, clustering of multiple normal-sized nodes (e.g. in the neck, the anterior mediastinum or the mesentery) has been described as a sign of early disease in some cases and should be viewed as suspicious and reported accordingly [2]. Bulky disease, defined in the Ann Arbor staging system as any lesion with a greatest diameter of >10 cm and designated by the subscript letter X, should also be reported, if present [5].

Extranodal disease. Organ involvement by lymphoma can take various forms and failure to properly detect it, is one of the main reasons for the lower sensitivity of CT compared with PET/CT in staging lymphoma. Extranodal disease can manifest as diffuse organ enlargement, as a single parenchymal mass or as multiple focal lesions [2]. *Diffuse* involvement of an organ manifesting as homogeneous enlargement (e.g. hepatomegaly, splenomegaly) may be overlooked at CT. Assessing splenic involvement non-invasively at initial staging can be challenging and is important for prognosis and treatment. This is especially true for HL patients, in whom splenic involvement is more likely to upstage disease, than in non-Hodgkin's lymphoma (NHL) patients who more often present with disseminated disease. Data regarding the value of CT in the detection of splenic disease often come from studies performed on older CT scanners, or from studies that suffer from suboptimal methodology (e.g. in properly defining splenic enlargement). In a large study using MDCT technology and i.v. contrast, it was found that the splenic index (length × thickness × height) was the easiest and most objective measurement of splenic size. When defining splenic involvement by lymphoma as either a splenic index greater than 725 cm^3 or the presence of hypoattenuating splenic nodules, sensitivity and specificity for CT were 91 % and 96 % respectively [10]. CT detection of organ involvement manifesting as *focal lesions* is aided by the administration of i.v. contrast as these lesions usually show less enhancement than the uninvolved parenchyma (liver, spleen, kidney). A significant drawback of CT regarding extranodal disease is its limited sensitivity, compared with both MRI and PET, for the detection of bone marrow disease, which may also manifest with diffuse or focal patterns of spread.

Diagnostic value of CT in staging. When reviewing multiple studies comparing CT and PET/CT in lymphoma staging, the following conclusions are consistent: (a) CT demonstrates high specificity in the range of 86–100 %, (b) Sensitivity of CT is somewhat lower than specificity (rarely over 90 %, has been reported as low as 77 %), (c) There is a relatively high level of concordance between the two methods, albeit with a consistent advantage for PET/CT in sensitivity [11]. Regarding histologic subtypes higher levels of concordance (80–90 %) are found in patients with DLBCL, follicular lymphoma and mantle cell lymphoma, whereas concordance is found in only about 60–80 % of HL patients [12].

The reasons for the lower sensitivity (i.e. the greater percentage of false negative results) of CT are its inability to detect disease in subcentimeter nodes and the lower rate of detection of extranodal sites (spleen, liver, bone marrow, skin)[2, 3, 11, 12]. An important question though, is in what percentage of patients the added information provided by PET/CT is clinically significant. While there is much published evidence that PET/CT identifies more lesions than CT alone, the frequency with which stage is changed with PET/CT is 10–30 % according to most studies, and the percentage of patients in whom this modification alters treatment or outcome is even lower [12, 13]. Furthermore, the value of FDG-PET for staging certain indolent lymphomas that are not FDG-avid (for example extranodal marginal zone lymphomas) may be limited. There is presently an overwhelming volume of published data regarding the most appropriate imaging approach to achieve accurate *and* cost-effective staging of the different histologic types of lymphoma (PET/CT alone, PET/CT combined with a separate fully diagnostic contrast-enhanced CT, PET/CT with the CT portion of the exam being fully diagnostic contrast-enhanced, rather than low-dose non contrast-enhanced). A brief discussion on imaging recommendations for initial staging of the various lymphoma types with emphasis on the role of PET is provided in Chaps. 33 and 35.

34.3 CT in Lymphoma Restaging

Response evaluation *after* completion of therapy is a field of great interest among physicians caring for lymphoma patients due to continuing advances in effective therapeutic regimens and the increasing use of experimental agents in clinical trials [3, 11, 12]. Recent research in lymphoma is also focusing in response evaluation with PET *during* therapy (interim PET).Interim PET will likely be helpful in the future in risk-adapted therapy modifications: abbreviation of therapy without compromising efficacy for patients with early responsive disease and adoption of more aggressive treatment regimens for patients with resistant disease [13]. The question of interim PET is addressed in the next chapter. The primary purpose of restaging lymphoma at the end of therapy is to confirm or exclude a complete response (CR). Persistent disease is associated with early relapse and poor clinical outcome, and additional therapy may be indicated [3]. Determining the need for additional treatment is especially significant for curable lymphomas like HL and DLBCL [11]. Establishing standardized response criteria is therefore very important, both in the context of clinical trials (permitting reliable comparison among studies) and everyday clinical practice. Until 1999 there was a great variability in response evaluation criteria for malignant lymphoma among various studies. Lack of uniformity existed with respect to many significant factors, including the definition of a normal-sized lymph node. In 1999 an International Working Group published guidelines for response evaluation, which were widely adopted by specialists [14]. These criteria were largely

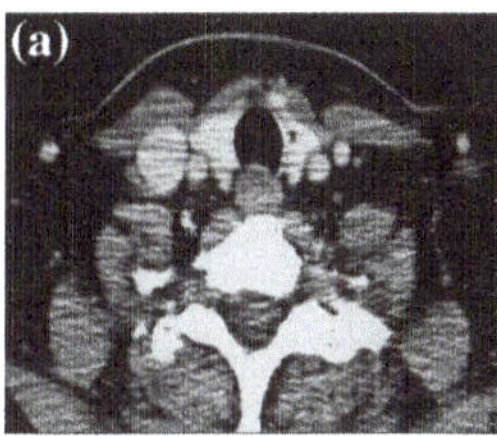

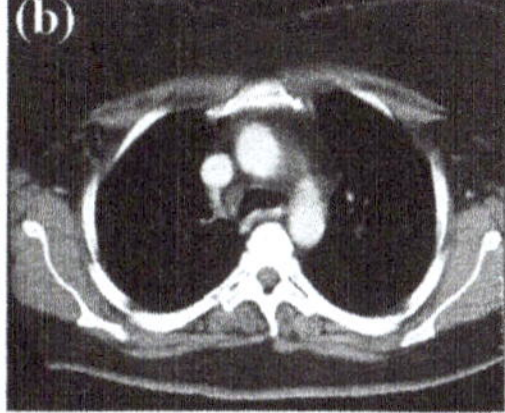

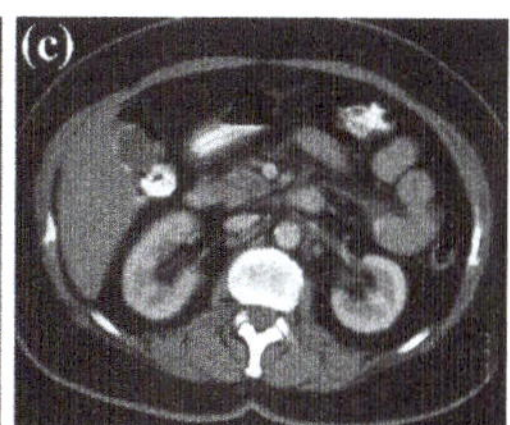

Fig. 34.3 CT of the neck (**a**), chest (**b**), and abdomen (**c**) in a patient with stage III Non-Hodgkin's lymphoma performed after the completion of therapy (same case and levels of imaging as Fig. 34.2). All previously enlarged lymph nodes have regressed to normal size, indicating a complete response by CT criteria

based on lymph-node size comparisons before and after treatment, performed with CT scans. A complete response required all lymph nodes regressing to normal size, as determined on the basis of a CT scan (Fig. 34.3). Assessing response based on CT has a major limitation though, which is the inability of CT to distinguish if a residual nodal mass represents viable tumor tissue or post-treatment fibrosis/necrosis [15]. Such residual masses are not uncommon in lymphoma patients following therapy and, although they are considered pathologic by CT-based size criteria, in many cases they are found to represent fibrosis and/or necrosis rather than viable tumor (Fig. 34.4). As a result of this, CT shows low-to-moderate specificity (i.e. an increased number of false positive results) in restaging lymphoma patients after completion of therapy [11, 12, 15]. PET on the other hand, is vastly superior to CT in differentiating viable tumor from post-treatment changes. Consequently, updated recommendations on response evaluation adding PET criteria (plus immunohistochemistry and flow cytometry parameters for bone marrow assessment) were published in 2007 by an International Harmonization Project [16]. The revised criteria incorporate an assessment of response based on both CT and FDG-PET imaging (see Chaps. 35, Table 35.1). In these recommendations a distinction is made between patients with typically FDG-avid lymphoma and patients with variably FDG-avid lymphoma or lymphoma of unknown FDG avidity. In the second group of patients CT-based size criteria are used to evaluate response. A CR in this patient population requires a CT scan showing the return of all lymph nodes to normal size and the complete resolution of extranodal disease.

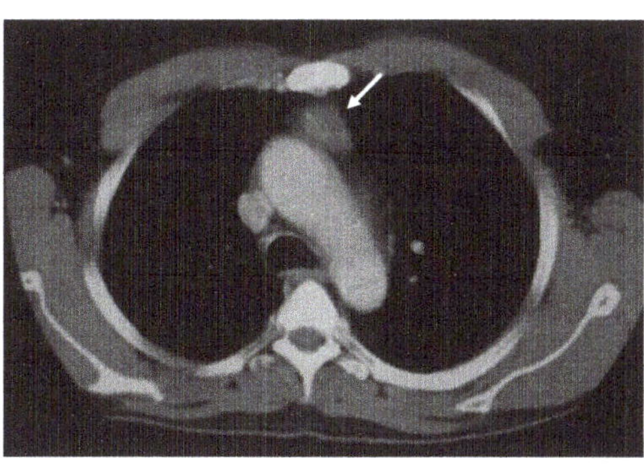

Fig. 34.4 CT of the chest in a patient with Non-Hodgkin's lymphoma performed after the completion of therapy. There is a residual mass measuring 3.5 × 2.2 cm in the anterior mediastinum (*arrow*). Subsequent PET/CT (*not shown*) demonstrated no metabolic activity in the mass, therefore establishing the presence of a complete response

34.4 MRI in Staging and Restaging

MRI is not routinely used for lymphoma staging and restaging, with the exception of Primary Central Nervous System Lymphoma (PCNSL), where it is the optimal modality for imaging the brain at initial staging and for evaluation of treatment response. Drawbacks of MRI compared with CT in staging lymphoma (apart from PCNSL) include higher cost and much longer scanning times. It must also be noted that when staging lymphoma with MRI, anatomic rather than functional imaging criteria are used for

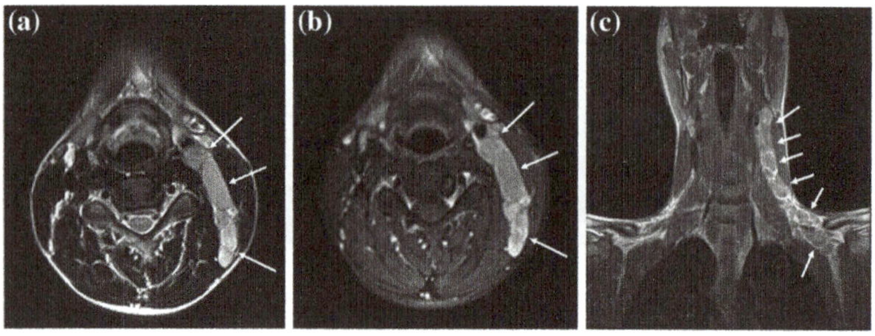

Fig. 34.5 MRI in a 16-year-old patient with Hodgkin lymphoma. T2 W axial image of the neck (**a**) shows enlarged left cervical lymph nodes (*arrows*). The nodes appear homogeneous, with increased signal intensity relative to muscle. On axial (**b**) and coronal (**c**) T1 W post-contrast images multiple enlarged left cervical, supraclavicular and infraclavicular lymph nodes with mild enhancement are seen (*arrows*)

detecting nodal and extranodal disease, similar to those described above with CT (Fig. 34.5). The use of functional MR techniques such as Diffusion-Weighted Imaging (DWI) is under investigation for possible improvement of lesion detection accuracy (e.g. detecting disease in subcentimeter nodes) but their results need to be validated in larger, well-designed studies [17]. On the other hand, an important advantage of MRI over both CT and PET is that it is a radiation-free imaging modality and could potentially be an attractive alternative for staging lymphoma patients, especially children and young adolescents [18]. This possibility has been investigated in studies using Whole-Body MRI technology [18–20]. Finally MRI has an important role in individual cases as a problem-solving tool, helping to characterize indeterminate lesions identified at CT or PET. A good example is its role in characterizing bone marrow lesions, at initial staging or after various treatment regimens causing changes in bone marrow composition. In patients with a negative staging bone marrow biopsy and focal areas of intense FDG uptake in the marrow, the discordancy should be further investigated with MRI if a treatment modification is planned based on these results [12].

MRI in CNS lymphoma. MR is the modality of choice for brain imaging at initial staging of patients with PCNSL as well as for response assessment after therapy [21]. PCNSL represents 1 % of all lymphomas with an increasing incidence since the 1980s, both in immunocompromised and immunocompetent populations [22]. 10–15 % of patients with systemic lymphoma have secondary CNS involvement, most often manifesting in the cerebrospinal fluid (CSF). PCNSL, on the other hand, is by definition restricted to the brain, eye and spinal cord. Once the diagnosis of CNS lymphoma is established by stereotactic biopsy or CSF cytology, staging for extent of disease should follow. Recommendations for initial staging and assessment of treatment response were formulated by the International Primary CNS Lymphoma Collaborative Group (IPCG) and published in 2005 [21]. According to these guidelines initial staging should include studies of the CNS, body, and bone marrow. Optimal imaging of the brain requires an MRI scan including post-contrast sequences. It should be supplemented with MRI of the total spine in patients with spinal symptoms. On brain MRI, most PCNSLs in immunocompetent patients appear iso- to hypointense relative to gray matter on T1 W and iso- to hypointense relative to gray matter on T2 W images. Typical locations include the periventricular white matter, the deep gray matter nuclei and the corpus callosum. The relatively low T2 signal seen in many cases is a distinguishing feature from most brain tumors, which are generally T2 hyperintense. In immunocompetent patients most PCNSLs show marked homogeneous contrast enhancement (Fig. 34.6). In the immunocompromised

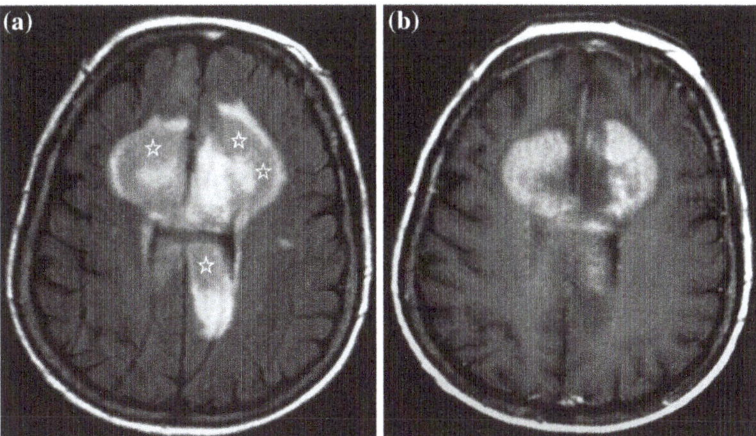

Fig. 34.6 Primary CNS lymphoma in an immunocompetent patient. Axial FLAIR MR image (**a**) shows a large isointense mass (*asterisks*) crossing the corpus callosum. Surrounding vasogenic edema is hyperintense. On the axial T1 post contrast MR image (**b**) the mass exhibits intense, homogeneous enhancement

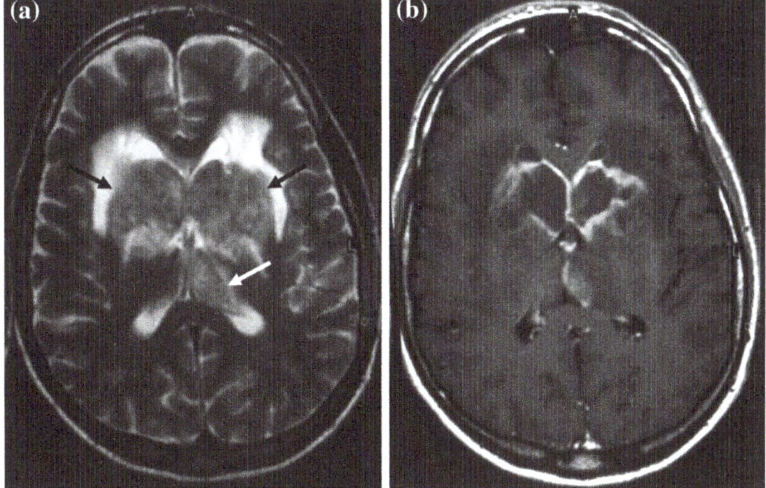

Fig. 34.7 Primary CNS lymphoma in an AIDS patient. Axial T2 W MR image (**a**) shows lesions in the basal ganglia bilaterally (*black arrows*) with surrounding edema, and in the left thalamus (*white arrow*). The lesions are inhomogeneous and mostly isointense to cortex. On the T1 post contrast image (**b**) they exhibit peripheral ring-like enhancement

population imaging features are more variable with many cases displaying heterogeneous (often ring-like) enhancement (Fig. 34.7). On Diffusion-Weighted images brain lymphomas are generally hyperintense with decreased Apparent Diffusion Coefficient (ADC) values. It has been reported in many studies that ADC values of PCNSLs are generally lower than those of high-grade gliomas, probably related to the dense cellularity and higher nuclear to cytoplasmic ratio of lymphomas, although many overlaps exist [23]. Systemic disease has been diagnosed in up to 8 % of cases initially thought to represent isolated PCNSL [21]. Baseline evaluation should therefore include CT scans of the chest, abdomen, and pelvis, and bone marrow biopsy. There is evidence from recent studies that FDG PET may be more sensitive in detecting concomitant subclinical systemic disease [24]. Contrast-enhanced MRI is also the optimal modality to assess treatment response in PCNSL. According to the IPCG response criteria, a CR requires the complete disappearance of all enhancing abnormalities on T1 post-contrast images [21]. An early CR, after the second of six scheduled methotrexate-based chemotherapy cycles, as evidenced by contrast-enhanced MRI, may be a strong and independent prognostic factor for PCNSL [25].

Whole-Body MRI for lymphoma staging and restaging. The use of MRI in lymphoma staging is limited in current clinical practice. Drawbacks of the method compared with CT include higher cost and long scanning times. In relation with PET, MRI shows the same limitations as CT: failure to detect disease in normal-sized lymph nodes, lower sensitivity for extranodal disease and inability to differentiate tumor from post-treatment fibrosis at restaging. Nonetheless, concern exists over long-term risks associated with the substantial radiation exposure of patients undergoing repeated CT and PET/CT exams. This is especially true in the case of pediatric lymphoma as well as lymphoma diagnosed in young adults [18]. In recent years advancements in MRI technology led to the concept of Whole-Body MRI (WBMRI) for evaluation of systemic diseases [17–20]. In WBMRI the whole body is covered in relatively fast scanning times, with good signal-to-noise ratio and spatial resolution. Protocols for WBMRI vary among studies. Sequences include Short TI Inversion Recovery (STIR) and T1-weighted fast spin echo sequences and images are usually acquired and displayed in the coronal plane. Also included in many protocols are whole-body diffusion-weighted images with background body signal suppression (DWIBBS) [20]. These diffusion-weighted images seem to provide superior visualization of lymph nodes compared with conventional sequences, although they are unhelpful for differentiating normal from involved nodes based on visual assessment alone. Published results about the diagnostic accuracy of WBMRI for lymphoma staging seem promising but they need to be validated further with larger, well-designed studies. Moreover, studies in which WBMRI is compared with FDG-PET/CT in response assessment are required in order to consider adopting WBMRI as an alternative modality for staging and restaging patients with lymphoma [18].

References

1. Matasar MJ, Zelenetz AD (2008) Overview of lymphoma diagnosis and management. Radiol Clin North Am 46(2):175–198
2. Kwee TC, Kwee RM, Nievelstein RA (2008) Imaging in staging of malignant lymphoma: a systematic review. Blood 111(2):504–516
3. Cronin CG, Swords R, Truong MT et al (2010) Clinical utility of PET/CT in lymphoma. AJR 194(1):W91–W103
4. Lister TA, Crowther D, Sutcliffe SB et al (1989) Report of a committee convened to discuss the evaluation and staging of patients with Hodgkin's disease: Cotswolds meeting. J Clin Oncol 7(11):1630–1636
5. American Joint Committee on Cancer (2010) Lymphoid neoplasms. In: AJCC Cancer Staging Manual (7th edn) Springer, New York Dordrecht Heidelberg London, pp 599–615
6. Aiken AH, Glastonbury C (2008) Imaging Hodgkin and non-Hodgkin lymphoma in the head and neck. Radiol Clin North Am 46(2):363–378
7. Bae YA, Lee KS (2008) Cross-sectional evaluation of thoracic lymphoma. Radiol Clin North Am 46(2):253–264
8. Schwartz LH, Bogaerts J, Ford R et al (2009) Evaluation of lymph nodes with RECIST 1.1. Eur J Cancer 45(2):261–267
9. Hricak H, Husband J, Panicek DM (2009) Essentials of reporting common cancers In: Oncologic Imaging. Saunders Elsevier, Philadelphia, p 12
10. de Jong PA, van Ufford HM, Baarslag HJ et al (2009) CT and 18F-FDG PET for noninvasive detection of splenic involvement in patients with malignant lymphoma. AJR 192(3):745–753
11. Cheson BD (2011) Role of functional imaging in the management of lymphoma. J Clin Oncol 29(14):1844–1854
12. Seam P, Juweid ME, Cheson BD (2007) The role of FDG-PET scans in patients with lymphoma. Blood 110(10):3507–3516
13. Cheson BD (2009) The case against heavy PETing. J Clin Oncol 27(11):1742–1743
14. Cheson BD, Horning SJ, Coiffier B et al (1999) Report of an international workshop to standardize response criteria for non-Hodgkin's lymphomas. J Clin Oncol 17(4):1244–1253

15. Juweid ME, Stroobants S, Hoekstra OS et al (2007) Use of positron emission tomography for response assessment of lymphoma: consensus of the Imaging Subcommittee of International Harmonization Project in Lymphoma. J Clin Oncol 25(5):571–578
16. Cheson BD, Pfistner B, Juweid ME et al (2007) Revised response criteria for malignant lymphoma. J Clin Oncol 25(5):579–586
17. Vermoolen MA, Kersten MJ, Fijnheer R et al (2011) Magnetic resonance imaging of malignant lymphoma. Expert Rev Hematol 4(2):161–171
18. Punwani S, Taylor SA, Bainbridge A et al (2010) Pediatric and adolescent lymphoma: comparison of whole-body STIR half-Fourier RARE MR imaging with an enhanced PET/CT reference for initial staging. Radiology 255(1):182–190
19. Brennan DD, Gleeson T, Coate LE et al (2005) A comparison of whole-body MRI and CT for the staging of lymphoma. AJR 185(3):711–716
20. Gu J, Chan T, Zhang J et al (2011) Whole-body diffusion-weighted imaging: the added value to whole-body MRI at initial diagnosis of lymphoma. AJR 197(3):W384–W391
21. Abrey LE, Batchelor TT, Ferreri AJ et al (2005) Report of an international workshop to standardize baseline evaluation and response criteria for primary CNS lymphoma. J Clin Oncol 23(22):5034–5043
22. Slone HW, Blake JJ, Shah R et al (2005) CT and MRI findings of intracranial lymphoma. AJR 184(5):1679–1685
23. Guo AC, Cummings TJ, Dash RC et al (2002) Lymphomas and high-grade astrocytomas: comparison of water diffusibility and histologic characteristics. Radiology 224(1):177–183
24. Mohile NA, Deangelis LM, Abrey LE (2008) The utility of body FDG PET in staging primary central nervous system lymphoma. Neuro Oncol 10(2):223–228
25. Pels H, Juergens A, Schirgens I et al (2010) Early complete response during chemotherapy predicts favorable outcome in patients with primary CNS lymphoma. Neuro Oncol 12(7):720–724

Clinical Implications of the Role of ^{18}FDG-PET/CT in Malignant Lymphomas

35

Theodoros P. Vassilakopoulos and Vassilios K. Prassopoulos

35.1 Introduction

PET/CT has a key role in final response assessment after chemotherapy in several types of malignant lymphomas, as well as in baseline staging and interim (mid-treatment) evaluation. Its application is widely established in Hodgkin lymphoma (HL) and aggressive B-cell lymphomas, including diffuse large B-cell lymphoma (DLBCL), primary mediastinal large B-cell lymphoma (PMLBCL) and other related subtypes. Its role in follicular lymphomas, mantle cell lymphoma (MCL), "nodal" T-cell lymphomas and Burkitt lymphoma is less well established, while it is much more controversial in other low-grade lymphomas and primary extranodal lymphomas other than DLBCL.

35.2 PET/CT in Initial Staging

The rationale of using FDG-PET in the initial staging of lymphomas is based on its improved accuracy in determining disease extend, as compared to conventional imaging [1]. FDG-PET is more sensitive than CT, mainly because it can detect disease in normal-sized lymph nodes or facilitate the evaluation of extranodal disease [1, 2]. PET has been reported to change disease stage in up to 40–59 % of the patients when compared to CT and alter therapeutic strategy in 14–23 % of adults and children suffering from HL or non-Hodgkin lymphomas (NHL) [1–3], but these are "global" figures, which may not be applicable in every specific lymphoma subtype.

35.2.1 Classification of Lymphomas According to FDG Avidity

Various lymphoma subtypes are not equally FDG-avid and this mainly depends on their histology and biologic characteristics. "Routinely FDG-avid lymphomas" include HL, DLBCL and other aggressive B-cell lymphomas, Burkitt lymphoma, follicular and MCL and the aggressive T-cell lymphomas (mainly the "nodal" types, such as peripheral T-cell, anaplastic large cell, and angioimmunoblastic lymphoma as well as extranodal NK/T-cell lymphomas), since they are almost invariably 18-FDG avid (>95–100 % of the cases) [2, 4–6]. In contrast, other indolent lymphomas are "variably 18-FDG-avid" or even not at all. Thus, several forms of extranodal lymphomas, including MALT and cutaneous B- and T-cell lymphomas, small lymphocytic, splenic marginal zone lymphoma as well as some rare lymphoma subtypes may not be satisfactorily evaluated by PET/CT.

T. P. Vassilakopoulos (✉)
Department of Haematology, National and Kapodistrian University of Athens, 17 Ag. Thoma Str, 11527 Athens, Greece
e-mail: theopvass@hotmail.com

V. K. Prassopoulos
Departments of Nuclear Medicine and PET/CT Departments, Hygeia Hospital, Athens, Greece

A. D. Gouliamos et al. (eds.), *Imaging in Clinical Oncology*,
DOI: 10.1007/978-88-470-5385-4_35, © Springer-Verlag Italia 2014

35.2.2 Role of PET in the Initial Staging of Lymphomas

Among the above named routinely FDG-avid lymphomas, baseline PET/CT for initial staging is not considered mandatory; however, it is strongly recommended as it can facilitate the interpretation of post-treatment PET/CT in HL and DLBCL, including PMLBCL [6] (Figs. 35.1a, 35.2a, 35.3a, 35.4a, 35.5a, and 35.7a). Interestingly, the current trend is to include baseline PET/CT as a mandatory imaging study in the near future [7]. In HL, where the number and density of Hodgkin-Reed-Sternberg cells in the tumor vary, FDG uptake occurs mainly by the inflammatory tumor microenvironment, while in NHL FDG uptake occurs mostly from the malignant cells. In HL, PET/CT identifies 25–30 % more lesions and leads to upstaging in 15–25 % of patients compared to conventional staging. Conversely, up to 10 % of the patients can be downstaged [1]. Such changes might lead to major treatment modification in half of these cases. In a more common scenario, the identification of more disease sites may affect irradiation fields, even in the absence of stage shift. However, current treatment approaches are based on conventional staging. Thus, it is not clear whether stage shift according to PET/CT should guide treatment decisions in HL. The situation is similar in DLBCL, the commonest form of aggressive B-cell lymphoma, but the effect on treatment decisions with standard Rituximab-based chemoimmunotherapy may be less important. The effect on potential irradiation fields may not be so relevant in DLBCL, since radiotherapy is not routinely applied in the majority of patients in many centers.

In the other routinely FDG-avid lymphomas, especially follicular lymphomas and MCL, PET/CT is considered mandatory only if PET-based criteria are going to be used for response evaluation [6]. However, this is not the case in the everyday practice and is mainly recommended within the context of clinical trials. Baseline PET evaluation is also not recommended in lymphoma subtypes which are not routinely FDG-avid [6] (Fig. 35.6).

In malignant lymphomas, the degree of FDG uptake has been proposed to correlate with tumor grade, proliferative activity and aggressiveness, and to be of prognostic value [2]. Studies using semiquantitative measurements based on SUVmax suggest that SUVmax >10 is usually seen in aggressive or transformed indolent lymphomas [2]. This may contribute to the identification and histologic confirmation of transformed disease in patients with known indolent lymphomas.

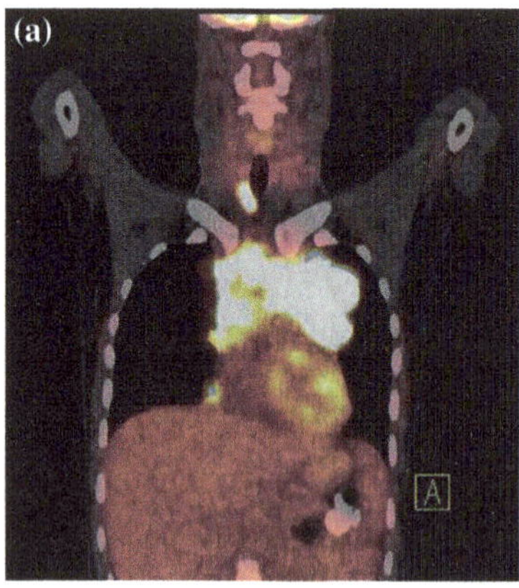

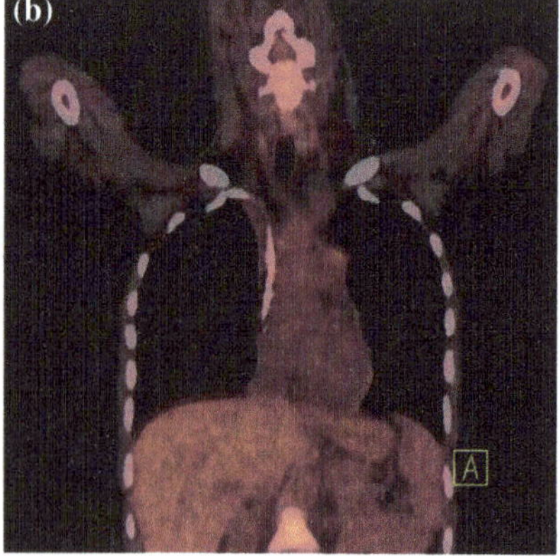

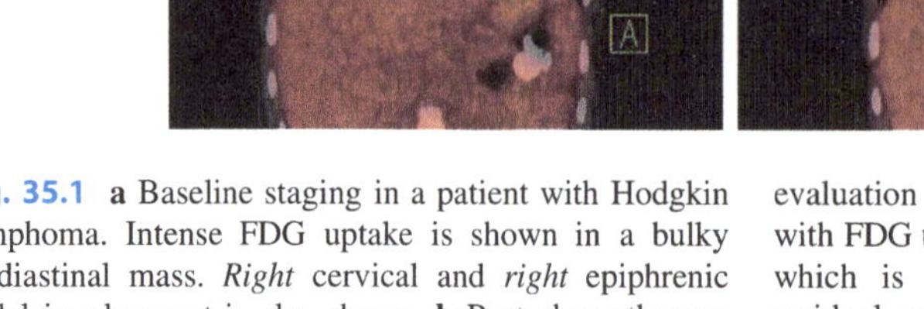

Fig. 35.1 **a** Baseline staging in a patient with Hodgkin lymphoma. Intense FDG uptake is shown in a bulky mediastinal mass. *Right* cervical and *right* epiphrenic nodal involvement is also shown. **b** Post chemotherapy evaluation revealed a residual madiastinal abnormality with FDG uptake higher than the mediastinal blood pool, which is interpreted as positive, i.e., suggestive of residual active disease

Fig. 35.2 **a** Baseline staging in a patient with diffuse large B-cell lymphoma. Disseminated lymphadenopathy including a left pelvic mass and multiple focal osseous/bone marrow lesions suggestive of bone marrow involvement are consistent with stage IV disease. **b** Interim PET after two cycles of R-CHOP is completely negative. **c** Post R-CHOP evaluation is also negative, as correctly predicted by the negative interim examination

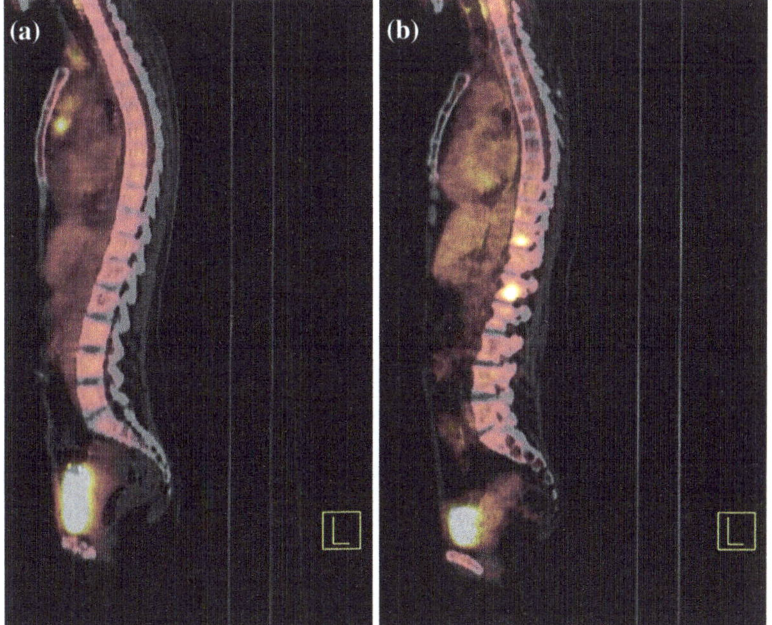

Fig. 35.3 **a** Baseline staging in a patient with Hodgkin lymphoma, indicating cervical and mediastinal involvement. Conventional staging had revealed mildly enlarged paraortic nodes, which were not demonstrable by PET/CT. Thus, the patient was downstaged from clinical stage IIIA to PET-stage IIA. **b** PET/CT at the time of relapse in the same patient. PET/CT had been normalized following ABVD × 6. Three months after the completion of involved field radiotherapy the patient presented with lumbar pain and elevated ESR and C-Reactive Protein levels. MRI revealed osseous abnormalities, which were confirmed by PET/CT. PET/CT normalized again after IGEV salvage chemotherapy and BEAM with autologous stem cell support

Finally, baseline PET/CT may be used to determine the metabolic tumor volume (MTV), which is a combined evaluation of both tumor burden and metabolic activity. Preliminary results suggest that higher MTV may be independently associated with the outcome in HL and DLBCL, but this needs further evaluation before the introduction in clinical use [8, 9].

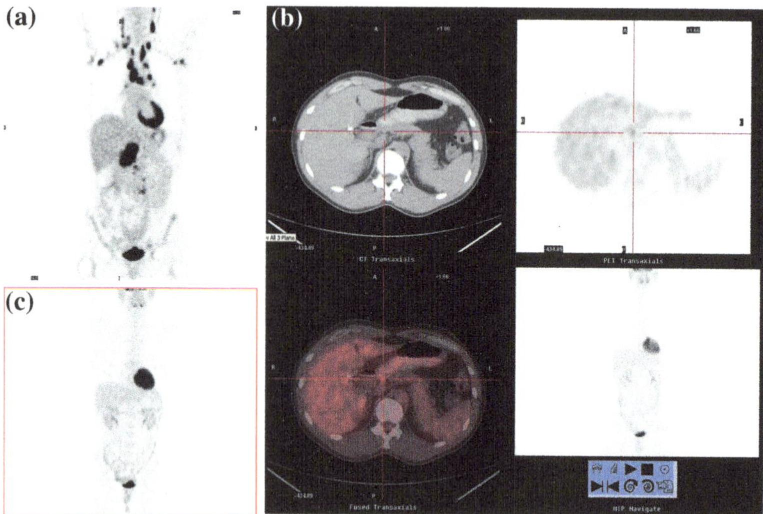

Fig. 35.4 **a** Baseline staging in a patient with Hodgkin lymphoma. The patient had disseminated nodal disease, including a mass at the hepatogastric junction, and a positive bone marrow biopsy (stage IVB). **b** Interim PET after two cycles of ABVD revealed complete resolution of FDG uptake except of the hepatogastric mass, which was reduced in size and had residual FDG uptake just above that of the liver. Interim PET was interpreted as positive, Deauville score 4. The patient received intensified chemotherapy with six cycles of BEACOPP-escalated. **c** Negative end-of-treatment PET in the same patient. He remains in complete remission 3 years after the positive interim PET/CT (Courtesy of Drs Datseris I and Rondogianni Ph, Department of Nuclear Medicine and PET/CT, Evangelismos General Hospital, Athens, Greece).

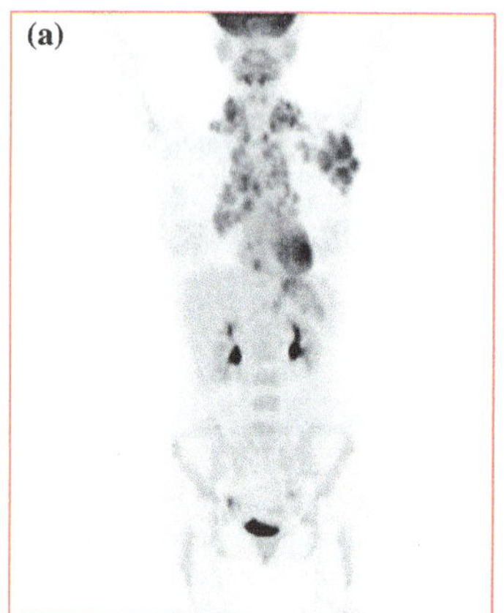

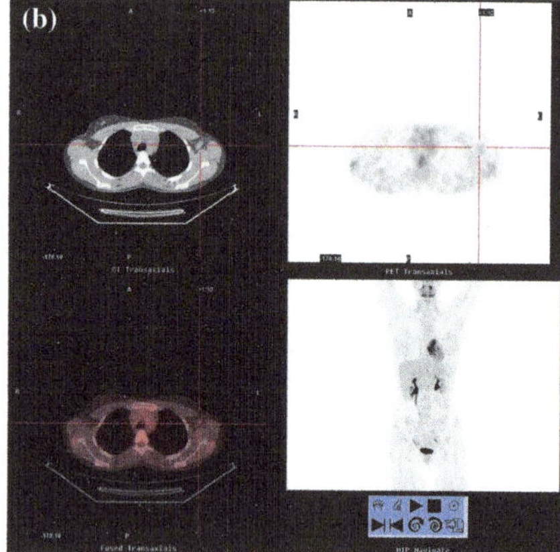

Fig. 35.5 **a** Baseline staging in a patient with Hodgkin lymphoma demonstrating stage IIB disease with extensive supradiaphragmatic nodal involvement. **b** Interim PET revealed a residual left axillary abnormality with FDG uptake above the surrounding background but below the mediastinal blood pool. Interim PET was interpreted as negative, Deauville score 2. The patient continued on ABVD. Posttreatment PET/CT was negative. Following involved field radiotherapy, the patient remains in complete remission 30 months after the negative interim PET/CT (Courtesy of Drs Datseris I and Rondogianni Ph, Department of Nuclear Medicine and PET/CT, Evangelismos General Hospital, Athens, Greece).

Fig. 35.6 Extranodal marginal zone lymphoma of the *left* eye. A mass with increased FDG uptake is shown. Marginal zone lymphomas are not routinely FDG-avid. According to current guidelines, PET/CT is not recommended either for baseline staging or for posttreatment evaluation in this entity

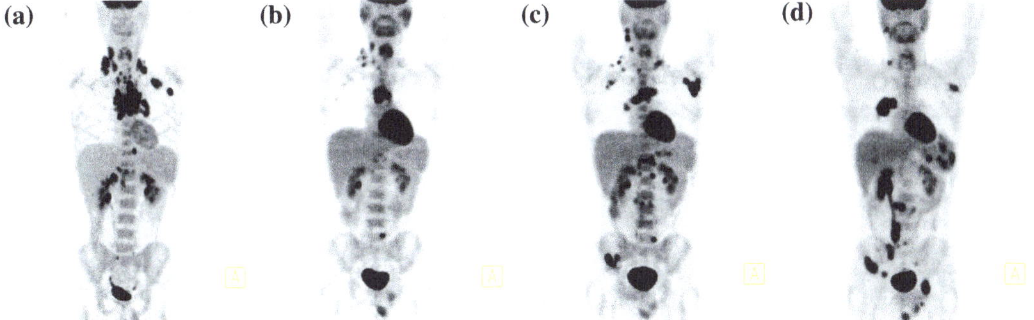

Fig. 35.7 **a** Baseline staging in a patient with Hodgkin lymphoma: Extensive supradiaphragmatic as well as infradiaphragmatic involvement consistent with stage IIIB disease. **b** Interim PET after two cycles of ABVD revealed persistence of multiple nodal sites on both sides of the diaphragm with FDG uptake markedly greater than that of the liver. A new focal osseous lesion is also seen. Interim PET was interpreted as positive, Deauville score 5. The patient continued on ABVD. **c** End-of-treatment PET after a total of six ABVD cycles demonstrated further progression. The patient had progressive disease by conventional restaging as well. **d** Further progression later on, during disease course in the same patient. Multiple focal splenic lesions are noted

35.2.3 PET in the Assessment of Bone Marrow Involvement

Several studies have investigated the role of PET in the identification of bone marrow involvement . In a meta-analysis including 587 lymphoma patients the reported sensitivity and specificity of PET against bone marrow biopsy was 51 and 91 %, which became 54 and 92 % if patients who were re-biopsied were included [10]. The comparative accuracy of PET/CT and bone marrow biopsy is highly depended on the specific lymphoma histologic type under evaluation.

In a recent large study, 454 HL patients were staged by both PET/CT and bone marrow biopsy [11] (Fig. 35.4a). As expected [12], 6 % (27 patients) had bone marrow involvement. However, 13 % (59 patients) had multi- ($n = 31$), bi- ($n = 9$), or unifocal ($n = 19$) PET/CT bone lesions and a negative bone marrow biopsy. Among 27 patients with a positive bone marrow biopsy, 4 (15 %) had no evidence of bone/bone marrow disease in PET/CT, 21 (77 %) had multifocal lesions, 1 (4 %) had bifocal, and 1 (4 %) had unifocal lesions. No cases of bone marrow involvement were detected among patients with diffusely increased 18 FDG-uptake. These data suggest that the main PET/CT pattern associated with bone marrow involvement in HL is the presence of multifocal bone/bone marrow lesions. Thus, PET/CT revealed more than double the cases of bone marrow involvement than detected by unilateral bone marrow biopsy alone. Patients with bone marrow involvement ($n = 27$) and those with multifocal PET/CT lesions ($n = 31$) had similar outcomes in terms of progression free survival (PFS). According to these data, the sensitivity of focal PET/CT lesions in predicting bone marrow disease, as reflected by bone marrow biopsy, is 85 and 86 %, while the positive and negative predictive value is 28 and 99 %, respectively. These results are similar to those reported in a relevant meta-analysis. However, when the gold standard for the detection of bone marrow disease was either focal PET/CT lesions or a positive biopsy, the sensitivity of PET/CT was 95 versus 31 % for bone marrow biopsy. According to the authors, bone marrow biopsy did not lead to treatment modification in any of the four patients with negative PET/CT findings, since all of them had already advanced disease (stage shift from III to IV). A recent study validated the above results and failed to identify any high-risk subgroup of patients, who might benefit from bone marrow biopsy in the absence of positive findings in PET/CT [13]. Bone marrow biopsy will probably be omitted in PET/CT-staged patients with HL in the near future [7]. Finally, PET/CT might facilitate the identification of foci of increased uptake in order to guide bone marrow biopsy, since bone marrow involvement can be patchy.

In DLBCL, the frequency of bone marrow involvement is 10–15 % (Fig. 35.2a). Bone marrow biopsy may be more informative, because more patients may have positive biopsies with negative PET/CT. Furthermore, in DLBCL, bone marrow involvement may be either concordant (large cell) or discordant (small cell) compared to lymph node histology [14]. This phenomenon, which is of prognostic significance, cannot be demonstrated by PET/CT. In a recent study of 89 patients with DLBCL, 7 were biopsy+/PET+, 7 were biopsy+/PET−, 10 were biopsy−/PET+ and 65 were negative by both methods [15]. Among the 10 biopsy−/PET+ patients, 9 had uni- or bifocal PET/CT findings and only 1 had more widespread findings. Among the 7 biopsy+/PET+ patients, 6 had multifocal or diffuse findings and 1 bifocal. A larger study has been reported in abstract form [16]: Among 374 patients with DLBCL, 95 (25 %) had bone marrow uptake; 18 % focal and 8 % diffuse. Only 16 patients (4.3 %) had a positive bone marrow biopsy in the presence of a negative PET/CT, but stage was already IV in half of them. Thus the authors proposed that PET/CT might replace biopsy in DLBCL, since upstaging to stage IV was missed in only 8/374 patients (2.1 %). These data deserve further verification with detailed PET findings and precise bone marrow histology reported. Similar findings were recently reported by other investigators as well [17,18].

In indolent lymphomas bone marrow biopsy is the gold standard for the evaluation of bone marrow disease, which is much more prevalent than in HL and DLBCL. PET/CT may not reveal bone marrow involvement by low-grade lymphoma [2]. Whatever the case, PET/CT is not currently considered mandatory for baseline staging of indolent lymphomas.

35.3 PET/CT in Response Assessment After Completion of Therapy

35.3.1 Criteria for Response Assessment and Definitions of PET Positivity

Response assessment has been traditionally based on the International Working Group Criteria described by Cheson et al., which were updated in 2007 in order to include PET findings, where appropriate [6]. The revised response criteria are summarized in Table 35.1 (Figs. 35.1b, 35.2c, 35.4c, 35.5c).

The most important information provided by PET, as far as response evaluation is concerned, is the differentiation between viable lymphomatous tissue and necrotic or fibrotic tissue at residual masses apparent on CT. Furthermore, PET/CT may uncover occult disease in normal-sized lymph nodes or bone marrow disease,

Table 35.1 Revised response criteria for malignant lymphoma in the PET era (adopted with modifications from Cheson et al. [6])

Complete remission (requires all of the following)

1. *Clinical findings*. Complete disappearance of all clinical evidence of disease and disease-related symptoms, if present at baseline

2. *Nodal disease*

- *Typically FDG-avid lymphoma or baseline PET positive:* PET negative. Residual mass of any size is permitted provided that PET is negative

- *Variably FDG-avid lymphoma or baseline PET negative:* Regression of all lymph nodes to normal size, i.e.: (a) ≤1.5 cm in greatest transverse diameter if it were >1.5 cm before therapy or (b) ≤1 cm in short axis, if 1.1–1.5 cm in long axis and >1 cm in short axis before treatment

3. *Splenic and liver disease*. Non-palpable organs and normal sized (if considered enlarged before treatment) and/or disappearance of nodules. However, splenic involvement cannot be reliably assessed based on its size

4. *Bone marrow*. No infiltration on repeat bone marrow biopsy of adequate size (preferably >2 cm). If morphology is indeterminate, immunohistochemistry should be negative

Partial remission (requires all of the following)

1. *Nodal disease*

- *Typically FDG-avid lymphoma or baseline PET positive:* Regression on CT (as described above and below for variably FDG-avid lymphoma), but at least one previously involved site PET positive (applicable to non-nodal disease as well)

- *Variably FDG-avid lymphoma or baseline PET negative:* ≥50 % decrease in the sum of the products (SPD) of up to six of the dominant nodes or masses and no increase in other nodes (dominant sites selected based on the following criteria: clearly measurable in at least two perpendicular dimensions, located at disparate body regions if possible, including mediastinal and retroperitoneal nodes if involved).

2. *Splenic and liver disease*. ≥50 % decrease in the SPD of nodules. In case of single nodule, ≥50 % decrease in its greatest transverse diameter. No increase in spleen or liver size

3. *Bone marrow*. Irrelevant if previously positive. Persistent bone marrow disease is classified as PR, if CR criteria are otherwise fulfilled. Clinical CR without bone marrow assessment in patients with baseline positive bone marrow is also classified as PR

Stable disease

1. *Failure to attain the criteria for CR/PR but not fulfilling the criteria of relapse/progression (see below)*:

- *Typically FDG-avid lymphoma or baseline PET positive:* PET should be positive at prior sites of disease without new areas of involvement in posttreatment CT or PET

- *Variably FDG-avid lymphoma or baseline PET negative:* No change in the size of previous lesions on the posttreatment CT scan

Relapsed/progressive disease (requires at least one of 1–3)

1. Appearance of any new lesion >1.5 cm in any axis during or at the end of therapy (even if other lesions are decreasing in size)

- Increased FDG uptake in a previously uninvolved site should be confirmed by other modalities in order to be considered as relapsed/progressive disease

- New lung nodules are mostly benign in the absence of prior history of pulmonary lymphoma. Therapeutic decisions should not be made solely on the basis of PET without histologic confirmation in such cases

2. ≥50 % increase from nadir in the SPD of any previously involved nodes, or in a single involved node or the size of other lesions (splenic or hepatic nodules). A node with a short axis of <1 cm should increase by ≥50 % and to a size 1.5 × 1.5 cm or >1.5 cm in the long axis

3. ≥50 % increase in the longest diameter of any single previously identified node >1 cm in short axis

4. Lesions should be PET-positive, if observed in a typical FDG-avid lymphoma or the lesion was PET-positive before therapy (unless the lesion is too small to be detected with current PET systems (long axis <1.5 cm by CT)

which may not be demonstrable by trephine biopsy. In 2005, Juweid et al. published a retrospective study in patients with aggressive NHL, predominantly DLBCL, who underwent PET and CT after 4–8 cycles of chemotherapy [15]. They noticed that patients otherwise categorized as CRu (Complete Response Unconfirmed) based on Cheson's 1999 criteria of response, were usually PET-negative, and, overall, had a favorable outcome with PFS similar to that of the CR group. Patients in PR had strikingly different outcomes when PET was negative or positive. Moreover, incorporation of PET in IWC (International Workshop Criteria) was reported as an independent prognostic factor for PFS [19].

Small studies and systematic reviews [20, 21] demonstrated and confirmed the high negative predictive value of PET for final response assessment. Based on such data, PET was incorporated in the revised criteria for assessment of response to therapy in malignant lymphoma in 2007 in the context of the International Harmonization Project (IHP) [6, 22], in which the CRu category was eliminated and PET-negativity is compatible with CR irrespectively of the conventional radiographic response status.

The definition of PET/CT positivity is an important issue. Final (end-of-treatment) response assessment criteria differ from those used for interim (mid-treatment) evaluation. Specific guidelines for final response assessment have been published in the context of the International Harmonization Project [22]. These data are summarized in Table 35.2 (Figs. 35.1b, 35.2c, 35.4c, 35.5c, 35.7c).

Table 35.2 Guidelines for the interpretation of end-of-treatment PET-scans in patients with malignant lymphomas (Modified from Juweid ME et al. J Clin Oncol. 2007; 25:571–578, [22])

(1) Visual assessment only (and not semi-quantitative or quantitative estimations, such as SUVmax) is required to determine if PET is positive after the end of treatment
(2) Based on visual assessment, a positive PET is defined as focal or diffuse FDG uptake above the background in a location, which is not compatible with normal anatomy/physiology, with the following exceptions
a. *If the residual mass is* ≥ 2 cm (regardless of its location), PET is defined as positive only if FDG uptake exceeds that of the mediastinal blood pool structures. Mild and diffuse uptake (between the background and the mediastinal blood pool structures) is considered negative for lymphoma. In contrast, smaller residual masses (<2 cm) or normal sized nodes are considered positive if their uptake exceeds the surrounding background, due to the effect of partial volume averaging
b. *New lung nodules* ≥ 1.5 cm—in the absence of baseline lung involvement—should be considered positive for lymphoma only if their FDG uptake exceeds that of the mediastinal blood pool structures. New lung nodules <1.5 cm may be PET-negative because of partial volume averaging effect; therefore active lymphoma cannot be excluded. However, new lung nodules in patients without baseline lung disease, who have achieved complete remission in all previously involved sites, should be considered negative (usually correspond to infectious or inflammatory changes)
c. *Residual splenic or hepatic lesions >1.5* cm are considered positive only if their uptake exceeds (or is equal to) that of the spleen or the liver respectively. *Smaller residual nodules (<1.5* cm*)* are considered positive, if their uptake exceeds that of the respective organ. *Diffusely increased splenic uptake* is considered positive, if exceeds that of the normal liver, unless cytokines have been recently administered
d. *Diffuse increase in bone marrow uptake* (even > liver) is usually due to post-treatment hyperplasia and should not be interpreted as lymphomatous infiltration. In contrast, *clearly increased (multi) focal bone or bone marrow uptake* is considered positive for lymphoma. Bone marrow biopsy should be repeated, if initially positive irrespective of PET result

35.3.2 Who Should Have PET-Based Response Assessment and When?

The use of PET/CT for final response assessment as well as accuracy parameters are highly depended on the histologic subtype of the lymphoma. PET/CT is routinely used for final response assessment in patients with HL and aggressive B-cell lymphomas. Its use in other FDG-avid subtypes is not recommended by current guidelines. However, FDG-avid T-cell lymphomas are usually restaged by PET/CT in everyday practice. In contrast, PET/CT restaging after immunochemotherapy may not be so informative in low-grade follicular lymphomas and MCL, since these diseases are incurable. In such cases, PET/CT is not generally recommended and should be preferably used within the context of clinical trials. When used in variably 18-FDG avid histologic subtypes, which is not also recommended as a general rule, it is essential to have a baseline PET/CT available in order to confirm that the tumor is 18-FDG avid (Fig. 35.6).

According to current guidelines, posttreatment PET/CT evaluation should preferably be performed 4–6 weeks (and at least 3 weeks) after chemotherapy and immunotherapy and 8–12 weeks after radiotherapy, in order to avoid false-positive findings due to inflammatory processes and false negative due to stunning from cytostatic drugs [6, 22]. As far as interim PET is concerned it should better be performed as close to the next chemotherapeutic cycle as possible (see next topic).

35.3.3 Clinical Data in Individual Lymphoma Subtypes

The positive and negative predictive values of post chemotherapy PET/CT depend on the histologic subtype (Hodgkin lymphoma vs. individual subtypes of non-Hodgkin lymphomas), the chemotherapy regimen applied, and the *a priori* probability of relapse, as reflected by clinical stage or even other prognostic factors.

Hodgkin Lymphoma

In patients with HL, a negative PET/CT after standard ABVD chemotherapy predicts a 5-year relapse free survival (RFS) of ~95 % in stages I/II (where ABVD is typically followed by radiotherapy) (Fig. 35.5) and ~80 % in stages III/IV (in which only few patients are irradiated) (Fig. 35.4c) [23]. These data may have important implications for the design of follow-up strategies. If advanced stage patients are treated with more aggressive chemotherapy such as BEACOPP-escalated, the 5-year RFS for patients with a residual mass of >2.5 cm and a negative post chemotherapy, PET/CT is approximately 90 % without radiotherapy [24]. In a large study, this was almost identical with the outcome of patients with CR or residual masses <2.5 cm, in whom PET/CT was not performed [24].

Despite additional radiotherapy, early stage patients who remain PET/CT positive after ABVD chemotherapy have a 5-year RFS of 40–65 % [25–27] (Fig. 35.1b). Higher 18-FDG uptake may be predictive of treatment failure in this setting and could have an impact on therapeutic strategies, but this needs further clarification [27]. In advanced stages, the figures are similar to early stages after ABVD, but it appears that, after more intensive chemotherapy such as BEACOPP-escalated, radiotherapy in >2.5 cm PET-positive residuals may be much more efficient for disease control with long-term RFS >80 % [24].

Primary Mediastinal Large B-cell Lymphoma

A negative PET/CT after R-CHOP is associated with >90 % cure rates in PMLBCL, even when radiotherapy is omitted in many patients [28–30]. If irradiated, PET/CT-positive residual masses are effectively controlled in ~70 % of cases [28–30] and the intensity of 18-FDG uptake may have a clinically meaningful prognostic role, since patients with higher uptake probably have significantly inferior outcomes [28,30]. These data need further verification, because of the limited number of patients due to the rarity of the disease.

Diffuse Large B-cell Lymphoma

On the other hand, a negative PET/CT after R-CHOP carries a lower negative predictive value in DLBCL. The long-term event free survival (EFS) in these patients after a negative post R-chemotherapy PET/CT is 75–80 % and the probability of relapse may depend on their baseline relapse risk, as reflected by the International Prognostic Index (IPI), similarly to what observed in HL, as well as to the depth of conventional radiographic response (Fig. 35.2c). Patients with DLBCL who remain PET/CT-positive after R-CHOP have a <40 % probability to remain disease-free [31, 32]. Some data suggest that PET/CT-positive patients suitable for radiotherapy may enjoy prolonged remissions. This is mainly applicable to patients with isolated PET/CT-positive lesions [33].

35.3.4 Impact on Clinical Practice: Randomized Trials

Although the prognostic significance and the diagnostic accuracy of PET/CT have already been established, studies evaluating PET-guided treatment decisions are few. In a randomized trial, evaluating radiotherapy versus observation according to PET results in bulky HL patients (defined as masses ≥5 cm) who had >75 % disease regression and persistent residual masses after six cycles of VEBEP chemotherapy, the relapse rate was higher for the observation group (11/80 or 14 % vs. 2/80 or 2.5 %) [34]. Thus, for the time being, radiotherapy cannot be safely omitted in HL patients with bulky (or relatively bulky) disease who have adequate response to conventional chemotherapy but still have residual radiographic abnormalities. However, as already mentioned, radiotherapy can probably be spared irrespectively of the initial bulk in advanced HL patients with a negative PET and >2.5 cm residual abnormalities (and those with smaller or no abnormalities), if this response has been achieved with more intensive chemotherapy with BEACOPP-escalated or similar regimens, because ~90 % of them remain disease-free at 5 years [24].

Finally, two recent randomized trials have focused to the possibility of omitting radiotherapy in early stage HL after a negative PET/CT following two or three cycles of ABVD. The design rather resembled an interim PET-, rather than an end-of-treatment-PET-driven trial and their preliminary results are interpreted as providing different messages [35, 36]: The preliminary results of the EORTC H10 trial have been recently reported and suggest that radiotherapy cannot be safely spared in patients with stage I/II HL, who become PET/CT-negative after two cycles of ABVD: Patients who became PET/CT-negative after ABVDx2 were randomized to receive: (1) one or two further ABVD cycles (according to the absence or presence of risk factors) plus 30 Gy involved node radiotherapy (standard arm) or (2) two or four further ABVD cycles (according to the absence or presence of risk factors) without radiotherapy (experimental arm). The study was prematurely terminated due to excess relapses in the no-radiotherapy arms [35]. In contrast, the British RAPID trial preliminarily suggested that radiotherapy could be spared in patients with clinical stage IA/IIA HL and no mediastinal bulk (<0.33 at T5/6) who become PET/CT-negative after three cycles of ABVD [36]: Patients who became PET/CT-negative 10–12 days after day 15 of the third ABVD cycle (Deauville categories 1 and 2; Table 35.3), were randomized to receive involved field radiotherapy or no further treatment. The 3-year PFS was 93.8 versus 90.7 % for irradiated versus non-irradiated patients. The difference was −2.9 % with 95 % confidence intervals, -10.7 to +1.4 % (the study allowed for a noninferiority margin of −7.0 %). However, the difference was greater in an "as treated" analysis, since a fraction of patients randomized to receive radiotherapy was not actually irradiated [37]. Further follow-up is obviously needed before concluding that omission of radiotherapy is feasible, although the difference between the two arms appears to be

Table 35.3 Five-point scale for the evaluation of interim PET/CT-scan in patients with malignant lymphomas (Deauville criteria). Interim PET-scans graded as 1, 2, or 3 are considered negative. Grades 4 and 5 define positive interim PET-scans

1. No abnormal FDG uptake
2. FDG uptake ≤ mediastinum
3. Mediastinum < FDG uptake ≤ liver
4. FDG uptake moderately increased above the liver at any site
5. FDG uptake markedly increased above the liver at any site and/or new sites of disease

small. Other randomized trials assessing similar questions as well as the impact of treatment intensification in PET/CT-positive patients are in progress.

35.4 Interim Response Assessment

Early prediction of response to therapy is of major importance, not only for prognostic reasons, but also as a potential basis for early treatment modification. CT, providing anatomic assessment, faces certain limitations, especially when bulky disease is present. Functional changes that precede anatomic ones could potentially be more accurate in predicting treatment response early in the course of therapy.

35.4.1 Who Might Benefit from Interim PET-Based Early Response Assessment?

Early response assessment has provided a major prognostic clue for patients with advanced Hodgkin lymphoma [38, 39]. The prognostic effect of interim PET is less marked, but still significant, for patients with diffuse large B-cell lymphoma. In the specific setting of primary mediastinal large B-cell lymphoma, interim PET does not appear to have an impact on the outcome [40]. Data on other lymphoma subtypes are sparse. However, the use of interim PET is not still recommended to guide treatment decisions.

35.4.2 Clinical Data in Individual Lymphoma Subtypes

Hodgkin Lymphoma

In HL, interim PET/CT positivity is evaluated according to the recently established Deauville criteria (Table 35.3). A negative interim PET/CT may not be nominally negative: Any positivity in previously involved sites with 18-FDG uptake up to that of the liver is acceptable as a favorable interim response (Deauville scores 1, 2, 3) (Fig. 35.5b). Any uptake higher than the liver is considered positive (scores 4, 5) (Figs. 35.4b, 35.7b). Using the criteria established in Deauville, the International Validation Study demonstrated that the 3-year PFS for patients with negative and positive interim PET/CT was 95 versus 28 % [41]. Such figures may apply not only to advanced HL, but also to intermediate stage HL (localized stages with ≥1 unfavorable features). However, the outcome of interim PET/CT-positive patients with localized disease and no adverse factors, especially no bulky disease, may be much better than the ~30 % reported above [26, 38, 42]. For the time being, the use of interim PET/CT is not recommended outside the setting of clinical trials. On the other hand, there are interesting data indicating that treatment intensification with BEACOPP-escalated in patients with advanced or even intermediate stage HL, who remain PET/CT-positive after two ABVD cycles, may produce long-term PFS rates of ~65 % (vs. ~30 % expected based on historical data) [43,44] (Fig. 35.4b).

Under BEACOPP-escalated, the negative predictive value of interim PET/CT is also >90 %; nevertheless, the positive predictive value is much lower compared with ABVD-treated patients, since the long-term PFS of interim PET/CT-positive patients may be up to 50–60 % [45].

Although major studies agree in that the negative predictive value of interim PET is at least 90 % irrespective of the chemotherapy regimen used, other series revealed less impressive values (for example, 80-85 % or even less) [44, 46, 47]. Whether the a priori risk of failure as reflected by stage IV or other prognostic factors may affect the negative predictive value of interim PET should be further investigated [39, 44, 47, 48].

Diffuse Large B-cell Lymphoma

In DLBCL, interim PET/CT is also predictive of the outcome after R-CHOP or similar immunochemotherapy, but differences are not so marked compared with HL. Deauville criteria are not so widely accepted in this setting, because of their moderate reproducibility and prognostic capacity [49, 50] (Fig. 35.2b). Alternatively, a satisfactory interim PET/CT response can be defined by a >66 % reduction in SUVmax between baseline and interim assessment. In the NHL International Validation Study , based on 120 DLBCL patients treated with standard R-CHOP-21 or intensified R-CHOP-14 or R-ACVBP-14, where no PET-driven treatment modification was made, the 2-year EFS was approximately 80 versus 41 % in patients with >66 and ≤66 % SUVmax reductions after two cycles of immunochemotherapy, while 2-year PFS was 83 versus 54 % [50]. In the LNH-2007 3B trial, higher risk, young DLBCL patients were randomly assigned to receive either R-CHOP-14 or R-ACVBP-14, and underwent interim PET assessments after two and four cycles, which modified subsequent treatment strategy. The study confirmed that visual analysis was not accurate enough. The cutoff for SUVmax reduction was set at 66 % for PET-2 and 70 % for PET-4. The 2-year PFS according to PET-2 was 77 versus 57 %, while it was 83 versus 40 % according to PET-4 [51]. Clinical trials are currently examining the potential role of treatment intensification in interim PET/CT-positive patients with DLBCL [52]. In the PETAL trial, preliminary results revealed a sixfold higher relapse rate in patients with aggressive NHL, mostly DLBCL, who had not achieved a 66 % SUVmax reduction after two cycles of R-CHOP as compared to those who had, despite treatment intensification with a protocol designed for Burkitt lymphoma in patients randomized to the experimental arm [52]. Such strategies are not justified outside the investigational setting for the time being.

Issues on Reproducibility of Interim PET Reading

The reproducibility of various criteria for interim PET-based response assessment is a major issue, which should be addressed before such strategies become widely adopted. Furthermore, when studies are evaluated—especially the initially published ones—the reader should take into account the definition of interim PET positivity used in each study, which may affect the magnitude of the difference in PFS between negative and positive cases [38, 39, 48, 53, 54].

In HL, the International Validation Study suggested that the concordance (paired among 6 reviewers) regarding whether interim PET was negative or positive (visual analysis, Deauville score 1, 2 or 3 vs. 4 or 5) ranged from substantial to almost perfect (Cohen's K 0.70–0.84). The impact of interim PET on PFS was much stronger if PET was centrally reviewed than after local interpretation. However, in DLBCL, both ECOG (Eastern Cooperative Oncology Group) and Deauville criteria display only moderate reproducibility among independent reviewers [49]. In the NHL International Validation Study, the concordance among three reviewers regarding whether interim PET was negative or positive (visual analysis, Deauville criteria) was substantial ($K = 0.65$) if liver was used as reference (Deauville 4,5 positive), or even moderate ($K = 0.49$), if reference was the mediastinal blood pool (Deauville 3, 4, 5 positive). However, if SUVmax-based assessment with a 66 % cutoff was used, concordance was upgraded to almost perfect ($K = 0.81$).

35.5 PET in Autologous Stem Cell Transplantation

The evaluation of PET in patients with lymphoma undergoing Autologous Stem Cell Transplantation (ASCT) was introduced early in the course of utilization of PET in clinical practice. Generally, published studies have included mixed (HL and NHL) patient populations: Patients with positive pre-transplant PET have inferior outcomes than those with negative studies. Pre-transplant PET appears to be an independent predictor from established clinical risk scores at the time of relapse/progression [55]. In a meta-analysis of 12 studies, incorporating 630 patients with HL and aggressive NHL who underwent ASCT and had been evaluated with pre high dose chemotherapy PET examination, Terasawa et al., reported a summary sensitivity of 69 %, summary specificity 81 %, similar prognostic accuracy among studies and shorter PFS for patients with positive PET-scan [56]. Another meta-analysis reported hazard ratios of 3.2 (for disease progression) and 4.5 (for death) for patients with positive versus negative pre-transplant PET [57].

In relapsed/refractory Hodgkin lymphoma, patients who become PET-negative with salvage chemotherapy and undergo ASCT have a long-term remission rate of 80–85 % versus 40–50 % for those who remain PET-positive [58, 59] (Fig. 35.8). These results demonstrate that failure to achieve a PET-negative status does not preclude ASCT in patients with HL, especially if they are chemosensitive by conventional imaging [58]. However, more standardized protocols are required for evaluation of pre-transplant PET/CT in patients undergoing ASCT: It is not clear whether pre-transplant PET should be evaluated under the rules of interim or end-of-treatment PET or even if SUVmax-based criteria should be implemented. As a general rule, the decision to proceed to ASCT in relapsed/refractory Hodgkin lymphoma should be based rather on conventional chemosensitivity criteria than on PET evaluation.

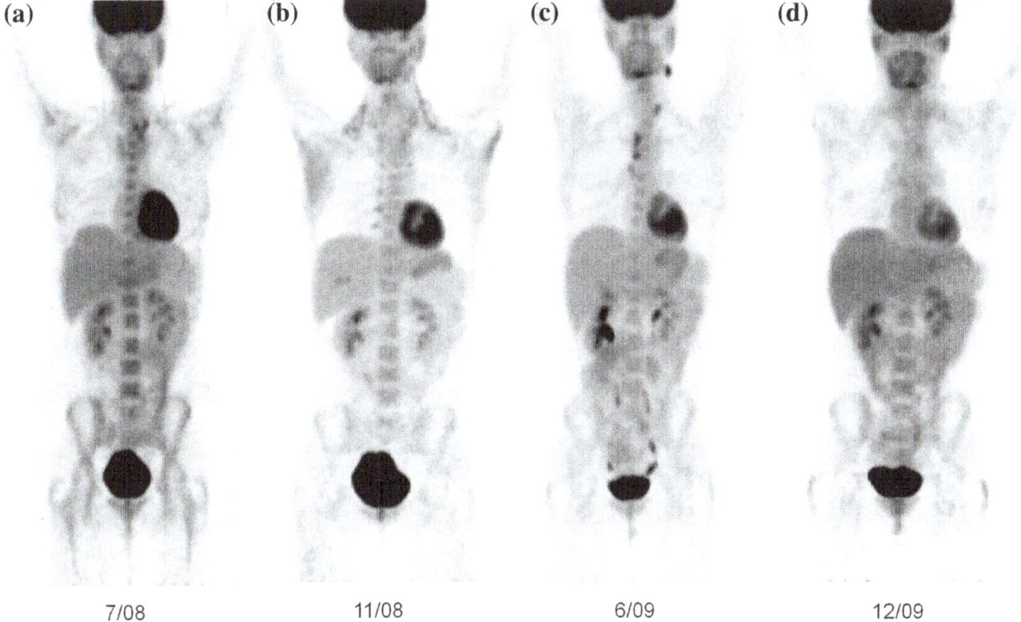

Fig. 35.8 **a** 18 FDG-PET before autologous transplantation in a patient with relapsed Hodgkin lymphoma: hypermetabolic lymph nodes at the upper mediastinum. **b** 18 FDG-PET 4 weeks after autologous transplantation: negative. **c** Relapsing disease 6 months later. **d** The patient received additional radiation treatment and reached CR (PET negative)

35.6 The Role of PET/CT in the Follow-up of Lymphomas

Once a negative PET/CT has been achieved, routine follow-up of patients with HL and aggressive B-cell lymphomas with PET/CT is not recommended, because the risk of false-positive findings outweighs any potential benefit of "earlier" identification of relapse and will lead to many unnecessary invasive procedures to exclude relapses. There is also no role for PET/CT in the follow-up of other lymphoma subtypes.

PET/CT is not a standard restaging procedure for relapsing lymphoma (Fig. 35.3b), but it may have a role in patients, mainly those with HL, who could be candidates for local treatment with curative intent.

35.7 Conclusions

FDG-PET is a unique equipment in the hands of hematologists, with high prognostic significance and accuracy, which has altered the definitions response to treatment and has already a major impact on the design of treatment and follow-up strategies. However, its exact role in guiding treatment decisions needs to be defined by randomized trials, many of which are ongoing. Questions under investigation include the role of PET to decide which patients should be irradiated, the potential of improving outcomes by early treatment intensification in interim PET-positive patients, or conversely, the possibility of treatment reduction in patients with negative interim PET. Evidence-based data on the appropriate use of PET in lymphomas are expected to be available shortly.

References

1. Hutchings M (2012) How does PET/CT help in selecting therapy for patients with Hodgkin lymphoma? Hematology. Am Soc Hematol Educ Program Book 2012:322–327
2. Ngeow JY, Quek RH, Ng DC et al (2009) High SUV uptake on FDG-PET/CT predicts for an aggressive B-cell lymphoma in a prospective study of primary FDG-PET/CT staging in lymphoma. Ann Oncol 20:1543–1547
3. Kabickova E, Sumerauer D, Cumlivska E et al (2006) Comparison of 18F-FDG-PET and standard procedures for the pretreatment staging of children and adolescents with Hodgkin's disease. Eur J Nucl Med Mol Imaging 33:1025–1031
4. Weiler-Sagie M, Bushelev O, Epelbaum R et al (2010) 18F-FDG avidity in lymphoma readdressed: a study of 766 patients. J Nucl Med 51:25–30
5. Tsukamoto N, Kojima M, Hasegawa M et al (2007) The usefulness of ^{18}F-fluorodeoxyglucose positron emission tomography (^{18}F-FDG-PET) and a comparison of ^{18}F-FDG-PET with ^{67}Gallium scintigraphy in the evaluation of lymphoma. Relation to histologic subtypes based on the World Health Organization classification. Cancer 110:652–659
6. Cheson BD, Pfistner B, Juweid ME et al (2007) Revised response criteria for malignant lymphoma. J Clin Oncol. 25:579–586
7. Cheson BD, Fisher RI, Barrington S, Zucca E, Cavalli F, Lister TA (2013) Follow-up of the 11-ICML workshop on lymphoma staging and restaging in the PET-CT era. Hematol Oncol 31(Suppl 1):139 (abstr. 128)
8. Kanoun S, Rossi C, Berriolo-Riedinger A et al (2012) Baseline metabolic tumor volume predicts patient's outcome in Hodgkin lymphoma. In: 4th international workshop on PET in lymphoma, Menton, France, 4–5th Oct 2012, abstract A1, p 2
9. Sasanelli MC, Itti E, Biggi A et al (2012) Prognostic value of pretherapy metabolic tumor volume (MTV) and early response assessment (two cycles) in diffuse large B-cell lymphoma (DLBCL). In: 4th international workshop on PET in lymphoma, Menton, France, 4–5th Oct 2012, abstract A10, p 11
10. Pakos EE, Fotopoulos AD, Ioannidis JP (2005) 18F-FDG PET for evaluation of bone marrow infiltration in staging of lymphoma: a meta-analysis. J Nucl Med 46:958–963
11. El-Galaly TC, d' Amore F, Mylam KJ et al (2012) Routine bone marrow biopsy has little or no therapeutic consequence for positron emission tomography/computed tomography-staged treatment-naïve patients with Hodgkin lymphoma. J Clin Oncol 30:4508–4514
12. Vassilakopoulos TP, Angelopoulou MK, Constantinou N et al (2005) Development and validation of a clinical prediction rule for bone marrow involvement in patients with Hodgkin lymphoma. Blood 105:1875–1880
13. Vassilakopoulos TP, Angelopoulou MK, Prassopoulos V et al (2013) Comparative assessment of bone marrow involvement by bone marrow biopsy or positron emission tomography in Hodgkin lymphoma. Hematol Oncol 31(Suppl 1):189 (abstr. 276)

14. Sehn LH, Scott DW, Chhanabhai M et al (2011) Impact of concordant and discordant bone marrow involvement on outcome in diffuse large B-cell lymphoma treated with R-CHOP. J Clin Oncol 29:1452–1457
15. Hong J, Lee Y, Park Y et al (2012) Role of FDG-PET/CT in detecting lymphomatous bone marrow involvement in patients with newly diagnosed diffuse large B-cell lymphoma. Ann Hematol 91:687–695
16. Cerci JJ, Gyorke T, Paez D et al (2012) Staging FDG-PET might replace bone marrow biopsy in diffuse large B-cell lymphoma. Results from a multicenter IAEA-sponsored study. In: 4th international workshop on PET in lymphoma, Menton, France, 4–5th Oct 2012, abstract B5, p 25
17. Berthet L, Cochet A, Kanoun S et al (2013) In newly diagnosed diffuse large B-cell lymphoma, determination of bone marrow involvement with 18F-FDG PET/CT provides better diagnostic performance and prognostic stratification than does biopsy. J Nucl Med. doi: 10.2967/jnumed.112.114710
18. Khan AB, Barrington SF, Mikhaeel NG et al (2013) PET-CT staging of DLBCL accurately identifies and provides new insight into the clinical significance of bone marrow involvement. Blood 122:61–67
19. Juweid ME, Wiseman GA, Vose JM et al (2005) Response assessment of aggressive non-Hodgkin's lymphoma by integrated International Workshop Criteria and fluorine-18-fluorodeoxyglucose positron emission tomography. J Clin Oncol 23:4652–4661
20. Terasawa T, Nihashi T, Hotta T, Nagai H (2008) 18F-FDG PET for posttherapy assessment of Hodgkin's disease and aggressive non-Hodgkin's lymphoma: a systematic review. J Nucl Med 49:13–21
21. Zijlstra JM, Lindauer-van der Werf G, Hoekstra OS et al (2006) 18F-fluoro-deoxyglucose positron emission tomography for post-treatment evaluation of malignant lymphoma: a systematic review. Haematologica 91:522–529
22. Juweid ME, Stroobants S, Hoekstra OS et al (2007) Use of positron emission tomography for response assessment of lymphoma: consensus of the Imaging Subcommittee of International Harmonization Project in Lymphoma. J Clin Oncol 25:571–578
23. Vassilakopoulos TP, Pangalis GA, Boutsikas G et al (2012). Prognostic factors in patients with Hodgkin lymphoma (HL) and a negative PET/CT after ABVD chemotherapy: Potential applications for the design of follow-up strategies. Haematologica/Hematol J 97(suppl 1):87 (abstr. 218)
24. Engert A, Haverkamp H, Kobe C et al (2012) Reduced-intensity chemotherapy and PET-guided radiotherapy in patients with advanced stage Hodgkin's lymphoma (HD15 trial): a randomised, open-label, phase 3 non-inferiority trial. Lancet 379:1791–1799
25. Barnes JA, LaCasce AS, Zukotynski K et al (2011) End-of-treatment but not interim PET scan predicts outcome in nonbulky limited stage Hodgkin's lymphoma. Ann Oncol 22:910–915
26. Sher DJ, Mauch PM, van den Abbeele A, LaCasce AS, Czerminski J, Ng AK (2009) Prognostic significance of mid- and post-ABVD PET imaging in Hodgkin's lymphoma: the importance of involved field radiotherapy. Ann Oncol 20:1848–1853
27. Vassilakopoulos TP, Rontogianni P, Pangalis GA et al (2012) Outcome and prognostic factors in patients with Hodgkin lymphoma (HL) who remain PET/CT-positive after ABVD combination chemotherapy: potential applications for the design of subsequent treatment. Haematologica/Hematol J 97(suppl 1):562 (abstr.1404)
28. Vassilakopoulos TP, Pangalis G, Masouridis S et al (2011) PET-Scan for response assessement after Rituximab-CHOP (R-CHOP) in primary mediastinal large B-cell lymphoma (PMLBCL): Prognostic significance and implications for subsequent radiotherapy (RT). Haematologica/Hematol J 96(Suppl 2):391 (abstr. 937)
29. Vassilakopoulos TP, Pangalis GA, Katsigiannis A et al (2012) Rituximab, cyclophosphamide, doxorubicin, vincristine, and prednisone with or without radiotherapy in primary mediastinal large B-cell lymphoma: The emerging standard of care. Oncologist 17:239–249
30. Ceriani L, Zucca E, Zinzani PL et al (2012) PET/CT response analysis in primary mediastinal diffuse large B-cell lymphoma (PMBL): results of the IELSG-26 study. In: 4th international workshop on PET in lymphoma, Menton, France, 4–5th Oct 2012, abstract B7, p 27
31. Dupuis J, Itti E, Rahmouni A et al (2009) Response assessment after an inductive CHOP or CHOP-like regimen with or without rituximab in 103 patients with diffuse large B-cell lymphoma: integrating 18 fluorodeoxyglucose positron emission tomography to the International Workshop Criteria. Ann Oncol 20:503–507
32. Thomas A, Gingrich RD, Smith BJ et al (2010) 18-fluoro-deoxyglucose positron emission tomography report interpretation as predictor of outcome in diffuse large B-cell lymphoma including analysis of "indeterminate" reports. Leuk Lymphoma 51:439–446
33. Sehn LH, Klasa R, Shenkier T et al (2013) Long-term experience with PET-guided consolidative radiation therapy (XRT) in patients with advanced stage diffuse large B-cell lymphoma (DLBCL) treated with R-CHOP. Hematol Oncol 31(Suppl 1):137 (abstr. 123)
34. Picardi M, De Renzo A, Pane F et al (2007) Randomized comparison of consolidation radiation versus observation in bulky Hodgkin's lymphoma with post-chemotherapy negative positron emission tomography scans. Leuk Lymphoma 48:1721–1727

35. Andre MPE, Reman O, Federico M et al (2012) Interim analysis of the randomized EORTC/LYSA/FIL Intergroup H10 trial on early PET-scan driven treatment adaptation in stage I/II Hodgkin lymphoma. Blood (ASH Annual Meeting Abstracts) 120:Abstract 549
36. Radford J, Barrington S, Counsell L et al (2012) Involved field radiotherapy versus no further treatment in patients with clinical stages IA and IIA Hodgkin lymphoma and a 'negative' PET scan after 3 cycles ABVD. Results of the UK NCRI RAPID trial. Blood (ASH Annual Meeting Abstracts) 120:Abstract 547
37. Illidge T (2013) Radiotherapy in early stage Hodgkin lymphoma. Hematol Oncol 31(Suppl 1):92-95
38. Hutchings M, Loft A, Hansen M et al (2006) FDG-PET after two cycles of chemotherapy predicts treatment failure and progression-free survival in Hodgkin lymphoma. Blood 107:52–59
39. Gallamini A, Hutchings M, Rigacci L et al (2007) Early interim 2-[18F]fluoro-2-deoxy-D-glucose positron emission tomography is prognostically superior to international prognostic score in advanced-stage Hodgkin's lymphoma: a report from a joint Italian-Danish study. J Clin Oncol 25:3746–3752
40. Moskowitz CH, Schoder H, Teruya-Feldstein J et al (2010) Risk-adapted dose-dense immunochemotherapy determined by interim FDG-PET in advanced-stage diffuse large B-cell lymphoma. J Clin Oncol 28:1896–1903
41. Gallamini A, Kostakoglou L (2012) Interim FDG-PET in Hodgkin lymphoma: a compass for a safe navigation in clinical trials? Blood 120:4913–4920
42. Kostakoglu L, Schoder H, Johnson JL et al (2012) Interim FDG PET imaging in stage I/II non bulky Hodgkin lymphoma: Would using combined PET and CT criteria better predict response than each test alone? Leuk Lymphoma 53:2143–2150
43. Gallamini A, Patti C, Viviani S et al (2011) Early chemotherapy intensification with BEACOPP in advanced-stage Hodgkin lymphoma patients with a interim-PET positive after two ABVD courses. Br J Haematol 152:551–560
44. Press OW, LeBlanc M, Rimsza LM et al (2013) A phase II trial of response adapted therapy of stages III-IV Hodgkin lymphoma using early interim FDG-PET imaging: US Intergroup S0816. Hematol Oncol 31(Suppl 1):137 (abstr. 124)
45. Markova J, Kobe C, Skopalova M et al (2009) FDG-PET for assessment of early treatment response after four cycles of chemotherapy in patients with advanced stage Hodgkin's lymphoma has a high negative predictive value. Ann Oncol 20:1270–1274
46. Rossi C, Kanoun S, Berriolo-Riedinger A et al (2012) Inerim PET SUVmax reduction is superior to visual analysis using 5-point scale criteria to predict patient's outcome in Hodgkin lymphoma. In: 4th international workshop on PET in lymphoma, Menton, France, 4–5th Oct 2012, abstract A2, p 3
47. Vassilakopoulos TP, Angelopoulou MK, Rondogianni P et al (2011) Interim PET-Scan for early response assessment and potential modification of treatment plan after 2 ABVD cycles in advanced stage Hodgkin lymphoma (HL). Haematologica/Hematol J 96(Suppl 2):322 (abstr. 772)
48. Cerci JJ, Pracchia LF, Linardi CCG et al (2010) 18 F-FDG PET after 2 cycles of ABVD predicts event-free survival in early and advanced Hodgkin lymphoma. J Nucl Med 51:1337–1343
49. Horning SJ, Juweid ME, Schoeder H et al (2010) Interim positron emission tomography scans in diffuse large B-cell lymphoma: an independent expert nuclear medicine evaluation of the Eastern Cooperative Oncology Group E3404 study. Blood 115:775–777
50. Meignan M, Gallamini A, Itti E, Barrington S, Haioun C, Polliack A (2012) Report on the third international workshop on interim positron emission tomography in lymphoma held in Menton, France, 26–27 September 2011 and Menton 2011 consensus. Leuk Lymphoma 53:1876–1881
51. Casasnovas RO, Meignan M, Berriolo-Riedinger A et al (2011) SUVmax reduction improves early prognosis value of interim positron emission tomography scans in diffuse large B-cell lymphoma. Blood 118:37–43
52. Dührsen U, Hüttmann A, Jöckel KH, Müller S (2009) Positron emission tomography guided therapy of aggressive non-Hodgkin lymphomas–the PETAL trial. Leuk Lymphoma 50:1757–1760
53. Zinzani PL, Rigacci L, Stefoni V et al (2010) Early interim 18F-FDG PET in Hodgkin's lymphoma: evaluation on 304 patients. Eur J Nucl Med Mol Imaging 39:4–12
54. Itti E, Juweid ME, Haioun C et al (2010) Improvement of early 18F-FDG-PET interpretation in diffuse large B-cell Lymphoma: importance of the reference background. J Nucl Med 51: 1857–1862
55. Schot BW, Zijlstra JM, Sluiter WJ et al (2007) Early FDG-PET assessment in combination with clinical risk scores determines prognosis in recurring lymphoma. Blood 109:486–491
56. Terasawa T, Dahabreh I, Nihashi T (2010) Fluorine-18-fluorodeoxyglycose positron emission tomography in response assessment before high-dose chemotherapy for lymphoma: a systematic review and meta-analysis. Oncologist 15:750–759
57. Poulou LS, Thanos L, Ziakas PD (2010) Unifying the predictive value of pretransplant FDG PET in patients with lymphoma: a review and meta-analysis of published trials. Eur J Nucl Med Mol Imaging 37:156–162

58. Angelopoulou MK, Moschogiannis M, Rondogianni P et al (2012) The prognostic significance of PET-Scan before and after high-dose therapy and autologous stem cell transplantation (ASCT) in relapsed/refractory Hodgkin lymphoma (HL) patients. Haematologica/Hematol J 97(suppl 1):178, abstract 443
59. Moskowitz AJ, Yahalom J, Kewalramani T et al (2010) Pretransplantation functional imaging predicts outcome following autologous stem cell transplantation for relapsed and refractory Hodgkin lymphoma. Blood 116:4934–4937

Part VII
Gynecologic Cancer

36 Introduction to Gynecologic Cancer

Georgios E. Hilaris

One of the key aspects in the assessment of the patient with suspected or known gynecologic cancer is imaging. Upon patient presentation, it is often the next step in its management following a thorough history and detailed physical examination. The role of imaging is equally crucial during the preoperative evaluation as well as during the postoperative surveillance period for the documentation of clinical remission or suspected tumor relapse and/or metastasis.

In this section, we summarize the main features of endometrial, ovarian, and cervical cancer. We will also point out the key clinical implications of the current imaging techniques tailored to each gynecologic cancer type. These clinical pearls can be equally helpful to the gynecologic oncologist, medical oncologist, radiation oncologist, pathologist, and radiologist in the everyday clinical setting.

G. E. Hilaris (✉)
Consultant Gynecologic Oncologist,
Hygeia and Mitera Hospitals and IASO Hospital,
Athens, Greece
e-mail: info@hilaris.org

G. E. Hilaris
Adjunct Clinical Instructor of Gynecology and Obstetrics, Stanford University School of Medicine,
Palo Alto, California, USA

36.1 Endometrial Cancer

It is the most common gynecologic malignancy and fourth overall malignancy in women in developed countries (in developing countries, it is the second most common gynecologic malignancy following cervical cancer) [1]. A woman's lifetime risk for endometrial cancer in western societies is 2.6 % [2].

There are two main types of endometrial cancer that differ: type I and type II.

Type I is the typical endometrioid adenocarcinoma grade 1 or 2, accounting for over 80 % of all endometrial cancer cases. In nearly 70 % of patients, it is diagnosed at an early stage (stage I or II) and carries a favorable prognosis. Type II is less common and encompasses grade 3 endometrioid tumors, serous or clear cell endometrial cancers, and other rarest high grade also histologic subtypes. Unfortunately, type II endometrial cancer is usually diagnosed at later stages and carries a poor prognosis [3].

Endometrial cancer is surgically staged (Table 36.1). Prognosis is directly related to surgical stage (Table 36.2). Besides stage, other risk factors for relapse and/or metastasis are histologic type and histologic grade, lymph-vascular space involvement (LVSI) as well as tumor size [4, 5].

Remission or cure is accomplished primarily with surgery and optimal debulking if deemed necessary. Adjuvant radiation therapy in the form of intracavitary or external beam radiation

A. D. Gouliamos et al. (eds.), *Imaging in Clinical Oncology*,
DOI: 10.1007/978-88-470-5385-4_36, © Springer-Verlag Italia 2014

Table 36.1 Endometrial Cancer Surgical Staging (FIGO 2009)

Stage I[a]	Tumor confined to the corpus uteri
IA[a]	None or less than half myometrial invasion
IB[a]	Invasion equal to or more than half of the myometrium
Stage II[a]	Tumor invades cervical stroma, but does not extend beyond the uterus[b]
Stage III[a]	Local and/or regional spread of the tumor
IIIA[a]	Tumor invades the serosa of the corpus uteri and/or adnexa[b]
IIIB[a]	Vaginal and/or parametrial involvement[c]
IIIC[a]	Metastases to pelvic and/or para-aortic lymph nodes[c]
IIIC1[a]	Positive pelvic nodes
IIIC2[a]	Positive para-aortic lymph nodes with or without positive pelvic lymph nodes
Stage IV[a]	Tumor invades bladder and/or bowel mucosa, and/or distant metastases
IVA[a]	Tumor invades bladder and/or bowel mucosa
IVB[a]	Distant metastases, including intra-abdominal metastases and/or inguinal lymph nodes

[a] Either G1, G2, or G3
[b] Endocervical glandular involvement should only be considered as stage I and no longer as stage II
[c] Positive cytology has to be reported separately without changing the stage

Table 36.2 Endometrial cancer FIGO surgical stage 5-year survival (%)

IA	90
IB	78
II	74
IIIA	56
IIIB	36
IIIC1	57
IIIC2	49
IVA	22
IVB	21

From SEER 1988–2006 patient data, adapted to the new 2010 FIGO staging

is often applied. Chemotherapy may also be instituted in later stages or high risk disease.

Metastasis and relapse in endometrial cancer are equally distributed in the pelvis, vagina, abdomen, and lungs.

Imaging holds a strong pivotal role in the preoperative assessment as well as in the confirmation of remission, cure, and in the documentation of relapse and metastasis.

36.2 Ovarian Cancer

Ovarian Cancer is the second most common gynecologic malignancy. It is the leading cause of death from gynecologic cancers and fifth overall from cancer death in women in developed countries. The lifetime risk of developing ovarian cancer in developed countries is 1.4 % [2, 6] (In developing countries, it is the third most common gynecologic cancer after cervical and endometrial cancers).

Nearly 95 % of all cases of ovarian cancer arise from the ovarian surface epithelium. These so called epithelial ovarian carcinomas (EOCs) include serous, mucinous, endometrioid, and clear cell subtypes and besides being most common they also exhibit an aggressive biologic behavior and tend to be diagnosed at a later stage. Unfortunately, less aggressive ovarian cancers are also less common and include those arising from germ cells, sex cord, or stromal cells as well as mixed types [7].

Overall, nearly three fourths of all cases are diagnosed at advanced stages when permanent cure is less feasible compared to earlier stages (I or II). Its indolent course at earlier stages, non-specific symptoms, and lack of successful screening strategies up to date, all contribute to the lethality of the disease. EOC is staged surgically (Table 36.3). Prognosis is directly related to stage (Table 36.4).

The gold standard in the management of ovarian cancer is still primary surgery and ideally primary optimal cytoreduction, followed in most instances by chemotherapy. Imaging plays a crucial role in both the preoperative evaluation as well as in the surveillance of remission and relapse.

Table 36.3 Ovarian Cancer Surgical Staging Classification

Stage	Characteristics
I	Growth limited to the ovaries
IA	Growth limited to one ovary; no ascites; no tumor on the external surfaces, capsule intact
IB	Growth limited to both ovaries; no ascites, no tumor on the external surfaces, capsule intact
IC	Tumor either stage IA or IB but on the surface of one or both ovaries; capsule ruptured; ascites containing malignant cells present; or positive peritoneal washings
II	Growth involving one or both ovaries with pelvic extension of disease
IIA	Extension of disease and/or metastases to the uterus and/or fallopian tubes
IIB	Extension of disease to other pelvic tissues
IIC	Tumor either stage IIA or IIB but on the surface of one or both ovaries; capsule(s) ruptured; ascites containing malignant cells present; or positive peritoneal washings
III	Tumor involving one or both ovaries with peritoneal implants outside the pelvis and/or positive retroperitoneal or inguinal nodes; superficial liver metastasis equals stage III; tumor is limited to the true pelvis but with histologically verified malignant extension to the small bowel or omentum
IIIA	Tumor grossly limited to the true pelvis with negative nodes but with histologically confirmed microscopic seeding of abdominal peritoneal surfaces
IIIB	Tumor of one or both ovaries; histologically confirmed implants on abdominal peritoneal surfaces, none >2 cm in diameter; nodes negative
IIIC	Abdominal implants >2 cm in diameter and/or positive retroperitoneal or inguinal nodes
IV	Growth involving one or both ovaries with distant metastases; if pleural effusion is present, there must be positive cytologic test results to allot a case to stage IV; parenchymal liver metastasis equal stage IV

FIGO International Federation of Gynecology and Obstetrics

Table 36.4 Ovarian cancer FIGO surgical stage and 2 year and 5-year survival (%)

Stage	2 year	5 year
IA	96.2	89.6
IB	93.9	86.1
IC	91.3	83.4
IIA	87.2	70.7
IIB	84.5	65.5
IIC	85.6	71.4
IIIA	72.6	46.7
IIIB	70.6	41.5
IIIC	64.5	32.5
IV	48.4	18.6

From: Heintz et al. [12]

36.3 Cervical Cancer

Cervical cancer is the third most common gynecologic cancer in developed countries and a relatively infrequent cause of cancer death overall. The lifetime risk of developing cervical cancer in the United States, based upon national data from 2000 to 2004, is 0.76 % [8, 9]. In developing countries, however, it is the most common gynecologic cancer as well as the second leading cause of cancer death in women [9].

The above figures reflect unfortunately the lack of cervical cancer screening with Papanicolaou smear in third world and developing nations.

Cervical cancer is caused by persistent infection from high-risk oncogenic HPV types in 99.7 % of all cases [10].

Diagnosis is made by histologic confirmation of cervical biopsies.

According to the international federation of gynecology and obstetrics, cervical cancer is still clinically staged (FIGO—Table 36.5).

In developed countries, however, various imaging studies are being used to assess nodal status or parametrial spread and tailor further management [11].

Table 36.5 Cervical cancer FIGO clinical stage (2009)

Stage I
Stage IA: Invasive cancer identified only microscopically. Invasion is limited to measured stromal invasion with a maximum depth of 5 mm and no wider than 7 mm
Stage IA1: Measured invasion of the stroma no greater than 3 mm in depth and no wider than 7 mm diameter
Stage IA2: Measured invasion of stroma greater than 3 mm but no greater than 5 mm in depth and no wider than 7 mm in diameter
Stage IB: Clinical lesions confined to the cervix or preclinical lesions greater than stage IA. All gross lesions even with superficial invasion are stage IB cancers
Stage IB1: Clinical lesions no greater than 4 cm in size
Stage IB2: Clinical lesions greater than 4 cm in size
Stage II
Stage IIA: No obvious parametrial involvement. Involvement of up to the upper two-thirds of the vagina
Stage IIB: Obvious parametrial involvement, but not into the pelvic sidewall
Stage III
Stage IIIA: No extension into the pelvic sidewall but involvement of the lower third of the vagina
Stage IIIB: Extension into the pelvic sidewall or hydronephrosis or non-functioning kidney
Stage IV
Stage IVA: Spread of the tumor into adjacent pelvic organs
Stage IVB: Spread to distant organs

Cervical cancer can be treated by both surgery and radiotherapy in stages up to IIA. Greater stages are being treated primarily by radiation therapy with concurrent chemosensitization. Sometimes adjuvant surgery may be used.

References

1. Jemal A, Bray F et al (2011) Global cancer statistics. CA Cancer J Clin 61:69
2. SEER cancer statistics. http://seer.cancer.gov
3. Felix AS, Weissfeld JL, Stone RA et al (2010) Cancer Causes Control 21(11):1851–1856
4. Lewin SN, Herzog TJ et al (2010) Comparative performance of the 2009 international Federation of gynecology and obstetrics' staging system for uterine corpus cancer. Obstet Gynecol 116(5):1141
5. Hilaris et al (2009) Feasibility safety and cost outcomes of laparoscopic management off early endometrial and cervical malignancy. J Soc Laparoendosc Surg 13(4):489–495
6. Siegel R, Naishadham D et al (2012) Cancer statistics. CA Cancer J Clin 62(1):10
7. Lacey JV, Sherman ME (2009) Ovarian neoplasia. In: Robboy SL, Mutter GL, Prat J et al (eds) Robboy's pathology of the female reproductive tract, 2nd edn. Elsevier, Oxford, p 601
8. Ries LAG, Melbert D et al (2007) SEER cancer statistics review, 1975–2004. National Cancer Institute, Bethesda
9. Siegel R, Ward E et al (2011) Cancer statistics: the impact of eliminating socioeconomic and racial disparities on premature cancer deaths. CA Cancer J Clin 61(4):212
10. Walboomers JM, Jacobs MV et al (1999) Human papillomavirus is a necessary cause of invasive cervical cancer worldwide. J Pathol 189(1):12
11. Pecorelli S et al (2009) Revised FIGO staging for carcinoma of the vulva, cervix, and endometrium. Int J Gynaecol Obstet 105(2):103
12. Heintz AP, Odicino F, Maisonneuve P et al (2006) Carcinoma of the ovary. Int J Gynaecol Obstet 95:S161

37 US Findings in Gynecologic Cancer

Charis I. Bourgioti and Aristeidis G. Antoniou

Ultrasonography (US) is regarded as the initial imaging method for the evaluation of the female pelvis. It is a noninvasive, easily repeatable, cheap, and widely available imaging modality, which provides a quick overview of the female reproductive system. Since it lacks ionization, it is a safe method for the evaluation of young females and pregnant patients [1, 2].

Bimanual clinical examination has low sensitivity in recognizing uterine and ovarian tumors [3]. On the contrary, US can easily detect and characterize pelvic masses of uterine or adnexal origin, predicting also their benign or malignant nature.

US is susceptible to pitfalls since it is dependent on the operator's experience, technical equipment, and patient's body mass index. In the last decades there is a particular improvement in technical quality parameters, so US can be used as a reliable tool in the depiction and classification of most gynecological tumors in pre- and postmenopausal women, in follow-up, and even in detection of recurrence in oncologic patients, especially when carried out by a sonographer specialized in gynecologic oncology [2].

C. I. Bourgioti (✉) · A. G. Antoniou
First Department of Radiology, Aretaieion Hospital, University of Athens Medical School,
76, Vasilissis Sofias Avenue, Athens, 11528, Greece
e-mail: charisbourgioti@yahoo.com

A. G. Antoniou
e-mail: aantoniou@med.uoa.gr

The purpose of this chapter is to describe the usual sonographic findings of uterine and ovarian malignancies in pre- and postmenopausal women and to review the diagnostic efficacy of ultrasound examination in such cases.

37.1 Uterine Cancers: US Evaluation

Uterine carcinomas primarily can be divided into endometrial cancer, uterine cervical cancer, and uterine sarcomas.

37.1.1 Endometrial Cancer

Endometrial cancer is the commonest malignant gynecological tumor and is predominately seen in postmenopausal women at the sixth and seventh decades of life. There is a high incidence rate in developed countries, probably because of increased life expectancy and obesity [1].

Transvaginal Ultrasound (TVUS) is the initial imaging method for the assessment of uterine endometrium and myometrium, especially in those patients.

The sonographic findings of endometrial cancer are not pathognomonic and there is a considerable overlap with other benign conditions. Endometrial cancer usually presents as a diffusely thickened endometrium with inhomogeneous echotexture and irregular or poorly defined margins. However, sometimes endometrial cancer

A. D. Gouliamos et al. (eds.), *Imaging in Clinical Oncology*,
DOI: 10.1007/978-88-470-5385-4_37, © Springer-Verlag Italia 2014

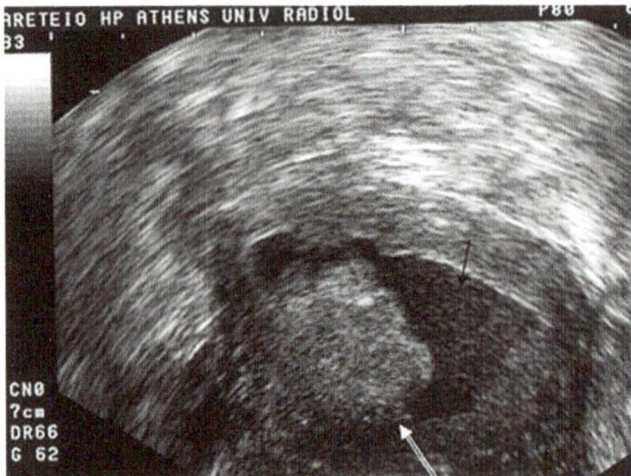

Fig. 37.1 Sagittal TVUS shows abnormal appearance of endometrium in a postmenopausal patient with biopsy confirmed endometrial carcinoma. Note a large broad based (*white arrow*) heterogeneous mass, with irregular borders protruding into the fluid-filled endometrial cavity (*black arrow*). The presence of echogenic debris within the endometrial fluid collection is highly indicative of hemorrhage

presents as a well-defined, uniformly thickened echogenic endometrium or as a polypoid mass and cannot be differentiated from endometrial hyperplasia or benign polyps (Fig. 37.1). Cystic changes may be found although they are not a usual finding in endometrial cancer. Hydrometra or hematometra may also occur in case of endometrial canal obstruction. The role of color and spectral Doppler still remains controversial. Fischerova [2] states that abnormal perfusion in tumors, which are isoechogenic with the myometrial stroma allows better delineation of the tumor borders.

TVUS may not be sensitive or specific for diagnosis of cancer but it has proved quite accurate in estimating endometrial thickness and in detecting other common sources of uterine bleeding, like polyps or leiomyomas, especially when combined with sonohysterography [1].

A clinical useful protocol based on US assessment of endometrial thickness has been proposed, for the initial management of postmenopausal patients with vaginal bleeding [4]. If measurement value is less than 4 mm, bleeding occurs probably due to endometrial atrophy and no further work-up is needed. If endometrium has thickness of more than 4 mm or if the endometrial thickness cannot be measured accurately, sonohysterography should be performed. Patients with thin endometrium (single layer less than 2 mm) need no further studies. Patients with focal thickening or polypoid mass should undergo hysteroscopic biopsy and those with diffuse thickening should be treated with conventional biopsy or dilatation and curettage.

In asymptomatic non-bleeding postmenopausal women or patients under hormonal replacement, endometrial thickness more than 8 mm is considered abnormal and further investigation should be made.

Patients who receive Tamoxifen as an adjuvant therapy for breast cancer may develop endometrial hyperplasia, polyps, or even endometrial cancer. Sonographic tamoxifen-related endometrial changes are usually nonspecific, but frequently cystic changes can be observed within the thickened endometrium. Serial sonographic examination for endometrial thickness evaluation is usually recommended in these patients.

The local extent of endometrial cancerous disease, especially the degree of myometrial and cervical invasion are important prognostic factors and can alter treatment planning. Although MR imaging is the modality of choice for endometrial cancer presurgical staging, TVUS seems also to be accurate in staging. Reported accuracies of TVUS for deep (more than half of the myometrium surface) myometrial infiltration range from 84 to 98.6 % and for cervical involvement from 93.5 to 95.65 %. Limitations in tumor measurement include diffuse infiltration of myometrium from cancerous tissue or compression and marked thinning of the normal myometrium due to quite large lesions [4].

Contrast-enhanced TVUS can increase the contrast between carcinoma and normal tissue, and may be very helpful in evaluating patients with thin endometrium after biopsy (Fig. 37.2). According to a recent study [5] contrast-enhanced sonography performs accuracy up to 85.3 % in estimating the depth of myometrial infiltration.

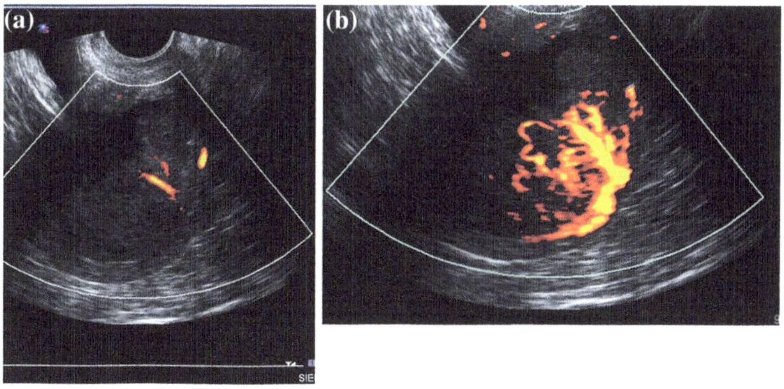

Fig. 37.2 Transvaginal US section of a postmenopausal woman with vaginal bleeding depicts a quite large endometrial tumor. **a** Power Doppler shows small internal vasculature of the tumor. **b** Note the increased abnormal vascularization of the same tumor demonstrated after the intravenous injection of contrast-enhanced agent. The presence of endometrial carcinoma was confirmed by biopsy

37.1.2 Cervical Cancer [1, 4, 6]

Cervical carcinoma is the third most common gynecologic malignancy and is typically seen in young sexually active population.

The diagnosis of cervical carcinoma is mainly clinical and the diagnostic modality of choice is MRI, so women are rarely referred for ultrasound evaluation. The cervix lies low in the pelvis and cannot be assessed adequately by transabdominal ultrasound (TAUS). TVUS offers better visualization but also has diagnostic limitations. In early cervical cancer, US may be negative and in case of advanced disease, sonography may demonstrate a diffusely enlarged and inhomogeneous cervix or a solid echogenic cervical mass, behind the urinary bladder without specific features.

Generally, in most gynecologic-oncology centers neither TAUS nor TVUS has a major role in depicting and staging of cervical carcinoma. The assessment of the tumor's local spread with US is considered suboptimal, due to small field of view and low soft tissue contrast resolution. However, some recent studies claim that US has a high detection rate (93–94 %) for cervical cancer and is an accurate presurgical staging method [7]. According to two studies, there was a specific correlation between US and surgicopathological tumor volume [7]. Also, three retrospective studies revealed sensitivity, specificity, and negative predictive value of US for parametrial assessment, ranging from 67 to 83 %, 56 to 100 %, and 89–99 %, respectively [7].

37.1.3 Uterine Sarcomas [1, 6, 8]

Sarcomas are rather uncommon uterine tumors of mesenchymal origin and include Malignant Mixed Mullerian Tumors (MMMTs), leiomyosarcomas, and the rare types of endometrial stromal sarcoma and adenosarcoma.

MMMTs (referred also as carcinosarcomas) have both carcinomatous and sarcomatous elements, are closely related to endometrial carcinomas, and mostly behave like carcinomas and not as sarcomas. They account for 50 % of primary uterine sarcomas. Sonographically, they appear as a bulky heterogeneous uterine mass of variable echogenity, with gross myometrial invasion and tumor vascularity, which can be detected with the use of power Doppler. Especially in case of a very large mass, US has limited role in tumor staging.

Adenosarcoma is a rare histological type of MMMT, which sonographically may present as a thickened inhomogeneous endometrium or as an ill-defined polypoid tumor causing expansion of the endometrial cavity and protruding through the external cervical os (Fig. 37.3). Also, small

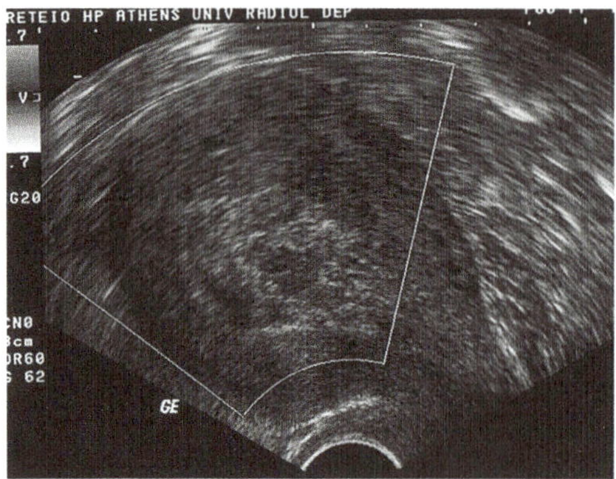

Fig. 37.3 TVUS sagittal image demonstrates a heterogeneous ill-defined endometrial mass expanding the endometrial cavity, which histologically proved to be adenosarcoma

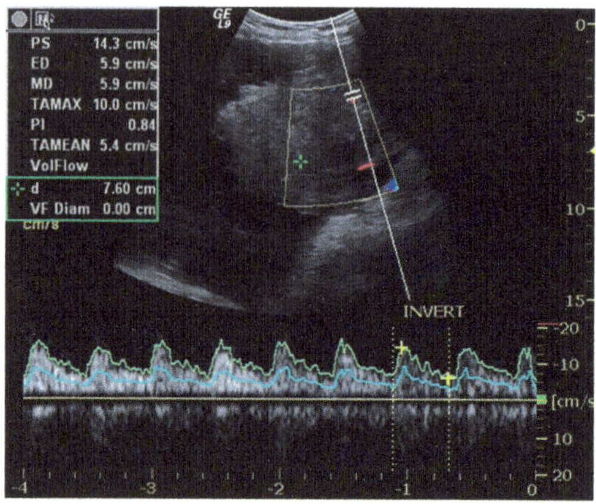

Fig. 37.4 Transabdominal axial US image of a postmenopausal woman demonstrates a left adnexal mass with cystic and solid components. Doppler spectral analysis shows a low resistance flow which is highly indicative of tumor's malignant nature. Serous-papillary adenocarcinoma of the left ovary was found on surgery

hypoechoic cystic spaces may be seen. In case of sarcomatous transformation of an adenomatous polyp, color Doppler can reveal a vascular pedicle entering the mass.

Leiomyosarcoma is the second most common histologic type of uterine sarcoma (30 %). Leiomyosarcomas behave aggressively and have poor prognosis. Benign leiomyomas rarely undergo sarcomatous degeneration (<1 %). However, early diagnosis of leiomyosarcoma is critical because tumor size proves to have the most impact in survival rates. Imaging differentiation between leiomyoma and low-grade leiomyosarcoma is quite difficult, since they have similar appearance. Sonographic findings include a uterine mass of heterogeneous echotexture (mostly because of necrosis or hemorrhage) which can be indistinguishable from benign leiomyoma. However, the rapid increase in size during serial imaging and the presence of increased vascularity are suggestive of malignancy and must be carefully evaluated by clinicians. In case of a quite large mass the role of US remains limited.

Endometrial stromal sarcoma is also a rare uterine tumor (0.2 % of all uterine malignancies) and commonly affects young women (mean 39 years). TVUS findings are not specific and usually include an endometrial-based mass, with mixed echogenity, poorly defined endometrial-myometrial interface, and increased vascularity. In advanced cases there is continuous extension to the adjacent structures, so adnexal solid masses may be visualized.

37.2 Ovarian and Fallopian Tubes Malignancies: US Evaluation

Ultrasound examination (transvaginal or transabdominal) is the modality of choice for the initial evaluation of a complex ovarian mass.

Morphologic analysis of an ovarian lesion with conventional US can detect potential malignancy with very high sensitivity [9]. Timmerman et al. [10] report sensitivity and specificity of 93 and 90 %, respectively, for the identification of malignant ovarian tumors.

Sonographic features of an adnexal mass which are suspicious for malignancy include the presence of solid components within a cystic mass, septa with thickness more than 3 mm, and Doppler flow within solid elements. Vascularity within the center of the solid part of the lesion and low resistance spectral waveform are indicative of neovascularization and are considered "worrisome" (Fig. 37.4). Resistive index (RI) less than 0.4 in postmenopausal populations is highly suspicious of malignancy but in premenopausal women has considerable overlap with other benign lesions such as corpus luteum cyst or inflammatory masses. If the mass has malignant features, additional US investigation of the whole abdomen should be made for the detection of potential metastatic disease like ascites, peritoneal implants, lymphadenopathy, and abdominal visceral metastasis [9, 11].

Three-dimensional TVUS can be used for a more detailed imaging of a neoplastic ovarian lesion and can detect tiny solid foci on lesion's internal wall [12]. The use of contrast-enhanced sonography seems to have higher sensitivity and specificity in defining the nature of an ovarian lesion than conventional US techniques, especially in case of early malignant ovarian disease. Marret et al. [13] referred sensitivity between 96 and 100 % and specificity between 83 and 98 % in differentiating malignant from benign ovarian mass, by estimating the kinetic parameters of the contrast agent. In particular, malignant tumors presented with significantly greater enhancement and rapid wash out times of contrast media compared with benign lesions [12, 13].

Careful interpretation of ovarian masses, especially in premenopausal women, is essential in order to avoid unnecessary surgeries.

Hemorrhagic corpus luteum can have a quite complex sonographic image and can mimic neoplasm, so a 6–12 week follow-up sonographic examination is usually recommended to confirm resolution. Also, benign lesions like peritoneal inclusion cysts, inflammatory pelvic process, or gastrointestinal masses can lead to false-positive findings.

MR imaging is the next imaging choice when US findings are controversial and can be very helpful in determining the origin and nature of a large pelvic mass.

The following text refers briefly to the commonest ovarian carcinomas and their usual sonographic features.

37.2.1 Ovarian Carcinomas [6, 8, 11]

Ovarian cancer is the second most common malignancy of the female reproductive system. Unfortunately, symptoms in early stages of the disease are subtle and usually the diagnosis is made at advanced stages, carrying an overall poor 5 year-survival rate (46 %) [1].

In general, the efficacy of screening programs using both serum cancer antigen CA125 and TVUS is not adequately established. These methods are considered more suitable for high risk patients, for example, patients with Lynch syndrome or BCRA mutations. According to a large Randomized Controlled Trial for Prostate, Lung, Colorectal, and Ovarian (PLCO) Cancer the use of both CA-125 and TVUS compared with usual gynecologic care did not decline ovarian cancer mortality. Also, false-positive screening test results lead to unnecessary interventions, which were associated with complications [14]. However, another large clinical trial running from the Ovarian Cancer Screening Research Program at the University of Kentucky states that women who were screened in this program and were diagnosed with ovarian cancer survived longer than women with ovarian cancer who did not receive screening, since with the screening program there was a decrease in stage at the time of the detection [15].

Primary ovarian malignant neoplasms can originate from surface epithelium of the ovary (70–75 %), from germ cells (10–15 %), or less frequently, from sex-cord stromal tissue.

Epithelial origin is the most common and tumors could be serous, mucinous, or endometrioid.

Benign serous lesions (cystadenomas) present as anechoic cystic structures, containing clear fluid and thin internal septa. Similar sonographic appearance may have their malignant counterparts (cystadenocarcinomas) (Fig. 37.5).

Mucinous cystadenocarcinoma is usually a large multiloculated cystic mass, with more echogenic internal fluid or fluid-debris levels due to mucus component. Solid mural nodules with increased vascular supply can also be seen. Rupture of these lesions can cause pseudomyxoma peritonei.

The commonest malignant germ cell tumor is dysgerminoma, usually demonstrating as a heterogeneous multilobulated solid mass, with

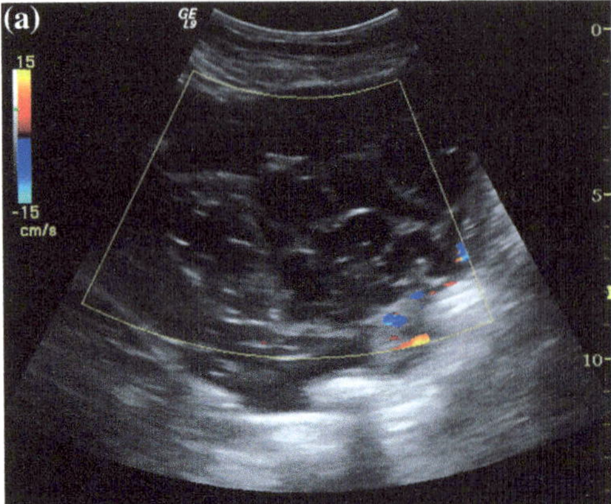

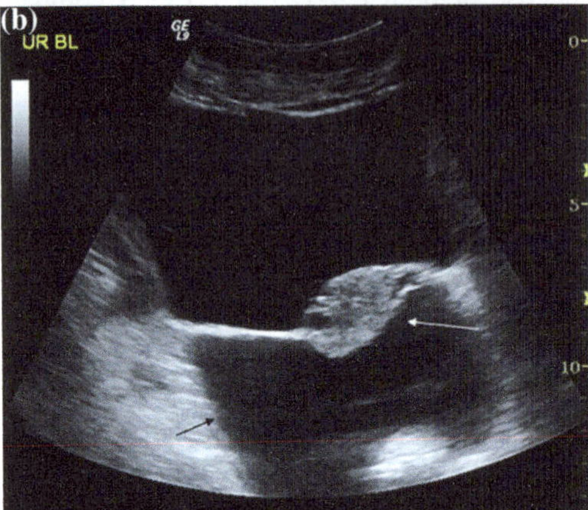

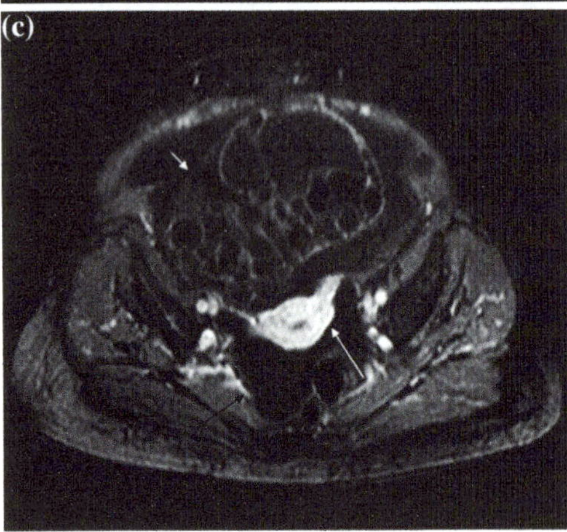

Fig. 37.5 Transabdominal US examination of a 57-year-old patient presenting with abdominal distention. US revealed a quite large multicystic mass with thick internal septa but no significant blood flow (**a**) and **b** a large amount of ascites (*black arrow*). Note the small postmenopausal uterus (*long white arrow in b and c*). **c** Contrast-enhanced T1 MR imaging with fat suppression (SPIR) in axial plane confirmed the presence of a right ovarian mass(*small white arrow*) and ascites (*black arrow*). Surgicopathological examination was consistent with a borderline malignant cystadenoneoplasm

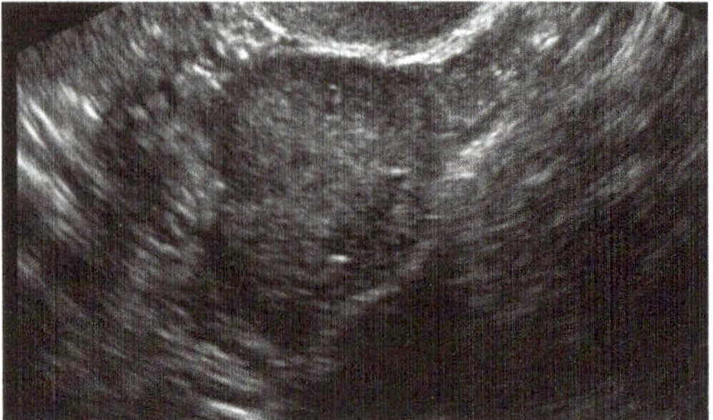

Fig. 37.6 TVUS image shows a diffusely enlarged right ovary in a 70-year-old patient with primary breast cancer. Biopsy confirmed the metastatic nature of the mass

cystic areas consistent with necrosis and with fibrovascular septa showing prominent Doppler blood flow. Malignant teratomas may demonstrate hyperechoic areas suggestive of fat or hemorrhage and large calcifications producing the characteristic posterior acoustic shadow.

Sex-cord tumors originate from ovarian mesenchyma and are hormonally active neoplasms. US findings are not specific and include a solid adnexal mass in most cases.

Finally, ovarian metastases are demonstrated mainly as bilateral solid masses with moderate or high vascularity and in many cases imaging findings overlap with primary ovarian cancer or lymphoma (Fig. 37.6). History of a known primary tumor (like breast, gastric, colon, or lung cancer) or the presence of extensive lymphadenopathy should aid diagnosis.

Exploratory laparotomy is regarded as the gold standard method for the diagnosis and staging of suspected ovarian cancer, according to International Federation of Gynecology and Obstetrics (FIGO) guidelines. Since surgical staging has restrictions in depicting microscopic tumor seedings, preoperative imaging can be very helpful in determining sites of potential dissemination for biopsy during surgery. Also, imaging assessment is helpful to determine the extent of disease and the need for primary cytoreduction or chemotherapy.

Generally, US is used as a complementary tool for cross-sectional modalities in ovarian cancer staging . MRI and CT proved more accurate than US in depicting peritoneal implants, especially those located in subdiaphragmatic and hepatic surfaces. Sensitivity for peritoneal seeding detection is 95 % for MRI, 92 % for CT, and 69 % for US, respectively [16]. Another study states that all three imaging modalities performed high diagnostic accuracy and US performed the highest specificity (96 %) in detecting advanced disease but had the lower sensitivity in staging (75 %). Therefore, even if no peritoneal dissemination or lymphadenopathy is detected at the initial sonographic examination of an ovarian malignancy, CT or MR imaging should be performed because of their higher sensitivity [17].

37.2.2 Fallopian Tube Carcinoma [1, 8]

Primary tubal carcinoma is a very rare tumor and the most common histologic type is papillary serous adenocarcinoma, which is histologically identical to ovarian serous carcinoma. Staging, treatment, and prognosis are similar to ovarian carcinoma. US findings may include a solid or partly solid and cystic adnexal mass, sometimes with tubular (like 'sausage') appearance. Color Doppler can demonstrate vasculature within solid components and spectral analysis reveals low resistance blood flow.

37.3 Lymph Nodes in Uterine Malignancies: US Evaluation [2]

The evaluation of lymph nodes' involvement in patients with gynecological malignancies is crucial for oncologists to determine prognosis and select the appropriate therapeutic treatment. The criteria of both CT and MRI for lymph nodes malignant infiltration are based on nodes size, with the normal minimum diameter (short axis) not exceeding 1 cm. US can estimate with high accuracy the morphology of a lymph node and its vascular pattern and can be useful in distinguishing between inflammation (reactive) and metastatic infiltration of a node.

However, there are technical restrictions in US depiction and assessment of abdominal lymph nodes, mainly due to patient's body shape and the existence of gastrointestinal air, which can degrade imaging quality.

Sonographically, normal lymph nodes have a characteristic bean-like shape with a prominent hyperechogenic hilum and peripheral hypoechoic lymphoid tissue. Normal nodes demonstrate vascularity only in the hilar region or appear avascular. Reactively enlarged lymph nodes have oval shape and distinct hilar vascularity, with radial (branch-like) configurations extending from the hilum. Inflammation results in lipomatous changes in the medulla and this makes the echogenic center to appear larger. These changes combined with the presence of hilar vessels only with longitudinal distribution account for hilum 'fat sign,' which is indicative of benign node changes.

A malignant lymph node is mainly rounded, inhomogeneous, with loss of hilum sign. An early malignant feature is peripheral or mixed (peripheral and central) vascularity, which remains even in the advanced stages of disease. Metastatic nodes from gynecological cancers are usually markedly hypoechoic and signs of necrosis or calcifications may be present. In advanced cases malignant nodes may be demonstrated with irregular margins, capsular disruption, and concomitant extranodular mass.

37.4 Distant Metastasis in Gynecological Malignancies: US Evaluation [2]

US is the initial imaging method for the evaluation of the abdominal organs in oncologic patients, especially for the liver (Fig. 37.7). Hematogenous metastases due to gynecological malignancies, are usually solid and hypoechoic, may contain necrotic areas, or they may be

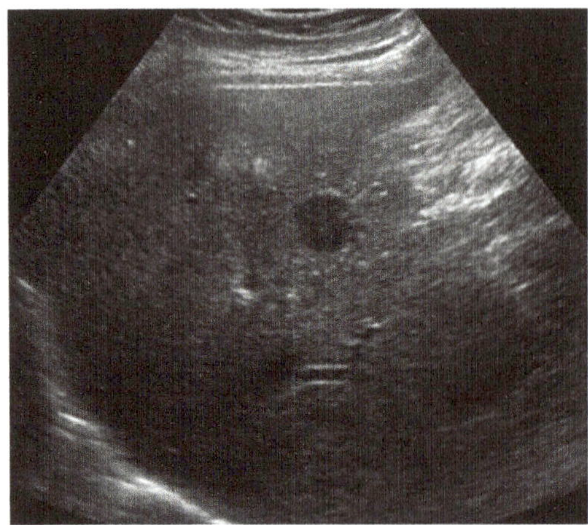

Fig. 37.7 Transabdominal sagittal section of the liver in a patient with biopsy confirmed endometrial carcinoma, shows a hypoechogenic hepatic lesion, highly suspicious for metastasis. CT imaging confirmed the diagnosis

cystic in case of ovarian carcinomas. Note that US usefulness is limited for small (<10 mm) or isoechogenic to the normal parenchyma lesions which can be easily missed. Furthermore, US has limitations in obese and non-compliant patients. Any suspicious lesion in US should be further evaluated with cross-sectional modalities.

Also, the presence of hydronephrosis can be easily and reliably detected and is an important factor in evaluating the extent of uterine and ovarian cancer.

37.5 US Postoperative/Therapeutic Evaluation in Patients with Gynecological Malignancies [11, 18]

US can be helpful in detecting post surgical complications such as free or lobulated fluid collections.

Sonography has a limited role in follow-up of uterine and ovarian cancer and the detection of potential recurrence in asymptomatic patients (Fig. 37.8). Cross-sectional imaging modalities (CT, MRI, PET/CT) perform better than US in depicting residual or recurrent cancerous disease in female pelvis. In daily practice, US is used as a supplementary tool in case of doubtful CT or MRI findings.

37.6 Conclusion

US is the initial imaging method for the evaluation of uterine endometrium and myometrium cancer. Although US findings are not specific for endometrial cancer diagnosis, TVUS has proved quite accurate in estimating endometrial thickness and has a major role in management of postmenopausal patients with vaginal bleeding. Furthermore, it is helpful in detecting other common sources of uterine bleeding.

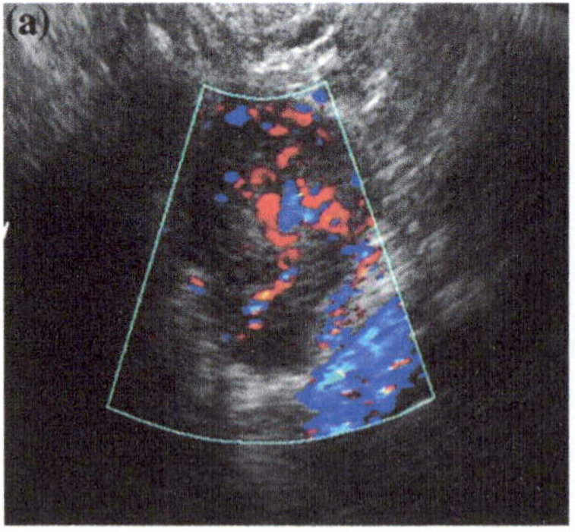

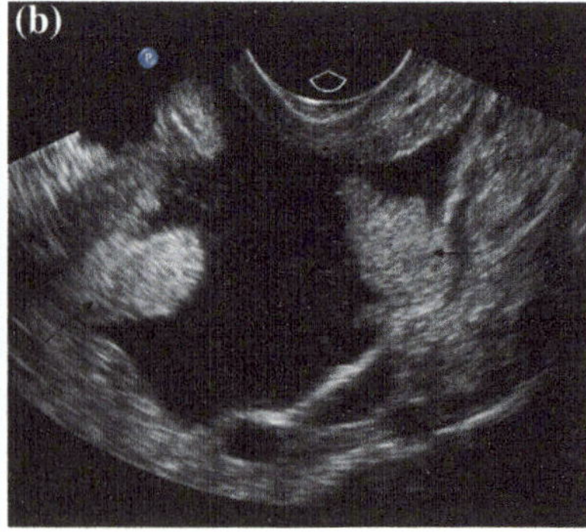

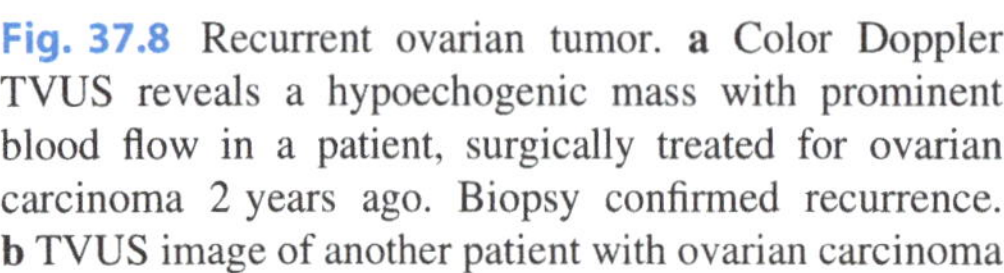

Fig. 37.8 Recurrent ovarian tumor. **a** Color Doppler TVUS reveals a hypoechogenic mass with prominent blood flow in a patient, surgically treated for ovarian carcinoma 2 years ago. Biopsy confirmed recurrence. **b** TVUS image of another patient with ovarian carcinoma relapse, shows multiple peritoneal masses, which are consistent with metastases (*black arrows*). Note the large peritoneal fluid collection with internal echoes, which proved to be hemoperitoneum

Sonography is very useful in depicting adnexal lesions and predicting their benign or malignant nature, but the role of TVUS as a screening method is still controversial. US is also helpful in detecting ascites, liver metastases, or evaluating lymph nodes morphology.

Although US is a safe modality for quick evaluation of female pelvis, it is an imaging study susceptible to diagnostic errors, mostly because it strongly depends on body type and operator's experience. It has restricted utility in evaluating uterine cervix or localizing quite large pelvic masses. Generally, sonography has limited role in staging and follow-up of uterine or adnexal malignant diseases or in detection of potential recurrence, where cross-sectional imaging performs better. The development of modern more sophisticated technologies, like contrast-enhanced or 3D US, may improve diagnostic efficacy in the future.

References

1. Fielding J, Brown D, Thurmond A (2011) Gynecologic imaging. Expert radiology series. Elsevier Saunders, Philadelphia
2. Fischerova D (2011) Ultrasound scanning of the pelvis and abdomen for staging of gynecological tumors: a review. Ultrasound Obstet Gynecol 38:246–266
3. Padilla LA, Radosevich DM, Milad MP (2000) Accuracy of the rectovaginal examination in detecting adnexal masses. Obstet Gynecol 96:593–598
4. Derchi L, Serafini G, Gandolfo N et al (2001) Ultrasound in gynecology. Eur Radiol 11:2137–2155
5. Liu ZZ, Jiang YX, Qing D et al (2011) Imaging in endometrial carcinoma using contrast-enhanced sonography. J Ultrasound Med 30(11):1519–1527
6. Rumack C, Wilson S, Chaborneau JW (1998) Diagnostic ultrasound, vol 1, 2nd edn. Mosby Inc., St.Louis, Missouri
7. Loubeyre P, Navarria I, Undurraga M et al (2012) Is imaging relevant for treatment choice in early stage cervical uterine cancer? Surg Oncol 21:e1–e6
8. Hricak H (2007) Diagnostic imaging. Gynecology. 1st edn. Amirsys Inc., Salt Lake City, Utah
9. Initial Evaluation and Referral Guidelines for Management of Pelvic/ Ovarian Masses (2009) JOGC JULY JUILLET No 230
10. Timmerman D, Testa AC, Bourne T et al (2008) Simple ultrasound-based rules for the diagnosis of ovarian cancer. Ultrasound Obstetrics Gynecol 31(6):681–690
11. Togashi K (2003) Ovarian cancer: the clinical role of US, CT, and MRI. Eur Radiol 13:L87–L104
12. Fleischer A, Lyshchik A, Hirari M et al (2012) Early detection of ovarian cancer and contrast-enhanced transvaginal sonography: recent advances and potential improvements. J Oncol 302858:11
13. Marret H, Sauget S, Giraudeau B et al (2004) Contrast-enhanced sonography helps in discrimination of benign from malignant adnexal masses. JUM 23(12):1629–1639
14. Buys SS, Partridge E, Black A et al (2011) Effect of screening on ovarian cancer mortality: the prostate, lung, colorectal and ovarian (PLCO) cancer screening randomized controlled trial. JAMA 305(22):2295–2303
15. Van Nagel JR, Pavlik EJ (2012) Ovarian cancer screening. Clin Obstet Gynecol 55(1):43–51
16. Tempany CM, Zou KH, Silverman SG et al (2000) Staging of advanced ovarian cancer: comparison of imaging modalities-report from the radiological diagnostic oncology group. Radiology 215:761–767
17. Kurtz AB, Tsimikas JV, Tempany CM et al (1999) Diagnosis and staging of ovarian cancer:comperative values of Doppler and conventional US, CT, and MR imaging correlated with surgery and histopathologic analysis- report from the radiological diagnostic oncology group. Radiology 212:19–27
18. Fehm T, Heller F, Kramer S et al (2005) Evaluation of CA125, physical and radiological findings in follow up of ovarian cancer patients. Anticancer Researce 25:1551–1554

38 CT-MR Findings in Cervical and Endometrial Cancer

Charis I. Bourgioti

It is widely accepted that the use of computed tomography (CT) and particularly of magnetic resonance imaging (MRI) increased in the last few years in the diagnosis, staging, therapy response assessment, and detection of potential recurrence in patients with gynecological malignancies. The aim of this chapter is to review the diagnostic efficacy of these imaging modalities in endometrial and uterine cervical cancer evaluation.

38.1 Endometrial Cancer

Worldwide, endometrial carcinoma staging is based upon International Federation of Gynecology and Obstetrics (FIGO) guidelines. It is a surgicopathological staging system, lately revised in 2009, and is independent of imaging assessment [1]. Differentiation between stages IA and IB is the critical clinical question and alters treatment planning. The estimation of endometrial tumor extension into uterine myometrium and cervix is the key prognostic factor, since the frequency of nodal metastasis is highly associated with myometrial (if tumor involves equal to or more than 50 % of myometrial thickness) and cervical infiltration [2].

Imaging cannot accurately distinguish between endometrial carcinoma and other benign conditions such as endometrial hyperplasia or polypoid lesions. However, it can estimate important prognostic factors in a histologically confirmed carcinoma, including the degree of myometrial and cervical stroma involvement, extrauterine metastases, and lymph nodes status.Preoperative assessment of these factors and especially the evaluation of myometrial infiltration can help clinicians to select candidates for primary lymphadenectomy and avoid unnecessary lymph nodes dissections. Imaging is also helpful in radiotherapy planning, in posttreatment response evaluation, and in clinically suspected cases of recurrence [3].

Although, recent FIGO guidelines do not recommend cross-sectional imaging modalities as routine methods for endometrial cancer staging [2], CT and pretty much MR imaging seem to have an increasing role among various centers in the management of those patients.

38.1.1 CT Evaluation: [3–5]

CT is not sensitive in depicting endometrial uterine cancer, due to low soft tissue contrast, so the evaluation of important morphological prognostic factors of the tumor such as size, myometrial infiltration, or extension to uterine cervix is limited, especially for small

C. I. Bourgioti (✉)
1st Department of Radiology, Aretaieion Hospital, University of Athens Medical School, 76, Vasilissis Sofias Avenue, Athens, 11528, Greece
e-mail: charisbourgioti@yahoo.com

A. D. Gouliamos et al. (eds.), *Imaging in Clinical Oncology*,
DOI: 10.1007/978-88-470-5385-4_38, © Springer-Verlag Italia 2014

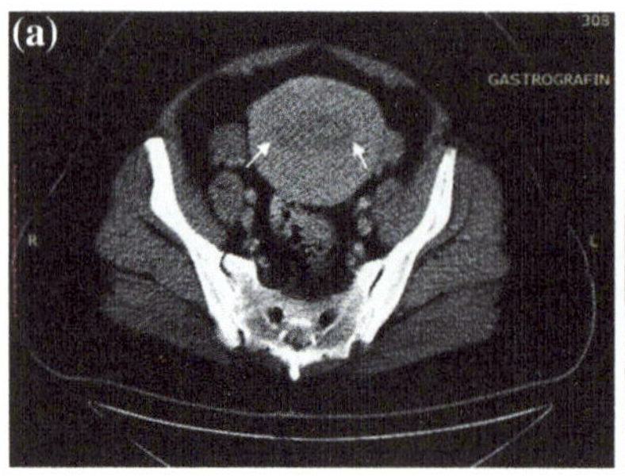

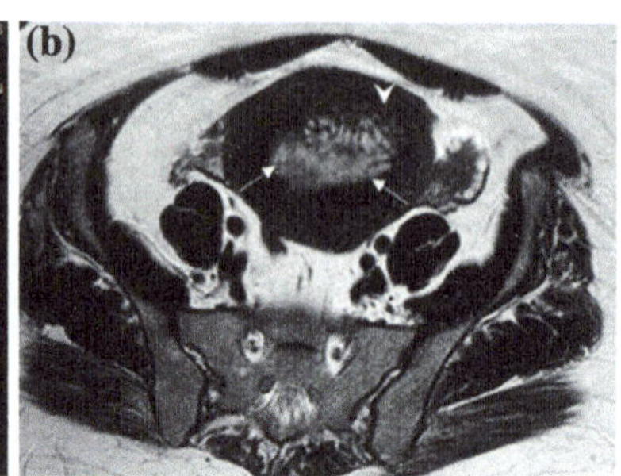

Fig. 38.1 Endometrial cancer, Figo stage IA. **a** Axial CT image with intravenous contrast enhancement reveals an enlarged uterus with a distended hypoattenuating endometrial cavity (*white arrows*). **b** Axial T2-weighted MR imaging of the same patient shows a rather low signal intensity mass expanding the endometrial cavity (*thin white arrows*). Surgicopathological examination was consistent with endometrioid adenocarcinoma. Multiple small high signal intensity foci seen on the left side of uterine fundus proved to be adenomyosis in histological specimen (*arrowhead*). Compared with CT, MR imaging provides better contrast resolution among the different tissues

endometrial carcinomas (Fig. 38.1). CT can be used as an alternative tool for local endometrial cancer staging in patients with contraindication to MR.

For the evaluation of deep myometrial invasion, conventional contrast-enhanced CT presents with sensitivity and specificity of 83 and 42 % respectively [3]. Some studies report CT accuracy for the detection of myometrial invasion from 58 to 61 % versus 69 % for US and 89 % for MRI [4]. The application of multidetector CT to presurgical evaluation of uterine myometrium and cervix in patients with endometrial cancer performed better diagnostic accuracies up to 95 and 81 % respectively [6].

Usually, CT is used to assess extrauterine disease as regional or paraortic lymphadenopathy, peritoneal implants, visceral, or bone metastases. Also CT has an overall accuracy of 92 % in the detection of recurrent endometrial cancer disease [3]. However, the differential diagnosis between recurrent tumor and postsurgical or radiation fibrosis can be quite challenging for the radiologists. The use of chest CT instead of the conventional chest radiography in the initial staging of endometrial malignancy remains controversial, since there is a significant radiation exposure for the patients. Chest CT should be performed in patients with abnormal radiography findings or those with high risk factors [4].

38.1.2 MRI Evaluation [3, 5, 7]

Although ultrasound, and particularly transvaginal ultrasound (TVUS), is the initial diagnostic examination to evaluate endometrium, MRI is the study of choice for endometrial cancer staging because of its excellent soft tissue resolution. Optimal diagnostic MRI protocols should be applied to avoid pitfalls and variability in interpretation.

In general, endometrial carcinoma presents with heterogeneous or low signal intensity compared with the normal endometrium on T2-weighted sequences and with rather high signal intensity compared with normal myometrium. Endometrial cancerous tissue is presented with early contrast enhancement in comparison to normal endometrium but it is enhanced later than surrounding myometrium. The optimal tumor to myometrium contrast is achieved about 50–120 s after intravenous injection. MRI criteria for myometrial invasion include a fully disrupted junctional zone or an irregular endometrium/junctional zone interface at T2-weighted and contrast-enhanced T1-weighted images or interruption of early subendometrial enhancement in dynamic contrast-enhanced sequence.

Pitfalls in endometrial carcinoma evaluation on MRI include cystic atrophy of endometrium, blood clots within endometrial cavity, quite large tumors which cause marked thinning of myometrium, poor contrast resolution between tumor and myometrium, adenomyosis and multiple leiomyomas.

Contrast-enhanced MRI performs better compared to TVUS and CT in estimating the depth of myometrial infiltration and the extension of the tumor within the cervix. In general MRI-staging accuracy values are between 85 and 93 %. Assessment of deep myometrial infiltration by MRI is good, with diagnostic accuracy varying from 83 to 96 %, although negative predictive value seems to be low, ranging between 42.2 and 49.2 % [4]. Frei et al. [8] claim that if MRI results are negative for myometrial involvement, the possibility of this pathology at final histological diagnosis decreases to less than 1 % for grade 1 to 5 % for grade 2, and to 10 % for grade 3 tumors. MR imaging is also reliable in depicting cervical os involvement, with accuracy ranging between 86 and 95 % (Fig. 38.2).

Diffusion weighted imaging (DWI) is a relatively newly established functional MR imaging technique which can be used for the demonstration of uterine malignancies. DWI performs excellently in detection of endometrial carcinoma and apparent diffusion coefficient (ADC) value can potentially detect the difference between normal and pathological tissue of the endometrium. High grade endometrial cancers show decreased ADC measurements unlike to those of lower grade, although characterization of histological grade according to ADC values is not advised because of significant overlap [5]. Also, a recent research [9] demonstrates that DWI has superior diagnostic accuracy in myometrial assessment compared with dynamic contrast-enhanced imaging (90 versus 71 %) and significantly higher staging accuracy in patients with endometrial cancer.

Routine follow-up is mainly recommended in patients with increased risk of recurrence, which usually occurs in vaginal vault or in lymph nodes and less frequently presents with distant metastasis (lung, liver, bone) or peritoneal infiltration. MRI can be useful in differentiating postoperative changes from recurrent disease and can determine the extent of the tumor spread and its surgical resectability. According to later studies, new functional techniques, including DWI and FDG-PET/CT seem to have more impact in detecting suspected recurrence [3].

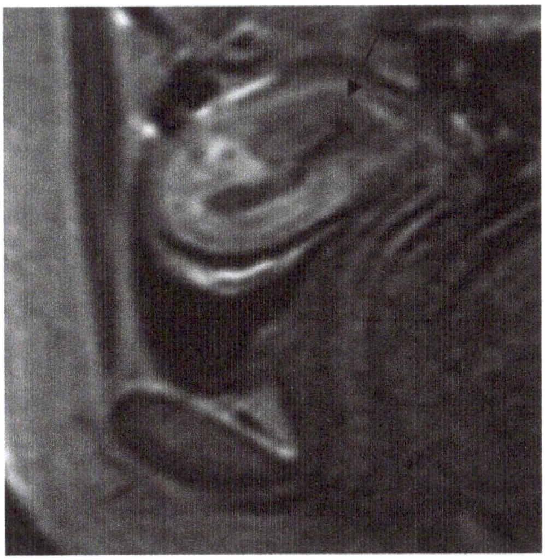

Fig. 38.2 Endometrial cancer, Figo stage II. Sagittal MR study of a patient with biopsy confirmed endometrial adenocarcinoma clearly shows invasion of the upper cervical stroma (*black arrow*)

38.2 Cervical Cancer

Cervical cancer staging is based upon FIGO criteria and it is completely clinical. Late FIGO revision (2009) encouraged the use of cross-sectional imaging (CT/MRI) in cervical cancer staging, where available [10].

Accurate staging of cervical cancer is not only important for patient's prognosis but is also crucial for patient's appropriate therapeutic options. The key point is whether or not the disease extends into the parametrial tissue. The detection of lymph nodes metastasis—although not incorporated in the FIGO staging—has also a significant impact in prognosis and treatment planning. Since cervical cancer has high incidence in young population [5], there is an increasing demand for fertility preserving options—like radical trachelectomy—in cases of non-advanced disease. Accurate estimation of tumor size, measurement of cervical canal length, and assessment of internal os and uterine myometrium are extremely important factors in planning radical trachelectomy surgery [11].

Clinical staging is sometimes inaccurate in estimating important tumor prognostic factors such as size (especially when located in endocervix), parametrial or pelvic side wall involvement, adjacent organs invasion, lymph nodes status, or distant metastasis. Overall, compared with surgery, FIGO staging underestimates the stage in 25–67 % of cases and overestimates the stage in 2 % [3].

MRI is now widely accepted from clinical oncologists as the imaging modality of choice in pretreatment evaluation of patients with cervical carcinoma.

38.2.1 CT Evaluation [3, 5, 12]

CT has inherently low soft tissue contrast, so it has a limited role in local staging of early cervical carcinoma because of the lack of difference between normal cervical parenchyma, tumor, and parametrial tissue (Fig. 38.3). The value of CT seems to increase in more advanced stages of the disease, mostly in assessing distant metastasis (peritoneal implants, abdominal organs, bones) or detecting lymph nodes involvement. Also, CT can be useful in radiotherapy planning and in the evaluation of postsurgical complications.

CT has sensitivity of 32–80 % in overall cervical cancer staging, and a particularly high sensitivity of 92 % in advanced cases of the disease. For parametrial evaluation, CT performs with sensitivity of 17–100 % (mean 64 %) and specificity of 50–100 % (mean 81 %) [12].

A multicentered trial (2007) run by the American College of Radiology Imaging Network (ACRIN) and Gynecologic Oncology Group (GOG) compared MRI and CT methods in patients with early invasive cervical carcinoma. According to this study, the multidetector contrast-enhanced CT was equivalent to MRI for overall preoperative staging, probably because of the low incidence of extra-cervical disease in study patients. CT revealed low sensitivity of 14-38 % andhigh specificity of 84-100 % in detectingadvanced stage cervical cancer, which werecomperable to MRI values [13].

38.2.2 MRI Evaluation [3, 5, 14]

Due to its excellent soft tissue delineation, MRI is considered as the most accurate imaging modality in initial staging of uterine cervical cancer. Since MRI combines high tissue contrast

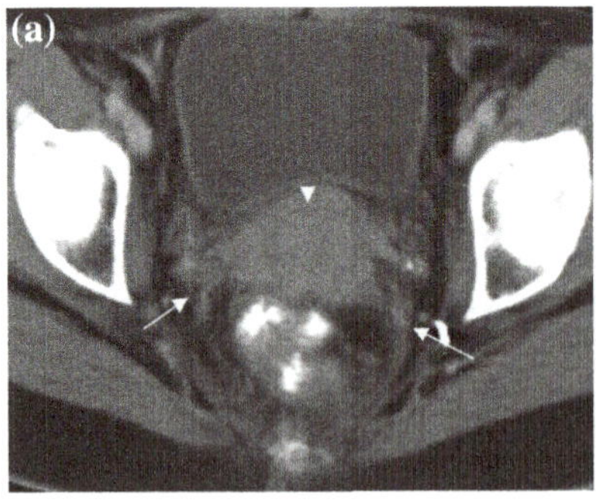

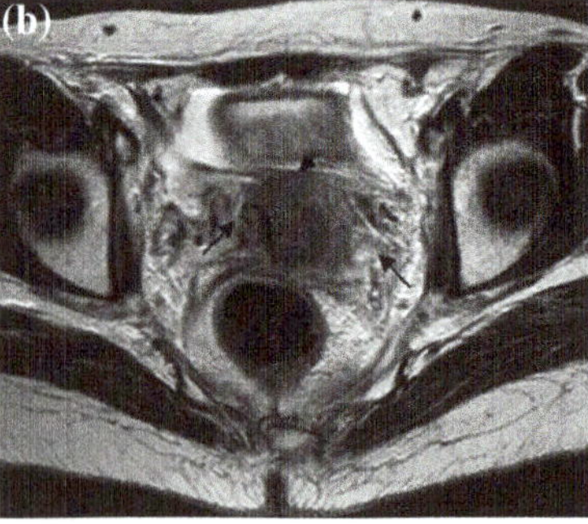

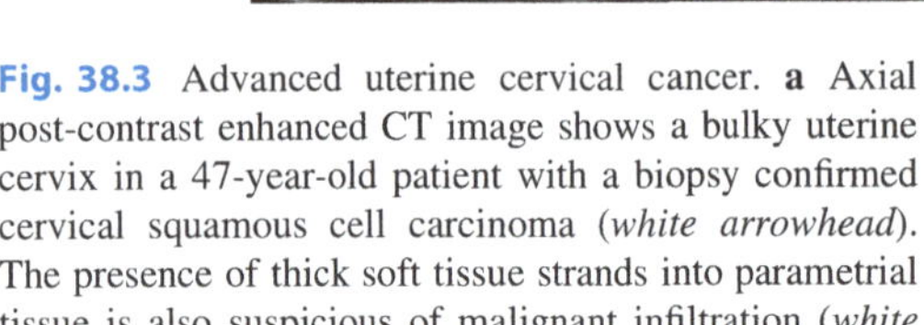

Fig. 38.3 Advanced uterine cervical cancer. **a** Axial post-contrast enhanced CT image shows a bulky uterine cervix in a 47-year-old patient with a biopsy confirmed cervical squamous cell carcinoma (*white arrowhead*). The presence of thick soft tissue strands into parametrial tissue is also suspicious of malignant infiltration (*white arrows*). **b** Axial T2-weighted MR imaging of the same patient demonstrates excellent the large cervical cancerous mass (*small black arrow*), the disruption of low intensity cervical ring, and the bilateral parametrial tissue involvement (*black arrows*). MRI is definitely superior to CT in depiction of uterine cervix pathology

with lack of radiation exposure, it is the imaging modality of choice in evaluating young patient candidates for trachelectomy and pregnant patients. MR imaging can also perform well in planning radiotherapy, evaluating treatment response, or detecting tumor recurrence. Furthermore, it is thought to be a cost-effective method since its use usually rules out the need for further diagnostic or endoscopic procedures.

Microinvasive tumors (Stage IA) are usually not detectable on T2-weighted images, but can be visualized on early arterial dynamic scans as an area of bright enhancement. In Stage IB, disease appears as high or intermediate signal intensity mass compared with the typical low intensity of normal fibrocervical stroma on T2-weighted images. In stage IIA disease, tumor infiltrates the upper two-thirds of vagina with disruption of normal low signal intensity vaginal wall. Parametrial infiltration features (stage IIB) include focal or diffuse loss of the normal hypointensity of the cervical stromal ring, irregular tumor-parametrium borders, extension of a soft tissue mass into parametrium space, or encircling of the periuterine vascular plexus from an abnormal soft tissue lesion (Fig. 38.4). An intact low signal intensity cervical stroma strongly indicates parametrial integrity and this feature is presented with an NPV of 94–100 %. Preservation of normal T2 hypointense signal of vaginal fornices in exophytic cervical tumors is usually suggestive of parametrial preservation. Extension of cervical mass into the lower third of vagina is considered as stage IIIA. Pelvic sidewall infiltration (stage IIIB) is defined as tumor extension to the pelvic muscles or iliac vessels. Thickening of uterosacral ligaments, which form part of the pelvic side wall, should also be evaluated carefully. Findings suggesting adjacent organs invasion (stage IV) are the loss (focal or diffuse) of the typical low signal intensity of bladder or rectal wall, irregular or nodular manifestation of the bladder or rectal muscle surface, intraluminal soft tissue lesions and, less specific, the mucosal thickening of bladder wall (bullous edema) [14].

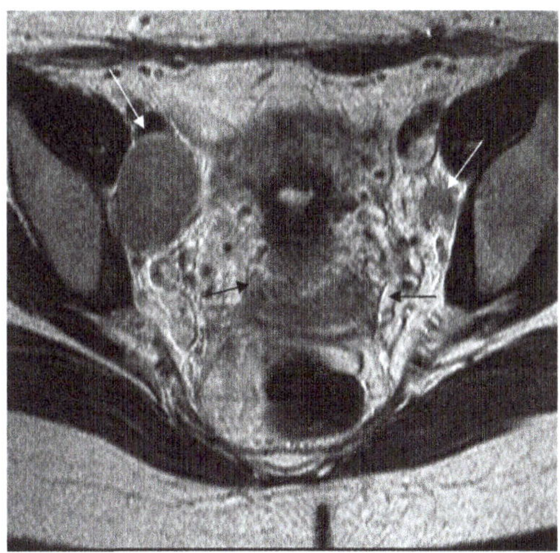

Fig. 38.4 Cervical cancer, Figo stage IIB. T2-weighted image in axial plane reveals a large cervical tumor, extending into parametrial tissues bilaterally. Note the absence of normal low signal intensity cervical ring at the lower cervical segment and the irregular surface between the tumor and the parametrial space (*black arrows*). A quite enlarged obturator lymph node is seen on the right and a smaller one on the left (*white arrows*)

Pitfalls in tumor's size estimation include false-positive results due to inflammatory reaction caused by cone biopsy. Also, superficial tumors may be not depictable due to very small size (<1 cm) or because of the coexistence of multiple nabothian cysts or cervical endometriosis. Adenoma malignum, a subtype of cervical adenocarcinoma, may be easily confused with multiple nabothian cysts, and usually only biopsy can confirmed the lesion's nature. Overestimation of parametrial infiltration can be seen in bulky large tumors, since tumor compression usually coalesce with local inflammation and stromal edema. Motion artifacts, bowel peristalsis, or wrong technical parameter settings can degrade imaging quality and obscure underlying tumor in some cases [14].

Accurate assessment of tumor size is important for patient management, since a lot of centers implement chemotherapy in case of bulky tumors even without parametrial invasion, with a critical value of 4 cm. MR imaging proves to be highly accurate to determine tumor size, with a variation of 5 mm from histological specimen, in 70–90 % of cases [15].

In the published literature, the accuracy of MRI for parametrial evaluation ranges from 88 to 97 %, the sensitivity ranges between 44 and 100 %, and the specificity ranges between 80 and 97 % [3]. MRI has high negative predictive value in parametrial invasion assessment, and can confidently identify suitable candidates for radical surgery. Also, MRI has great sensitivity in depicting vaginal infiltration, which ranges from 86 to 93 %. Internal cervical os is not accessible in clinical examination but it can be reliably assessed by MR imaging especially in young patients, who are candidates for trachelectomy. MRI is presented with extremely high sensitivity (100 %) and specificity (96 %) in internal cervical os evaluation [14]. Note that the extension of tumor beyond internal os and myometrial invasion, although not incorporated in FIGO staging system, is an important prognostic factor, since it increases the probability of nodal metastasis [3].

MRI has shown high sensitivity and specificity in the evaluation of bladder and rectal involvement, ranging from 71 to 100 % and 88 to 91 % respectively. Also, it has an extreme NPV of 100 % in excluding urinary bladder invasion, so there is little need for endoscopic staging procedures [14].

The new high field MRI systems (3T) can increase the signal-to-noise ratio (SNR) compared with the 1.5T MR systems and improve the quality of image although some technical issues can cause limitations. Hori et al. [16] support that 3T MRI in preoperative staging of cervical carcinoma has improved tumor SNR approximately 15 % compared with that of 1.5T but nevertheless, the accuracy was not found to be considerably higher compared to 1.5T imaging [5]. Also, endovaginal MR imaging in combination with DWI in 3T magnet seems to have better results in visualization of microinvasive cervical tumors [17].

New functional techniques like DWI are expected to be important in the evaluation of gynecological malignancies, although additional long-term studies should be performed in the future [5]. Median ADC values in cervical carcinoma are significantly lower compared with normal cervical tissue, and this finding can be helpful in tumor depiction and staging (Fig. 38.5). Also, median ADC values of

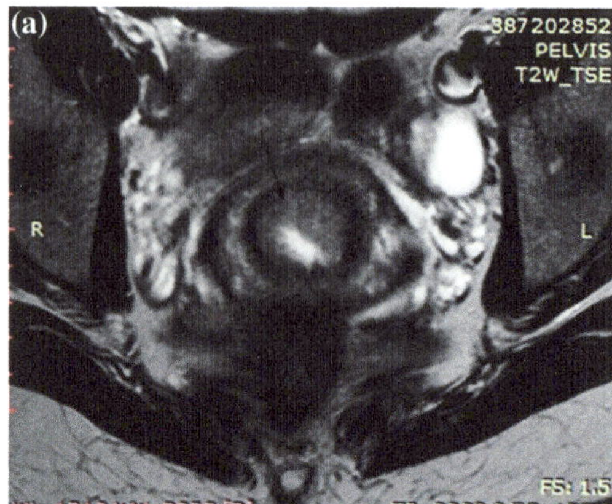

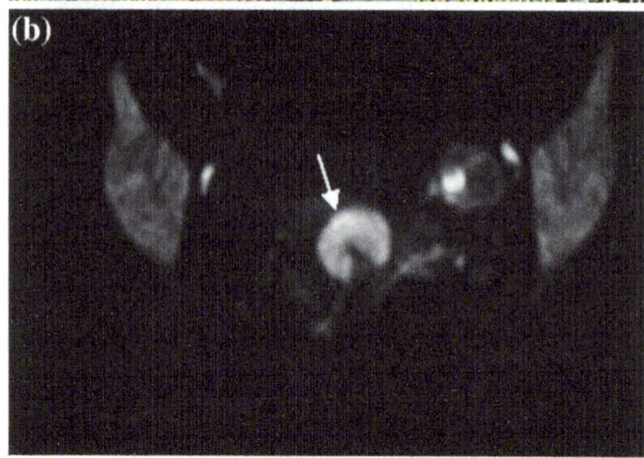

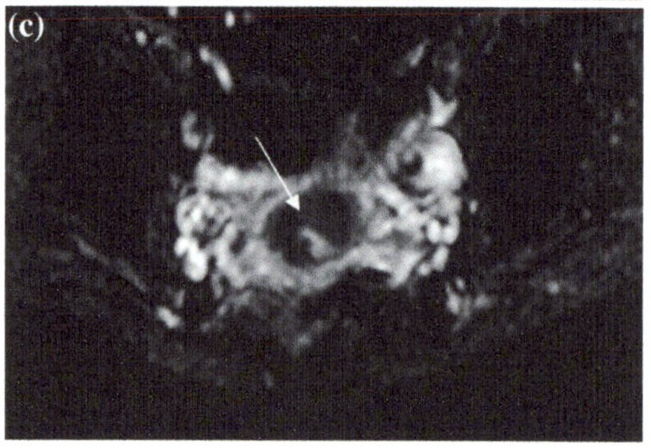

Fig. 38.5 **a** Axial T2-weighted image reveals a low-to intermediate signal intensity exophytic cervical mass (*black arrow*), which proved to be adenosquamous cell cancer in biopsy. **b** The same cervical mass presents with high signal intensity on DW image (b = 1,000) and **c** with marked low intensity on ADC map, findings indicative of restricted diffusion (*white arrow*). Note the excellent delineation of tumor margins in DWI/ADC images

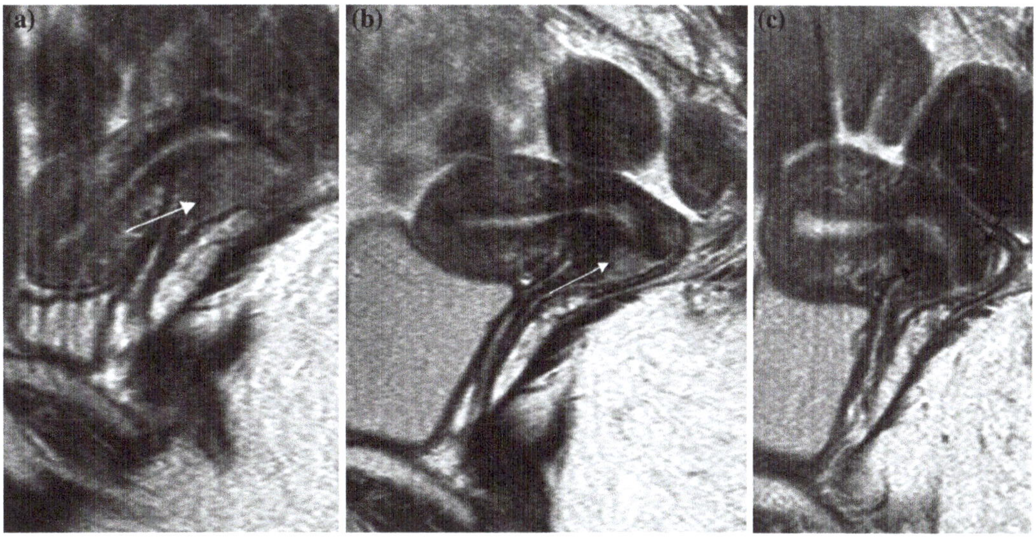

Fig. 38.6 Advanced cervical carcinoma fully responded to radiotherapy. T2-weighted images in sagittal plane of the same patient. **a** before **b** two months and **c** six months after brachytherapy and external irradiation treatment. Note (*white arrow*) the decrease of tumor size (more than 50 %) in image (**b**) and the complete remission of cervical mass in image (**c**). Complete restitution of low signal intensity cervical stroma (*black arrows* **c**) is a reliable sign of successful response to radiotherapy

cervical cancer seem to be highly increased after radiotherapy or chemotherapy, and this can be used to evaluate the response to treatment [5]. Lin et al. [18] state that the use of DWI/ADC has performed accuracy of 85 % in the differentiation between cervical adenocarcinomas and endometrial carcinomas, since the previous ones have significantly higher ADC values.

Complete restitution of normal cervical anatomy and of low signal intensity of cervical stroma in T2-weighted images (Fig. 38.6) is a reliable sign of successful response to radiotherapy with a negative predictive value more than 95 % [19]. Recurrence usually occurs within the pelvis, especially in vaginal vault. T2-weighted images are highly sensitive (90 %) in depiction of a high signal soft tissue cancerous mass but referred with low specificity (22–38 %) and accuracy (68 %). Especially for the first 6 months after treatment, differentiation between residual disease and inflammation/edema due to postsurgical or radiation fibrosis is rather difficult. Usually, a serial imaging or even imaging guided biopsies may be required to confirm diagnosis. Dynamic contrast-enhanced sequences improve specificity (67 %) and accuracy (83 %), although new functional imaging modalities (FDG-PET/CT, DWI) reported to be more sensitive and accurate in detecting recurrent disease [3].

38.3 Lymph Nodes Evaluation in Endometrial and Cervical Cancer

Surgical assessment of lymph nodes is the gold method for the confirmation of nodal metastasis, but it is related to an increased risk of complications. Alternatively, noninvasive cross-sectional modalities can be used for lymph nodes evaluation.

The diagnosis of nodal metastasis on cross-sectional images is based, almost exclusively, on size criteria, with a nodal short axis diameter of 1 cm or less to be considered as normal. Therefore, both CT and MRI are inaccurate in detecting microscopic nodal invasion and cannot differentiate between inflammatory (reactive) lymph node enlargement or enlargement due to malignant involvement.

Note that the presence of nodal central necrosis, which is demonstrated as a hypoattenuating area in CT images or an area of T2 high signal intensity in MR images, is considered pathognomonic for lymph node metastatic infiltration, with PPV of 100 % [3]. Sometimes, it is possible for a necrotic lymph node to be misinterpretated as a normal ovarian tissue with cystic follicles, and radiologists should be aware to avoid such pitfall [5]. Also, malignant nodal features include round shaped, spiculated nodal margins or extranodal mass.

CT assessment of pelvic and paraortic lymphadenopathy in endometrial cancer presents with sensitivity and specificity of 52 and 92 % respectively [4]. MRI assessment of lymph nodes status is equivalent to CT with sensitivity values between 44 and 66 % and specificity values between 73 and 98 % [3].

In patients with uterine cervical carcinoma, CT and MRI have similar sensitivity and specificity in lymph nodes assessment. CT performed sensitivity between 31 and 65 % and NPV between 86 and 96 % in malignant lymph nodes evaluation [13]. Also, MRI presents with a low sensitivity (43–73 %) but relatively high accuracy (86–90 %) in lymph nodes evaluation.

DWI demonstrates higher sensitivity than conventional MRI in lymph nodes detection. The application of DWI for the distinction between malignant and non-malignant lymph nodes may be promising in the future, but current results remain controversial [5]. The use of special contrast agents like USPIO (ultra small super paramagnetic iron oxide contrast agent) seems to increase diagnostic performance, although their use is limited in clinical practice [3].

38.4 Conclusion

MR imaging is an excellent noninvasive modality, which complements clinical examination in localizing and staging endometrial and cervical cancer. It performs high accuracy in differentiating between FIGO stage IA and stage IB endometrial cancer, and between early (FIGO $<$ IIB) and advanced (FIGO $\geq$ IIB) cervical carcinoma. Also, it is an excellent modality for the evaluation of young patients who want to preserve their fertility and for pregnant patients. Therefore, MRI is a useful tool for gynecologists for selecting surgical candidates and planning the optimal surgical procedure. Although, MRI study is not officially incorporated into the FIGO classification system, the revised FIGO criteria (2009) encourage MRI use for the assessment of cervical cancer, where available. Knowledge of potential pitfalls and optimization of MR imaging protocols may limit diagnostic errors in the future. CT can be used as an alternative imaging modality in endometrial and cervical cancer staging, mostly for the evaluation of extrauterine disease.

References

1. Creasman W (2009) Revised FIGO staging for carcinoma of the endometrium. Int J Gynaecol Obstet 105(2):109
2. Amant F, Moerman P, Timmerman D et al (2005) Endometrial cancer. Lancet 366(9484):491–505
3. Patel S, Liyanage S, Sahdev A et al (2010) Imaging of endometrial and cervical cancer. Insights Imaging I:309–328
4. Lee HJ, Dubinsky T, Andreotti R et al (2011) ACR appropriateness criteria preatreatment evaluation and follow-up of endometrial cancer of the uterus. Ultrasound Q 27:139–145
5. Fielding J, Brown D, Thurmond A (2011) Gynecologic imaging. Expert radiology series. Elsevier Saunders, Philadelphia
6. Tsili AC, Tsampoulas C, Dalkalitsis N et al (2008) Local staging of endometrial carcinoma: role of multidetector CT. Eur Radiol 18(5) :1043–8
7. Kinkel K, Forstner R, Danza FM et al (2009) Staging of endometrial cancer with MRI: guidelines of European society of urogenital imaging. Eur Radiol 19:1565–1574
8. Frei KA, Kinkel K (2001) Staging endometrial cancer: role of magnetic resonance imaging. J Magn Reson Imaging 13(6):850–855
9. Beddy P, Moyle P, Kataoka M et al (2012) Evaluation of depth of myometrial invasion and overall staging in endometrial cancer: comparison of diffusion-weighted and dynamic contrast-enhanced MR imaging. Radiology 262(2):530–537

10. Pecorelli S, Zigliani L, Odicino F (2009) Revised FIGO staging for carcinoma of the cervix. Int J Gynaecol Obstet 105(2):107–108
11. Plante M, Roy M (2006) Fertility preserving options in cervical cancer. Oncology 20:479
12. Ozsarlak O, Tjalma W, Schepens E et al (2003) The correlation of preoperative CT, MR Imaging and clinical staging (FIGO) with histopathology findings in primary cervical carcinoma. Eur Radiol 13:2338–2345
13. Hricak H, Gatsonis C, Coakley F et al (2007) Early invasive cervical cancer: CT and MR imaging in preoperative evaluation-ACRIN/GOG comperative study of diagnostic performance and interobserver variability. Radiology 245:491–498
14. Sala E, Wakely S, Senior E et al (2007) MRI of malignant neoplasms of the uterine corpus and cervix. AJR 188:1577–1587
15. Mitchell DG, Snyder B, Coakley F et al (2006) Early invasive cervical cancer: tumor delineation by magnetic resonance imaging, computed tomography, and clinical examination, verified by pathologic results, in the ACRIN 6651/GOG 183 intergroup study. J Clin Onc 24(36):5687–5694
16. Hori M, Kim T, Murakami T et al (2009) Uterine cervical carcinoma: preoperative staging with 3.0-T MR imaging- comparison with 1.5-T MR imaging. Radiology 251:96–104
17. Charles-Edwards EM, Messiou C, Morgan VA et al (2008) Diffusion-weighted imaging in cervical cancer with an endovaginal technique: potential value for improving tumour detection in stage Ia and Ib1 disease. Radiology 249:541–550
18. Lin YC, Lin G, Chen YR et al (2011) Role of magnetic resonsnce imaging and apparent diffusion coefficient at 3T in distiguishing between adenocarcinoma of the uterine cervix and endometrium. Chang Gung Med J 34:93–100
19. Zand KR, Reinhold C, Abe H et al (2007) Magnetic resonance imaging of the cervix. Cancer Imaging 7:69–76

CT-MR Findings in Ovarian Cancer

39

Dimitra G. Loggitsi

39.1 Introduction

Ovarian cancer accounts for 4 % of all female cancers worldwide. Since the majority of patients will have advanced disease at time of presentation (stage III and IV), the most important determinant of survival for ovarian cancer patients is the disease stage at diagnosis and maximum residual disease after cytoreductive surgery. Cross-sectional imaging provides staging information which can assist in surgical planning and in selection of treatment options.

39.2 Indications-Imaging Findings

If ultrasound (US) is technically limited or findings are indeterminate (in up to 20 % of patients), further imaging characterization is required. Computed tomography (CT) is not routinely used as the first approach for the evaluation of adnexal mass lesions due to the poor soft tissue discrimination compared to magnetic resonance imaging (MRI). MRI on the other hand has been proven to be superior compared to other imaging modalities for the characterization of ovarian tumors especially when gadolinium injection is performed, and facilitates differentiation between adnexal and uterine origin masses.

MRI can exclude typical benign ovarian tumors which may have a complex appearance in US such as endometriomas, dermoids, and uterine fibromas, based on the recognition of blood products, lipid contents, and fibrous tissue, respectively.

Primary MR imaging features suggestive of malignancy are (a) ovarian mass size greater then 5 cm, (b) bilateral masses, (c) papillary projections (vegetations), (d) cystic lesion with irregular thickening of wall or septal thickness greater than 3 mm, (e) partially cystic and partially solid mass, and (f) predominantly solid masses or necrosis within a solid mass.

Serous tumors are usually unilocular cystic masses, while mucinous tumors commonly present as multilocular cystic tumors. Papillary projections can protrude either inside the cystic mass (Fig. 39.1) or on its surface, and are markedly enhanced on contrast-enhanced images in both CT and MRI. Stained-glass appearances and daughter cysts are well-known imaging findings of mucinous tumors (Fig. 39.2).

Dynamic contrast-enhanced MRI (DCE-MRI) can be used to distinguish benign, borderline, and invasive ovarian tumors by their distinct enhancement patterns. The maximal slope of dynamic enhancement was found to be steeper for invasive tumors than for benign and borderline tumors [1].

Secondary features of malignancy include ascites, peritoneal/mesenteric/omental disease, and lymphadenopathy.

D. G. Loggitsi (✉)
CT/MRI Department, Mitera Hospital, 6, Erythrou Stavrou, 15123 Marousi, Athens, Greece
e-mail: loggitsi@med.uoa.gr

A. D. Gouliamos et al. (eds.), *Imaging in Clinical Oncology*,
DOI: 10.1007/978-88-470-5385-4_39, © Springer-Verlag Italia 2014

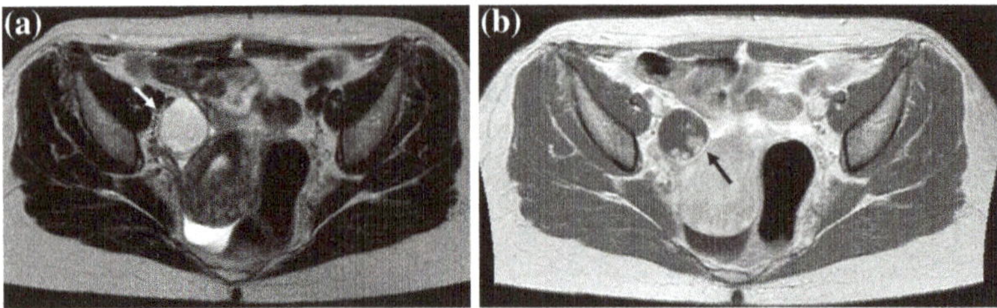

Fig. 39.1 Adnexal mass on MRI with malignant characteristics. **a** T2 weighted image shows a cystic lesion arising from the right ovary (*arrow*) with subtle focal thickening on its posterior wall. **b** Axial T1 weighted image post-gadolinium reveals multiple solid papillary mural nodules (*arrow*). The mass was proven to be a serous cystadenocarcinoma

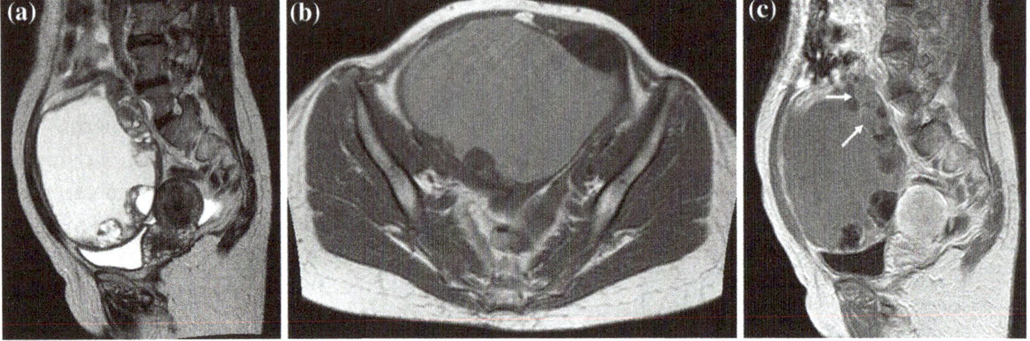

Fig. 39.2 A 49-year-old woman with a pelvic mass. **a** Sagittal T2 weighted image demonstrates a large complex mass with extensive cystic and smaller solid components. **b** Axial T1 weighted image shows the different signal intensities between the locules, which gives a "murano glass effect" suggestive of a mucinous tumor. **c** Sagittal T1 weighted image post-gadolinium shows the enhancing solid components (*arrows*). Final histology confirmed a grade II mucinous cystadenocarcinoma

39.3 Staging

Ovarian cancer is most commonly staged using the International Federation of Gynecology and Obstetrics (FIGO) surgical-pathological staging system. A Tumor, Nodes, Metastasis (TNM) classification has also been defined by the American Joint Committee on Cancer (AJCC). The definitions of the T stage categories correspond to several stages accepted by FIGO. Stages I and II are considered early disease, with the tumor confined to the ovaries (stage I) or pelvis (stage II). Stages III and IV are advanced disease, with the tumor limited to the abdomen (stage III) or extending beyond the abdomen, or with parenchymal liver metastases (stage IV).

CT is the imaging modality of choice for noninvasive staging and follow-up in ovarian cancer because it is quick, widely available, and reproducible. The reported accuracy for all stages ranges from 70 to 90 % [2].

In order of decreasing frequency, ovarian carcinoma spreads via locoregional extension, peritoneal, and lymphatic pathways, and hematogenously. The fat planes surrounding the primary tumor should be carefully evaluated for the detection of local tumor spread. Local dissemination involves the adnexal structures, the uterus, the contralateral ovary, the muscular pelvic sidewalls, the pelvic side wall vessels, the rectosigmoid colon, and the bladder. A distance <3 mm between tumor and pelvic side wall indicates pelvic side wall invasion. Distortion or encasement of the iliac vessels and obliteration of the fat plane by the solid component of an ovarian mass in relation with the rectosigmoid colon and the bladder wall should be assessed. Local disease extent is more accurately delineated by MRI than CT due to greater tissue contrast with MRI [3].

Peritoneal seeding is found in approximately 70 % at initial diagnosis and is the most common pathway of dissemination in ovarian cancer as tumor cells are distributed within the normal circulation of peritoneal fluid around the abdomen and pelvis. Large volumes of ascites usually indicate peritoneal metastases even if cytology from the ascetic fluid is negative. The commonest sites of peritoneal deposits are the greater omentum, paracolic gutters, pouch of Douglas, liver, diaphragmatic, and bowel surfaces. There is a preferential flow along the right paracolic gutter and hence the right side of the peritoneum and diaphragm. Peritoneal metastases may have a variable appearance from nodular soft tissue lesions to linear or plaque-like thickening of the parietal or visceral peritoneum. Tiny calcified peritoneal deposits can be easily detected by CT. Omental disease may have a fine reticular pattern appearance, focal nodular thickening or extensive thickening, the so-called "omental cake" (Fig. 39.3). The detection of peritoneal implants depends on location, presence of ascites, and implant size. The overall sensitivity of gadolinium-enhanced MRI in depicting peritoneal disease is found to be equal to CT (95 and 92 %, respectively) when peritoneal implants larger than 2 cm in diameter are encountered [4]. Sensitivity significantly decreases to 7–28 % for both modalities though, when the maximal diameter of the deposits is <1 cm. MRI may be advantageous in the detection of small implants with the administration of oral contrast media for the opacification of the gastrointestinal tract; however, the high cost and lengthy scan duration have prevented the wide acceptance of MRI as a staging modality for ovarian cancer. Diffusion-weighted imaging (DWI) can reveal foci of omental and serosal disease of the order of 5 mm, even in complex anatomic locations such as the right subdiaphragmatic space, omentum, root of mesentery, and serosal surface of the mesentery. Malignant deposits retain high signal with increasing b-values, whereas signal in normal adjacent structures including mesenteric fat, bowel loops, and ascites, is strongly suppressed [5].

Lymph node involvement primarily follows the ovarian vessels to the upper common iliac and para aortic lymph nodes. A secondary lymphatic spread is along the broad ligament and parametria to the external and iliac obturator nodes and rarely, drainage to the external iliac and inguinal nodes via the round ligament is seen. Recognizing the location of metastatic nodes is particularly important for direct selective nodal dissection in the subcohort of patients with exclusively nodal stage IIIC disease. With a threshold of 1 cm diameter in short axis, CT and MRI are both problematic in detecting metastases in smaller lymph nodes and in discriminating hyperplastic lymph nodes from metastases. CT and MRI have similar diagnostic performance for detecting metastatic lymph nodes [6] with a suboptimal sensitivity of 30 %. New lymph node-specific contrast media in MRI have shown promising results in other gynecologic cancers but are no longer available for routine clinical use. However, when DWI-MRI is combined with conventional anatomic imaging, detection of nodal metastases increases between 17 and 21 % [7]. Malignant lymph nodes have restricted diffusion with signal intensity similar to that of the primary tumor or other metastatic sites on high b-value images.

Hematogenous spread is a late occurrence representing stage IV ovarian cancer. Stage IV is defined by seeding to abdominal solid organs such as the liver, spleen, kidneys, and adrenals, or outside the abdominal cavity with the most common manifestation being malignant pleural effusion, followed by lung parenchymal, brain, and bone disease. Special attention should be given when assessing liver lesions. Liver parenchymal metastases (stage IV) are very rare at the time of the initial diagnosis and have indistinct margins and an infiltrative appearance. Liver surface metastases on the other hand are a

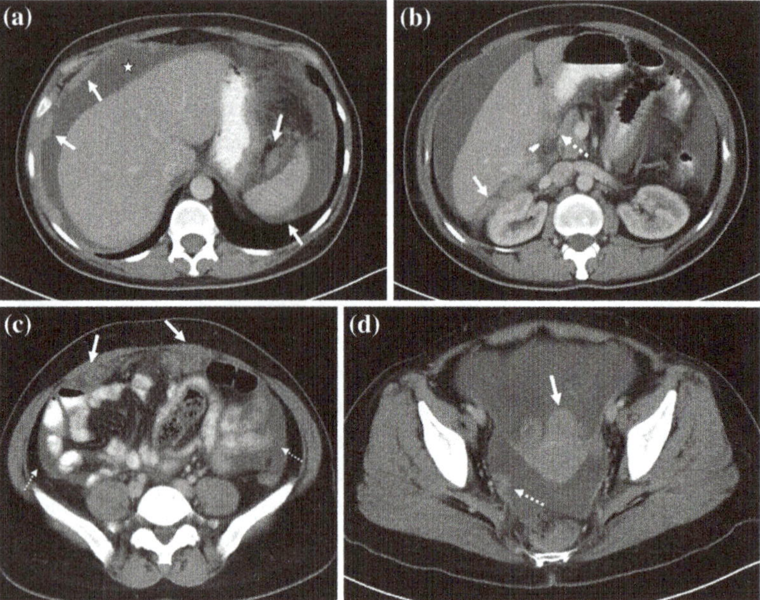

Fig. 39.3 Abdominal peritoneal metastases in various patients with stage III ovarian cancer. **a** Peritoneal implants along the diaphragm and in the gastrosplenic fossa (*arrows*) well visualized due to ascites (*star*). **b** Peritoneal implants in the hepatorenal fossa (*arrow*) and the hepatic hilum (*dashed arrow*), along with ascites. **c** Plaque-like thickening of the omentum (omental cake) between abdominal wall and bowel loops (*arrows*) and a small amount of ascites in both paracolic gutters (*thin dashed arrows*). **d** Solid masses in the cul-de-sac (*arrow*) and nodular peritoneal metastases in the pelvis (*thin dashed arrow*)

typical feature of stage III disease. They are smooth, crescent shaped, and may cause scalloping of the liver surface. Differentiation of the above liver lesions influences the surgical management.

Follow up after primary therapy in ovarian cancer is poorly defined as there is no routine post-operative imaging protocol. Clinical findings from the bimanual pelvic examination or serial increases in the serum levels of tumor marker CA-125 should alert imaging to identify the site of recurrence and assess a patient's suitability for secondary surgical cytoreduction. It is important to consider the anatomic sites of relapse in order to early detect recurrent ovarian cancer. The commonest sites of relapse are with a pelvic mass (48 %), peritoneal disease-diffuse carcinomatosis (45 %), large or small bowel serosal disease (45 %), and nodal disease (33 %) most commonly in the para aortic region [8]. The imaging study of choice to assess recurrence is usually CT scan. MRI is reserved as a problem-solving technique for the evaluation of suspicious lesions in the vaginal vault, the cul-de-sac, and the bladder base. Vaginal apex nodularity can be easily missed by CT scans and multiplanar reconstructions should always be performed. Hydronephrosis and pelvic side wall invasion are predictors of nonresectability. CT scan and MRI are generally unable to detect peritoneal disease less that 1–2 cm. DWI may be useful for characterizing postsurgical findings, with high ADC values being more likely to represent areas of edema or inflammation and low ADC values being suggestive of the presence of active tumor cells.

39.4 Conclusion

Cross-sectional imaging has an invaluable role in the preoperative surgical and management planning in patients with ovarian cancer. Contrast-enhanced CT is the imaging modality of choice for preoperative staging and detection of recurrence because it provides all the required information in a short examination time and is widely available and reproducible. MRI is a problem-solving tool in the characterization of the origin and morphologic features of indeterminate ovarian masses and is particularly useful for local staging. DWI seems a new promising technique for the depiction of peritoneal metastases, when combined with conventional imaging [9].

References

1. Thomassin-Naggara I, Bazot M, Daraï E, Callard P, Thomassin J, Cuenod CA (2008) Epithelial ovarian tumors: value of dynamic contrast-enhanced MR imaging and correlation with tumor angiogenesis. Radiology 248:148–159
2. Moyle P, Addley HC, Sala E (2010) Radiological staging of ovarian carcinoma. Semin Ultrasound CT MRI 31:388–398
3. Forstner R (2007) Radiological staging of ovarian cancer: imaging findings and contribution of CT and MRI. Eur Radiol 17:3223–3246
4. Tempany CM, Zou KH, Silverman SG et al (2000) Staging of advanced ovarian cancer: comparison of imaging modalities—report from the radiology oncology group. Radiology 215:761–767
5. Kyriazi S, Kaye SB, DeSouza NM (2010) Imaging ovarian cancer and peritoneal metastases—current and emerging techniques. Nat Rev Clin Oncol 7(7):381–393
6. Yuana Y, Gub ZX, Taoa XF, Liua SY (2012) Computer tomography, magnetic resonance imaging, and positron emission tomography or positron emission tomography/computer tomography for detection of metastatic lymph nodes in patients with ovarian cancer: a meta-analysis. Eur J Radiol 81:1002–1006
7. Low RN, Gurney J (2007) Diffusion-weighted MRI (DWI) in the oncology patient: value of breathhold DWI compared to unenhanced and gadolinium-enhanced MRI. J Magn Reson Imaging 25(4):848–858
8. Bharwani N, Reznek RH, Rockall AG (2011) Ovarian cancer management: the role of imaging and diagnostic challenges. Eur J Radiol 78(2011):41–51
9. Forstner R, Sala E, Kinkel K, Spencer JA (2010) ESUR guidelines: ovarian cancer staging and follow-up. Eur Radiol 20:2773–2780

40 PET/CT with [^{18}F]FDG in Cervical Cancer

Evangelia V. Skoura and Ioannis E. Datseris

40.1 Initial Diagnosis and Prognosis

Imaging with [^{18}F]FDG-PET/CT is not routinely used for the initial diagnosis of cervical cancer although the primary tumor is generally [^{18}F]FDG avid, because of the lack of precise anatomic information which limits its clinical utility.

[^{18}F]FDG uptake of the primary cervical tumor, as measured by SUVmax, provides valuable prognostic information for predicting lymph node involvement, treatment response, and overall survival. Although there is no standard SUVmax cut-off value defining the prognosis in patients with cervical cancer, cervical tumors with a higher SUVmax are more likely to be poorly differentiated and have an increased risk of lymph node involvement. Median preoperative SUVmax values in the primary tumours were significantly higher in patients with higher FIGO stages ($p = 0.0149$), pelvic lymph node metastasis ($p = 0.0068$), parametrial involvement ($p = 0.0002$), large (>4 cm) tumour size ($p = 0.0022$), presence of lymphovascular space invasion ($p = 0.0055$), and deep cervical stromal invasion ($p < 0.0001$) [1].

E. V. Skoura · I. E. Datseris (✉)
Nuclear Medicine Department, Evangelismos General Hospital, Ipsilantou 45–47, 10676 Athens, Greece
e-mail: datseris@otenet.gr

E. V. Skoura
e-mail: lskoura@yahoo.gr

40.2 Initial Staging

Most primary tumors over 1 cm are easily detectable with [^{18}F]FDG-PET/CT but due to the relatively poor spatial resolution of this modality, it is not considered suitable for T staging. However, [^{18}F]FDG-PET/CT is quite helpful in delineating the margins in cases that an invasive tumor extents superiorly into the uterine cavity and inferiorly into the vaginal cuffs.

[^{18}F]FDG-PET/CT has an important role in staging cervical cancer and it aids particularly in identifying the involvement of lymph nodes and distant metastases. Although the assessment of lymph nodes is not a part of the FIGO staging, it is generally performed during the initial workup of patients with cervical cancer as an important component of treatment planning, since the survival rates for patients with nodal metastases are significantly lower than those without. Recently, PET/CT scan has been increasingly used for staging work up [2–4]. [^{18}F]FDG-PET/CT shows a significant benefit to assess the metabolic activities of the tumor, especially for distant metastases, taking advantage from the whole body cross-sectional images. [^{18}F]FDG-PET/CT demonstrates a specific benefit to assess the pelvic and paraaortic lymph node involvement with equivocal size and morphology on CT or MRI.

In studies where [^{18}F]FDG-PET/CT was evaluated in patients with negative CT/MR, the sensitivity and specificity of [^{18}F]FDG-PET/CT

A. D. Gouliamos et al. (eds.), *Imaging in Clinical Oncology*,
DOI: 10.1007/978-88-470-5385-4_40, © Springer-Verlag Italia 2014

for detection of metastases have been found 83.3–85.7 % and 94.4–96.7 %, respectively [5, 6]. In recent meta-analyses, [^{18}F]FDG-PET or [^{18}F]FDG-PET/CT showed the highest pooled sensitivity (79–84 %) and specificity (95–99 %), compared with 47–50 % and 92–97 %, respectively, for CT and 56–72 % and 90–96 %, respectively, for MR imaging [7–12]. [^{18}F]FDG-PET/CT positivity for lymph node metastases correlates well with survival and is highly predictive of progression-free survival. A multivariate analysis demonstrated that the most significant prognostic factor for progression-free survival was the presence of positive para-aortic lymph nodes as detected by PET imaging ($p = 0.025$) [8] Concerning para-aortal nodal disease [^{18}F]FDG-PET/CT demonstrated a sensitivity of 100 % and specificity of 99 % despite another study that demonstrated lower values (50 and 83.3 %, respectively [13, 14].

According to American College of Radiology appropriateness criteria, [^{18}F]FDG-PET/CT with concurrent abdomino-pelvic CT is considered highly appropriate in assessing nodal disease at stage II or higher and in patients with suspected tumor recurrence [15]. Also, for detecting distant metastases [^{18}F]FDG-PET/CT demonstrated a sensitivity of 100 %, and specificity 94 % [14].

40.3 Radiotherapy Planning

[^{18}F]FDG-PET/CT has been shown to impact external-beam radiotherapy planning by modifying the treatment field and customizing the radiation dose. This particularly applies to detection of previously uncovered para-aortic and inguinal nodal metastases.

[^{18}F]FDG-PET/CT-based brachytherapy optimization allows improved tumor-volume dose distribution and detailed 3D dosimetric evaluation of risk organs.

Furthermore, [^{18}F]FDG-PET/CT guided intensity-modulated radiation therapy (IMRT) allows delivery of higher doses of radiation to the primary tumor and to grossly involved nodal disease while minimizing treatment-related toxicity. IMRT use in cervical cancer has been demonstrated to produce equivalent or better results [16].

40.4 Restaging After Treatment

The current literature supports the use of [^{18}F]FDG-PET/CT for evaluating response after chemoradiation for locally advanced carcinoma of the cervix.

The posttreatment metabolic response is predictive of both cause-specific and progression-free survival after chemoradiation for cervical cancer. These results have been validated in a prospective cohort study [17]. [^{18}F]FDG-PET/CT was performed about 3 months after the completion of chemoradiation and demonstrated that it can provide reliable long-term prognostic information and may be used to guide early interventions for patients with less than a complete metabolic response [17].

Abnormal [^{18}F]FDG uptake in the cervix or lymph nodes after completion of radiotherapy is associated with poor survival outcomes. The optimal timing to obtain [^{18}F]FDG-PET/CT scans during RT for cervical cancer is unclear. FDG activity tends to show an initial increase followed by a steady decline after treatment. Early elevation of FDG activity may be associated with acute inflammation in normal tissue or elevated metabolic activity within the tumor cells; the later reduction in FDG uptake is a reflection of a decrease in the number of viable tumor cells or a reduction in tumor metabolic activity.

40.5 Tumor Recurrence

[^{18}F]FDG-PET/CT appears to have an acceptable diagnostic performance in suspected recurrent cervical cancer and it may affect patient management. Furthermore, FDG avidity may predict the prognosis of recurrent cervical cancer (Figures 40.1, 40.2).

For the detection of combined local and metastatic recurrence of cervical cancer, according to several studies, the sensitivity of [^{18}F]FDG-PET/CT ranges from 92 to 93 %, the

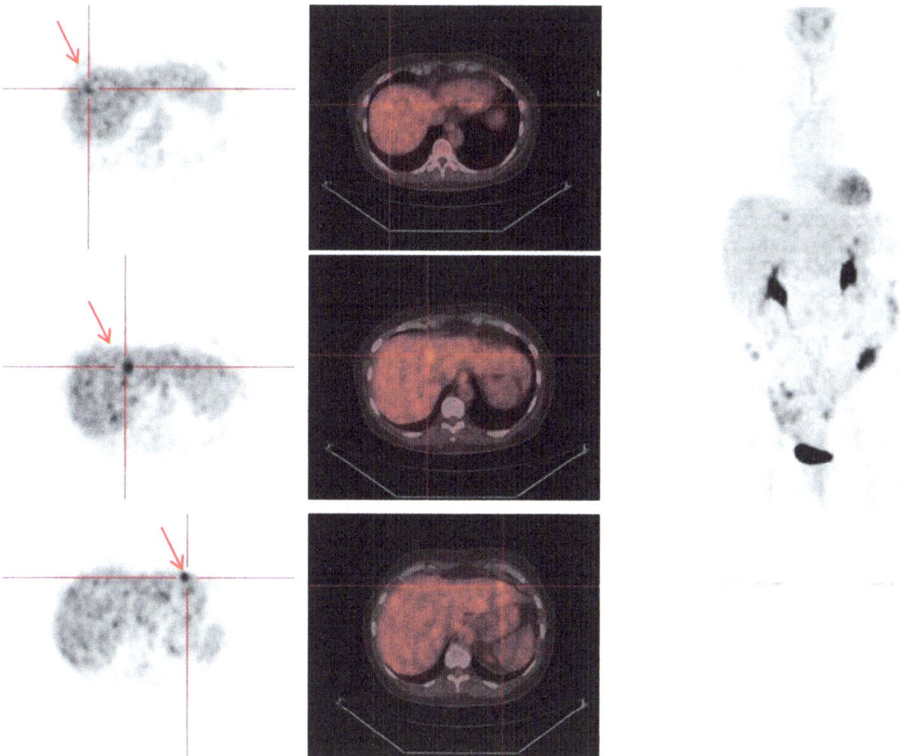

Figs. 40.1 56-year-old woman, with previously treated cervical cancer, presenting with increased serum tumor markers and equivocal findings in conventional imaging. [^{18}F]FDG-PET/CT showed increased [^{18}F]FDG uptake in multiple lesions in liver

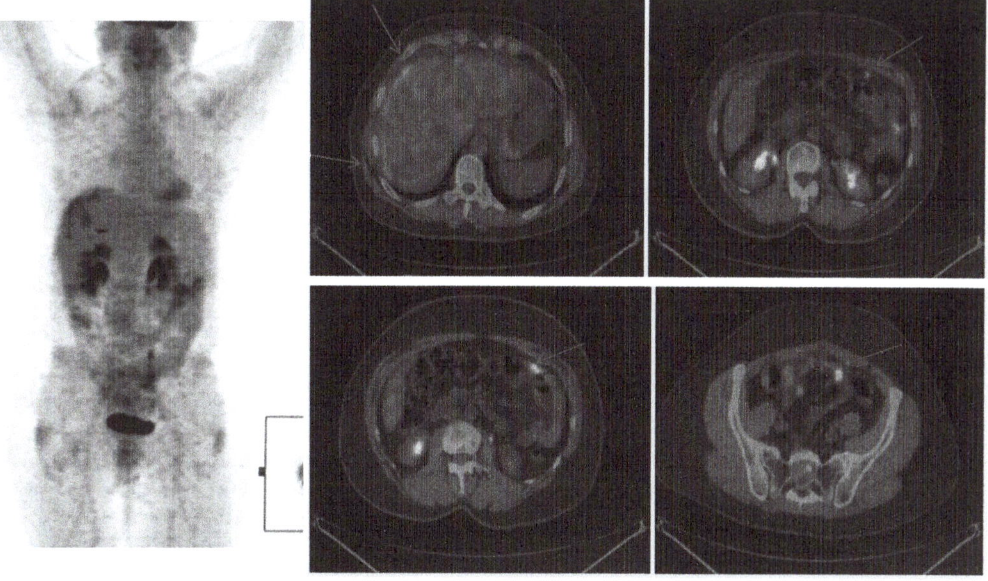

Figs. 40.2 51-year-old woman, with previously treated cervical cancer presenting with elevated CEA serum levels and negative findings on CT and MRI imaging. [^{18}F]FDG-PET/CT showed several areas of increased metabolic activity in the peritoneum (peritoneal implants)

specificity from 81 to 100 %, and the accuracy from 87 to 96 % [18–21]. [^{18}F]FDG-PET/CT was strongly predictive of overall survival [18]. The results of another study were in accordance with the above and [^{18}F]FDG-PET/CT for the evaluation of local recurrence showed sensitivity, specificity, positive predictive value, and negative predictive value of 93, 93, 86, and 96 %, respectively and for metastatic disease showed sensitivity, specificity, positive predictive value, and negative predictive value of 96, 95, 96, and 95 %, respectively [22].

The low rate of false-positive results and high prognostic value suggest that [^{18}F]FDG-PET/CT is an important diagnostic tool for detecting recurrent cervical cancer in clinically equivocal patients. For treatment planning, it is reported that [^{18}F]FDG-PET/CT may change management in 23.1–48 % of cases in suspected recurrent cervical cancer [18, 19]. Because of its high sensitivity and positive predictive value, [^{18}F]FDG-PET/CT should be the imaging technique of choice for evaluating extrapelvic disease prior to performing pelvic exenteration. It seems to be useful in identifying recurrent cervical cancer in both asymptomatic and symptomatic patients with elevated tumor markers and negative imaging findings (squamous cell carcinoma antigen >1.5 ng/mL) [23].

40.6 Conclusion

[^{18}F]FDG-PET/CT provides pretreatment prognostic information concerning the aggressiveness of cervical tumors which may contribute to optimizing and individualizing patient therapy. Although [^{18}F]FDG-PET/CT is not considered suitable for T staging, it has an important role in staging cervical cancer and it aids particularly in identifying the involvement of lymph nodes and distant metastases. In this context it is helpful in targeted radiotherapy planning. Finally, [^{18}F]FDG-PET/CT is an important diagnostic tool for detecting recurrent cervical cancer in clinically equivocal patients.

References

1. Chung HH, Nam BH, Kim JW, Kang KW, Park NH, Song YS, Chung JK, Kang SB (2010) Preoperative [18F]FDG PET/CT maximum standardized uptake value predicts recurrence of uterine cervical cancer. Eur J Nucl Med Mol Imaging 37:1467–1473
2. Haie-Meder C, Mazeron R, Magne N (2010) Clinical evidence on PET-CT for radiation therapy planning in cervix and endometrial cancers. Radiother Oncol 96:351–355
3. Petsuksiri J, Jaishuen A, Pattaranutaporn P, Chansilpa Y (2012) Advanced imaging applications for locally advanced cervical cancer. Asian Pac J Cancer Prev 13:1713–1718
4. Yoon MS, Ahn SJ, Nah BS, Chung WK, Song HC, Yoo SW, Song JY, Jeong JU, Nam TK (2012) Metabolic response of lymph nodes immediately after RT is related with survival outcome of patients with pelvic node-positive cervical cancer using consecutive [(18)F]fluorodeoxyglucose-positron emission tomography/computed tomography. Int J Radiat Oncol Biol Phys 84:e491–e497
5. Lin WC, Hung YC, Yeh LS, Kao CH, Yen RF, Shen YY (2003) Usefulness of (18)F-fluorodeoxyglucose positron emission tomography to detect para-aortic lymph nodal metastasis in advanced cervical cancer with negative computed tomography findings. Gynecol Oncol 89:73–76
6. Yeh LS, Hung YC, Shen YY, Kao CH, Lin CC, Lee CC (2002) Detecting para-aortic lymph nodal metastasis by positron emission tomography of 18F-fluorodeoxyglucose in advanced cervical cancer with negative magnetic resonance imaging findings. Oncol Rep 9:1289–1292
7. Grigsby PW (2005) 4th international cervical cancer conference: update on PET and cervical cancer. Gynecol Oncol 99(3 suppl 1):S173–S175
8. Sugawara Y, Eisbruch A, Kosuda S, Recker BE, Kison PV, Wahl RL (1999) Evaluation of FDG PET in patients with cervical cancer. J Nucl Med 40:1125–1131
9. Choi HJ, Roh JW, Seo SS et al (2006) Comparison of the accuracy of magnetic resonance imaging and positron emission tomography/computed tomography in the presurgical detection of lymph node metastases in patients with uterine cervical carcinoma: a prospective study. Cancer 106:914–922
10. Havrilesky LJ, Kulasingam SL, Matchar DB, Myers ER (2005) FDG-PET for management of cervical and ovarian cancer. Gynecol Oncol 97:183–191
11. Kim SK, Choi HJ, Park SY et al (2009) Additional value of MR/PET fusion compared with PET/CT in the detection of lymph node metastases in cervical cancer patients. Eur J Cancer 45:2103–2109
12. Choi HJ, Ju W, Myung SK, Kim Y (2010) Diagnostic performance of computer tomography, magnetic

resonance imaging, and positron emission tomography or positron emission tomography/computer tomography for detection of metastatic lymph nodes in patients with cervical cancer: meta-analysis. Cancer Sci 101:1471–1479
13. Loft A, Berthelsen AK, Roed H, Ottosen C, Lundvall L, Knudsen J, Nedergaard L, Højgaard L, Engelholm SA (2007) The diagnostic value of PET/CT scanning in patients with cervical cancer: a prospective study. Gynecol Oncol 106:29–34
14. Yildirim Y, Sehirali S, Avci ME, Yilmaz C, Ertopcu K, Tinar S, Duman Y, Sayhan S (2008) Integrated PET/CT for the evaluation of para-aortic nodal metastasis in locally advanced cervical cancer patients with negative conventional CT findings. Gynecol Oncol 108:154–159
15. American College of Radiology (2010) ACR appropriateness criteria. Women's imaging: staging of invasive cancer of the cervix. http://www.acr.org/. Accessed 20 Mar 2010
16. Kizer NT, Zighelboim I, Case AS, Dewdney SB, Thaker PH, Massad LS (2009) The role of PET/CT in the management of patients with cervical cancer: practice patterns of the members of the society of gynecologic oncologists. Gynecol Oncol 114:310–314
17. Antoch G, Freudenberg LS, Beyer T, Bockisch A, Debatin JF (2004) To enhance or not to enhance? 18F-FDG and CT contrast agents in dual-modality 18F-FDG PET/CT. J Nucl Med 45(suppl 1):56S–65S
18. van der Veldt AA, Buist MR, van Baal MW, Comans EF, Hoekstra OS, Molthoff CF (2008) Clarifying the diagnosis of clinically suspected recurrence of cervical cancer: impact of 18F-FDG PET. J Nucl Med 49:1936–1943
19. Chung HH, Jo H, Kang WJ et al (2007) Clinical impact of integrated PET/CT on the management of suspected cervical cancer recurrence. Gynecol Oncol 104:529–534
20. Kitajima K, Murakami K, Yamasaki E, Domeki Y, Kaji Y, Sugimura K (2008) Performance of FDG-PET/CT for diagnosis of recurrent uterine cervical cancer. Eur Radiol 18:2040–2047
21. Sironi S, Picchio M, Landoni C, Galimberti S, Signorelli M, Bettinardi V et al (2007) Post-therapy surveillance of patients with uterine cancers: value of integrated FDG PET/CT in the detection of recurrence. Eur J Nucl Med Mol Imaging 34:472–479
22. Mittra E, El-Maghraby T, Rodriguez CA, Quon A, McDougall IR, Gambhir SS, Iagaru A (2009) Efficacy of 18F-FDG PET/CT in the evaluation of patients with recurrent cervical carcinoma. Eur J Nucl Med Mol Imaging 36:1952–1959
23. Jover R, Lourido D, Gonzalez C, Rojo A, Gorospe L, Alfonso JM (2008) Role of PET/CT in the evaluation of cervical cancer. Gynecol Oncol 110(3 suppl 2):S55–S59

PET/CT with [^{18}F]FDG in Ovarian Cancer 41

Evangelia V. Skoura and Ioannis E. Datseris

41.1 Initial Diagnosis-Differentiation Between Malignant and Benign Ovarian Tumors and Prognosis

The role of [^{18}F]FDG-PET/CT for differentiating between malignant and benign ovarian tumors remains controversial, and false-negative and false-positive cases have been reported. Concerning the prognostic value of [^{18}F]FDG-PET/CT there have been reports that a high (>13.15) pretreatment SUVmax of the primary tumor in patients with ovarian cancer was associated with a poor prognosis [15]. The SUVmax of the primary tumor had a statistically significant association with stage ($p = 0.010$) and histology ($p = 0.001$) [1].

41.2 Initial Staging

In ovarian cancer [^{18}F]FDG-PET/CT has an effective role in staging patients with advanced disease, providing useful information about extrapelvic sites, such as supraclavicular and paraaortic nodular involvement, peritoneum and omentum implants, bone and muscle metastases. A recent meta-analysis, including data from 882 patients with ovarian cancer, showed that [^{18}F]FDG-PET or [^{18}F]FDG-PET/CT was a more accurate modality for detecting metastatic lymph nodes [2]. Approximately 70 % of metastatic lymph nodes and 97 % of negative lymph nodes could be correctly diagnosed by [^{18}F]FDG-PET or [^{18}F]FDG-PET/CT. Though significantly better than those of CT and MR imaging, the sensitivity of [^{18}F]FDG-PET or [^{18}F]FDG-PET/CT was moderate [2]. A possible explanation is that this method can only detect lesions with sufficient malignant cells to change the glucose metabolism and that FDG uptake may not be increased in low-grade tumors.

The main effect of [^{18}F]FDG-PET/CT seems to be the detection of metastases outside the pelvis as it may detect distant metastasis in the liver, pleura, mediastinum, and supraclavicular lymph nodes that had been missed on CT imaging. It has been shown that [^{18}F]FDG-PET/CT may increase the pretreatment staging accuracy to 69–87 % compared with 53–55 % with CT alone [3, 4]. [^{18}F]FDG-PET/CT is particularly useful in distinguishing patients with stages IIIC–IV cancer from those with stages I–IIIB. For this classification, the specificity, sensitivity, and accuracy of [^{18}F]FDG-PET/CT was 91, 100, and 98 %, respectively, in comparison with 64, 97, and 88 % for CT [5].

E. V. Skoura · I. E. Datseris (✉)
Nuclear Medicine Department, Evangelismos General Hospital, Ipsilantou 45–47, 10676 Athens, Greece
e-mail: datseris@otenet.gr

E. V. Skoura
e-mail: lskoura@yahoo.gr

A. D. Gouliamos et al. (eds.), *Imaging in Clinical Oncology*,
DOI: 10.1007/978-88-470-5385-4_41, © Springer-Verlag Italia 2014

41.3 Radiotherapy Planning

In the literature there is only one report about the role of [^{18}F]FDG-PET/CT on intensity-modulated radiation therapy (IMRT) planning that showed that [^{18}F]FDG-PET/CT information seems that may change gross tumor volume (GTV) delineation in 35 % of cases. In these patients, the average increase in GTV was 21.6 %, due to the incorporation of additional lymph node metastases, minimal recurrent nodularity, and extension of the metastatic tumor beyond the frame defined by CT [6].

41.4 Restaging After Treatment

Several studies have demonstrated that [^{18}F]FDG-PET/CT derived parameters, including SUV and percentage change, have the potential to predict response to therapy in patients with ovarian cancer (Fig. 41.1).

When an arbitrary SUV of 3.8 was taken as the cut-off for differentiating between responders and nonresponders after therapy, [^{18}F]FDG-PET/CT showed a sensitivity of 90 % and specificity of 63.6 %. When an arbitrary percentage change of 65 % was taken as the cut-off, the sensitivity was 90 % and specificity 81.8 % [7].

41.5 Tumor Recurrence

Potential advantages of the use of integrated [^{18}F]FDG-PET/CT for evaluation of recurrent ovarian cancer include increased lesion detection with the use of a metabolic tracer, simultaneous acquisition of anatomic reference points to determine the exact location of lesions, and, in most cases, differentiation of disease processes from physiologic processes. Moreover, [^{18}F]FDG-PET/CT may survey the entire body in one examination. These superior qualities may help identify which patients are eligible for secondary surgical cytoreduction. There have been many reports discussing the usefulness of [^{18}F]FDG-PET/CT for detecting ovarian cancer recurrence. When the gold standard was clinical follow-up including radiological imaging, the diagnostic accuracy of [^{18}F]FDG-PET/CT was very high with 73–100 % sensitivity, 71–100 % specificity, and 83–100 % accuracy in patient-based analysis

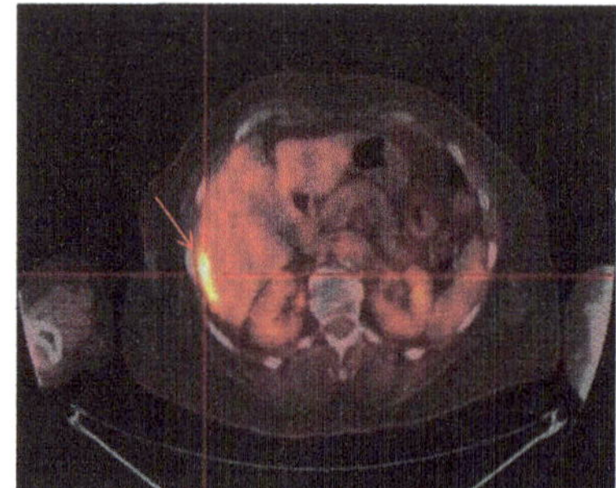

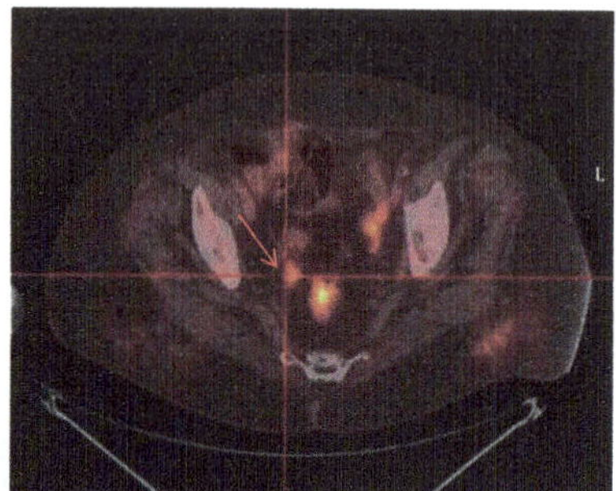

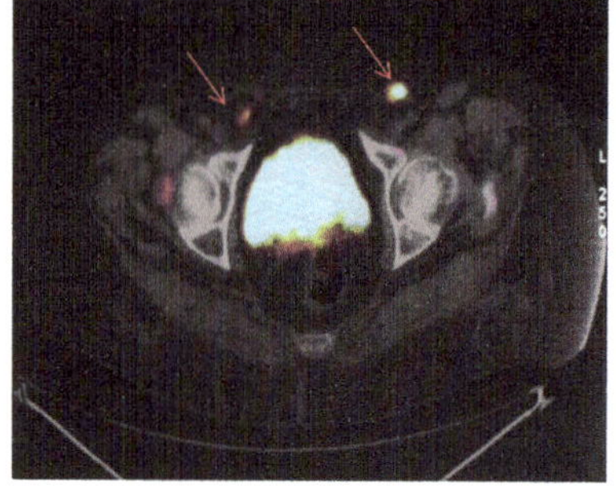

Fig. 41.1 78-year-old woman post-treatment for ovarian carcinoma, presenting with rising tumor serum markers and negative findings on recent CT imaging. [^{18}F]FDG-PET/CT revealed increased [^{18}F]FDG uptake in the peritoneum and in bilateral inguinal lymph nodes

[5, 8–18]. However, when the gold standard was histopathology by surgery, the diagnostic accuracy of [^{18}F]FDG-PET/CT tended to be poorer and it was reported that the sensitivity, specificity, and accuracy of patient-based analysis were 53–83, 40–86, and 63–82 %, respectively [19–21]. The discrepancies in these values between the clinical follow-up and the surgical histopathology as a gold standard may partly depend on the resolution of the [^{18}F]FDG-PET/CT systems used and partly on the size of microscopically small lesions. The spatial resolution of PET is approximately 6–10 mm; therefore, its sensitivity for depicting lesions smaller than 1 cm is lower than that for larger lesions [22] (Figs. 41.2, 41.3).

Several studies and a meta-analysis has compared techniques for detection of recurrence and demonstrated that [^{18}F]FDG-PET/CT was better (sensitivity 91 % and specificity 88 %) than CT (sensitivity 79 %, specificity 84 %) or MRI (sensitivity 75 %, specificity 78 %) [5, 9, 15, 23, 24]. In addition, [^{18}F]FDG-PET/CT had the highest positive predictive value (89–98 %) for recurrence of ovarian cancer when compared with other modalities [25, 26].

A major indication for [^{18}F]FDG-PET/CT is the evaluation of ovarian cancer recurrence after first-line therapy in patients in which CA-125 levels are rising and conventional imaging studies show negative or equivocal findings [8, 27]. Investigators have reported that [^{18}F]FDG-PET or PET/CT has a sensitivity of 96 % for localizing recurrent disease in patients with rising CA-125 levels and that PET evidence of recurrent ovarian cancer preceded CT findings by 6 months, allowing earlier reintroduction of therapy [28, 29].

Concerning the detection of peritoneal implants in a recent study, the sensitivity and specificity of [^{18}F]FDG-PET/CT were 97.5 and 100 % whereas those of MRI were 95 and 85.7 %, respectively. For the small-to-medium-sized (0.5–2 cm) peritoneal implants diagnostic accuracy values of [^{18}F]FDG-PET/CT were significantly better than those of MRI ($p < 0.05$) [30].

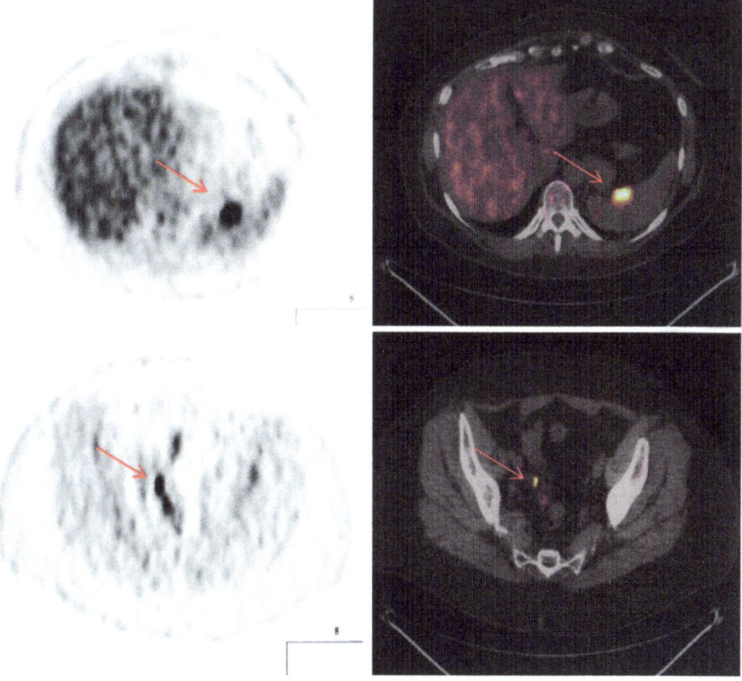

Fig. 41.2 52-year-old woman with a history of bilateral ovarian carcinoma presenting with slight but persistent elevation of tumor marker serum levels and negative findings on MRI imaging. [^{18}F]FDG-PET/CT revealed two [^{18}F]FDG avid lesions in the peritoneum

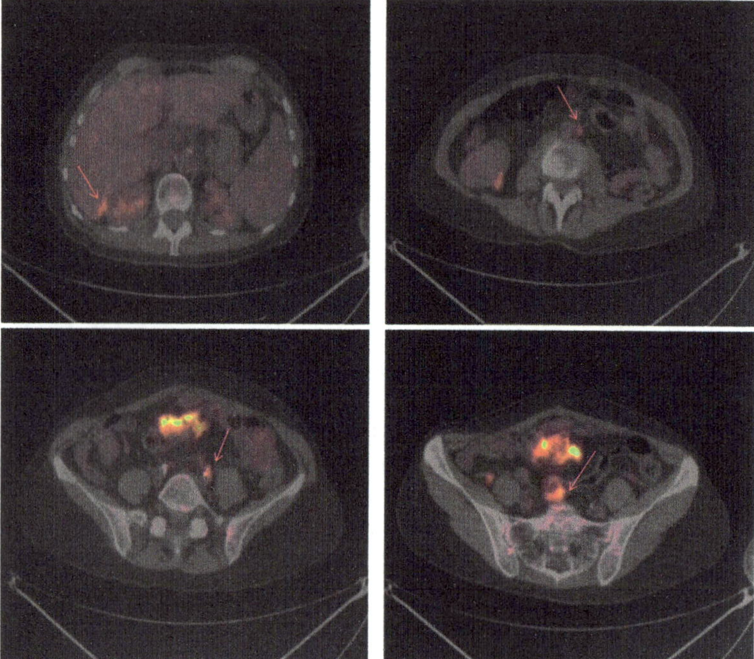

Fig. 41.3 66-year-old woman, status post-treatment for ovarian carcinoma, presenting with progressively elevated CA-125 antigen and negative conventional imaging evaluation. [^{18}F]FDG-PET/CT revealed several foci of increased [^{18}F]FDG uptake in the peritoneum. Abnormal metabolic activity was also present in a small left paraaortic and a small left common iliac lymph node

41.6 Conclusion

[^{18}F]FDG-PET/CT has an effective role in the detection of metastases outside the pelvis as it may detect distant metastasis in the liver, pleura, mediastinum, and supraclavicular lymph nodes that may missed on CT imaging. Another major indication of the modality is the evaluation of ovarian cancer recurrence after first-line therapy in patients in which CA-125 levels are rising and conventional imaging studies show negative or equivocal findings.

References

1. Nakamura K, Hongo A, Kodama J, Hiramatsu Y (2012) The pretreatment of maximum standardized uptake values (SUVmax) of the primary tumor is predictor for poor prognosis for patients with epithelial ovarian cancer. Acta Med Okayama 66:53–60
2. Yuan Y, Gu ZX, Tao XF, Liu SY (2012) Computer tomography, magnetic resonance imaging, and positron emission tomography or positron emission tomography/computer tomography for detection of metastatic lymph nodes in patients with ovarian cancer: a meta-analysis. Eur J Radiol 81:1002–1006
3. Castelluci P, Perrone AM, Picchio M, Ghi T, Farsad M, Nanni C et al (2007) Diagnostic accuracy of 18F-FDG PET/CT in characterizing ovarian lesions and staging ovarian cancer: correlation with transvaginal ultrasonography, computed tomography, and histology. Nucl Med Commun 28:589–595
4. Yoshida Y, Kurokawa T, Kawahara K, Tsuchida T, Okazawa H, Fujibayashi Y, Yonekura Y, Kotsuji F (2004) Incremental benefits of FDG positron emission tomography over CT alone for the preoperative staging of ovarian cancer. AJR Am J Roentgenol 182:227–233
5. Kitajima K, Murakami K, Yamasaki E (2008) Diagnostic accuracy of integrated FDG-PET/contrast-enhanced CT in staging ovarian cancer: comparison with enhanced CT. Eur J Nucl Med Mol Imaging 35:1912–1920
6. Du XL, Jiang T, Sheng XG, Li QS, Wang C, Yu H (2012) PET/CT scanning guided intensity-modulated radiotherapy in treatment of recurrent ovarian cancer. Eur J Radiol 81:3551–3556
7. Nishiyama Y, Yamamoto Y, Kaneishi K, Ohno M, Hata T, Kushida Y et al (2008) Monitoring the neoadjuvant therapy response in gynecological cancer patients using FDG PET. Eur J Nucl Med Mol Imaging 35:287–295
8. Chung HH, Kang WJ, Kim JW, Park NH, Song YS, Chung JK, Kang SB, Lee HP (2007) Role of [18F]FDG PET/CT in the assessment of suspected recurrent ovarian cancer: correlation with clinical or

histological findings. Eur J Nucl Med Mol Imaging 34:480–486
9. Hauth EA, Antoch G, Stattaus J, Kuehl H, Veit P, Bosckisch A et al (2005) Evaluation of integrated whole-body PET/CT in the detection of recurrent ovarian cancer. Eur J Radiol 56:263–268
10. Nanni C, Rubello D, Farsad M, De Iaco P, Sansovini M, Erba P et al (2005) 18F-FDG PET/CT in the evaluation of recurrent ovarian cancer: a prospective study on forty-one patients. Eur J Surg Oncol 31:792–797
11. Simcock B, Neesham D, Quinn M, Drummond E, Milner A, Hicks RJ (2006) The impact of PET/CT in the management of recurrent ovarian cancer. Gynecol Oncol 103:271–276
12. Mangili G, Picchio M, Sironi S, Vigano R, Rabaiotti E, Bornaghi D et al (2007) Integrated PET/CT as a first-line re-staging modality in patients with suspected recurrence of ovarian cancer. Eur J Nucl Med Mol Imaging 34:658–666
13. Thrall MM, DeLoia JA, Gallion H, Avril N (2007) Clinical use of combined positron emission tomography and computed tomography (FDG-PET/CT) in recurrent ovarian cancer. Gynecol Oncol 105:17–22
14. Kim CK, Park BK, Choi JY, Kim BG, Han H (2007) Detection of recurrent ovarian cancer at MRI: comparison with integrated PET/CT. J Comput Assist Tomogr 31:868–875
15. Sebastian S, Lee SI, Horowitz NS, Scott JA, Fischman AJ, Simeone JF et al (2008) PET-CT vs. CT alone in ovarian cancer recurrence. Abdom Imaging 33:112–118
16. Iagaru AH, Mittra ES, McDougall IR, Quon A, Gambhir SS (2008) 18FFDG PET/CT evaluation of patients with ovarian carcinoma. Nucl Med Commun 29:1046–1051
17. Soussan M, Wartski M, Cherel P, Fourme E, Goupil A, Le Stanc E et al (2008) Impact of FDG PET/CT imaging on the decision making in the biologic suspicion of ovarian carcinoma recurrence. Gynecol Oncol 108:160–165
18. Fulham MJ, Carter J, Baldey A, Hicks RJ, Ramshaw JE, Gibson M (2009) The impact of PET/CT in suspected recurrent ovarian cancer: a prospective multi-centre study as part of the Australian PET data collection project. Gynecol Oncol 112:462–468
19. Makhija S, Howden N, Edwards R, Kelley J, Townsend DW, Meltzer CC (2002) Positron emission tomography/computed tomography imaging for the detection of recurrent ovarian and fallopian tube carcinoma: a retrospective review. Gynecol Oncol 85:53–58
20. Bristow RE, DelCarmen MG, Pannu HK, Cohade C, Zahurak ML, Fishman EK et al (2003) Clinically occult recurrent ovarian cancer: patient selection for secondary cytoreductive surgery using combined PET/CT. Gynecol Oncol 90:519–528
21. Sironi S, Messa C, Mangili G, Zangheri B, Aletti G, Garevaglia E et al (2004) Integrated FDG-PET/CT in patients with persistent ovarian cancer: correlation with histologic findings. Radiology 233:433–440
22. Torizuka T, Nobezawa S, Kanno T et al (2002) Ovarian cancer recurrence: role of whole-body positron emission tomography using 2-[fluorine-18]-fluoro-2-deoxy-D-glucose. Eur J Nucl Med Mol Imaging 29:797–803
23. Gu P, Pan LL, Wu SQ, Sun L, Huang G (2009) CA125, PET alone, PET-CT, CT and MRI in diagnosing recurrent ovarian carcinoma: a systematic review and meta-analysis. Eur J Radiol 71:164–174
24. Nakamoto Y, Saga T, Ishimori T et al (2001) Clinical value of positron emission tomography with FDG for recurrent ovarian cancer. Am J Roentgenol 176:1449–1454
25. Prakash P, Cronin CG, Blake MA (2010) Role of PET/CT in ovarian cancer. AJR Am J Roentgenol 194:W464–W470
26. Antunovic L, Cimitan M, Borsatti E, Baresic T, Sorio R, Giorda G, Steffan A, Balestreri L, Tatta R, Pepe G, Rubello D, Cecchin D, Canzonieri V (2012) Revisiting the clinical value of 18F-FDG PET/CT in detection of recurrent epithelial ovarian carcinomas: correlation with histology, serum CA-125 assay, and conventional radiological modalities. Clin Nucl Med 37:e184–e188
27. Kitajima K, Murakami K, Sakamoto S, Kaji Y, Sugimura K (2011) Present and future of FDG-PET/CT in ovarian cancer. Ann Nucl Med 25:155–164
28. Son H, Khan SM, Rahaman J, Cameron KL, Prasad-Hayes M, Chuang L, Machac J, Heiba S, Kostakoglu L (2011) Role of FDG PET/CT in staging of recurrent ovarian cancer. Radio Graph 31:569–583
29. Zimny M, Siggelkow W, Schrφder W et al (2001) 2-[Fluorine-18]-fluoro-2-deoxy-D-glucose positron emission tomography in the diagnosis of recurrent ovarian cancer. Gynecol Oncol 83:310–315
30. Sanli Y, Turkmen C, Bakir B, Iyibozkurt C, Ozel S, Has D, Yilmaz E, Topuz S, Yavuz E, Unal SN, Mudun A (2012) Diagnostic value of PET/CT is similar to that of conventional MRI and even better for detecting small peritoneal implants in patients with recurrent ovarian cancer. Nucl Med Commun 33:509–515

42 PET/CT with [^{18}F]FDG in Endometrial Cancer

Evangelia V. Skoura and Ioannis E. Datseris

42.1 Initial Diagnosis and Prognosis

Like most neoplasms, endometrial carcinoma does demonstrate an increased rate of glycolysis and takes up [^{18}F]FDG. Imaging with [^{18}F]FDG-PET/CT seems that may play role as a prognostic factor in endometrium cancer. Several studies have shown that there is statistically significant correlation between SUVmax and FIGO stage, histological grade, depth of myometrial invasion, lymph node metastasis, lymphovascular space involvement and tumour size. Also, they have demonstrated that high SUVmax was an independent prognostic factor for both disease-free survival (DFS) and overall survival (OS), $p < 0.05$ [1–3].

42.2 Initial Staging

There have been several reports demonstrating the accuracy of [^{18}F]FDG-PET/CT for detecting lymph node metastasis in endometrial cancer. The referred sensitivity and specificity of [^{18}F]FDG-PET/CT on region-specific analyses are 36–72 % and 88–99 %, respectively, and that corresponding values for patient-based analyses were 41–100 % and 56–100 %, respectively [4–13]. It seems that [^{18}F]FDG-PET/CT tends to show low sensitivity and high specificity. It is primarily limited by its inability to detect microscopic metastasis. As tiny lymph nodes tend to show smaller SUV than real values due to the partial volume effect, it is difficult to use the usual cut-off point (2.5–3.0) for differentiating malignant from benign lymph nodes [14]. A study has shown that in metastatic lymph nodes with a short axis diameter of 4 mm or less, [^{18}F]FDG-PET/CT had a detection sensitivity of 12.5 %, with a diameter between 5 and 9 mm the sensitivity was 66.7 % and with a diameter of 10 mm or greater it was 100.0 % [5].

A recent study that compared the diagnostic performance of [^{18}F]FDG-PET/CT, MRI and two-dimensional ultrasound (2DUS) found that all three methods were comparable in predicting myometrial invasion [15]. For cervical invasion and lymph node metastases, however, [^{18}F]FDG-PET/CT was more accurate [15]. It seems that compared to MRI, [^{18}F]FDG-PET/CT has a limited role for local staging of primary cancer, whereas it is a useful technique for assessing distant metastases throughout the whole body in a single examination in patients with advanced-stage disease [16].

E. V. Skoura · I. E. Datseris (✉)
Nuclear Medicine Department, Evangelismos General Hospital, Ipsilantou 45–47, 10676 Athens, Greece
e-mail: datseris@otenet.gr

E. Skoura
e-mail: lskoura@yahoo.gr

A. D. Gouliamos et al. (eds.), *Imaging in Clinical Oncology*,
DOI: 10.1007/978-88-470-5385-4_42, © Springer-Verlag Italia 2014

42.3 Tumour Recurrence

Unlike conventional imaging modalities which provide morphological information, PET with [^{18}F]FDG is able to identify viable tumour lesions based on the increased glucose metabolism of malignant tissue. [^{18}F]FDG-PET/CT can detect recurrent lesions otherwise missed or misinterpreted on conventional imaging studies and several studies support this.

A recent meta-analysis of the literature and several studies demonstrated that the patient-based sensitivity and specificity for detection of endometrial cancer recurrence were 91–100 % and 83–100 %, respectively [5, 14, 17–20]. A previous study showed that the overall lesion site-based sensitivity and specificity of [^{18}F]FDG-PET/CT were 94.7 and 99.5 %, respectively [17]. The lesion site-based sensitivity and specificity of [^{18}F]FDG-PET/CT for the detection of pelvic recurrence were 92.3 and 97.3 %, while for the detection of extra-pelvic recurrence the indices were all 100 % [17].

42.4 Conclusion

[^{18}F]FDG-PET/CT has a limited role for local staging of primary cancer, whereas it is a useful technique for assessing lymph node and distant metastases throughout the whole body in a single examination in patients with advanced-stage disease. Its main role is in detecting recurrent lesions otherwise missed or misinterpreted on conventional imaging studies.

References

1. Nakamura K, Joja I, Fukushima C, Haruma T, Hayashi C, Kusumoto T, Seki N, Hongo A, Hiramatsu Y (2013) The preoperative SUVmax is superior to ADCmin of the primary tumour as a predictor of disease recurrence and survival in patients with endometrial cancer. Eur J Nucl Med Mol Imaging 40:52–60
2. Kitajima K, Kita M, Suzuki K, Senda M, Nakamoto Y, Sugimura K (2012) Prognostic significance of SUVmax (maximum standardized uptake value) measured by [^{18}F]FDG PET/CT in endometrial cancer. Eur J Nucl Med Mol Imaging 39:840–845
3. Nakamura K, Hongo A, Kodama J, Hiramatsu Y (2011) The measurement of SUVmax of the primary tumor is predictive of prognosis for patients with endometrial cancer. Gynecol Oncol 123:82–87
4. Kitajima K, Murakami K, Yamasaki E et al (2008) Accuracy of FDG PET/CT in detecting pelvic and paraortic lymph node metastasis in patients with endometrial cancer. AJR Am J Roentgenol 190:1652–1658
5. Kitajima K, Murakami K, Yamasaki E, Kaji Y, Sugimura K (2009) Accuracy of integrated FDG-PET/contrast-enhanced CT in detecting pelvic and paraaortic lymph node metastasis in patients with uterine cancer. Eur Radiol 19:1529–1536
6. Choi HJ, Roh JW, Seo SS et al (2006) Comparison of the accuracy of magnetic resonance imaging and positron emission tomography/computed tomography in the presurgical detection of lymph node metastases in patients with uterine cervical carcinoma: a prospective study. Cancer 106:914–922
7. Kitajima K, Yamasaki E, Kaji Y, Murakami K, Sugimura K (2012) Comparison of DWI and PET/CT in evaluation of lymph node metastasis in uterine cancer. World J Radiol 4:207–214
8. Sironi S, Buda A, Picchio M, Perego P, Moreni R, Pellegrino A, Colombo M, Mangioni C, Messa C, Fazio F (2006) Lymph node metastasis in patients with clinical early-stage cervical cancer: detection with integrated FDG PET/CT. Radiology 238:272–279
9. Park JY, Kim EN, Kim DY, Suh DS, Kim JH, Kim YM, Kim YT, Nam JH (2008) Comparison of the validity of magnetic resonance imaging and positron emission tomography/computed tomography in the preoperative evaluation of patients with uterine corpus cancer. Gynecol Oncol 108:486–492
10. Chung HH, Park NH, Kim JW, Song YS, Chung JK, Kang SB (2009) Role of integrated PET-CT in pelvic lymph node staging of cervical cancer before radical hysterectomy. Gynecol Obstet Invest 67:61–66
11. Signorelli M, Guerra L, Buda A, Picchio M, Mangili G, Dell'Anna T, Sironi S, Messa C (2009) Role of the integrated FDG PET/CT in the surgical management of patients with high risk clinical early stage endometrial cancer: detection of pelvic nodal metastases. Gynecol Oncol 115:231–235
12. Picchio M, Mangili G, Samanes Gajate AM et al (2010) High-grade endometrial cancer: value of 18F-FDG PET/CT in preoperative staging. Nucl Med Commun 31:506–512
13. Nayot D, Kwon JS, Carey MS et al (2008) Does preoperative positron emission tomography with computed tomography predict nodal status in endometrial cancer? A pilot study. Curr Oncol 15:123–125
14. Kitajima K, Murakami K, Yamasaki E et al (2008) Performance of FDG-PET/CT in the diagnosis of recurrent endometrial cancer. Ann Nucl Med 22:103–109

15. Antonsen SL, Jensen LN, Loft A, Berthelsen AK, Costa J, Tabor A, et al (2013) MRI, PET/CT and ultrasound in the preoperative staging of endometrial cancer—a multicenter prospective comparative study. Gynecol Oncol 128:300–308
16. Kitajima K, Murakami K, Kaji Y, Sugimura K (2010) Spectrum of FDG PET/CT findings of uterine tumors. AJR Am J Roentgenol 195:737–743
17. Sironi S, Picchio M, Landoni C, Galimberti S, Signorelli M, Bettinardi V et al (2007) Post-therapy surveillance of patients with uterine cancers: value of integrated FDG PET/CT in the detection of recurrence. Eur J Nucl Med Mol Imaging 34:472–479
18. Chung HH, Kang WJ, Kim JW et al (2008) The clinical impact of [18F]FDG PET/CT for the management of recurrent endometrial cancer: correlation with clinical and histological findings. Eur J Nucl Med Mol Imaging 35:1081–1088
19. Park JY, Kim EN, Kim DY et al (2008) Clinical impact of positron emission tomography or positron emission tomography/computed tomography in the posttherapy surveillance of endometrial carcinoma: evaluation of 88 patients. Int J Gynecol Cancer 18:1332–1338
20. Kadkhodayan S, Shahriari S, Treglia G, Yousefi Z, Sadeghi R (2013) Accuracy of 18-F-FDG PET imaging in the follow up of endometrial cancer patients: systematic review and meta-analysis of the literature. Gynecol Oncol 128:397–404

43 Clinical Implications of Gynecologic Cancer

Georgios E. Hilaris

43.1 Endometrial Cancer

The postmenopausal patient with new onset vaginal bleeding should be assessed with transvaginal pelvic sonography. An endometrial thickness ≤4 mm (ACOG) (or 5 mm by other societies) is a safe cutoff to defer endometrial sampling as the risk or endometrial malignancy is 1 % unless the patient has persistent or intermittent bleeding where the risk may be higher [1].

Contrast-enhanced MRI is superior when compared to nonenhanced MRI, ultrasound, or Computed Tomography (CT) in the assessment of myometrial invasion or cervical involvement [2], although a negative study does not exclude microscopic involvement.

MRI is also as sensitive and specific in the preoperative assessment of pelvic or para-aortic lymph nodes compared to FDG PET-CT which possibly performs best for evaluation of distant metastasis [3].

According to international federation of gynecology and obstetrics (FIGO), endometrial cancer is surgically staged [4]. This includes evaluation of lymph node status by lymphadenectomy or lymph node sampling and histologic confirmation.

MRI and/or PET-CT should be reserved mainly for post-treatment surveillance and detection of relapse and distant metastasis when clinically indicated. Alternatively, these modalities may be reserved for incompletely staged patients, where lymph nodes were not or could not be removed, or for selected patients who are poor surgical candidates [3].

Surveillance in the post-treatment period is mainly clinical, including a detailed history and physical exam every 3–4 months for the first 2 years followed by semiannual exam for 3–5 years. Some groups order a Ca-125 in every visit as well.

There is still disagreement as to the frequency of imaging during the post-treatment surveillance period since frequent imaging has not been linked to any survival advantage. In addition, more than 70 % of relapses occur in symptomatic patients [4].

Most societies suggest imaging once a year or more frequently as clinically indicated. In our institution, we order a post-surgery CT or MRI to serve as an imaging reference. We then conduct surveillance CT or MRI once or twice a year depending on risk factors, including annual chest CT for the first 2 years followed by yearly CT or MRI of the abdomen and pelvis for the next 3 years, unless clinically indicated.

G. E. Hilaris (✉)
Consultant Gynecologic Oncologist, Hygeia and Mitera Hospitals and IASO Hospital, Athens, Greece
e-mail: info@hilaris.org

G. E. Hilaris
Adjunct Clinical Instructor of Gynecology and Obstetrics, Stanford University School of Medicine, Palo Alto, California, USA

A. D. Gouliamos et al. (eds.), *Imaging in Clinical Oncology*,
DOI: 10.1007/978-88-470-5385-4_43, © Springer-Verlag Italia 2014

43.2 Ovarian Cancer

Ovarian cancer is surgically staged according to the FIGO [5].

According to most expert groups in North America and Europe, universal screening of the general population (at average risk) for ovarian cancer is not currently recommended [6, 7]. Data from recent prospective trials illustrates this [8, 9]. Other trials, however, have shown more favorable results of screening, especially in low risk women [10, 11].

Pelvic ultrasound is the first step in the evaluation of the adnexal mass. Its high sensitivity and specificity can point toward expectant management, further imaging or surgical intervention.

MRI may follow ultrasonographic evaluation of a suspicious complex adnexal mass. It has the advantage of providing an overall assessment of the abdomen, pelvis, and retroperitoneal space.

CT is less sensitive than MRI and U/S in the assessment of the adnexae.

Overall, CT, contrast-enhanced MRI, and or FGD, PET-CT are best reserved for post-treatment surveillance and detection of relapse and distant metastasis. Alternatively they may be used in incompletely staged patients, where lymph nodes were not or could not be removed, or for selected patients who are poor surgical candidates.

There is still disagreement as to the frequency of imaging during the post-treatment surveillance period since frequent imaging has not been linked to any survival advantage. Most societies suggest imaging as clinically indicated.

We recommend a post-surgery CT (or MRI) to serve as an imaging reference. We also obtain a baseline prechemotherapy and post-surgical Ca-125. We then conduct surveillance CT or MRI twice a year for the first 2 years including annual chest CT followed by yearly CT or MRI of the abdomen and pelvis for the next 3 years, unless clinically indicated. We also recommend history and physical examination and Ca-125 every 3–6 months for 5 years and yearly thereafter which is in line with most expert groups [12].

43.3 Cervical Cancer

According to FIGO, cancer of the cervix is clinically staged [13]. Several reasons justify this recommendation even nowadays: clinical staging is more accessible in low resource countries where cervical cancer is also the most common gynecologic cancer; it may be better in assessing locally advanced disease (tumor size, vaginal/parametrial involvement); it also helps avoid unnecessary surgery in women who are poor surgical candidates. On the other hand in developed countries, more expensive imaging techniques are often preferred for more accurate selection of surgical candidates as well as in post-treatment surveillance. For example, a preoperative MRI is often helpful in the assessment of cervical stroma invasion and/or parametrial extension and may also reveal enlarged lymph nodes. In this event, some centers prefer a CT-guided biopsy of enlarged nodes or alternatively a PET-CT. Still other groups perform a targeted laparoscopic lymph node excision of enlarged nodes and histologic examination. In either case, all these modalities—when available—assist in better assignment of patients in the primary surgical or chemoradiation arm, respectively.

Post-treatment surveillance typically involves physical examination every 3–4 months for the first 2 years followed by exams every 6 months for the rest 3 years. In addition to annual Papanicolaou smear, a chest X-ray is also being done yearly for up to 5 years.

There is insufficient data to support routine use of imaging such as CT, PET-CT, or MRI in the surveillance period and should be reserved for suspected recurrence or as clinically indicated [12, 14, 15].

We recommend, however, a post-treatment CT or MRI to serve as a baseline reference. We have found that it helps the clinician avoid future mis/over diagnosis from postradiation or post-surgical changes.

References

1. Smith-Bindman R, Kerlikowske K et al (1998) Ultrasound to exclude endometrial cancer and other endometrial abnormalities. JAMA 280(17):1510
2. Beddy P, Moyle P et al (2012) Evaluation of depth of myometrial invasion and overall staging in endometrial cancer: comparison of diffusion-weighted and dynamic contrast-enhanced MR imaging. Radiology 262(2):530
3. Park JY, Kim EN et al (2008) Comparison of the validity of magnetic resonance imaging and positron emission tomography/computed tomography in the preoperative evaluation of patients with uterine corpus cancer. Gynecol Oncol 108(3):486
4. Fung-Kee-Fung M, Dodge J et al (2006) Follow-up after primary therapy for endometrial cancer: a systematic review. Cancer care ontario program in evidence-based care gynecology cancer disease site group. Gynecol Oncol 101(3):520
5. American Joint Committee on Cancer (2010) Corpus uteri. In: AJCC staging manual 7th edn. Springer, New York, p 403
6. www.cancer.gov/cancertopics/pdq/screening/ovarian/healthprofessional/allpages
7. National Comprehensive Cancer Network (NCCN)
8. Buys SS, Partridge E et al (2011) Effect of screening on ovarian cancer mortality: the prostate, lung, colorectal and ovarian (PLCO) cancer screening randomized controlled trial. PLCO project team. JAMA 305(22):2295
9. Kobayashi H, Yamada Y et al (2008) A randomized study of screening for ovarian cancer: a multicenter study in Japan. Int J Gynecol Cancer 18(3):414
10. Menon U, Gentry-Maharaj A, Hallett R, Ryan A et al (2009) Sensitivity and specificity of multimodal and ultrasound screening for ovarian cancer, and stage distribution of detected cancers: results of the prevalence screen of the UK collaborative trial of ovarian cancer screening (UKCTOCS). Lancet Oncol 10(4):327
11. Van Nagell JR Jr, Miller RW et al (2011) Long-term survival of women with epithelial ovarian cancer detected by ultrasonographic screening. Obstet Gynecol 118(6):1212
12. NCCN Guidelines Version 2.2012: Epithelial ovarian cancer/fallopian tube cancer/primary peritoneal cancer. http://www.nccn.org.laneproxy.stanford.edu/professionals/physician_gls/pdf/ovarian.pdf
13. Benedet JL, Bender H et al (2000) FIGO staging classifications and clinical practice guidelines in the management of gynecologic cancers. FIGO committee on gynecologic oncology. Int J Gynaecol Obstet 70(2):209
14. Elit L, Fyles AW et al (2009) Follow-up for women after treatment for cervical cancer: a systematic review. Gynecology cancer disease site group. Gynecol Oncol 114(3):528
15. Salani R, Backes FJ et al (2011) Posttreatment surveillance and diagnosis of recurrence in women with gynecologic malignancies: society of gynecologic oncologists recommendations. Am J Obstet Gynecol 204(6):466

Part VIII
Breast Cancer

Breast Cancer

44

Dimitris-Andrew D. Tsiftsis

44.1 Introduction

In the USA for 2012 estimated are 229,060 new cases of breast cancer (BC) and 39,920 deaths. These figures make BC the leading malignancy in females with a 29 % share and second in morbidity with 14 % behind only lung cancer. The picture is similar in most western and developed countries. Although the annual incidence of BC in the USA has a 2 % decline between years 1999 and 2005, it is still increasing in developing countries. Encouraging though is the fact that since 1990 death rates decrease worldwide, reflecting the progress made in early diagnosis and treatment. We live in an era where technological advancement in breast imaging and individualized treatments can and will take this achievement a step further.

Due to the elevated awareness of women in relation to BC and the resulting adoption of preventive strategies, we witness a decrease in the mean diameter of invasive cancers with less axillary involvement, more in situ carcinomas and a steep increase in non-palpable image detected lesions. This poses more problems as to the more accurate BI-RADS classification, non-invasive tissue sampling, and less invasive staging. In addition to that, the spectacular advances in molecular biology have enabled us to classify BC to molecular subtypes according to gene expression profiles, to develop marker targeted therapies and identify a population in genetic predisposition to cancer development. Combined with information from patient's family and past history we can fairly accurately calculate her risk. In this setting, imaging oncology has a pivotal role to play in prevention protocols competing with chemoprevention and prophylactic surgery.

Critical to the employment of imaging modalities in breast oncology seems to be its rational and sensible use. Recently voices caution the overuse of high cost imaging especially in stage IV patients [1]. This is attributed to many factors such as easy access to high end technology, defensive practices, patients demand, treatment predicament, etc. If this trend continuous it will not only cause unnecessary harassment and anxiety to seriously ill patients but will waste funds and effort much needed from other actions. To combat this, health care providers must religiously adhere to evidence-based practice guidelines. In this context, new mammographic

D.-A. D. Tsiftsis (✉)
Hygeia Diagnostic and Therapeutic Center
of Athens, Er. Stavrou 4, 15123 Marousi, Greece
e-mail: d.d.tsiftsis@gmail.com

A. D. Gouliamos et al. (eds.), *Imaging in Clinical Oncology*,
DOI: 10.1007/978-88-470-5385-4_44, © Springer-Verlag Italia 2014

(Mm) techniques like photon-counting, contrast enhanced, positron emission, tomosynthesis and others, as breast specific gamma imaging, enhanced MRI, etc., have to be very carefully evaluated for their added diagnostic value as compared to cost and availability.

Reference

1. Yabroff KR, Warren JL (2012) High-cost imaging in elderly patients with stage IV cancer: challenges for research, policy, and practice. J Natl Cancer Inst 104:1113–1114

Mammographic Diagnosis of Breast Cancer

45

Evangelia C. Panourgias

Early diagnosis of breast cancer and successful treatment has resulted in a significant decrease in death from breast cancer. For a screening test to be effective it should lead to an earlier diagnosis, in the case of mammography, of breast cancer. The end result of primary or secondary prevention is to reduce mortality from the disease. Finding a cancer earlier may not always benefit the patient. Some women may be diagnosed with metastatic disease, but have such small primary tumors, that they are hard to detect even pathologically. On the other end of the spectrum, autopsy studies have shown that some women who died from other causes were incidentally diagnosed with breast cancer, post-mortem.

The advantage of using mammography as a screening tool is that it detects breast cancer in a presymptomatic stage, when the tumor has a smaller size and is more often lymph node negative, in comparison to palpable malignancies. The goal of screening with mammography is to detect more small non-palpable malignancies, in situ cancers and invasive breast lesions less than 15 mm in diameter. Data from randomized controlled trials and ongoing population screening programs have demonstrated that the most effective way to control breast cancer is to prevent it from proceeding to advanced stages by delaying its growth with early detection (secondary prevention). The reduction in death rate from breast cancer attributed to screening is in the range of 20–30 % [1].

According to an editorial by Cady and Michelson consider that the results from Sweden are a major public health achievement and secondary to numerous technical factors that require improvement [2].

Although screening women between 40 and 49 remains a controversial subject, the results from numerous studies show that screening women in their forties may reduce mortality from the disease. According to several large studies, the survival rate in the screened group was significantly higher than in the group where the women presented with palpable tumors, concluding that the results support regular screening with mammography for women aged 40–49 [3].

There is no consensus as to how often women should be screened. In the UK, triennial screening mammography is undertaken in women 50-years old and up. The Dutch screening program screens women between 50 and 75 years of age, every 2 years.

The ultimate solution to breast cancer is primary prevention of the disease. Until such a day or a universal cure is discovered, periodic mammographic screening, clinical breast examination, and monthly breast self-examination is the best way to prevent death from breast cancer. Because mammography may miss tumors, especially in younger women with dense

E. C. Panourgias (✉)
Department of Radiology, University of Athens, Medical School, Areteion Hospital, 76 Vasilisis Sofias Avenue, 11528, Athens, Greece
e-mail: epanourgias@yahoo.com

A. D. Gouliamos et al. (eds.), *Imaging in Clinical Oncology*,
DOI: 10.1007/978-88-470-5385-4_45, © Springer-Verlag Italia 2014

breasts, a palpable lesion must be clinically evaluated, despite a negative mammogram. Identifying an abnormality on a mammogram is the first step in diagnosing a malignancy.

An asymmetric density with spiculated or irregular margins on a mammogram is highly suggestive of breast cancer. Architectural distortion and pleiomorphic calcifications are mammographic findings that are consistent with breast malignancy.

Unfortunately, a significant number of tumors display atypical radiological characteristics. In addition, there is considerable radiological overlap between benign and malignant lesions.

Clustered or pleiomorphic microcalcifications on a mammogram are signs of breast cancer.

The development of new imaging tools such as digital mammography and tomosynthesis of the breast have made an impact lately on radiological diagnosis of breast cancer.

Clinical trials have compared digital mammography to screen film mammography. Digital mammography demonstrated an increased number of clinically relevant cancers, but demonstrates a slightly higher recall rate. In addition to this, lower radiation dose with these systems is now feasible. Currently, the major limitation of digital mammography is high cost of new equipment, but in time, filmless reporting using this screening tool may prove cost-effective.

Digital mammography and CAD aim to reduce the false negative rate, particularly for screening mammography by marking an electronically perceived abnormality and directing the attention of the interpreting radiologist toward it. The results of a recent study reported an increased cancer detection rate by 26–58.7 %. However, a significant limitation of this study was that it included cancer-only cases and therefore the specificity of the method could not be calculated [4].

Breast tomosynthesis is a new problem solving tool in women with dense breasts and lesions obscured by overlying breast tissue (Fig. 45.1). According to a recent study, this technique seems to increase the specificity of mammography and spot magnification may be unnecessary when using digital breast imaging.

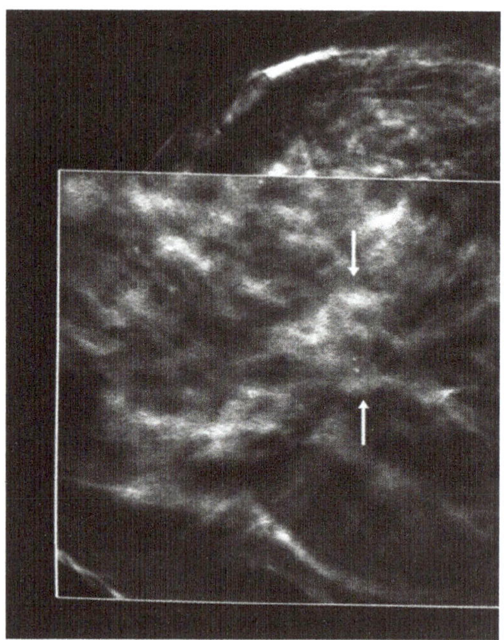

Fig. 45.1 The spicules of this small cancer are seen on this digital breast tomosynthesis (DBT) slice

45.1 Spiculated Density on a Mammogram

The majority of invasive malignant breast tumors present as stellate lesions on a mammogram. Occasionally, benign lesions such as postsurgical scars, fat necrosis, radial scars, sclerosing adenosis, and very rarely, granular cell tumors will appear as a stellate lesion on mammography.

The individual spicules are straight and dense, consisting primarily of collagen. They are seen clearly when the malignancy is embedded in fat, or almost invisible when surrounded by dense breast tissue (Figs. 45.2, 45.3). The spiculations radiate from a central solid mass and their length is determined by the size of the tumor. On mammography, these lesions tend to be stable from view to view.

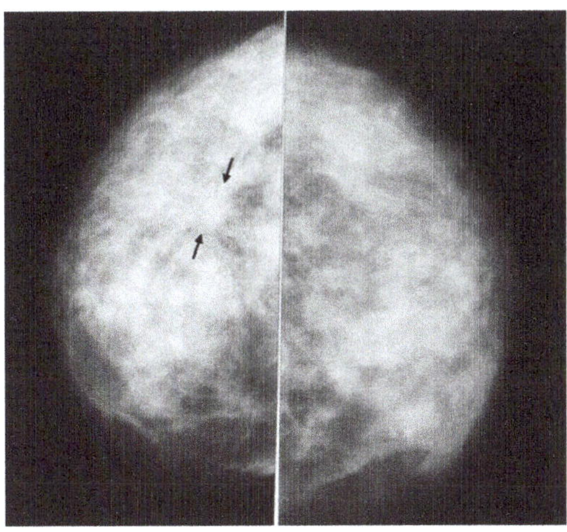

Fig. 45.2 Dense fibroglandular tissue in the craniocaudal views partially obscures a spiculated lesion in the lateral half of the right breast (*arrow*)

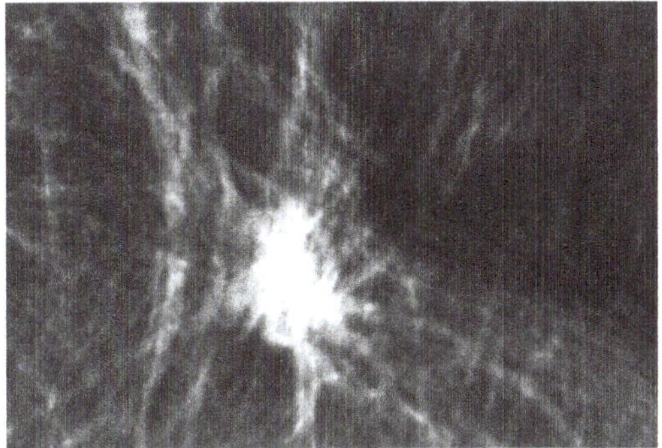

Fig. 45.3 Enlarged image of a typical stellate lesion with irregular margins

A spiculated lesion should be viewed with suspicion even when mammographically stable for a number of years. When analyzing a stellate lesion on a mammogram it is imperative to determine it really exists and not the result of overlapping normal breast tissue (pseudostellate structure). Spot compression and micro focus magnification views assist in making this decision.

If the additional views reveal lucencies in the central mass and, if the lesion changes its appearance from one view to the next, then the possibility of a radial scar should be considered.

Radial scars represent an idiopathic scarring process and is unrelated to known trauma. The mammographic appearance of such a lesion is not specific enough to permit reliable differentiation from cancer, surgical excision is recommended. It has been reported that FNAB and large core needle biopsy may result in under- or overdiagnosis, as about 30 % of the cases, are associated with atypia, low-grade DCIS, or tubular carcinoma. However, a recent study shows that patients who displayed benign biopsy results in cases of radial scars, did not reveal any signs of malignancy on surgical excision. Routine follow-up has been suggested in these patients [5].

A postsurgical scar may on occasion appear as a stellate mass on a mammogram. Frequently it looks different between projections, suspicious in one, and not clearly visible in the other.

Markers can be placed on the skin to relate to the incision of the underlying postsurgical scar. Postsurgical change usually diminishes over a period of 12–18 months.

45.2 Lesions with Irregular or Microlobulated Margins

Once a density is identified on a mammogram, it should be clarified if it is seen consistently in all projections or if it represents an asymmetry. Lesions with an ill-defined margin contour suggest a malignant process. Tumor infiltration is evident mammographically as an unsharp border because the cancer invades the surrounding breast tissue. A mass that is partially obscured by the surrounding parenchyma then further evaluation is required to distinguish between a well-circumscribed lesion and an ill-defined mass.

Digital breast tomosynthesis usually aids in margin assessment. If the margins are sharp then the mass should be examined sonographically. In the case of an ill-defined mass biopsy is indicated. The density of the mass should also be analyzed. If the mass has higher X-ray attenuation than the surrounding fibroglandular tissue then it should be viewed with suspicion. Tumors have increased density centrally, with the attenuation fading in the periphery. There are exceptions to this rule, especially in cases of colloid cancers where the attenuation is often lower than the surrounding parenchyma.

Many well-defined lesions display a degree of lobulation. However, multiple microlobulations are a sign of malignancy and the lesion should be examined pathologically.

Although sharply circumscribed lesions are most likely due to benign masses, there can be a differential diagnostic problem in cases of cancers appearing as circular masses with well-defined margins [6]. These include colloid, medullary cancers, and intracystic tumors. Adjunctive diagnostic tools such as ultrasound examination and biopsy should be used to arrive at an accurate diagnosis.

45.3 Focal Asymmetric Densities

An asymmetric density has many etiologies. The majority of lesions are due to asymmetric normal breast parenchyma. Benign causes include accessory breast tissue, asymmetric involution of breast parenchyma, or an area of fibrosis.

A mammographically suspicious focal asymmetry usually has ill-defined margins and is seen in both views. The lesion will have a dense core with fading density in the periphery (Fig. 45.4). Coned-down compression with microfocus magnification or digital breast tomosynthesis clarifies the image, since summation is eliminated. Once an asymmetry is characterized as a mass ultrasound may help to determine its nature. If it represents a solid lesion then biopsy should be considered.

Breast parenchyma gradually involutes over time, even though it may persist in many older women. The density of breast parenchyma may appear increased on the mammogram in women who lose a significant amount of weight or are on hormone replacement therapy (HRT). However, an increasing focal density when compared to prior studies should be evaluated carefully.

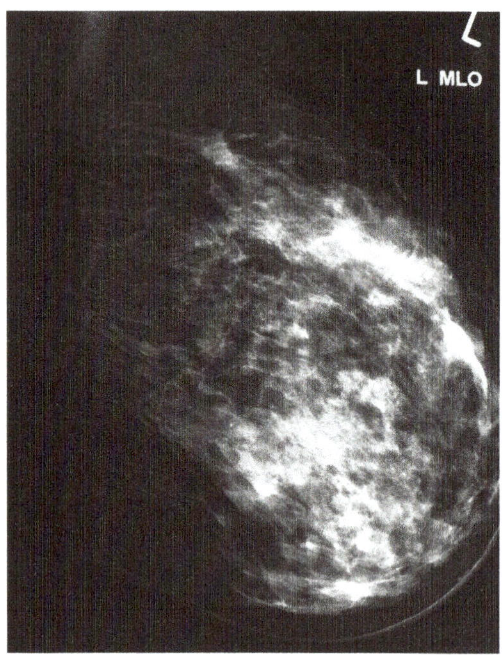

Fig. 45.4 An ill-defined density on the left mediolateral oblique projection

45.4 Architectural Distortion

Breast cancer does not always produce a lesion of increased density on a mammogram, but it may distort the normal tissues causing retraction, straightening, or flattening of the parenchymal contour. Perception of this subtle sign of malignancy is more difficult in women with denser breast tissue. Recognizing the normal breast anatomy makes characterization of architectural distortion possible.

On the mammogram Cooper's ligaments form a scalloped edge with the subcutaneous fat and concave toward the skin. A malignancy developing at the edge of the breast parenchyma causes peripheral architectural distortion. Lesions may cause retraction, flattening, straightening, or bulging of the parenchyma. A bulge or convexity is often due to cancer, but it may also indicate the presence of a cyst or fibroadenoma. The "tent sign" refers to retraction of the posterior edge of the breast tissue and is a specific mammographic sign of malignancy. On a mammogram tissue retraction produces a V-shaped border, resembling the peak of a tent.

Additional mammographic views are necessary to verify that an area of distortion exists. Oblique views clarify the location if the mammographic sign is initially seen in only one view. Magnification and spot compression may demonstrate associated microcalcifications or the presence of a mass.

Benign causes of architectural distortion include postsurgical scarring and fat necrosis.

A permanent mammographically visible scar is not common. The imager must correlate the region of previous surgery with the underlying architectural distortion. Unless architectural distortion clearly coincides with a site of previous surgery, it should be biopsied. Radial scars often have thin spicules converging on a lucent or partially lucent center. This characteristic is suggestive of a radial scar, but because it cannot be reliably differentiated from a malignancy, a biopsy is warranted to provide a reliable diagnosis [7].

45.5 Calcifications

Mammography remains to this day, the most important method of detecting microcalcifications. There are a wide variety of calcifications in the breast. Most of them have typical morphologies and are due to benign lesions. Excluding calcifications of benign etiology is the first step of the analysis. Densities that mimic microcalcifications should be effectively excluded. These include technical artifacts such as screen scratches, specks of dust between the screen and film, and skin ointments.

All other cases of breast calcifications on a mammogram should be studied and divided into categories according to their number, size, shape, and distribution. Evaluation of microcalcifications should include the presence of an associated tumor. If they cannot be reliably classified, then they should be further analyzed with magnification views.

The first characteristic to analyze is size. Malignant microcalcifications are usually less than 0.5 mm in diameter. A cluster is defined as five or more calcifications within a 1 cm^3 volume of the breast. Groups of calcifications containing less than five calcifications are most likely due to a benign process [8].

The probability of malignancy increases when the calcifications are heterogeneous in size and shape and when the number of particles is increased in a specific volume of breast tissue.

The shape of microcalcifications can be categorized into the following patterns: (1) round or punctuate, (2) amorphous or indistinct, (3) pleiomorphic or heterogeneous, and (4) fine linear, branching, or casting calcifications. The first type usually indicates a benign process. If a cluster of round microcalcifications appears for the first time, then they are probably benign and should be followed up on 6-monthly basis for a year and yearly for 3 years after that to establish stability of the finding. If these calcifications change in any way, then a biopsy is suggested.

Amorphous or hazy calcifications are moderately suspicious. Benign conditions in which they can be encountered are adenosis, fibroadenomas, and fat necrosis. If they appear in clusters and tend to be heterogeneous, they should be biopsied.

Pleiomorphic or heterogeneous microcalcifications, sometimes referred to as "crushed stone" or "granular type", are suspicious for malignancy. The more irregular the individual particles in size and shape, the more suspicious they are. The malignant epithelial cells accumulate in the duct and expand it. The cells in the center of the duct have minimal blood supply and central necrosis occurs. Because this occurs in an irregular fashion at the center of the intraductal cancer, the resulting microcalcifications are irregular in shape and size [9].

Fine linear casting calcifications are thin, irregular calcifications that occasionally branch. High grade ductal carcinoma causes extensive necrosis interspersed with amorphous calcifications. These fragmented calcifications appear on the mammogram as linear, branching casts of the duct lumen, termed as casting-type calcifications. This is a reliable sign of malignancy, having a positive predictive value of 92 % [10].

A subtype of the casting-type calcifications is the dotted castings pattern. When the cancer cells in the duct have a micropapillary architecture, these protrusions may break off, undergo

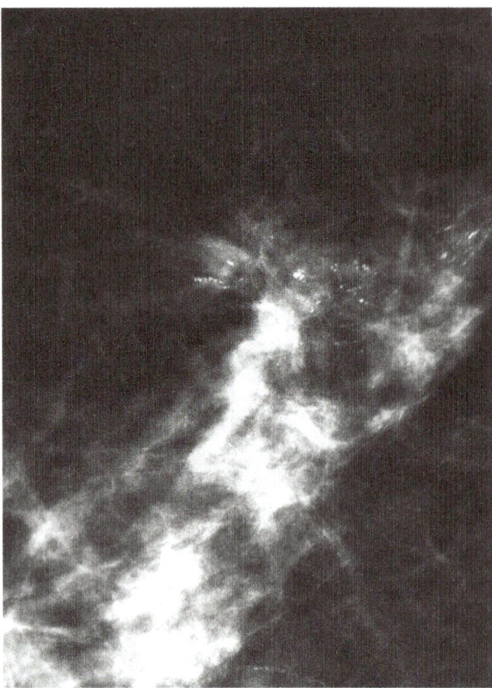

Fig. 45.5 An enlarged view of a spiculated lesion associated with fine, linear, heterogeneous calcifications in the lateral portion of the right breast

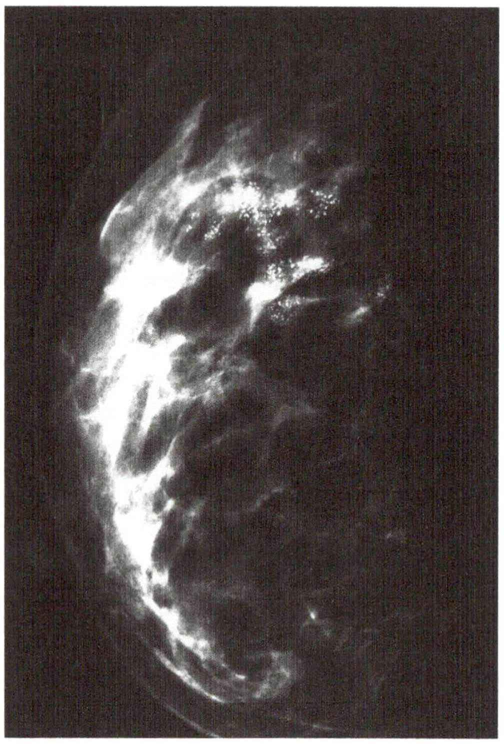

Fig. 45.6 Segmentally distributed irregular, heterogeneous calcifications in the right breast, on the craniocaudal (**a**) and (**b**) mediolateral projection

necrosis, and calcify within the lumen. The lumen is then filled with a plethora of tiny calcifications, giving the cast a dotted appearance.

Five patterns of distribution have been described by the American College of Radiolgy BIRADS:

1. clustered
2. linear
3. segmental
4. regional
5. diffusely scattered

Clustered calcifications are the most difficult to analyze and the cause of most benign biopsies. Aetiologies include adenosis, papillomas, atypical hyperplasia, as well as low-grade carcinoma. Biopsy is often warranted to establish the diagnosis.

Linearly distributed calcifications within ducts, pleiomorphic in morphology are almost always due to a malignant process (Fig. 45.5).

Segmental distribution represents calcifications within a single duct or lobe. This distribution descriptor is highly predictive of malignancy.

Anatomically, it is defined by a major duct and its branches spreading into the breast, beginning in the terminal ductal lobules of the breast (Fig. 45.6a, b). Malignant processes include extensive DCIS unilaterally or less often, bilaterally. Mammographically, multiple, heterogeneous calcifications confined to a large segment of the breast are observed. Benign lesions are less common and usually associated with adenosis. In most cases, biopsy is necessary.

Calcifications that appear randomly or diffusely distributed throughout the breast are mainly due to benign processes. Differential diagnosis of the diffuse pattern as opposed to extensive segmental distribution is imperative. The latter are highly suspicious and need to be biopsied.

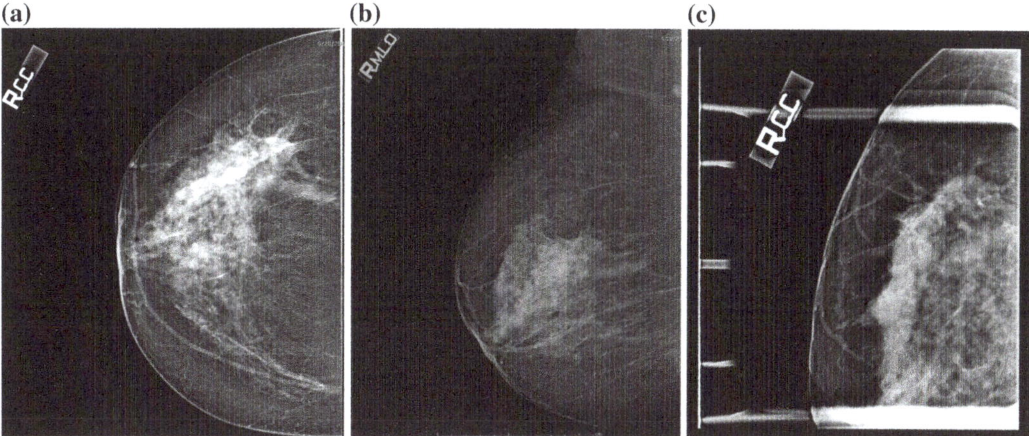

Fig. 45.7 Skin retraction and local thickening in the upper outer quadrant of the right breast is seen. **a** Right craniocaudal, and (**b**) mediolateral projection. On the spot compression of the right breast (**c**) an area of spiculated architectural distortion at the edge of the parenchyma is apparent, causing retraction of the skin

The stability of intermediate or suspicious microcalcifications is not a reassuring sign of benignity. Short interval follow-up for these cases is suggested for a period of 2 years and if the calcifications remain stable in number and morphology, then the woman may return to routine screening. Suspicious microcalcifications associated with a mass usually indicate an invasive cancer with an associated intraductal component. These lesions are becoming less common now that breast cancer is being discovered at an earlier stage.

There are several less commonly seen findings that could be associated with breast cancer.

45.6 Skin Changes and Trabecular Thickening

Skin changes that are associated with malignancy occur late in the disease, either with direct invasion by the tumor or obstruction of the lymphatic return. Skin is better evaluated clinically. The mammogram mainly evaluates the underlying tissues and not the skin.

Skin retraction usually occurs because of a tumor lying close to the overlying skin (Fig. 45.7a, b, c).

Diffuse skin thickening is usually associated with trabecular coarsening and diffuse increased density of the breast tissue is a late manifestation of breast cancer. These mammographic signs are rather specific of inflammatory cancer, even though rarely, inflammatory changes may be observed in benign cases. These include infection, granulomatous mastitis, congestive heart disease, and superficial thrombophlebitis.

Enlarged axillary lymph nodes indicate a progressed stage of the disease and have a negative impact on survival. In cases of occult breast carcinoma presenting with axillary lymph node metastases, a primary tumor was found pathologically in 75 % of the cases.

References

1. Tabár L, Vitak B, Chen TH, Yen AM, Cohen A, Tot T, Chiu SY, Chen SL, Fann JC, Rosell J, Fohlin H, Smith RA, Duffy SW (2011) Swedish two-county trial: impact of mammographic screening on breast cancer mortality during 3 decades. Radiology 260(3):658–663
2. Cady B, Michaelson JS (2001) The life-sparing potential of mammographic screening. Cancer 1(9):1699–1703
3. Shen N, Hammonds LS, Madsen D, Dale P (2011) Mammography in 40-year-old women: what difference does it make? The potential impact of the U.S. preventative services task force (USPSTF) mammography guidelines. Ann Surg Oncol 18(11):3066–3071
4. Cole EB, Zhang Z, Marques HS, Nishikawa RM, Hendrick RE, Yaffe MJ, Padungchaichote W,

Kuzmiak C, Chayakulkheeree J, Conant EF, Fajardo LL, Baum J, Gatsonis C, Pisano E. (2012). Assessing the stand-alone sensitivity of computer-aided detection with cancer cases from the digital mammographic imaging screening trial. AJR Am J Roentgenol 199(3):W392–401

5. Karen A Lee, Margarita L Zuley, Mamatha Chivukula, Neha Desai Choksi, Marie A Ganott, Jules H Sumkin. (2012) Original research: risk of malignancy when microscopic radial scars and microscopic papillomas are found at percutaneous biopsy. AJR198:141–145
6. Swann CA, Kopans DB, Koerner FC, McCarthy KA, White G, Hall DA (1987) The halo sign and malignant breast lesions. AJR Am J Roentgenol 149(6):1145–1147
7. Mitnick JS, Vazquez MF, Harris MN, Roses DF (1989) Differentiation of radial scar from scirrhous carcinoma of the breast: mammographic-pathologic correlation. Radiology 173:697–700
8. Thomas DB, Whitehead J, Dorse C, Threatt BA, Gilbert FI Jr, Present AJ, Carlile T (1993) Mammographic calcifications and risk of subsequent breast cancer. J Natl Cancer Inst 85(3):230–235
9. Yamada T, Mori N, Watanabe M, Kimijima I, Okumoto T, Seiji K, Takahashi S (2010) Radiologic-pathologic correlation of ductal carcinoma in situ. Radiographics 30(5):1183–1198
10. Bent CK, Bassett LW, D' Orsi CJ, Sayre JW (2010) The positive predictive value of BI-RADS microcalcification descriptors and final assessment categories. AJR Am J Roentgenol 194(5):1378–1383

US Findings in Breast Cancer

46

Elias C. Primetis and Irene S. Vraka

46.1 Introduction

Breast ultrasound is an important diagnostic tool complementary to mammography, especially in women with mammographically dense breasts. Breast ultrasound technology evolves continuously. Currently, with the introduction of the new high resolution probes (11–14 MHz), investigators evaluate a possible role of the breast ultrasound for screening purposes.

46.2 Indications and Findings

Despite of the marked improvements in technology and image quality over the past decade, ultrasound remains primarily a method for differentiating cystic lesions from solid masses and for guiding interventional procedures (aspiration, localization, and core biopsies). It is also used as an adjunct diagnostic tool to further investigate and characterize suspicious findings in mammography. A classification system (BI-RADS for breast ultrasound) similar to that of mammography has been developed for assessment of mass lesions, based on the following lesion characteristics [1]:

1. *Echogenicity*: Anechoic, hyperechoic, isoechoic, hypoechoic, or mixed echogenicicy
2. *Shape*: Oval, round, irregular
3. *Orientation*: Parallel, non parallel
4. *Margin*: Circumscribed, not circumscribed (indistinct, angular, microlobulated, spiculated)
5. *Lesion boundary*: Abrupt interface, thick echogenic rim
6. *Posterior acoustic features*: Posterior acoustic enhancement, posterior acoustic shadowing
7. *Surrounding structures*: Cooper ligaments, ducts, skin.

The suspicious sonographic features can be thought of as "hard", "soft", and "mixed". The "hard" findings suggest the presence of invasive cancer. The "soft" findings tend to represent ductal carcinoma in situ (DCIS) components of the lesion. The "mixed" findings can represent either invasive or DCIS component [2] (Table 46.1), (Fig. 46.1).

A controversial issue is the use of ultrasound for breast cancer screening using either the established technique of handheld whole breast ultrasound or the newer development of volumetric—Automated Breast Ultrasound (ABUS). There is only one randomized control study that addresses the possible role of ABUS as a screening tool for cancer detection [3].

An additional potential use of ultrasound is lymph nodes staging by localizing and aspirate or biopsy axillary lymph nodes with sonographic

E. C. Primetis (✉) · I. S. Vraka
Department of Radiology, University of Athens Medical School, Aretaieion Hospital, 76, Vas. Sofias Avenue, 11528, Athens, Greece
e-mail: elprimetis@yahoo.gr

I. S. Vraka
e-mail: irenevraka@yahoo.gr

A. D. Gouliamos et al. (eds.), *Imaging in Clinical Oncology*,
DOI: 10.1007/978-88-470-5385-4_46, © Springer-Verlag Italia 2014

Table 46.1 Hard versus soft suspicious sonographic findings for malignancy

	Finding
Hard	Spiculation/thick hyperechoic halo
	Angular margins
	Acoustic shadowing
Mixed	Taller than wide (not parallel)
	Hypoechoic appearance
	Microlobulation
Soft	Calcifications
	Duct extension
	Branch pattern

features indicative of metastatic disease [4] (Fig. 46.2). Ultrasound is a valuable diagnostic tool in localizing, evaluate and biopsy additional lesions depicted by breast MRI (targeted or second—look ultrasound).

46.3 Results

Breast ultrasound differentiates cystic from solid lesions. According to a landmark study by Stavros et al. [5], it has also a high sensitivity (approximately 93 %) in characterizing a lesion as malignant or not benign and a high negative predictive value (99.5 %). On the other hand,

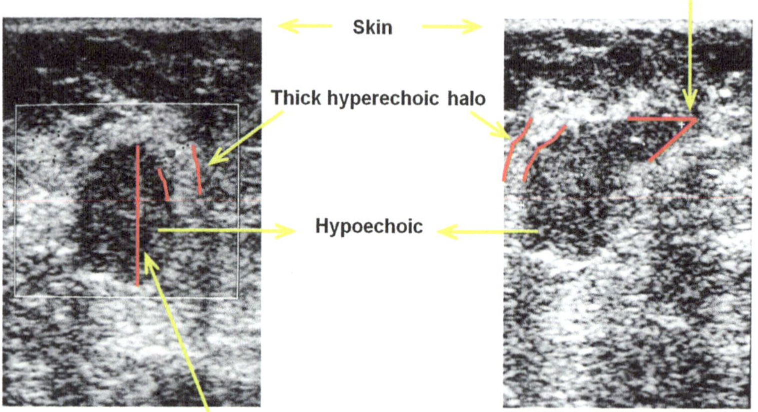

Fig. 46.1 Ultrasound images in two different sites of the same cancerous nodule and its BI-RADS descriptors

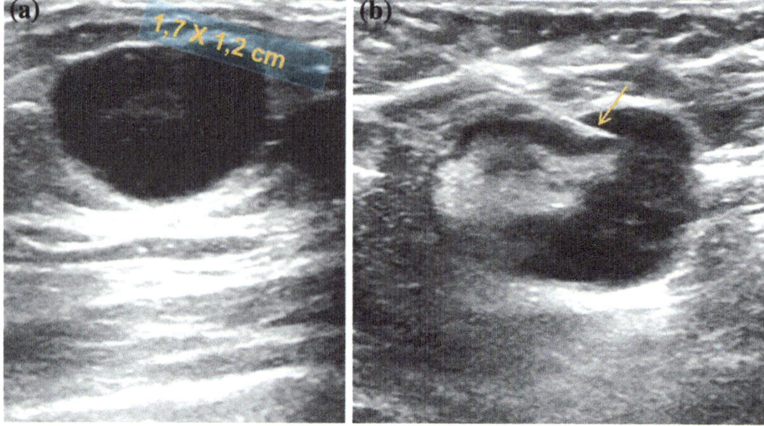

Fig. 46.2 Enlarged intramammary lymph node with cortical thickening and indistinct fatty hilum (**a**). Enlarged axillary lymph node with cortical thickening. Aspiration needle (*arrow*)

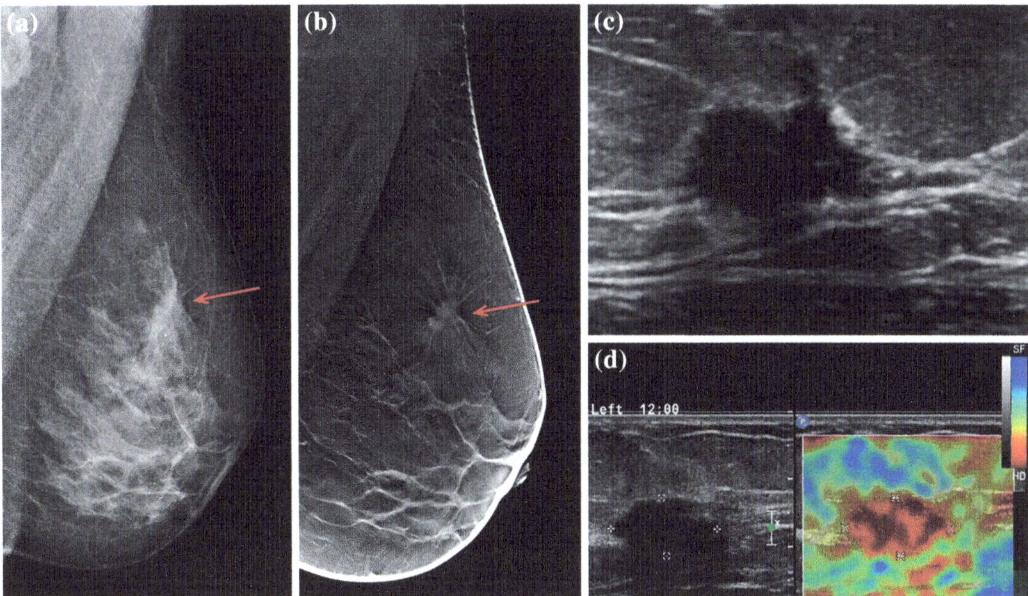

Fig. 46.3 16 mm invasive ductal cancer in a 42-year-old woman. Mammography (**a**) shows an architectural distortion. Tomosynthesis −1 mm slice (**b**) reveals a spiculated mass. Ultrasound (**c**) shows a solid hypoechoic spiculated mass with mild acoustic shadowing. Lesion is hard on elastography (**d**), a characteristic feature of cancerous lesions (hard depicted as *red* in color mapping)

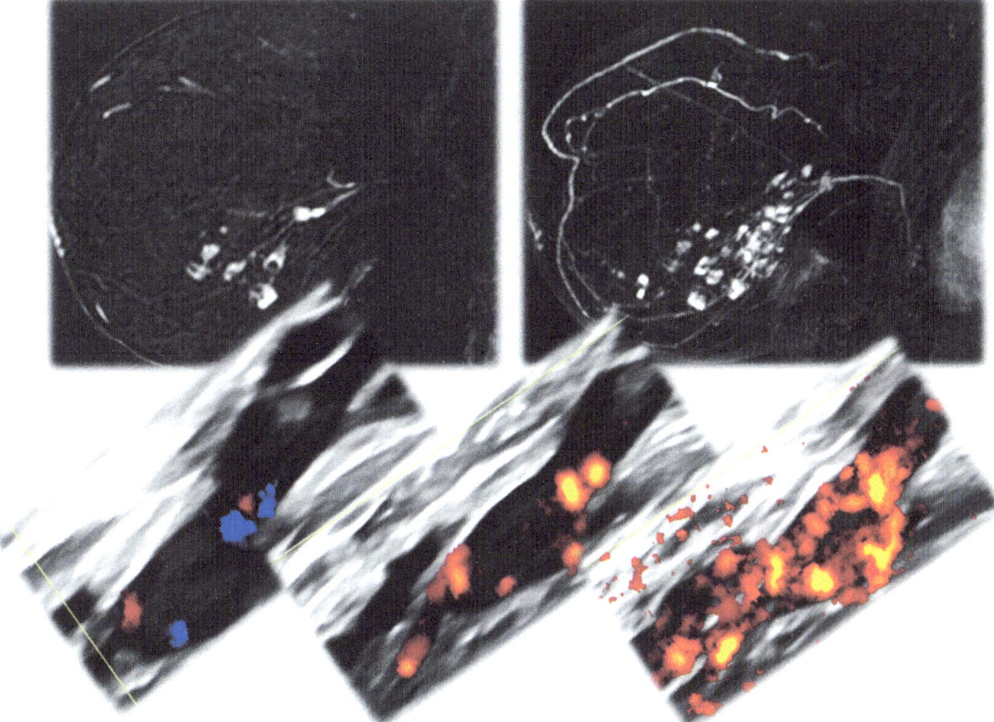

Fig. 46.4 DCIS: MRI shows regional stippled enhancement. Targeted ultrasound reveals intraductal hypervascular tissue

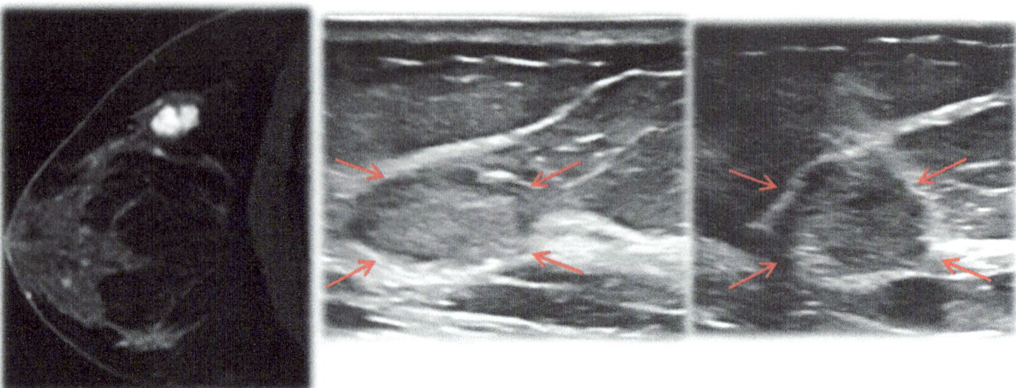

Fig. 46.5 Mixed mucinous carcinoma: MRI shows an enhancing lesion. Targeted ultrasound revealed an isoechoic (easily overlooked) lesion

ultrasound lead in unnecessary biopsies, as its specificity and positive predictive value are low (20.2 and 38.7 %, respectively). Combined conventional ultrasound and elastography was more specific than conventional ultrasound alone. Combining elastography with ultrasound improved specificity and positive predictive value (33.3 and 45.1 %, respectively) [6, 7] (Fig. 46.3). Targeted or second—look ultrasound can identify as many as 89 % of the additional detected lesions on breast MRI and is a reliable method to correlate, further evaluate and biopsy suspicious additional MRI abnormalities [8] (Figs. 46.4, 46.5).

46.4 Conclusions

Breast ultrasound helps in differentiating cystic from solid lesions and in further characterizing solid nodules. Sonographic features of malignancy include speculations, hypoechogenicity, microlobulation, shadowing, vertical orientation of lesion (taller than wide), and angular margins. Ultrasound is a reliable diagnostic tool in evaluation of the axillary lymph node status and in identifying additional abnormalities initially detected on breast MRI. The ability of ultrasound to localize and characterize lesions affects decision making in clinical patient management and contributes to improve patient care.

References

1. American College of Radiology (2003) BI-RADS-US. In: ACR BI-RADS breast imaging reporting and data system breast imaging atlas. American College of Radiology, Reston
2. Stavros TA, Rapp CL, Kaske TI, Parker SH (2005) Hard and soft sonographic findings of malignancy. In: Feig SA (ed) Syllabus, breast imaging, categorical course in diagnostic radiology. Radiological Society of North America, Oak Brook, pp 125–142
3. Kelly KM, Dean J, Lee SJ, Comulada WS (2010) Breast cancer detection: radiologists' performance using mammography with and without automated whole-breast ultrasound. Eur Radiol 20:2557–2564
4. Garcia-Ortega MJ, Benito MA, Vahamonde EF et al (2011) Pretreatment axillary ultrasonography and core biopsy in patients with suspected breast cancer: diagnostic accuracy and impact on management. Eur J Radiol 79:64–72
5. Stavros AT, Thickman D, Rapp CL et al (1995) Solid breast nodules: use of sonography to distinguish between benign and malignant lesions. Radiology 196:123–134
6. Itoh A, Ueno E, Tohno E et al (2006) Breast disease: clinical application of US elastography for diagnosis. Radiology 239:341–350
7. Yoon JH, Kim MH, Kim EK et al (2011) Interobserver variability of ultrasound elastography: how it affects the diagnosis of breast lesions. AJR Am J Roentgenol 196:730–736
8. Beran L, Liang W, Nims T et al (2005) Correlation of targeted ultrasound with magnetic resonance imaging abnormalities of the breast. Am J Surg 190:592–594

MR Mammography

47

Arkadios Chr. Rousakis and Dimitrios G. Spigos

Early attempts to study the breast with magnetic resonance imaging (MRI) were not successful. In the late 1980s, however, the introduction of the intravenous use of paramagnetic contrast agents (CA) dramatically increased the diagnostic accuracy of MRI and made it clinically relevant. The concept of using CA for the detection of breast cancer relies on the fact that malignant neoplasms grow faster and invade adjacent normal tissues. Thus, they develop new blood supply called neovascularity. Because the blood flow of tumors is different than that of normal tissues, it can be analyzed either visually or with the aid of computers.

Today, MRI of the breast or MR mammography (MRM) is an established method in the diagnostic armamentarium of most medical centers. However, its wider use is hindered due its expense, and also because most clinicians are not well acquainted with its indications.

D. G. Spigos (✉)
Radiology Hygeia Hospital, Erythrou Stavrou 4,
Athens, 15123, Attica, Greece
e-mail: Spigos.1@osu.edu

A. Chr. Rousakis
Radiology Hygeia Hospital, Erythrou Stavrou 4,
Marousi, 15123 Attica, Greece
e-mail: a.rousakis@hygeia.gr

47.1 Choice of Equipment and Imaging Techniques for MRM

As in other MRI studies, the diagnosis of malignant and benign tumors is dependent on intravenous injection of gadolinium chelates CA. After the contrast is injected, it accumulates in the extracellular space of tissues and causes variations of T1 and T2 relaxation times that last a few minutes. The contrast leaks out faster from tumors than normal tissues, allowing for their differentiation. The usual contrast dose for MRM is 0.1 mmol per kilogram of body weight. The contrast is commonly injected in an antecubital fossa vein with a power injector at a rate of 3 ml per second, and is traced by a 20–30 ml normal saline flush.

MRM should be performed with equipment that provides strong magnetic field, possesses strong gradients, and has advanced software for the application of adequate imaging sequences. Magnets with field strength less than 1.5 Tesla (T), are not suitable for MRM as their signal-to-noise ratio is low. Although different imaging protocols can be successfully used on different magnets, they should all satisfy certain criteria. Effective fat suppression is essential, as fatty tissue is prevalent in most breasts. Superior spatial resolution is mandatory, so that the lesions' morphology can be depicted and studied in detail. Finally, high temporal resolution (fast imaging sequences) is needed for successful

A. D. Gouliamos et al. (eds.), *Imaging in Clinical Oncology*,
DOI: 10.1007/978-88-470-5385-4_47, © Springer-Verlag Italia 2014

"dynamic studies," as the contrast tends to transit quickly in malignant tumors and washes out. The best time for their maximal detection is the early post contrast phase between 60 and 120 s [1, 2].

Diffusion-weighted imaging (DWI) displays the apparent diffusion (free motion) of water molecules in tissues, where the movement of water is modified by its interaction with cell membranes and macromolecules. In the extracellular space of dense cellular tissues, such as tumors, the diffusion of water is restricted. DWI is evaluated either qualitatively as an "apparent diffusion coefficient (ADC) map", or quantitatively based on ADC measurements. ADC measurements can be magnet specific and also depend on the DWI sequence that is used (b values) [3].

MR spectroscopy (MRS) is a noninvasive method of obtaining metabolic information in vivo and, thus, can help in tissue characterization. Protons are commonly used in clinical MRS because of their high nuclear abundance and sensitivity. The metabolite used to diagnose breast cancer is choline, which is detected at 3.2 ppm. If MRS is to be employed, high field strength is needed to acquire enough signal within a reasonable period of time. This can be done better with 3T magnets.

In our institution, MRM studies are performed either in a 1.5T or a 3T magnet. Both breasts are always imaged simultaneously, placed symmetrically within a dedicated surface coil, with the patient in prone position. After obtaining a three-plane localizer scan, the first acquisition is an axial turbo spin echo T2-weighted sequence with a field of view (FOV) of 330 mm and slice thickness of 2.5 mm (1.5T) or 4 mm (3T). The next acquisition is a dynamic series that consists of a repetitive T1-weighted three-dimensional gradient echo (GE) sequence, with a FOV of 330 mm and slice thickness of 2.5 mm. Each acquisition lasts 81–87 s. We obtain one acquisition before the injection of CA and three following the bolus contrast injection. Fat suppression is used in the 3T protocol, while non-fat suppressed images are obtained with the 1.5T dynamic series. A high spatial resolution axial fat suppressed T1-weighted GE sequence with a slice thickness of 1.2 mm (1.5T) or 0.7 mm (3T), is interposed between the second and third postcontrast scan of the dynamic series. Finally, we obtain an axial DWI sequence with b values 0, 400, and 800 (1.5T) or 0, 750, and 1,200 (3T). In selected cases, we perform proton MRS of lesions with a diameter more than 1.5 cm, exclusively in the 3T magnet.

Postprocessing is routinely performed in a computer-aided detection (CAD) system, which provides subtraction images of the postcontrast scans of dynamic series and maximum intensity projection (MIP) reconstructions of each set of subtracted images. It also enables immediate pixel-by-pixel measurements of the signal intensity (SI) of detected breast lesions. On the images of the dynamic study, it automatically provides the kinetic curves and permits measurements of ADC values. Also, it offers accurate localization of each lesion in relation to the nipple, skin, and thoracic wall. Finally, it incorporates a standard reporting format according to the guidelines of American College of Radiology Imaging Network (ACRIN). We find the postprocessing station very useful for accelerating the workflow of interpreting MRM studies, and also for better presentation of the results to the breast surgeons. When MRM is performed for evaluation of breast implants, we incorporate in the imaging protocol additional "dual-inversion recovery" and "silicon-only" sequences on the axial and sagittal planes.

47.2 Diagnostic Criteria of MRM

When interpreting an MRM, one should first determine if a focus or region of abnormal contrast enhancement is a lesion. When a lesion is found, it has to be decided if it is benign or malignant. The differential diagnosis is based on the lesion's morphology and its kinetics (hemodynamic behavior) [1, 2]. Specifically, we have to decide if the contrast enhancement is a focus, a mass, or a non-mass enhancement.

An enhancing lesion that is 5 mm or less is defined as a focus. Foci are too small to characterize and are overwhelmingly benign. In a

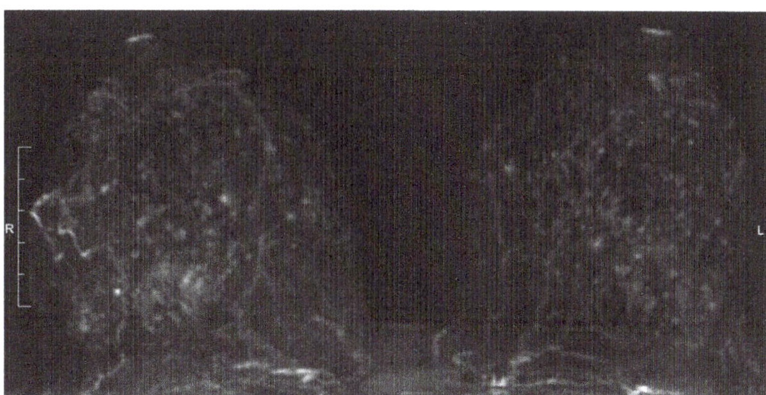

Fig. 47.1 Focal enhancement: on this MIP reconstruction of subtracted post contrast images, multiple tiny foci of contrast uptake (diameter <5 mm) with a symmetric distribution are seen in both breasts

study, only 1 out of 37 foci was found to be malignant [4] (Fig. 47.1).

A mass is a space-occupying lesion that, as in mammography, can be described in three dimensions (Fig. 47.2). A non-mass enhancement has no correlate in precontrast sequences and is non-specific (Fig. 47.3). The differential diagnosis of non-mass enhancement abnormalities includes DCIS, lobular breast cancer, inflammatory changes, and changes due to hormonal stimulation either from external sources or from physiologic hormonal fluctuations during the woman's menstrual cycle. Then, the extent, shape, and morphology of the enhancing lesion or area have to be evaluated.

In the case of a mass lesion, its shape, border, and internal structure (homogenous or heterogeneous enhancement, peripheral "ring-like" enhancement, presence of internal septations showing or not contrast enhancement) and SI on T1 and T2-weighted images need to be assessed. The hemodynamic behavior of an enhancing lesion is defined by the speed of contrast uptake (time to reach the peak contrast enhancement), the intensity of enhancement (the percentile of increase of the SI of the lesion), and the

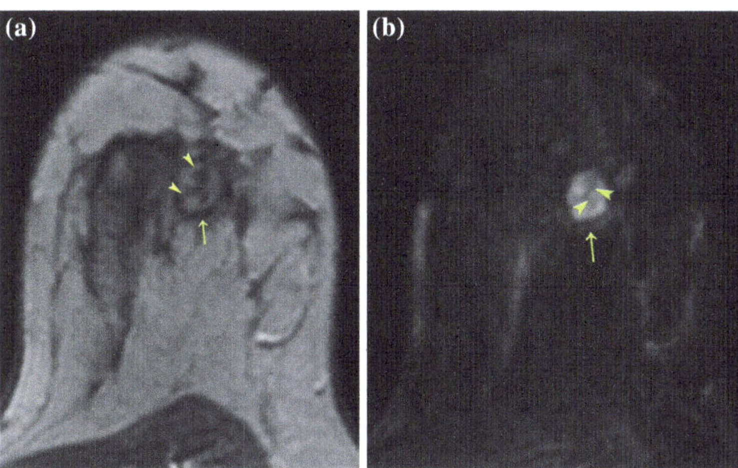

Fig. 47.2 Mass enhancement . **a** Axial T1-w. post contrast image, where a well-defined round-shaped mass is seen in the central part of left breast, easily demarcated from the surrounding normal mammary parenchyma (*arrow*). **b** Corresponding subtracted image, on which the mass-like enhancing lesion (a typical fibroadenoma) is better delineated (*arrow*). Note the characteristic internal septations which do not show any contrast uptake (*arrowheads*)

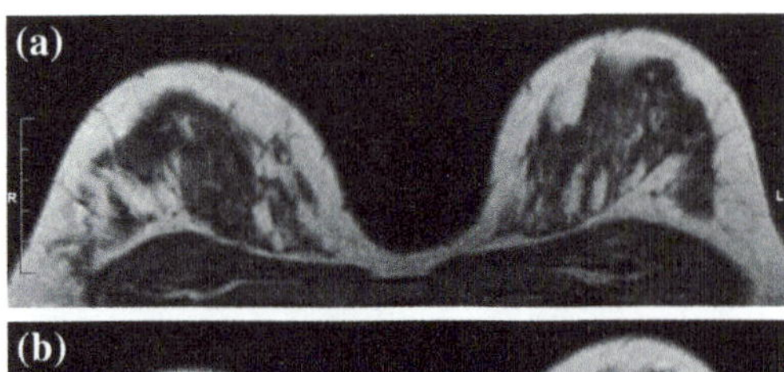

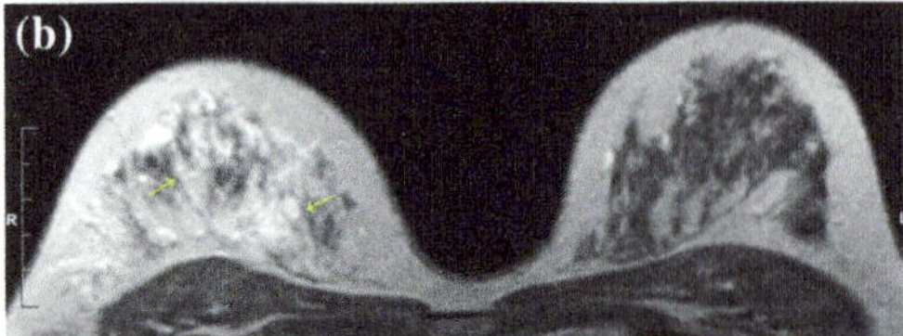

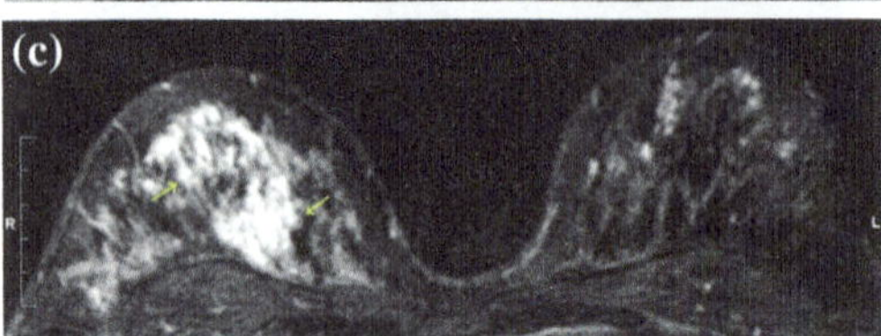

Fig. 47.3 Non-mass like enhancement . Axial T1-w. images pre contrast injection (**a**), late post contrast (**b**) and corresponding subtraction image (**c**). There are multiple confluent foci and areas of abnormal contrast uptake in the right breast (*arrows*), which cannot be anatomically separated from the adjacent parenchyma

retention or washout of the contrast medium from the lesion. These basic hemodynamic features are represented by the "hemodynamic curve" (derived if the SI of a lesion, after the bolus IV injection of contrast, is plotted against time), which may have three main types: Type 1 curve is characterized by a continuous increase of the SI during the dynamic study and is usually associated with benign lesions. Type 2 curve shows a steep early increase of the SI, reaching its peak value during the first two dynamic scans post contrast, and then a stable horizontal course (plateau). Type 2 curves are the least specific of the three types. Type 3 curve resembles the type 2 regarding the steep early increase of the SI, but it exhibits a fast decrease due to "wash-out" of the contrast. It is commonly associated with malignant lesions (Fig. 47.4).

47.3 Imaging of Malignant Neoplasms with MRM

Infiltrating breast carcinoma is typically imaged on MRM as a mass lesion with intense inhomogeneous contrast uptake. It usually has ill-defined and irregular borders, occasionally with spiculated margins. It is often accompanied by contrast enhancement along lactiferous ducts, a sign of co-existing intraductal neoplasia. Regarding its kinetic curve, it is typically of type 3 and occasionally the non-specific type 2. However, there are malignancies such as lobular cancers and DCIS, which show type 1 curve and/or may have smooth margins and well-defined borders. Myeloid and mucinous cancers may mimic benign lesions such as mastopathy and fibroadenomas [1]. If the tumor is very large, it may have areas of necrosis, usually in its central portions, and may exhibit the characteristic peripheral "ring-like" enhancement pattern. Other secondary findings associated with breast

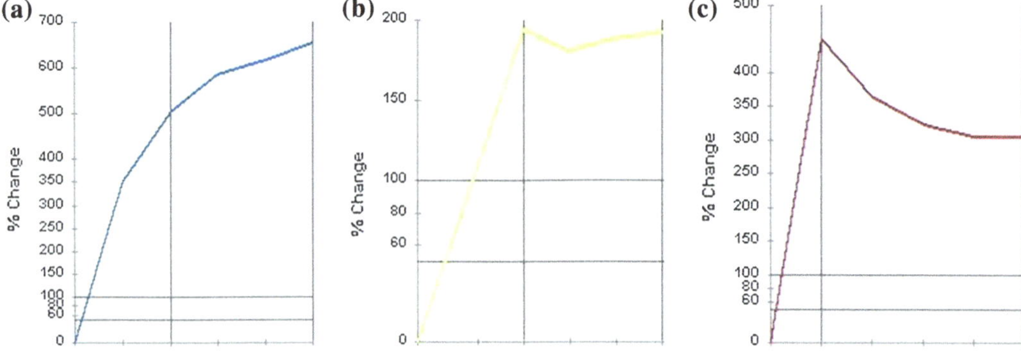

Fig. 47.4 Kinetic *curves* of type 1 (**a**), 2 (**b**), and 3 (**c**)

cancer are skin thickening, nipple retraction, prominent veins, metastatic axillary lymph nodes, and distant metastases in structures of the thorax such as in ribs, vertebrae, or the lungs (Fig. 47.5).

DCIS has variable enhancement; it grows in a linear fashion along the ductal system from its periphery and toward the nipple. If abnormal calcifications are detected in the same location by mammography, the diagnosis can be suggested with certainty. As in other malignancies, the grade and aggressiveness of this disease varies. Thus, the kinetic curves may be of benign or malignant type (Fig. 47.6). Also, 10–25 % of DCIS cases are diagnosed because of microcalcifications on mammography, they may not show any contrast enhancement and, thus, remain undetected by MRM.

Inflammatory breast cancer, as the name implies, can mimic diseases of infectious etiology. It often develops without a palpable mass. Most patients are diagnosed after they fail to respond to antibiotic treatment. Mammograms (MG), ultrasound (US), and MRM are helpful in establishing the diagnosis. Multiple small, confluent, heterogeneously enhancing masses and global skin thickening are key MRM features of inflammatory breast cancer (Fig. 47.7). In a study of 88 patients with inflammatory breast cancer, MRM established the diagnosis correctly in 98 % of the cases versus 68 % for MG and 94 % for US [5].

47.4 Imaging of Benign Lesions with MRM

Although breast cancer is the most common cancer in women in western countries, benign lesions of the breast are far more frequent [1, 2]. Detailed description of their imaging features on MRM is beyond the scope of this chapter. Inflammatory conditions, such as acute mastitis, usually occur in the first three post partum months, and are primarily a clinical diagnosis. Granulomatous mastitis is secondary to systemic autoimmune diseases, such as sarcoidosis. Identification of its etiology requires microbiologic, immunologic, and histopathologic evaluations, as the findings from MRM are non-specific.

Benign tumors such as fibroadenomas appear as space occupying lesions with well-defined margins. The internal enhancement of these lesions is typically homogeneous with type 1 curve and, quite often, have characteristic non-enhancing internal septation (Fig. 47.2). Myxoid fibroadenomas are more common in young women. They are hypervascular, and usually show fast and intense contrast enhancement with

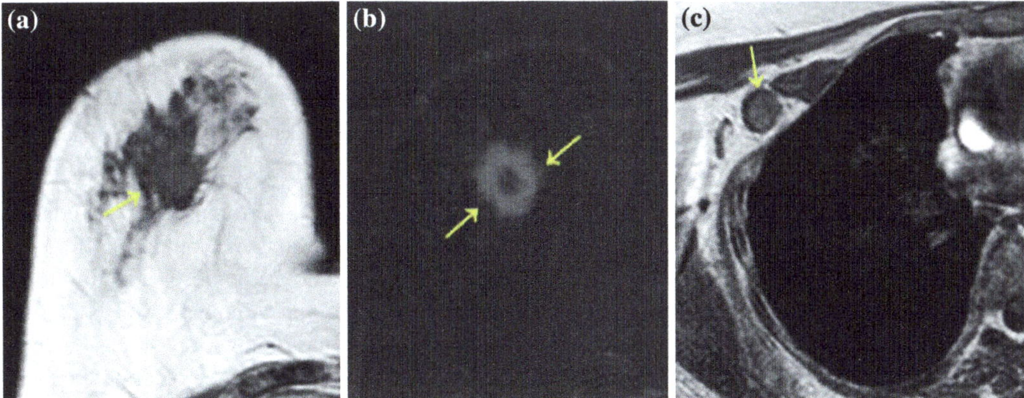

Fig. 47.5 Infiltrating cancer of the right breast. **a** Axial T1-w. pre contrast image and (**b**) corresponding subtracted early post contrast axial image, on which a mass lesion is detected (*arrow* on **a**), with peripheral "ring-like" enhancement and irregular, partially spiculated, borders (*arrows* on **b**). **c** axial T1-w. pre contrast image, on which an enlarged lymph node is seen in the right axilla (*arrow*)

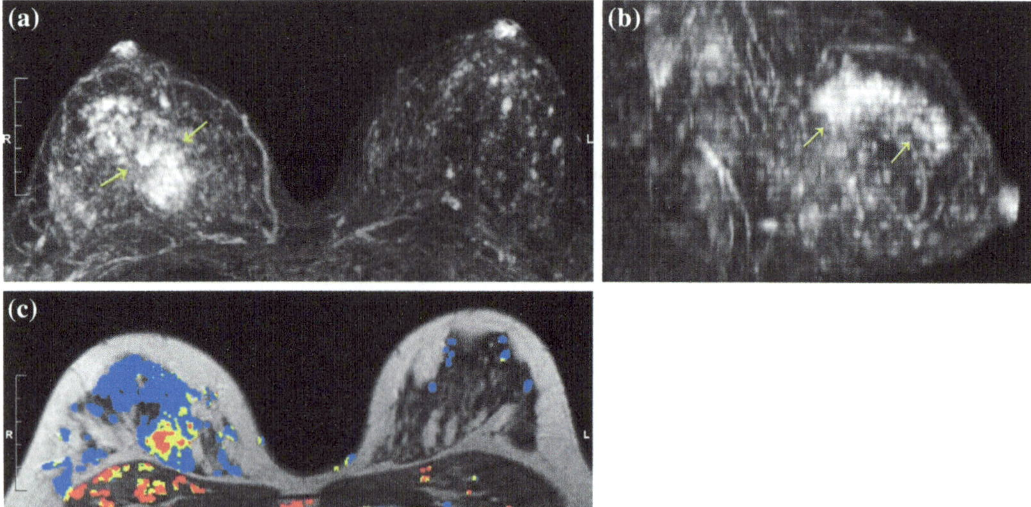

Fig. 47.6 DCIS in the left breast. **a** MIP reconstruction of the subtracted images of the late postcontrast T1-w. sequence of the dynamic scan. There is a large area of asymmetric abnormal non-mass like enhancement, which on the left lateral MIP reconstruction, **b** shows a distribution pattern along the lactiferous ducts and toward the nipple (*arrows*). **c** Color map superimposed on a postcontrast T1-w. image, shows that the greater part of the neoplasia exhibits progressive contrast uptake (type-1 *curve*, *blue color*), while smaller areas exhibit intense early contrast uptake with type-2 (*yellow color*) or type-3 *curve* (*red color*). Same case as in Fig. 47.3

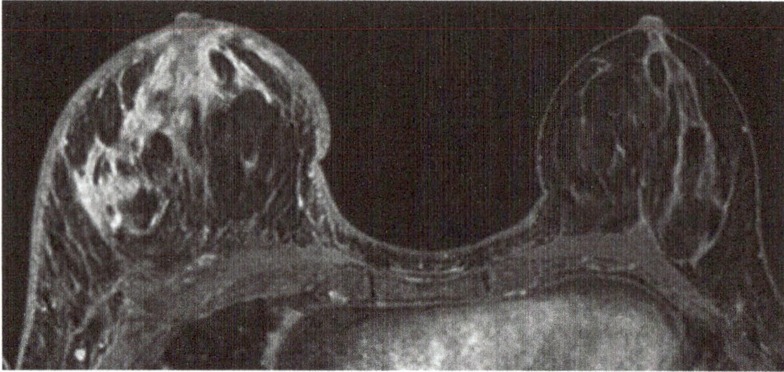

Fig. 47.7 Inflammatory cancer of the right breast. High spatial resolution T1-w. fat suppressed postcontrast image. Note enlargement of the right breast, extensive contrast uptake, and diffusely thickened and enhancing skin

type 2 or 3 curves. Most of fibroadenomas tend to grow while patients are young and regress during the postmenopausal period. MG and targeted US are invaluable in making the diagnosis. Phyllodes (from the Greek word phyllon, which means leaf) is a tumor that is difficult to differentiate from fibroadenomas. On MRM, it demonstrates high SI on T2 imaging and contrast enhancement. Since some of these tumors may have malignant potential, tissue sampling is recommended. Hamartomas are uncommon benign tumor-like masses, composed of varying amounts of glandular, adipose, and fibrous tissue. The classic appearance on MG is that of a circumscribed mass known as "breast within a breast". On MRM, they demonstrate characteristics and kinetics similar to that of normal breast. Other benign conditions frequently seen in breast are cysts, fat necrosis , papillomas, fibrocystic breast disease, radial scars, and

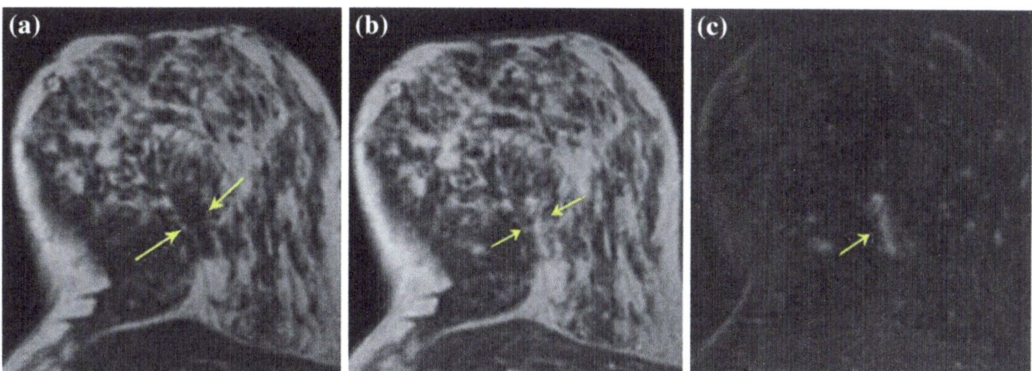

Fig. 47.8 Sclerosing adenosis (surgically confirmed) mimicking DCIS. Axial T1-w. **a** precontrast, **b** late postcontrast, and **c** corresponding subtraction images. An ill-defined linear enhancing lesion is detected deeply in the right breast (*arrows*). On mammography (not shown) suspicious confluent microcalcifications were present in the same region

pseudoangiomatous stromal hyperplasia (PASH). Benign cysts can be easily diagnosed on T2-weighted and DWI sequences. Fat necrosis and papillomas are enhancing lesions on MRM that commonly show kinetic curves as in cancer. Fat necrosis can be easily diagnosed if the typical "dystrophic" calcifications are present on MG, especially if a history of trauma, such as prior operation or seat belt injury is elicited. Patients with papillomas usually present with bloody nipple discharge. Abnormal enhancement due to fibrocystic breast disease is typically of "non-mass" type, with type 1 curve and symmetric distribution in both breasts. However, occasionally may show atypical features, such as intense mass-like or regional enhancement with type 2 or 3 curves. Focused US can provide invaluable information regarding the presence or absence of disease in the region of concern. Sites of benign dysplastic changes, like sclerosing adenosis and apocrine metaplasia, may appear on MRM as focal lesions with irregular borders and variable enhancement, mimicking the features of invasive breast cancer or DCIS (Fig. 47.8).

Usual causes of false positive (FP) findings for Breast Cancer on MRM.

1. Inverted nipple.
2. Focal adenosis, usually in women of reproductive age and/or under hormonal therapy. In order to decrease the FP findings, it is recommended to perform MRM during the second week of the menstrual cycle or 6–8 weeks after discontinuation of any hormonal therapy.
3. Pregnancy and lactation.
4. Mastitis and abscess.
5. Benign lesions mimicking breast cancer such as hypervascular myxoid fibroadenomas (common in young women), recent fat necrosis, sclerosing adenosis (Fig. 47.8).
6. Postsurgical changes. To minimize the FP findings from that cause, it is advised to perform MRM not earlier than 3 months from a previous surgical operation in the breast.
7. Postradiation changes, which may show variable and occasionally intense and confusing contrast enhancement of the irradiated breast. For that reason, baseline MRM should be performed 12–18 months after completion of radiotherapy.

Usual causes of false negative (FN) findings for Breast Cancer on MRM.

1. Technical failure.
2. Diagnostic error: e.g., breast cancers with well-defined border, mimicking fibroadenomas (Fig. 47.9).
3. Focal lesion, with a diameter smaller than the double of slice thickness of MRM images.
4. DCIS, presenting only with microcalcifications on MG: occasionally, it does not show any contrast enhancement on MRM.

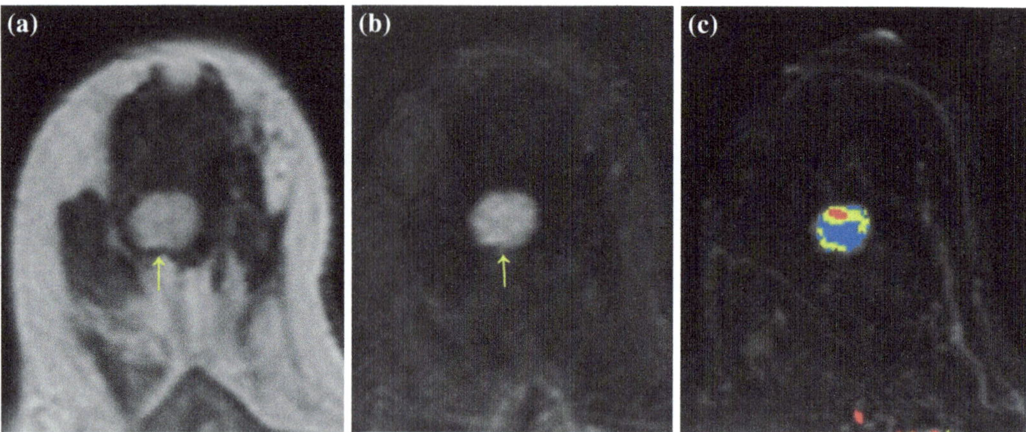

Fig. 47.9 Invasive ductal cancer of the right breast, mimicking fibroadenoma. Axial T1-w. early post contrast (**a**), corresponding subtraction image (**b**) and MIP reconstruction of the subtracted images. There is a round mass in the right breast with sharp, partially lobulated, border (*arrows*). These benign-looking morphological features may be misleading, suggesting the diagnosis of a myxoid fibroadenoma. The color map of contrast uptake, superimposed on the MIP reconstruction, shows areas of early intense contrast enhancement in the mass, with type-2 (*yellow*) and type-3 (*red*) *curves*

47.5 Sensitivity and Specificity

According to several studies, MRM has high sensitivity ranging between 89 and 100 % in the diagnosis of breast cancer. Its sensitivity for detecting DCIS, however, is only 85–90 %. Its specificity varies between 30 and 90 % because the modality often results in FP diagnoses, especially in young women. This is due to the significant overlapping of the imaging findings of benign and malignant breast lesions.

47.6 Indications for MRM

1. MRM is the study of choice in the screening of women at high-risk of developing breast cancer [2, 6]. Given that breast cancers in young women have a faster growth rate, their mean diameter is 1.7 cm at the time of diagnosis and 50 % have metastasized to the axillary lymph nodes. According to the guidelines issued by the American Cancer Society (ACS) in 2007, MRM is recommended as an annual screening test for women whose life-time risk for developing breast cancer is estimated to be 25 % and higher [7]. This group includes women with: BRCA 1 and 2 mutations or with first degree relatives with such mutations; two or more first degree relatives with breast or ovarian cancer; history of radiation therapy to the chest (e.g., for Hodgkin's disease) at young age; other rare syndromes mostly related to PTEN, TP53, and CHECK gene mutations in which breast cancer is prevalent. Other risk factors justifying annual screening with MRM include women with biopsy proven intraductal or lobular breast cancers or DCIS, or atypical ductal hyperplasia (ADH) before the age of 40. Finally, those with male relatives with breast cancer (Fig. 47.10). Another indication less agreed upon includes young women with dense breasts, for whom mammographic screening is challenging, as its sensitivity is lower than 50 %.

During the past 15 years, many studies compared the diagnostic performance of annual screening in women at high-risk between MRM to that of "conventional screening" that includes clinical breast examination (CBE), MG, and US [8]. In these studies, the sensitivity of MRM (79–98 %) is significantly higher than that of MG and/or US (<50 %), and CBE (about 30 %). Kriege et al. [9] screened 1,909 women and

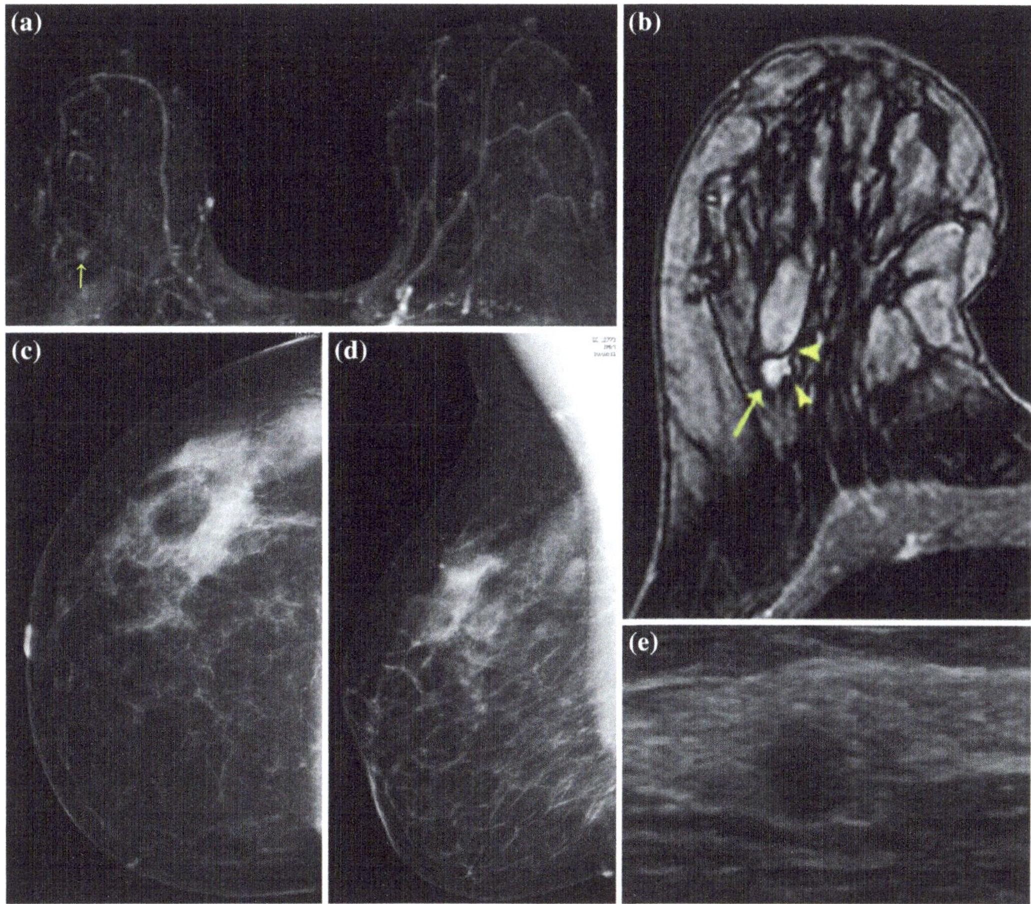

Fig. 47.10 Small invasive breast cancer in a high-risk woman, detected by MRM (**a**, **b**). On the MIP reconstruction (**a**) of MRM, a small enhancing lesion (*arrow*), less than 5 mm in diameter, is detected in the right breast. On the high resolution T1-w. fat suppressed post contrast image (**b**), the lesion shows partially ill-defined border (*arrow*) and small spiculations (*arrowheads*). On the digital MG of the right breast (**c**, craniocaudal view and (**d**), lateral oblique view) there is no abnormal finding detected. A focused US (**e**), performed after MRM, detected the small neoplastic lesion and guided a biopsy

diagnosed 51 breast cancers (44 invasive). The sensitivity of CBE, MG, and MRM for detecting invasive breast cancer was 17.9, 33.3, and 79.5 % while their specificity was 98.1, 95, and 89.8 %, respectively. Although the positive predictive value (PPV) of 35–64 % of MRM is suboptimal, it is still considered acceptable given the very low sensitivity of the other screening methods. The major limitation of MRM is the high rate of FP findings, which was shown to decrease as the experience of the radiologists (learning curve) increases.

2. MRM should be considered in the preoperative work up when breast-conserving surgery is contemplated in women with dense breast parenchyma [2]. Several studies have shown that MRM is more sensitive than MG, US, and CBE for depicting the full extent of breast cancer, the coexistence of intraductal component, and the presence of multicentricity or multifocality in the affected or contralateral breast. Finally, it is more effective in diagnosing the invasion of pectoralis muscles. Specifically, the sensitivity of MRM

for detecting breast cancer in the contralateral breast is ranging between 88 and 100 %, while that of MG and US is 30–38 % [10] (Fig. 47.11). The additional findings of MRM may lead to a modification of the operative approach in 15–27 % of patients, and has resulted in an increase of the number of mastectomies, a concern among surgeons. The availability of MR-guided percutaneous biopsy, or wire-localization of the additional suspicious lesions, is mandatory for making MRM useful in making evidence-based clinical decisions [2]. Although there is some evidence that preoperative MRM may lead to a lower rate of local recurrences, there are still no convincing data supporting improvement in the overall survival of patients with breast cancer.

3. In cases of questionable breast cancer in order to decide further management [2]. The most common reasons for using MRM are: (a) Differential diagnosis of a post-therapy scar versus breast cancer recurrence. In women with previous breast-conserving surgery, the sensitivity of MRM in the detection of recurrence is almost 100 %, compared to 70 % for MG and 30 % for CBE. The accuracy of MRM is highest when it is performed after at least 3–6 months post surgery and 12–18 months post completion of radiotherapy (Fig. 47.12). (b) Differential diagnosis of atypical benign breast lesions (e.g., cysts with hemorrhagic or inflamed content, fibroadenomas) from breast cancer. (c) Evaluation of a focal or regional asymmetry of breast tissue or of an area of architectural distortion, without suspicious microcalcifications, detected on MG. (d) Evaluation of any suspicious density detected on only one MG projection, in order to clarify if it represents a true lesion. (e) Further evaluation of an area of suspicious microcalcifications on MG.

In the above clinical situations a–d, the excellent negative predictive value (NPV) of MRM for invasive breast cancer (99 %) may help to avoid further investigation and unnecessary biopsies. In the case of microcalcifications, further management must be decided exclusively on their MG features, even if MRM is negative. This is due to the results of several studies that have shown that MRM may be FN in 6–15 % of the cases of DCIS that are obvious on MG only, as a cluster of suspicious

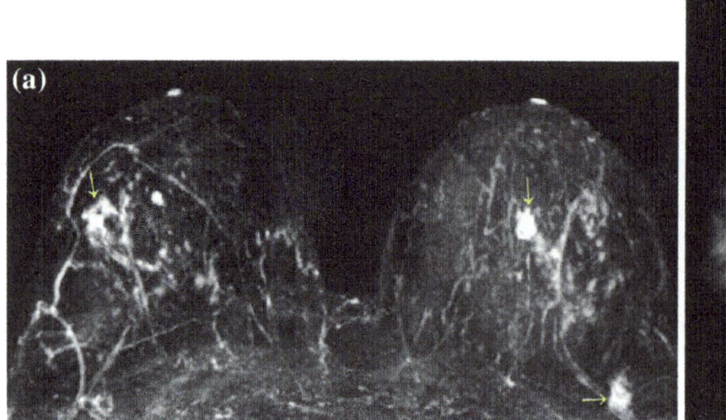

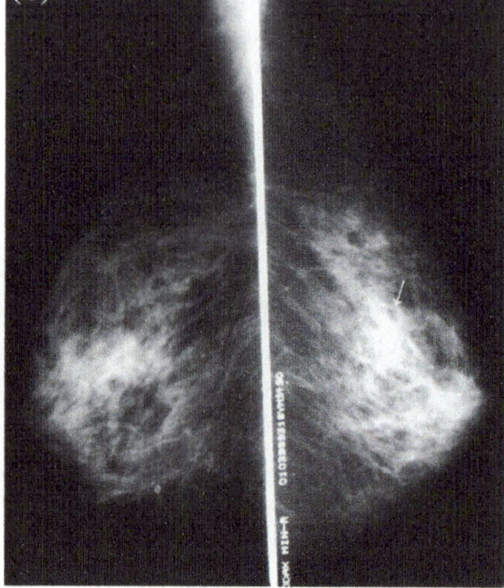

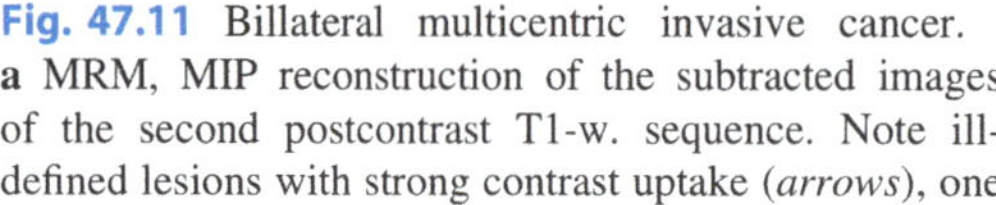

Fig. 47.11 Billateral multicentric invasive cancer. **a** MRM, MIP reconstruction of the subtracted images of the second postcontrast T1-w. sequence. Note ill-defined lesions with strong contrast uptake (*arrows*), one in the lateral part of the right breast and two in the left breast (central and posterior part). On the lateral oblique mammogram (**b**) only the lesion in the central part of left breast (*arrow*) could be detected

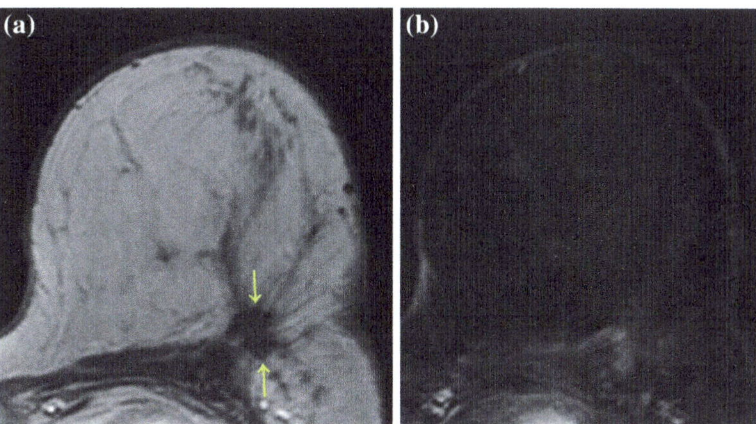

Fig. 47.12 Typical appearance of a scar, 20 months post lumpectomy and radiation therapy for invasive cancer of the left breast. **a** Axial T1-w. postcontrast image and (**b**) corresponding subtraction image. At the posterior part of the left breast, almost in contact with the major pectoral muscle, there is an ill-defined mass with irregular shape and low SI, without any obvious contrast uptake (*arrows*)

microcalcifications. However, many studies have shown that MRM, despite its inability to image the microcalcifications, may play a complementary role to MG. It has been shown that MRM is more accurate than MG for depicting the full extent of DCIS (especially those of high-grade histology). About 40 % of all cases of DCIS are depicted only on MRM. Additionally, MRM is capable to depict possibly coexisting, MG occult, invasive breast cancers.

4. When breast cancer is suspected clinically, while MG and US are inconclusive [2]: (a) Women with metastatic adenocarcinoma of unknown primary origin: (b) Women with bloody nipple discharge, in whom the conventional imaging studies are negative. MRM may help to diagnose an intraductal lesion. However, in most cases, it cannot differentiate a papilloma from a small invasive ductal carcinoma or DCIS.
5. Detection of residual cancer status post lumpectomy: MRM is indicated when the margins of the surgical specimen are positive or the resected cancer extends close to the margins. Also, if lobular cancer is found as it is known to be often multicentric (Fig. 47.13).
6. Recently, MRM has been used for evaluating the response to neoadjuvant chemotherapy. There is evidence that ADC measurements can be used as a quantitative marker to determine the response to treatment [3]. However, the sensitivity of MRM for detecting residual cancer after the completion of chemotherapy is dependent on the hormonal status of the disease, being more sensitive in "triple-negative" and Her2/neu-positive and less sensitive in ER-positive/HER2-negative breast cancers. The overall sensitivity and specificity of MRM for detecting residual cancer are 63 and 100 %, respectively. The sensitivity is lower when patients are treated with taxane-based chemotherapy (Fig. 47.14).
7. Evaluation of breast implants [2]. MRM is the examination of choice for the diagnosis of implant rupture, with sensitivity, and specificity reported between 90 and 100 %. It is highly accurate (>90 %) for detecting inflammation around the implant, as well.

47.7 MR-Guided Interventional Procedures in the Breast

Aproximately 40 % of the suspicious lesions found by MRM are not detectable with either MG or second-look US. This fact makes the availability of MR-guided biopsies and/or wire-localization of such lesions essential [2, 8].

Fig. 47.13 MRM performed 30 days post lumpectomy in the right breast. Histological examination of the surgical specimen detected invasive lobular cancer. On the MIP reconstruction (**a**) of the subtracted postcontrast images and on the axial high resolution T1-w. fat suppressed post contrast image (**b**), two additional enhancing lesions are detected (*arrows*). They have morphological features highly suspicious for cancer (irregular shape, ill-defined, and spiculated borders), a diagnosis that was confirmed in the histological examination of the subsequent right mastectomy

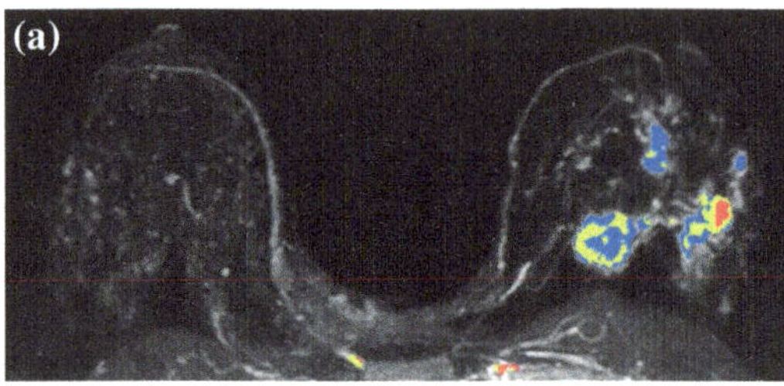

Fig. 47.14 Locally advanced multicentric invasive cancer of the left breast. MIP reconstructions of the subtracted post contrast images of MRM examinations that were performed at the time of diagnosis (**a**) and after two cycles of neoadjuvant chemotherapy (**b**). All the cancerous lesions (marked with color, according to the contrast uptake) on (**a**), have almost resolved in the second examination (**b**)

Preoperative histological diagnosis is best accomplished when vacuum assisted biopsies are performed. Proposed therapy for MR-guided thermal ablation of small breast tumors is still under evaluation.

47.8 Conclusion

MRI of the Breast is the most sensitive currently available technique for the detection of breast cancer. Although it does not use ionizing radiation, it is a lengthy and expensive study. To improve its diagnostic accuracy, it should be performed at 1.5T or higher field magnets and be interpreted by experienced radiologists. Since its specificity can be low, it should be used when clinically indicated only, and correlated with the findings from clinical breast examination, mammography, and breast US. It can be used as a sole study only in young women who are at high-risk for breast cancer.

References

1. Kuhl C (2007) The current status of breast MR imaging. Part I. Choice of technique, image interpretation, diagnostic accuracy and transfer to clinical practice. Radiology 244(2):356–367
2. Kuhl C (2007) The current status of breast MR imaging. Part II. Clinical applications. Radiology 244(3):672–691

3. Woodhams R, Kakita S, Hata H et al (2010) Identification of residual breast carcinoma following neoadjuvant chemotherapy: diffusion-weighted imaging-comparison with contrast-enhancent MR imaging and pathologic findings. Radiology 254:357–366
4. Liberman L, Mason G, Morris EA, Dershaw DD (2006) Does size really matters? Positive predictive value of MRI-detected lesions as a function of lesion size. Am J Roentgenol 186:426–430
5. Le-Petross HT, Cristofanilli M, Carkaci S, et al (2011) MRI features of inflammatory breast cancer. Am J Roentgenol 197(4):W769–W776
6. Warner E, Messersmith H, Causer P et al (2008) Systematic review: using MRI to screen women at high risk for breast cancer. Ann Intern Med 148(9):671–679
7. Saslow D, Boetes C, Burke W et al (2007) American Cancer Society guidelines for breast screening with MRI as an adjunct to mammography. CA Cancer J Clin 57:75–89
8. Berg WA, Zhang Z, Lehrer D et al (2012) Detection of breast cancer with addition of annual screening ultrasound or a single screening MRI to mammography in women with elevated cancer risk. JAMA 307(13):1394–1404
9. Kriege M, Brekelmans C, Boetes C (2004) Efficacy of MRI and mammography for breast-cancer screening in women with a familial or genetic predisposition. N Engl J Med 351:427–437
10. Lehman CD, Gatsonis C, Kuhl CK et al (2007) MRI evaluation of the contralateral breast in women with recently diagnosed breast cancer. N Engl J Med 356:1295–1303

48 Breast Cancer: PET/CT Imaging

Vasiliki P. Philippi

PET/CT is a hybrid method that combines anatomical imaging with metabolic information in a single examination. The combination of these two methods has the advantage of precise localization of foci of pathologically increased metabolic activity. Pathological metabolic activity in malignant tissue often precedes anatomical changes and in some cases, due to previous surgery or radiotherapy, anatomical findings alone are not specific for recurrence or dissemination of disease.

Fluorodeoxyglucose (FDG) is a tracer, analog to glucose, that is mainly used, currently, for PET and PET/CT imaging. FDG uptake by metabolically active tissue is related to the fact that malignant cells have proportionally increased demand for glucose [1].

FDG/PET has a limited role in the detection of primary breast cancer (Fig. 48.1). The overall sensitivity of the method is 64–96 % and specificity is 73–100 %. The reported accuracy is 70–97 %, the positive predictive value 81–100 % and the negative predictive value is 52–89 % [2].

The limitations of the method are due to the low sensitivity of the method in detection of small lesions (<1 cm), and to low FDG uptake in specific histological types (such as lobular carcinomas, and ductal carcinoma in situ) and well-differentiated tumors. Taking into account these limitations, as well as the low availability and the high cost, FDG PET is not currently indicated as a screening test for breast cancer [3].

In order to improve the efficacy of the method the development of dedicated breast positron emission mammography (PEM) units seems promising. Possible applications of PEM are detection of small primary breast tumors, local staging and restaging, and evaluation of tumor response to therapy. So far, the method is not validated in large trials [4].

Accurate locoregional staging of the disease is very useful in patient management, as it is related to patient prognosis. For early stage breast cancer patients FDG PET has relatively low sensitivity in axillary staging, and is not recommended by the literature for this purpose. However, in patients with advanced disease, FDG PET may provide additional information such as distant occult metastases, or pathological internal mammary lymph nodes [4].

FDG PET may be useful in assessment of tumor response to therapy, since metabolic changes precede morphological regression. A decrease in the level of FDG uptake-compared to the baseline scan-following even the first or second cycle of chemotherapy, can predict response to chemotherapy treatment (accuracy 64–91 %). Not responders are obviously benefited by avoiding useless, toxic treatment [5].

V. P. Philippi (✉)
MRI, CT and PET/CT Departments, Hygeia and Mitera Hospitals, Erythrou Stavrou 4, 15123, Maroussi, Greece
e-mail: vicky.filippi@gmail.com

A. D. Gouliamos et al. (eds.), *Imaging in Clinical Oncology*,
DOI: 10.1007/978-88-470-5385-4_48, © Springer-Verlag Italia 2014

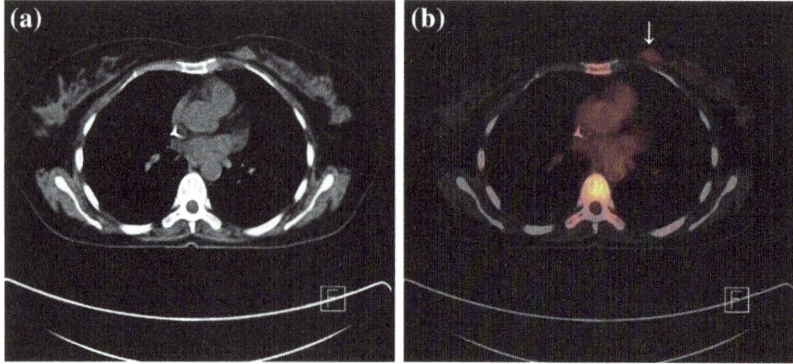

Fig. 48.1 **a** CT image within normal limits. **b** PET/CT image shows an area with increased metabolic activity in the left breast (*arrow*), finding suspicious for malignancy, as an incidental finding

On the basis of scientific results obtained to date, there is not enough evidence to substitute anatomical imaging methods with molecular imaging modalities. However, FDG PET may play a complementary role in assessment of possible disease progression [6].

Recurrence of disease is frequent in patients with breast cancer, after completion of initial treatment. Early detection of tumor recurrences is beneficial for breast cancer patients, and is associated both with prognosis as well as appropriate treatment choice. Estimation of the true extend may sometimes be quite challenging, due to occult recurrences. This may be correlated to the small size of a lesion, that is considered normal with anatomical–morphological criteria, e.g., a lymph node, or inconclusive findings in areas that coexist post treatment findings, e.g., scar tissue post radiotherapy (Fig. 48.2).

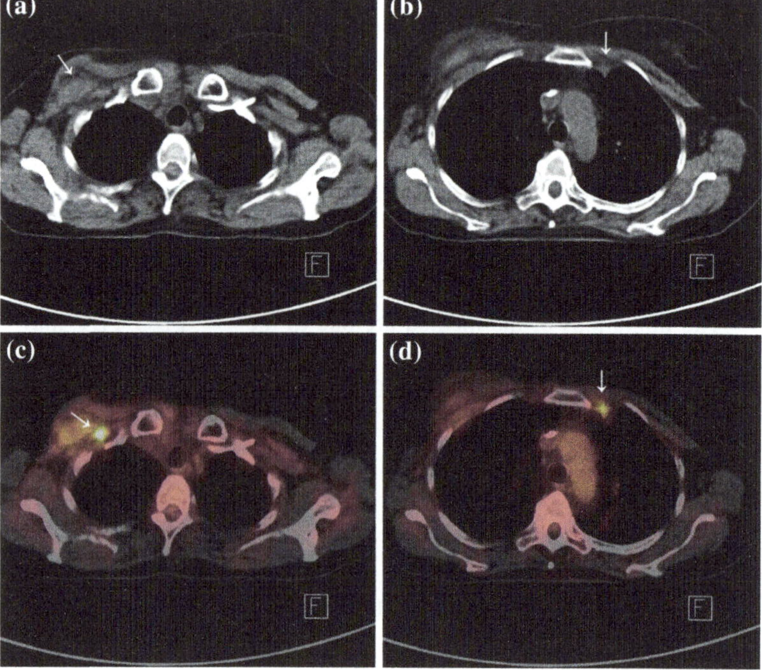

Fig. 48.2 Patient with suspicious recurrence in the right breast after surgery. CT images show abnormal soft tissue at the surgical region (**a**, *arrow*) and a borderline left internal mammary lymph node (**b**, *arrow*). PET/CT images confirm the local recurrence (**c**, *arrow*) and additionally show increased uptake in the left internal mammary lymph node (**d**, *arrow*)

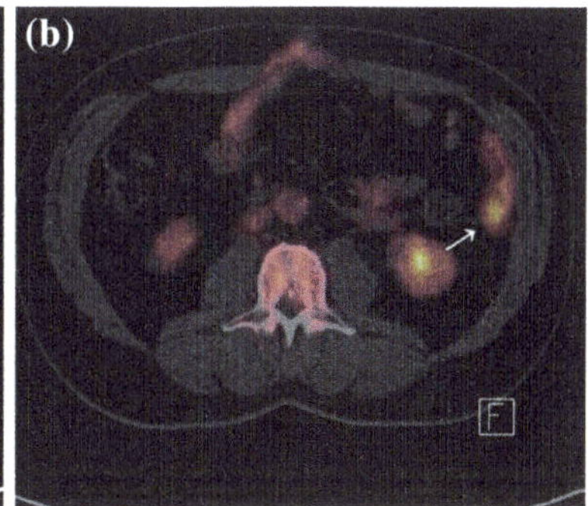

Fig. 48.3 **a** Equivocal findings on CT (obliteration of the left paracolic fat, *arrow*) in a patient with breast cancer history and elevated tumor markers. **b** PET/CT image shows a focus of increased metabolic activity (*arrow*), suspicious for peritoneal implantation

FDG PET has been shown to be effective in early accurate restaging of patients with breast cancer, as it detects pathologic metabolic activity of tumors, which usually can be detected earlier than anatomic–morphologic alterations. FDG PET is considered an effective diagnostic tool and is recommended in the follow-up of breast cancer patients. Isasi et al. estimated the diagnostic performance of FDG PET using meta-analysis. Among the studies with patient-based data, median sensitivity was 92.7 % and median specificity was 81.6 % [7].

The higher sensitivity of the method, compared to Computed Tomography, especially in detecting lymphatic dissemination of the disease is the main advantage of the method [8].

FDG PET/CT has an even greater diagnostic accuracy compared to PET alone, since lesions are better localized and false positive findings, attributed to physiological FDG uptake, are avoided.

Moreover, FDG PET/CT is of great importance in patients with elevated tumor markers and negative or equivocal findings on conventional imaging techniques, as it provides information about the disease status in terms of localization of recurrence. In these patients it seems that although tumor markers levels may strongly indicate that there is occult tumor

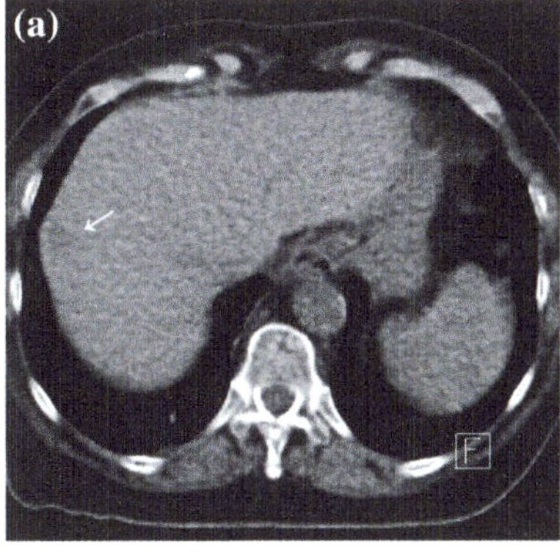

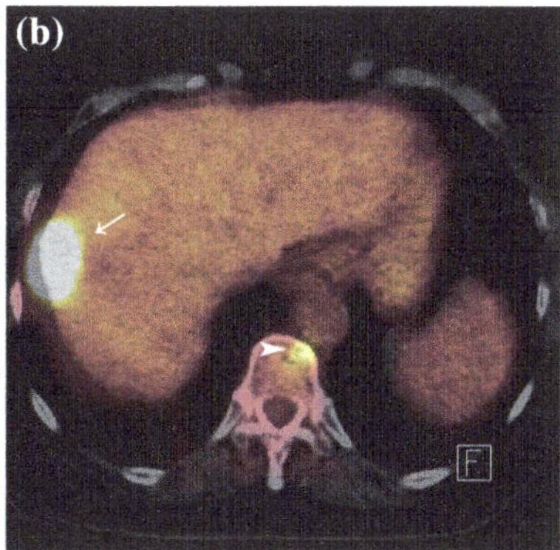

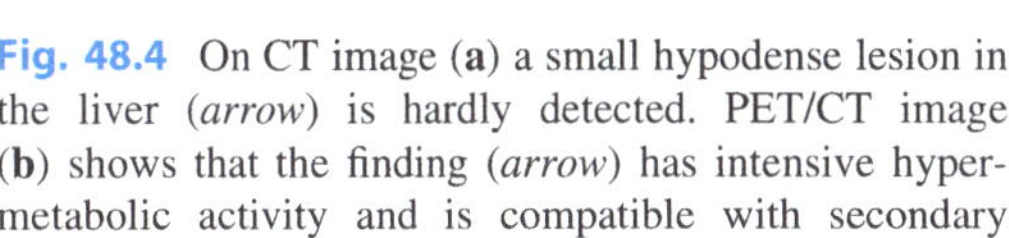

Fig. 48.4 On CT image (**a**) a small hypodense lesion in the liver (*arrow*) is hardly detected. PET/CT image (**b**) shows that the finding (*arrow*) has intensive hypermetabolic activity and is compatible with secondary deposit. Additionally, in the same image (**b**), a hypermetabolic focus (*arrowhead*) is seen in the anterior aspect of the 11th thoracic vertebra

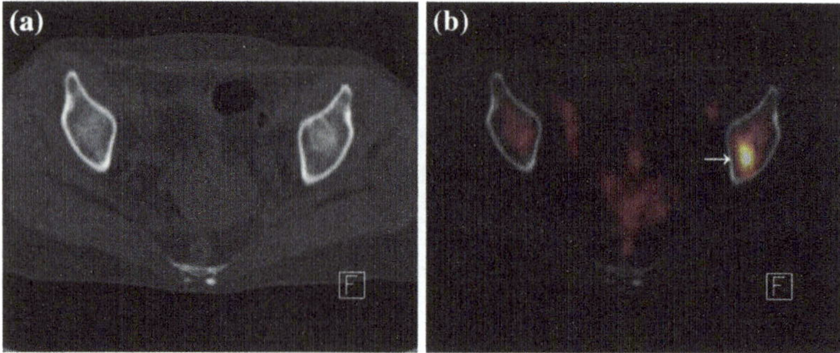

Fig. 48.5 CT image (**a**) shows no abnormal findings. PET/CT image (**b**) shows a lesion of increased uptake in the left ilium (*arrow*), consistent with bone metastases

recurrence, conventional imaging methods cannot always estimate the true extent of the disease. FDG PET/CT in this population has a sensitivity of 86.8 %, specificity 87.5 %, and accuracy of 86.9 % (Figs. 48.3, 48.4). The positive prognostic value is 97 % and the negative prognostic value 58.3 % [9].

Bone metastases are very common in breast cancer patients. FDG PET and bone scintigraphy are methods complementary to each other, since FDG PET is more sensitive in detection of lytic and intramedullary secondary deposits and bone scintigraphy is superior in detection of osteoblastic lesions [10].

FDG PET has an important clinical impact in the management of breast cancer patients. By altering, which is more often upgrading, the stage of the disease, clinical management decisions are usually influenced. FDG PET has been shown to change the clinical stage of the patients examined in 36 %. Even if the stage of the disease is not changed by FDG PET results, information about the true extend of the disease provided, may result in differentiation in treatment options. Physicians seem rely on FDG PET results, thus altering clinical management in 58 % of cases. This fact is of proof that FDG PET is already considered as in important diagnostic tool among physicians [11].

Currently, FDG is the radiopharmaceutical in clinical use. New tracers like fluorothymidine (FLT), fluoroestradiol, methionine, and choline seem promising, especially in the field of monitoring tumor response to therapy [12].

In conclusion, the role of FDG PET/CT is complementary to conventional imaging methods and should not replace them. The main indication currently is to provide additional information in selected cases in the restaging of breast cancer patients and in evaluation of response to treatment (Fig. 48.5).

References

1. Kapoor K, McCook B, Torok FS (2004) An introduction to PET-CT imaging. Radiographics 24:523–543
2. Scheidhauer K, Walter C, Seemann MD (2004) FDG PET and other imaging modalities in the primary diagnosis of suspicious breast lesions. Eur J Nucl Med Mol Imaging 31(1):70–79
3. Kumar R, Chauhan A, Zhuang H, Chandra P, Schnall M, Alavi A (2006) Clinicopathologic factors associated with false negative FDG-PET in primary breast cancer. Breast Cancer Res Treat 98(3):267–274
4. Rosen E, Eubank W, Mankoff D (2007) FDG PET, PET/CT and breast cancer imaging. Radiographics 27:S215–S229
5. Avril N, Sassen S, Roylance R (2009) Response to therapy in breast cancer. J Nucl Med 50:55S–63S
6. Eisenhauera EA, Therasseb P, Bogaertsc J, Schwartzd LH, Sargente D, Fordf R, Danceyg J, Arbuckh S, Gwytheri S, Mooneyg M, Rubinsteing L, Shankarg L, Doddg L, Kaplanj R, Lacombec D, Verweijk J (2009) New response evaluation criteria in solid tumours: revised RECIST guideline (version 1.1). Eur J Cancer 45:228–247
7. Isasi C, Moadel R, Blaufox M (2005) A meta-analysis of FDG-PET for the evaluation of breast cancer recurrence and metastases. Breast Cancer Res Treat 90:105–112

8. Eubank W, Mankoff D, Vessele H, Eary J, Schubert E, Dunnwald L, lindsley S, Grallow J, Austin-Seymour M, Ellis G, Livingston R (2002) Detection of locoregional and distant recurrences in breast cancer patients by using FDG PET. Radiographics 22:5
9. Filippi V, Malamitsi J, Vlachou F, Laspas F, Georgiou E, Prassopoulos V, Andreou J (2011) The impact of FDG-PET/CT on the management of breast cancer patients with elevated tumor markers and negative or equivocal conventional imaging modalities. Nucl Med Commun 32(2):85–90
10. Lee J, Rosen E, Maankoff D (2009) The role of radiotracer imaging in the diagnosis and management of patients with breast cancer: part 1-overview detection, and staging. J Nucl Med 50(4):569–581
11. Yap S, Seltze M, Schiepers C, Gambhir S, Rao J, Phelps M, Valk P, Czernin J (2001) Impact of whole body 18F-FDG PET on staging and managing patients with breast cancer: the referring physician's perspective. J Nucl Med 42(9):1334–1337
12. Kenny L, Al-Nahhas A, Aboagye E (2011) Novel PET biomarkers for breast cancer imaging. Nucl Med Commun 32:333–335

Clinical Implications of Breast Cancer 49

Dimitris-Andrew D. Tsiftsis

Breast cancer (BC) has advanced by strides the last few years reaching the stage of functional molecular imaging. The objectives though remain the same: detection of tumors at the earliest phase, reliable pre- and post-treatment staging, and correlation of image characteristics to prognosis.

49.1 Early Diagnosis and Preoperative Planning

It is well-documented that early diagnosis of BC tenders less disfiguring treatments and thus improved quality of life. The crucial step to a woman's striving for early diagnosis is to have her risk assessed. For low to moderate risk, the accepted guideline is from age 40 to 70 digital mammography (dMm) every 2–3 years. In high risk women MRI of upgraded specifications to increase its specificity is introduced as a reliable screening, with better tumor yield even at a higher biopsy rate. MRI is also indicated in dense breasts and diffuse micro calcifications. It is imperative for centers using MRI to have available MRI-guided interventions like core biopsy and J-wire placement. In confirmed genetic predisposition, MRI breast screening protocols have to compete against prophylactic surgery that holds the leading role [1].

Another open to debate subject pertains to the routine use of MRI on all women with newly diagnosed BC preoperatively in an effort to detect multicentricity, contralateral disease, and the extend of the reference tumor. Meta-analysis have shown a rise of 16 % in additional tumors detected at the cost of more radical surgery that does not translate into better survival or fewer re-excisions and recurrences. RCTs are needed to settle the argument and until then this practice is not recommended [2].

49.2 Accurate Diagnosis of Breast Lesions

The cornerstone of the evaluation of a breast finding is the triple assessment. Central component of the triad is Mm and the clinician is bound to take further action or not on the BI-RADS classification of the finding. The same applies to US and MRI.

Category 3 is assigned to very few reports (2.34 %) and the probability of malignancy remains low (0.81 %). Short-term follow-up (FU) covers the patient sufficiently. In categories 4 and 5, a definite tissue diagnosis of the lesion is mandatory. In palpable lesions this is accomplished either by FNA or core biopsy. The use of US helps to select the proper site of the mass to take the sample. In non-palpable lesions the sample has to be taken under the guidance of the imaging modality that has revealed the lesion. Core needle is used to secure a dissent specimen. Today, we have automated stereotactic apparatus

D.-A. D. Tsiftsis (✉)
Hygeia Diagnostic and Therapeutic Center
of Athens, Er. Stavrou 4, 15123 Marousi, Greece
e-mail: d.d.tsiftsis@gmail.com

A. D. Gouliamos et al. (eds.), *Imaging in Clinical Oncology*,
DOI: 10.1007/978-88-470-5385-4_49,

that can approach safely almost any part of the breast and cut specimens of a size that combines biopsy and cure. If sampling is unsuccessful or not feasible, a J-wire or a tracer is left in place for a guided open biopsy. The patient has the right to be fully informed and consulted of the nature of her finding and the treatment options available to her. Open surgical biopsy is not the first choice.

In cases where a patient has disease in her axilla with a negative Mm, MRI may reveal the index tumor in the breast and allow a sample of it. The surgical treatment of the axilla in patients with BC has become less extensive with the introduction of sentinel lymph node (SLN) biopsy. Further, clinical N1 nodes can be assessed preoperatively by US and sampled by guided FNA. To locate the SLN during surgery the patient usually has a radioisotope lymphoscintigraphy beforehand and in theater the surgeon with a handheld probe spots the "hot" node. There are patients with unusual, complex, or delayed drainage and those with extra axillary drainage. In these cases, the use of SPECT/CT gives excellent results with 3D images and a clear map of the lymphatic route [3].

49.3 Evaluation of Response to Therapy

Accurately measuring the response to therapies of the index tumor or of the metastatic disease is a difficult but inescapable endeavor for many reasons. The size of the tumor does not correspond to the tumor cells volume. The criteria used (RECIST or WHO) have application limitations. Each treatment modality has different response time. Targeted treatment aims mainly at stabilizing and not decreasing the tumor burden. Different imaging studies have better yield in different organs. Technological evolution and the introduction of new methods are so rapid that the added value of each cannot be assessed in the long run. This reflects to the fact that there are not published guidelines.

For the evaluation of the primary breast tumor to induction chemotherapy conventional means like clinical examination still hold strong. Mm and US are used widely correlating well with the pathology specimen. Modalities like quantified DW/PW MRI and dynamic PET can not only measure response accurately but also tumor function and can predict if it will respond to given treatment. Another functional study is diffuse optical spectroscopy promising better prediction of response with early application in the treatment course.

For the evaluation of systemic disease, FDG-PET seems more accurate. Early results from trials using new imaging agents like amino acid analogs and choline fair even better [4]. As for the assessment of residual disease after breast conserving surgery (BCS), MRI is the study of choice especially if the breast has been augmented with implants.

49.4 Preoperative Staging

A patient with confirmed BC needs clinical TNM staging and detailed review of her pathology report. For clinical stages I–IIB, additional imaging studies are not indicated unless directed by signs and symptoms. For stage IIIA or locally advanced disease when preoperative chemotherapy is scheduled chest CT, abdominal ± pelvic CT or MRI, bone scan, and FDG-PET/CT are recommended (NCCN, NICE, ESMO, BASO guidelines). In this clinical setting, RCTs are still trying to define which combination of imaging studies is best to detect metastatic disease being cost-effective at the same time and most importantly whether this additional information has any gain for the patient in terms of DFS or OS. Take into account that preoperative staging is the phase where a high proportion of patients undergo unnecessary, costly, high-end investigations to no avail.

49.5 Post-Treatment Surveillance

Women after BCS may develop ipsilateral recurrence or a new metachronous primary in the operated or contralateral breast as well as systemic disease. Ipsilateral recurrence is known to affect survival. Women with a second tumor ≥2.0 cm are at greater risk of death compared to those with tumors ≤1.0 cm or no recurrence. So, early detection seems to be beneficial to the patient's outcome. Of the potentially treatable relapses almost half are detected by Mm, 15 % at clinical visits and the rest by the patient. From the surveillance studies Mm seems to have been adopted as the preferred method by the majority of clinicians (87 %) and scientific bodies. Issued guidelines (ASCO, ESMO, NICE) differ in frequency, protocol, and duration. They agree on closer FU the first 2–3 years. We must keep in mind that though relapses are indeed more often the first 2–3 years, they never cease to appear and that metachronous tumors occur latter. Mm is a widely available, reliable, time-honored study with a sensitivity of about 65 % and a specificity of 85–97 % [5]. A new array of technological improvements (tomosynthesis, spectral Mm, dye enhanced, etc.) is expected to increase its performance. MRI fares better and is a useful tool in dubious cases. The length of FU should be 10 years for the average case. We do need though robust evidence from RCTs that would allow us to categorize patients according to their risk for relapse and tailor surveillance protocols to meet their needs.

49.6 DCIS

As a result of breast screening the incidence of DCIS has increased disproportionately to other tumors. Age-adjusted incidence rate is 32.5 per 100,000 women. The average size is 1.0–1.5 cm, 50 % is high grade and the usual histologic type is "non-comedo". In 2005 the estimated prevalence in the US was 500,000 cases. This number is expected to double by 2020. The 10 year survival rate is 96–98 %. A substantial proportion will remain "in situ" and will never progress to invasive. It is easily concluded that a tumor of fairly good prognosis is very often treated aggressively to a great psychological and physical cost for the woman.

MRI is more often employed today pretreatment to evaluate the local extent, multicentricity, and contralateral disease. Comparison to dMm gives inconsistent results. Therefore, if there could ever be an imaging study that combined with the findings of the core biopsy could safely distinguish patients in need only of FU it would had provided women and healthcare system with a miraculous service.

References

1. Kurian AW, Sigal BM, Plevritis SK (2010) Survival analysis of cancer risk reduction strategies for BRCA ½ mutation carriers. J Clin Oncol 28:222–231
2. Houssami N, Hayes DF (2009) Review of preoperative magnetic resonance imaging (MRI) in breast cancer. CA Cancer J Clin 59:290–302
3. Wagner T, Buscombe J, Gnanasegaran G, Navalkissoor S (2013) SPECT/CT in sentinel node imaging. Nucl Med Commun 34:191–202
4. Zhu A, Lee D, Shim H (2011) Metabolic positron emission tomography imaging in cancer detection and therapy response. Semin Oncol 38:55–69
5. Robertson C, Arcot Ragupathy SK, Boachie C et al (2011) The clinical effectiveness and cost-effectiveness of different surveillance mammography regiments after the treatment for primary breast cancer. Health Technol Assess 15:1–322

Part IX
Gastrointestinal Cancer

Esophageal and Gastric Tumors Where the Clinician Requires Imaging

50

Ioannis K. Danielides and Antonis N. Nikolopoulos

50.1 Introduction

There are 2 different histological types of **esophageal carcinoma** (squamous cell- and adenocarcinoma) with different characteristics such as location (primarily upper esophagus for SCC and lower for adenocarcinoma) and risk factors (alcohol and smoking for SCC vs. gastroesophageal reflux and Barretts esophagus for adenocarcinoma) [1]. As adenocarcinoma is the commonest, discussion is referring mainly to this particular histological type [2].

Esophageal adenocarcinoma presents with solid food dysphagia and weight loss and is diagnosed with upper gastrointestinal endoscopy and biopsies.

Both prognosis, which unfortunately remains poor [3] and therapeutic algorithm (neoadjuvant therapy before surgery, endoscopic resection vs. surgery) depends on staging.

With regards to **gastric cancer**, the majority of patients has limited symptoms (weight loss and abdominal pain) or is completely asymptomatic and present with advanced, metastatic and thus incurable disease.

I. K. Danielides (✉) · A. N. Nikolopoulos
Gastroenterology Department, Hygeia Hospital,
Erythrou Stavrou Street 4, 15123,
Marousi, Athens, Greece
e-mail: iodaniel@hol.gr

A. N. Nikolopoulos
e-mail: dra.nikolopoulos@yahoo.com

The diagnosis is made with upper gastrointestinal endoscopy and biopsies where at least 7 biopsies are thought to be needed to increase diagnostic accuracy [4]. In a particular type of diffuse-gastric cancer (**linitis plastica**) apart from sufficient number, a specific endoscopic biopsy technique is advocated to ensure adequate tissue sample (strip and bite biopsy technique). In these cases, Barium study is a useful diagnostic tool with the characteristic "leather flask" appearance of the stomach due to poor distensibility.

MALT is one of the most common histologic types of gastric lymphoma which is diagnosed with endoscopy and biopsies.

Staging investigations include CT chest, abdomen and pelvis (distant disease-M stage) and EUS (depth of invasion-perigastric lymph nodes-T and N stage).

GISTs are stromal or mesenchymal tumors that can present as subepithelial masses anywhere in the gastrointestinal tract (more often in the stomach rather than the esophagus where leiomyomas are the commonest) including rarely mesentery, omentum and peritoneum. The majority are sporadic with a mutation in the KIT or much less frequently in the PDGFRA gene [5].

They affect predominantly middle-aged or older individuals and typically present with no or nonspecific symptoms (bloating, early satiety) unless they are complicated by ulceration, bleeding or intestinal obstruction.

A. D. Gouliamos et al. (eds.), *Imaging in Clinical Oncology*,
DOI: 10.1007/978-88-470-5385-4_50, © Springer-Verlag Italia 2014

References

1. Engel LS, Chow WH, Vaughan TL, et al (2003) Population attributable risks of esophageal and gastric cancers. J Natl Cancer Inst 95:1404–1413
2. Jemal A, Bray F, Center MM et al (2011) Global cancer statistics. Cancer J Clin 61:69–90
3. Daly JM, Karnell LH, Menck HR (1996) National cancer data base report on esophageal carcinoma. Cancer 78:1820–1828
4. Graham DY, Schwartz JT, Cain GD et al (1982) Prospective evaluation of biopsy number in the diagnosis of esophageal and gastric carcinoma. Gastroenterology 82:228–231
5. Medeiros F, Corless CL, Duensing A et al (2004) KIT-negative gastrointestinal stromal tumors: proof of concept and therapeutic implications. Am J Surg Pathol 28:889–894

51 Imaging Findings in Gastrointestinal Cancer: Esophagus, Stomach

Spyros D. Yarmenitis

51.1 Esophageal Cancer

According to the TNM staging system, described elsewhere in this section, the goal of imaging is to determine the local primary disease stage (T) represented by the depth of the cancer invasion through the esophageal wall, the presence (N1) or absence (N0) of locoregional nodal involvement along the esophageal course and to depict distant disease (M).

51.2 T Stage

51.2.1 Endoscopic US

With EUS, a well-described pattern of five alternating hyperechoic and hypoechoic layers—from inner superficial mucosa to outer serosa—illustrates the normal sonographic appearance of the intact esophageal wall. Hence EUS is currently the most accurate modality to discriminate T1, T2 and T3 disease. Even more so, some reports claim that high-frequency EUS can distinguish mucosal from submucosal involvement. An overall average accuracy of EUS for T staging of esophageal cancer is reported to be 84 % and compared to CT, EUS is found more accurate (EUS: 76–89 %, CT: 49–59 %) [1].

51.2.2 Computed Tomography

The most important role of CT is the exclusion of T4 stage [2]. The CT criteria of invasion of adjacent structures/organs are mediastinal fat planes obliteration and displacement or indentation of neighboring mediastinal structures (Fig. 51.1).

An 88–100 % sensitivity and 85–100 % specificity of CT is reported for detecting mediastinal invasion [3].

In particular if a 90° or more of the aortic circumference is in contact with the tumor or an obliteration of the triangular fat between the esophagus, spine and aorta is observed, aortic invasion should be considered [4] (Fig. 51.2).

Displacement of the trachea or bronchus or indentation of the posterior tracheal wall is accurately indicative of tracheobronchial invasion [3].

Pericardial effusion and thickening of the pericardium or indentation of the heart margin and obliteration of fat plane are suggestive of pericardial invasion.

CT compared to EUS is limited in determining the exact depth of wall infiltration by the tumor [5]. However, a wall thickness of more than 5 mm is considered abnormal whenever the esophagus is illustrated distended. Also any asymmetric thickening of the wall is a major but non-specific finding of esophageal cancer.

S. D. Yarmenitis (✉)
Department of Diagnostic radiology, Hygeia Hospital, 4, Erythrou Stavrou St, 15123, Maroussi, Greece
e-mail: spyros.yarmenitis@hotmail.com

A. D. Gouliamos et al. (eds.), *Imaging in Clinical Oncology*,
DOI: 10.1007/978-88-470-5385-4_51, © Springer-Verlag Italia 2014

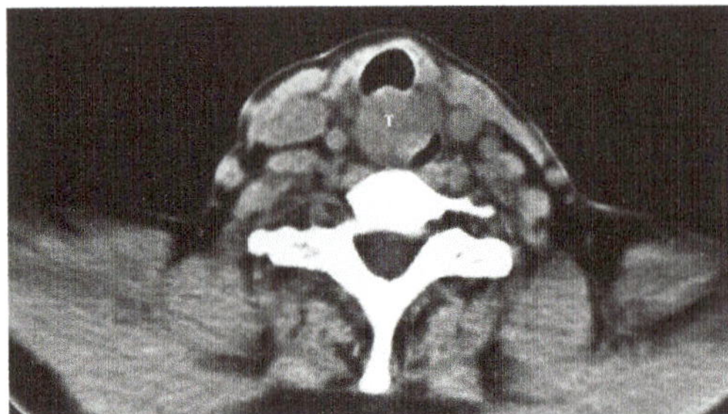

Fig. 51.1 Cancer of the upper third of the esophagus (T) in contact with the tracheal border provoking indentation of the posterior tracheal wall

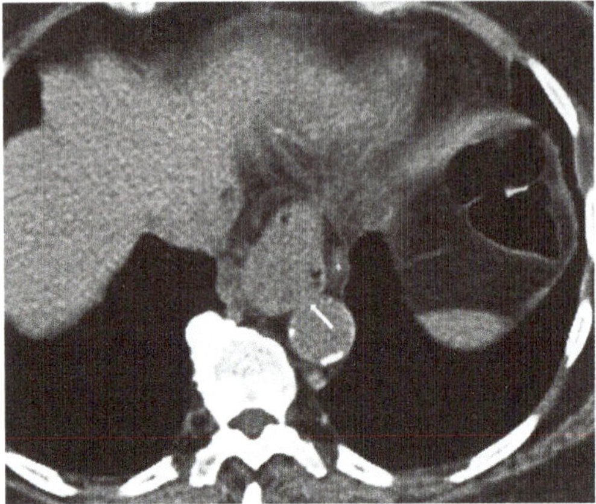

Fig. 51.2 Esophageal cancer at the lower third of the organ that extends beyond the esophageal wall invading the mediastinal fat. Less than 90 degrees of the aortic circumference is in contact with the tumor (*arrow*). Enlarged lymph node is observed at the same level (*asterisk*)

A major contribution of CT with the capability of multiplanar reconstructions is the more accurate assessment of the upper and lower margins of the esophageal tumor in planning curative resection (Fig. 51.3). The multiplanar reformatted images are also useful in the evaluation of esophageal cancer of the abdominal part of the organ, since most of these tumors are now considered gastric cancers according to the revised TNM staging.

51.2.3 FDG PET

PET has been found to have better sensitivity than CT in the detection of primary esophageal cancer, however, it shows limited performance in T staging since it cannot offer useful information on the extent of tumor invasion [6].

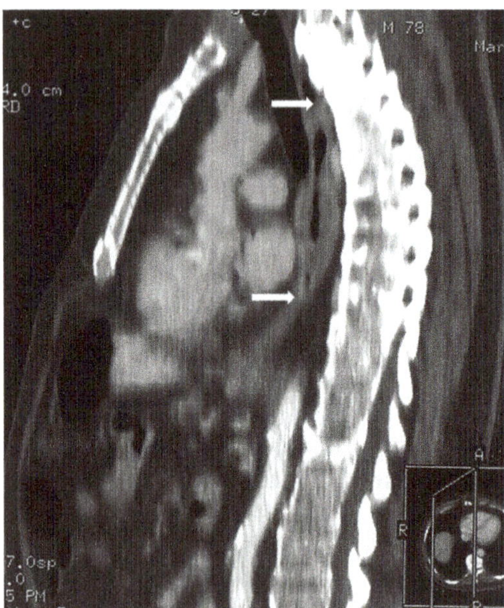

Fig. 51.3 CT scan sagittal reconstruction illustrates the upper and lower extension of a middle esophagus carcinoma (*arrows*). Image courtesy of Dr. Ch. Triantopoulou

51.3 N Stage

Detection of metastatic lymph nodes by US and CT depend on size criteria.

51.3.1 Endoscopic US

Malignant characteristics of a lymph node are a short axis of >10 mm, round shape, homogeneous hypoechoic center and clear border [7]. EUS shows better accuracy values than CT on N stage (EUS: 72–80 %, CT: 46–58 %) [8].

EUS accuracy rates increase when combined with fine needle aspiration of lymph nodes guided by EUS. This is more effective at the celiac axis region, which is also an area of better diagnostic performance of EUS [9].

51.3.2 Computed Tomography

Lymph nodes at intrathoracic and abdominal locations are diagnosed as pathologic when greater than 1 cm in diameter (Fig. 51.2). Supraclavicular lymph nodes are considered pathologic when their short axis measures more than 5 mm [10, 11].

The most important limitation of CT is its poor sensitivity and specifity to diagnose metastatic foci into normal-sized lymph nodes or to distinguish benign enlarged lymph nodes [3].

Multiplanar reformatted images are significantly useful in depicting resectable left gastric nodes or unresectable celiac axis nodes.

51.3.3 FDG PET

Low sensitivity (51 %) and specificity (84 %) is reported in regard with locoregional metastases as a result of the strong uptake of FDG by the primary tumor, which obscures the adjacent lymph nodes [12]. The combined PET/CT improves these rates by the anatomic details illustrated by CT Sensitivities increase considerably up to 90 % at distal sites [13, 14].

51.4 M Stage

CT or FDG PET is the first-line study for the detection of distant metastatic disease. EUS is of limited value with the exception of the detection of metastatic lymph nodes at the celiac axis.

CT is the preferred modality for liver evaluation. The reported sensitivity of contrast enhanced multidetector CT is 90 % for the detection of focal liver lesions 1 cm or larger. The fact that only 50 % of lesions less than 1.5 cm and 12 % of lesions less than 1 cm are metastases should be taken in mind [15, 16].

The pooled sensitivity and specificity of FDG PET is reported to be 67 % for the detection of distal lymph nodes metastases and 97 % for the detection of hematogenous metastases [12].

There is recent evidence that PET may detect metastatic disease that was remaining undiagnosed by the other imaging modalities in up to 15 % of cases of esophageal cancer. However, this has not been proven in cases of early-stage (Tis, T1) disease [6].

51.5 Assessment of Therapeutic Response

FDG PET is considered the best imaging modality for the assessment of neoadjuvant treatment response [17].

The quantitative drop of FDG uptake observed after neoadjuvant treatment seems to correlate with pathologic response to treatment and with survival rates.

There is also evidence that FDG PET can detect interval distant metastases that are found in 8–17 % of patients [18] (Figs. 51.4, 51.5).

There are no guidelines, so far, for the optimal timing of the FDG PET post-treatment assessment.

EUS have shown similar results to that of FDG PET and higher than that of conventional CT [17].

The exact role of multidetector CT has to be defined by further investigation.

51.5.1 Gastric Cancer

As with esophageal cancer, imaging provides a method for local tumor, lymph nodes and distant metastatic assessment of gastric cancer.

CT, EUS, MRI and PET are the imaging modalities currently in use for the management of gastric cancer. However a clear tendency towards CT is present in the literature to be considered as the all-in-one method for gastric cancer.

Major attempts have been made with multidetector CT to illustrate the discrete stages of Early and Advanced gastric cancer as categorized by the latest revision of TNM system.

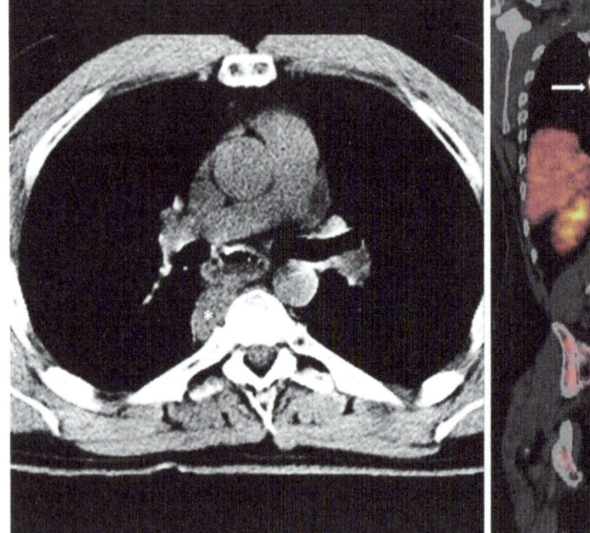

Fig. 51.4 Post-surgical treatment follow-up assessment of esophageal cancer. CT scan: a right paraspinal mass is observed at the level of T6-T8 vertebrae (*asterisk*). FDG PETCT scan uptake confirms the presence of neoplastic tissue (*arrow*)

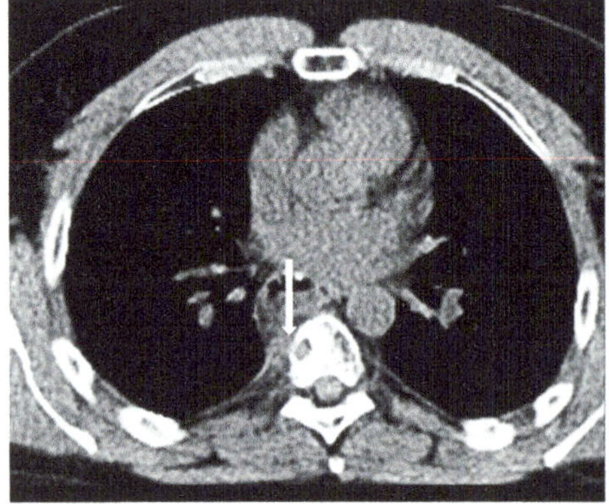

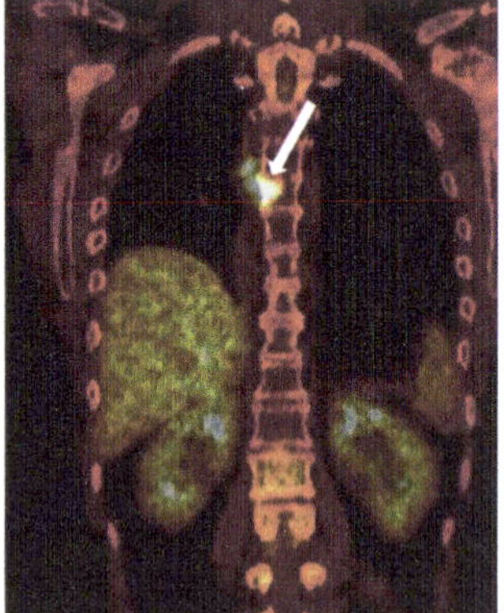

Fig. 51.5 Further post-surgical follow-up of the Fig. 51.4 case, after a 6 months period, reveals decrease of the paraspinal mass. However, invasion of the bony structures of the thoracic vertebrae is observed in both CT scan and FDG PETCT (*arrows*)

51.6 T Stage

CT gastrography based on 2D and 3D image analysis yields a 73–96 % detection rate of early gastric cancer with good depiction of T1b and T2 stages. T1a is rarely visualized in 2D images [19, 20].

Discrimination of T3 and T4a on CT images is very difficult. Furthermore the perigastric infiltration and inflammation or fibrosis may provoke a T2 over-staging as T3 or even T4 tumor [21, 22].

T4b tumors correspond to direct extension and invasion of the primary tumor to adjoining organs/structures (Figs. 51.6, 51.7).

51.7 N Stage

A short axis >6 mm for perigastric and >8 mm for extra-perigastric lymph nodes denotes tumor infiltration.

Multidetector CT has achieved improved pre-operative N staging for advanced gastric cancer but without much impact on early gastric carcinoma [19, 23, 24].

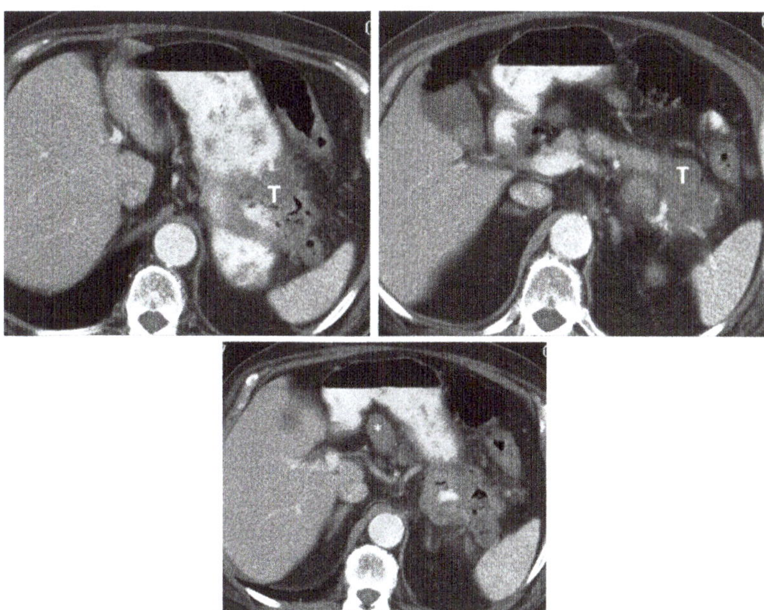

Fig. 51.6 GIST tumor (T) of the gastric greater curvature. The mass extends to the perigastric fat and invades the pancreatic tail. Lymph node enlargement at the hepatogastric ligament (*asterisk*)

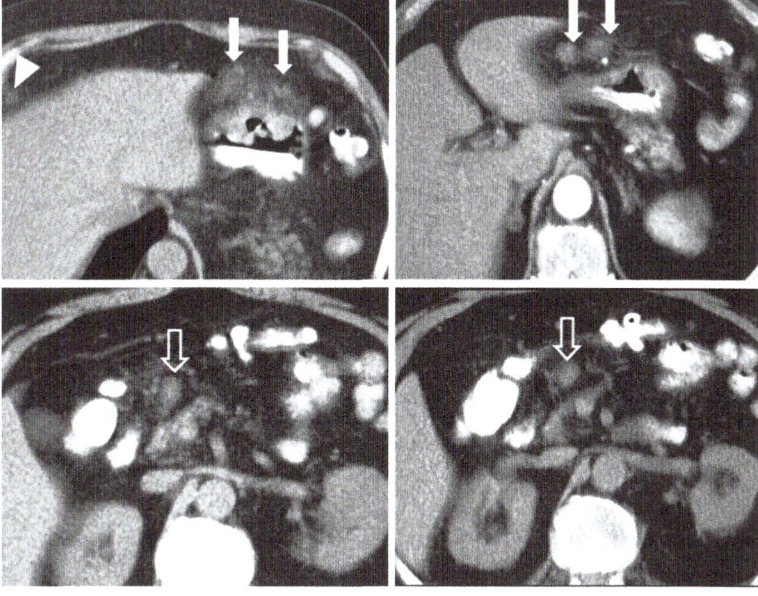

Fig. 51.7 Gastric carcinoma of the greater curvature and anterior wall. The tumor invades the anterior perigastric fat with characteristic fat stranding and deposits (*arrows*). A peritoneal deposit is also seen at the prehepatic area (*arrowhead*). An enlarged extraperigastric lymph node is illustrated anteriorly to the superior mesenteric vein (*open arrows*)

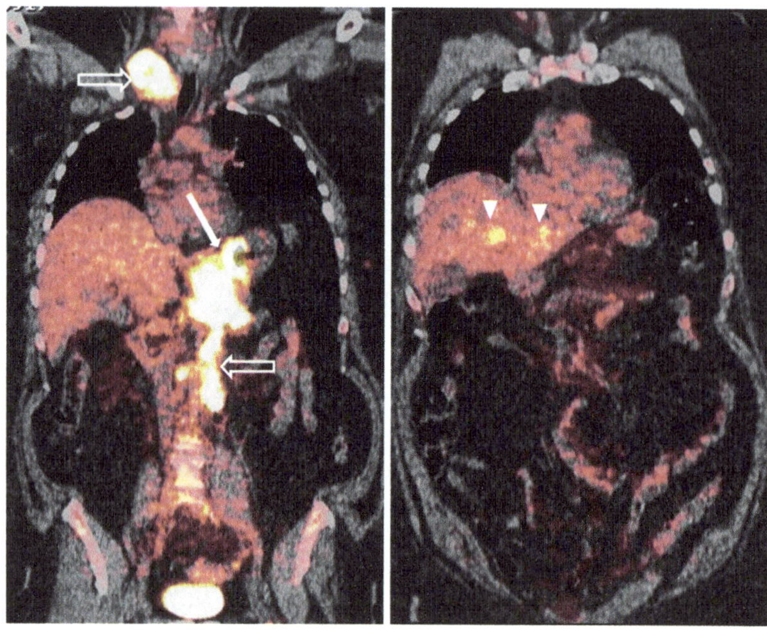

Fig. 51.8 FDG PETCT in the staging of a gastroesophageal junction carcinoma (*white arrow*). M1 stage: Distal disease is confirmed by depicting both right supraclavicular and abdominal para-aortic nodal involvement (*open arrows*) and liver metastases (*arrowheads*)

Lack of consensus regarding the CT criteria for metastatic lymph nodes is the reason of wide ranges of sensitivity (62.5–91.9 %) [25].

51.8 M Stage

Hematogenous metastases involve the liver and less frequently the lungs, adrenal glands, kidneys, bones, brain and other areas of the gastrointestinal tract.

Lymphatic metastases beyond the perigastric region are considered M1 disease.

Advanced gastric cancer can spread into the peritoneum, a fact that is correlated with tumor size and T staging [26].

The group of findings indicating peritoneal metastases are: ascites, soft tissue nodules or plaques on the peritoneal surfaces, small bowel wall thickening and nodularity, intra-abdominal fat stranding and peritoneal thickening and/or enhancement [27]. Ascites is the most important predicting factor for the possibility of existing peritoneal metastases. In the presence of $\geq$50 ml of ascites peritoneal carcinomatosis is found in 75–100 % of patients [28].

FDG PETCT offers considerable advantage in depicting distant disease in both the solid organ sites and the distant lymph nodes (Fig. 51.8)

References

1. Reed CE, Eloubeidi MA (2002) New techniques for staging for esophageal cancer. Surg Clin North Am 82:697–710
2. Rice TW (2000) Clinical staging of esophageal carcinoma. CT, EUS, and PET. Chest Surg Clin N Am 10:471–485
3. Picus D, Balfe DM, Koehler RE et al (1983) Computed tomography in the staging of esophageal carcinoma. Radiology 146:433–438
4. Takashima S, Takeuchi N, Shiozaki H et al (1991) Carcinoma of the esophagus: CT vs MR imaging in determining resectability. AJR Am J Roentgenol 156:297–302
5. Berger AC, Scott WJ (2004) Noninvasive staging of esophageal carcinoma. J Surg Res 117:127–133
6. Flamen P, Lerut A, Van Cutsem E (2000) Utility of positron emission tomography for the staging of patients with potentially operable esophageal carcinoma. Clin Oncol 18:3202–3210
7. Tio TL, Cohen P, Coene PP et al (1989) Endosonography and computed tomography of esophageal carcinoma: preoperative classification compared to the new (1987) TNM system. Gastroenterology 96:1478–1486.

8. Souquet JC, Napoleon B, Pujol B et al (1994) Endoscopic ultrasonography in the preoperative staging of esophageal cancer. Endoscopy 26:764–766
9. Parmar KS, Zwischenberger JB, Reeves AL, Waxman I (2002) Clinical impact of endoscopic ultrasound- guided fine needle aspiration of celiac axis lymph nodes (M1a disease) in esophageal cancer. Ann Thorac Surg 73:916–920
10. Dorfman RE, Alpern MB, Gross BH, Sandler MA (1991) Upper abdominal lymph nodes: criteria for normal size determined with CT. Radiology 180:319–322
11. Fultz PJ, Feins RH, Strang JG et al (2002) Detection and diagnosis of nonpalpable supraclavicular lymph nodes in lung cancer at CT and US. Radiology 222:245–251
12. van Westreenen HL, Westerterp M, Bossuyt PM et al (2004) Systematic review of the staging performance of 18F fluorodeoxyglucose positron emission tomography in esophageal cancer. J Clin Oncol 22:3805–3812
13. Kato H, Kuwano H, Nakajima M et al (2002) Comparison between positron emission tomography and computed tomography in the use of the assessment of esophageal carcinoma. Cancer 94:921–928
14. Lerut T, Flamen P, Ectors N et al (2000) Histopathologic validation of lymph node staging with FDG-PET scan in cancer of the esophagus and gastroesophageal junction: a prospective study based on primary surgery with extensive lymphadenectomy. Ann Surg 232:743–752
15. Kuszyk BS, Bluemke DA, Urban BA et al (1996) Portal-phase contrast-enhanced helical CT for the detection of malignant hepatic tumors: sensitivity based on comparison with intraoperative and pathologic findings. AJR Am J Roentgenol 166:91–95
16. Schwartz LH, Gandras EJ, Colangelo SM, Ercolani MC, Panicek DM (1999) Prevalence and importance of small hepatic lesions found at CT in patients with cancer. Radiology 210:71–74
17. Westerterp M, van Westreenen HL, Reitsma JB et al (2005) Esophageal cancer: CT, endoscopic US, and FDG PET for assessment of response to neoadjuvant therapy—systematic review. Radiology 236:841–851
18. Weber WA, Ott K, Becker K et al (2001) Prediction of response to preoperative chemotherapy in adenocarcinomas of the esophagogastric junction by metabolic imaging. J Clin Oncol 19:3058–3065
19. Kim YN, Choi D, Kim SH et al (2009) Gastric cancer staging at isotropic MDCT including coronal and sagittal MPR images: endoscopically diagnosed early vs. advanced gastric cancer. Abdom Imaging 34:26–34
20. Yang DM, Kim HC, Jin W et al (2007) 64 multidetector-row computed tomography for preoperative evaluation of gastric cancer: histological correlation. J Comput Assist Tomogr 31:98–103
21. Lee IJ, Lee JM, Kim SH et al (2010) Diagnostic performance of 64-channel multidetector CT in the evaluation of gastric cancer: differentiation of mucosal cancer (T1a) from submucosal involvement (T1b and T2). Radiology 255:805–814
22. Kim AY, Kim HJ, Ha HK (2005) Gastric cancer by multidetector row CT: preoperative staging. Abdom Imaging 30:465–472
23. Ba-Ssalamah A, Prokop M, Uffmann M et al (2003) Dedicated multidetector CT of the stomach: spectrum of diseases. Radiographics 23:625–644
24. Husband JE, Reznek R (2004) Imaging in oncology. In: Mclean A (ed) Gastric cancer. Taylor and Francis, London, pp 189–215
25. Kwee RM, Kwee TC (2009) Imaging in assessing lymph node status in gastric cancer. Gastric Cancer 12:6–22
26. Kim SJ, Kim HH, Kim YH et al (2009) Peritoneal metastasis: detection with 16- or 64-detector row CT in patients undergoing surgery for gastric cancer. Radiology 253:407–415
27. Jacquet P, Jelinek JS, Steves MA, Sugarbaker PH (1993) Evaluation of computed tomography in patients with peritoneal carcinomatosis. Cancer 72:1631–1636
28. Chang DK, Kim JW, Kim BK et al (2005) Clinical significance of CT-defined minimal ascites in patients with gastric cancer. World J Gastroenterol 11:6587–6592

Clinical Implications

52

Ioannis K. Danielides and Antonis N. Nikolopoulos

Therapeutic decisions and clinical outcome of all different types of esophageal and gastric cancers depends largely on staging of the disease.

Staging process comprises apart from clinical evaluation, radiological, and endoscopic tests.

The main staging system for both esophageal and gastric cancers is the *TNM system* of the American Joint Committee on Cancer (AJCC) and the International Union Against Cancer (UICC) which was revised in 2010 [1] and the most important differences from the previous classification are listed in Table 52.1.

Early esophageal cancers (T1) are more often seen during endoscopy, with the use of high definition scopes, in the context of Barrett's esophagus surveillance. After histological confirmation and appropriate staging to exclude lymph node involvement (with CT chest, abdomen, and in selected cases Endoscopic Ultrasound with or more often without the use of through the scope ultrasound probes), they can be removed endoscopically. The mucosal resection specimen itself serves the purpose of staging [2].

In the revised 2010 AJCC/UICC, TNM Staging, T1 has been subdivided to T1a (epithelium, lamina propria, muscularis mucosa) and T1b (submucosa). T1a early cancers (even when involving up to the upper third of submucosa) resected during endoscopy are likely to have more favorable prognosis as free submucosa implies very small chance of positive lymph nodes. Another endoscopic treatment modality is radiofrequency ablation (*HALO*) used to treat dysplastic Barrett (without macroscopically visible lesions) as well as nondysplastic Barrett surrounding dysplastic focus.

Endoscopy showing a bulky exophytic esophageal lesion suggests *an advanced tumor*. After histological confirmation, staging and therapeutic decisions depend mainly upon *imaging* which helps:

1. To rule out distant metastases that will preclude an aggressive surgical approach.
2. To assess locoregional spread (i.e., T and N stage) and decide whether to proceed directly to surgery or start therapy with neoadjuvant chemoradiation.
3. In cases of borderline resectability, where neoadjuvant chemoradiation can potentially downstage the disease and make it amenable to surgery.

Imaging tests include *CT chest, upper/lower abdomen* which is particularly useful in detecting mainly distant metastasis (M stage) and is rather poor in celiac axis and peritoneal deposits. *EUS* is helpful in locoregional tumor staging (T, N, and M stage) especially in differentiating

I. K. Danielides (✉) · A. N. Nikolopoulos
Gastroenterology Department, Hygeia Hospital,
Erythrou Stavrou Street 4, Marousi, 15123,
Athens, Greece
e-mail: iodaniel@hol.gr

A. N. Nikolopoulos
e-mail: dra.nikolopoulos@yahoo.com

A. D. Gouliamos et al. (eds.), *Imaging in Clinical Oncology*,
DOI: 10.1007/978-88-470-5385-4_52, © Springer-Verlag Italia 2014

Table 52.1 Main differences of **TNM 2010 AJCC/UICC** with previous TNM classifications

Esophagus	Gastric	GIST
All gastric tumors which extend from the EGJ and up to 5 cm into the stomach are considered esophageal neoplasms	Gastric tumors that extend >5 cm from the EGJ into the stomach or any size that do not extend in the EGJ are considered gastric	T stage still based on size of tumor (T1: <2 cm, T2: 2–5 cm, T3: 5–10 cm, T4: >10 cm)
Tis is classified as high grade dysplasia and not as carcinoma in situ. T1 is subdivided in T1a (tumor invades lamina propria or muscularis mucosae) and T2b (tumor invades submucosa)	T stage is similar to esophageal with emphasis in the depth of tumor invasion rather than the size	N stage only states existence or not of metastatic nodes (N0: no nodes, N1: regional lymph node metastasis)
T4 is subdivided in a (potential resectability despite involvement of adjacent organs) and b (not resectable tumor)	T4 is subdivided in a (potential resectability despite involvement of adjacent organs) and b (not resectable tumor)	Existence of G grade (histologic) with G1:low grade (mitotic rate <5/50HPF) and G2: high grade (mitotic rate >5/50 HPF)
Emphasis in the number of involved lymph nodes rather than location (N1: 1–2 lymph nodes, N2: 3–6 lymph nodes, N3: >6 lymph nodes)	Similar to esophageal (importance to number rather than location). Additional N3a: metastasis in 7–15 lymph nodes, N3b: Metastasis >16 lymph nodes	
Addition of histologic grade differentiation (GX, G1, G2, G3, G4)	M1: positive peritoneal cytology	

between T1 and T2 and less so between T3 and T4. It enables the clinician to measure tumor *thickness*, an independent prognostic predictor factor as well as with the use of *fine needle aspiration* (*FNA*) to tissue sample clinically suspicious lymph nodes (affects the decision about neoadjuvant chemo radiotherapy). Stenotic tumors add a clinical dilemma between an endoscopic dilatation prior to EUS and the small risk of perforation or using *miniature EUS probes* (with limited depth of penetration <3 cm). Finally, EUS is of limited use in restaging esophageal cancer postradiotherapy with problems both due to under and over-staging. *PET or PET/CT* is a more novel imaging modality which might be helpful in detecting metastatic disease especially in the scenario where radical surgery is contemplated and can change management strategy in up to 20 % of patients [3]. It is also of use in post neoadjuvant treatment evaluation. Finally, *diagnostic laparoscopy* might be helpful mainly in T3 and T4, especially, detecting peritoneal deposits and thus precluding a fruitless operation. During a diagnostic laparoscopy *peritoneal washings* can be obtained (positive washings could lead to neoadjuvant treatment and after potential negative subsequent washing result to a surgical resection of the primary esophageal tumor).

The cornerstone of treatment of esophageal adenocarcinoma remains *surgical resection* of the tumor. The type of operation depends on Siewert type classification (type 1, 2, 3) at the initial diagnostic endoscopy. Total gastrectomy and distal esophagectomy is contemplated for Siewert type 2, 3 where a subtotal gastrectomy and subtotal esophagectomy with Thoracotomy for Siewert 1. Regional lymphadenectomy should be performed in all types.

Similarly, treatment strategy of *gastric cancer* depends on staging where TNM criteria were also revised in 2010, with differences depending on the site of the tumor, number of lymph nodes, and stage groupings.

Locoregional (stage 1–3) is potentially resectable disease. Palliative therapy is contemplated for stage 4. The only widely accepted criteria of unresectability are distant metastases and invasion of major vessels (hepatic artery encasement, celiac axis, and proximal splenic, aorta, whereas distal splenic involvement might be amenable to major resection). Lymphadenopathy in the mediastinum, porta hepatis, aortocaval area, nodes behind/inferior to pancreas constitutes metastatic and thus inoperable disease.

Imaging modalities which are used in staging of gastric cancer include *CT chest, upper/lower abdomen* for detecting hepatic, adnexal metastases, ascites, and distal nodal spread (M stage). CT scan has poor sensitivity for peritoneal and smaller than 5 mm metastases as well as determining the depth of invasion of the primary gastric tumor (T stage) [4]. If there is no evidence of metastatic disease *EUS* is useful in locoregional stage evaluation (T and N stage). Direct assessment of the depth of invasion of the primary tumor could potentially offer (for superficial tumors) endoscopic resection as an alternative treatment option as well as consideration of neoadjuvant chemotherapy or chemoradiotherapy for lesions T2 or higher. In addition, suspicious nodal involvement could be assessed with or without *FNA* and potentially instigate neoadjuvant chemoradiotherapy [5]. The role for *PET scan* in the gastric cancer staging pathway is evolving as it is more sensitive from CT in detection of distant metastases but still poor for peritoneal carcinomatosis (positive only in 50 %) as well as for histologically diffuse cancer (not FDG avid). Finally, *Staging laparoscopy* is useful especially for T3 and T4, despite negative CT, as 20–30 % of patients have peritoneal metastases which are not detected with other imaging modalities. It also offers ability to perform *peritoneal cytology* even in patient without macroscopic peritoneal metastases (positive cytology would lead to neoadjuvant therapy followed by reassessment) [6].

There are different types of operations depending on the position of the gastric tumor. Gastric cancers within the upper third of the stomach require a total gastrectomy and Roux anastomosis, tumors in the lower two-thirds subtotal gastrectomy (large midgastric tumors may require total gastrectomy) whereas linitis plastica if operable, would also need a total gastrectomy. Hepatic metastasectomy is very rare since only 0.5 % have an isolated liver metastasis.

Early gastric cancer invades no more deeply than the submucosa irrespective of lymph node metastasis and similar approach in staging with CT and EUS is followed once diagnosed.

Treatment options include endoscopic resection (*Endoscopic Mucosal Resection or Endoscopic Submucosal Dissection*) for patients without lymph node involvement, who are low risk for nodal metastasis. It is important that the resection is performed 'en bloc' (especially with regard to the vertical margins) and requires specialized endoscopic expertise in high volume centers [7].

For patients with low probability of en bloc endoscopic resection, larger tumor size, ulceration, or less favorable histological characteristics (diffuse adenocarcinoma, evidence of lymphovascular invasion) *gastrectomy* should be considered.

Antibiotic treatment with Helicobacter Pylori eradication may reduce the risk of metachronous cancers [8].

Post treatment surveillance is less clear with *annual endoscopy* being a reasonable measure.

Treatment of *MALT lymphoma* also depends on *the disease stage* but also the presence or absence of a concomitant *Helicobacter pylori* infection (present in 90 % of cases) [9].

Patients with MALT lymphoma should be tested for Helicobacter pylori (H pylori), which can be detected primarily by histologic specimen microscopy but also biopsy urease test, urea breath test, stool antigen test, or serology. In addition, testing for t(11;18) should be performed [10].

Patients with *early stage H pylori positive* gastric MALT lymphoma without t(11;18) should receive initial H pylori eradication therapy rather than radiation therapy. On the contrary patients with *early stage H pylori negative* gastric MALT lymphoma or those with t(11;18) should have local radiotherapy (RT) [11]. For patients with *advanced stage* gastric MALT lymphoma, treatment with H pylori eradication therapy if H pylori positive should be followed by observation until the development of symptoms at which time chemotherapy is initiated. Finally, gastric resection is reserved for patients with complications such as perforation or obstruction.

Gastrointestinal stromal tumors (*GISTs*) are diagnosed with upper endoscopy (size of intraluminal component can be measured but as they are subepithelial tumors, seldom standard endoscopic biopsies are useful) or radiological imaging tests (ultrasound, CT, or MRI) commonly as an 'incidentaloma'. EUS is another important diagnostic test that helps both delineating the wall layer the tumor arise from (muscularis propria for GISTs) and giving an idea about the relative prognosis (irregular extraluminal margins, cystic spaces, and enlarged lymph nodes are thought to be more common features of malignant GISTs). PET scan using FDG can be useful for clarifying inconclusive CT scan findings.

The clinical behavior of GISTs depends on tumor size (larger tumors have worse prognosis), anatomic location (intestinal have worse prognosis compared to gastric), and mitotic rate (>5/50 hpf have worse prognosis) [12, 13].

Similarly, to other gastrointestinal tumors, there is a TNM (tumor-node-metastases) staging system for GISTs (AJCC and UICC 2010).

Surgical resection is the cornerstone of treatment for highly suspicious for GIST lesions on CT (all GISTs >2 cm should be resected) without the need for a preoperative biopsy [14]. A biopsy might be needed in a patient with locally advanced or metastatic GIST who is due to have *medical therapy* with a tyrosine kinase inhibitor (such as imatinib) either as a 'downstaging measure' or in more advanced disease, as a sole treatment. Should chemotherapy with imatinib is decided (not in PDGFRA exon 18 D842 V mutation which is insensitive to imatinib altogether), the usual daily dose is 400 mg with dose escalation to 800 mg (KIT exon 9 mutation) [15].

References

1. AJCC Cancer Staging Manual, Seventh Edition (2010) Springer, New York
2. Pech O, Behrens A, May A et al (2008) Long-term results and risk factor analysis for recurrence after curative endoscopic therapy in 349 patients with high-grade intraepithelial neoplasia and mucosal adenocarcinoma in Barrett's oesophagus. Gut 57:1200–1206
3. Van Westreenen HL, Heeren PA, van Dullemen HM et al (2005) Positron emission tomography with F-18-fluorodeoxyglucose in a combined staging strategy of esophageal cancer prevents unnecessary surgical explorations. J Gastrointest Surg 9:54–61
4. Kim SJ, Kim HH, Kim YH et al (2009) Peritoneal metastasis: detection with 16- or 64-detector row CT in patients undergoing surgery for gastric cancer. Radiology 253:407–415
5. Pollack BJ, Chak A, Sivak MV Jr (1996) Endoscopic ultrasonography. Semin Oncol 23:336–346
6. Lowy AM, Mansfield PF, Leach SD et al (1996) Laparoscopic staging for gastric cancer. Surgery 119:611–614
7. Hiki Y, Shimao H, Mieno H et al (1995) Modified treatment of early gastric cancer: evaluation of endoscopic treatment of early gastric cancers with respect to treatment indication groups. World J Surg 19:517–522
8. Fukase K, Kato M, Kikuchi S et al (2008) Effect of eradication of Helicobacter pylori on incidence of metachronous gastric carcinoma after endoscopic resection of early gastric cancer: an open-label, randomised controlled trial. Japan Gast Study Group Lancet 372:392–397
9. Bayerdörffer E, Neubauer A, Rudolph B et al (1995) Regression of primary gastric lymphoma of mucosa-associated lymphoid tissue type after cure of Helicobacter pylori infection. MALT Lymphoma Study Group. Lancet 345:1591–1594
10. Ye H, Liu H, Raderer MI et al (2003) High incidence of t(11;18)(q21;q21) in Helicobacter pylori-negative gastric MALT lymphoma. Blood 101:2547–2550
11. Tomita N, Kodaira T, Tachibana H et al (2009) Favorable outcomes of radiotherapy for early-stage mucosa-associated lymphoid tissue lymphoma. Radiother Oncol 90:231–235
12. Fletcher CD, Berman JJ, Corless C et al (2002) Diagnosis of gastrointestinal stromal tumors: a consensus approach. Hum Pathol 33:459–465
13. Miettinen M, Sobin LH, Lasota J (2005) Gastrointestinal stro mal tumors of the stomach: a clinicopathologic, immunohistochemical, and molecular genetic study of 1765 cases with long-term follow-up. Am J Surg Pathol 29:52–68
14. Tio TL, Tytgat GN, den Hartog Jager FC (1990) Endoscopic ultrasonography for the evaluation of smooth muscle tumors in the upper gastrointestinal

tract: an experience with 42 cases. Gastrointest Endosc 36:342–350
15. Blanke CD, Demetri GD, von Mehren M et al (2008) Long-term results from a randomized phase II trial of standard- versus higher-dose imatinib mesylate for patients with unresectable or metastatic gastrointestinal stromal tumors expressing KIT. J Clin Oncol 26:620–625

53 Introduction to Liver Cancer

Georgios P. Fragulidis

Imaging of the liver is carried out for the detection and characterization of suspected primary or secondary neoplasms prior to planning surgery or chemotherapy for the staging of neoplasms, for assessing treatment response, for evaluating biliary pathology and for screening liver neoplasms in high-risk patients. Imaging also provides the assessment of vascular anatomy of the liver for surgical scheduling, and diagnosis and treatment by guided procedures including percutaneous biopsy, radiofrequency ablation (RFA), hepatic artery infusion therapy and transarterial chemoembolization (TACE).

Although liver ultrasonography (US) is still the first choice investigation, the role of CT and MRI has been recognized as the main imaging modalities. Contrast-enhanced CT and magnetic resonance imaging (MRI) are frequently used to estimate the tumor burden, vascular or biliary invasion, residual normal liver volume and for evaluating patients with preexisting liver disease (chronic hepatitis or cirrhosis) to search for development of potential primary malignancies. Further, the advances in 18-fluorodeoxyglucose positron emission tomography (18-FDG-PET) have also added a new dimension to functional liver imaging.

A primary objective in liver carcinoma imaging is to distinguish metastatic from primary malignant tumors. Liver metastases are 18–40 times more common than primary liver tumors. Most metastases are hypovascular, such as the extremely common of colorectal primaries, and therefore liver imaging protocols benefit from the use of intravenous contrast agents. Hypervascular liver metastases are seen in primary breast, renal cell, thyroid carcinomas, pancreatic neuroendocrine tumors, pheochromocytoma, malignant melanoma, carcinoid tumor, and sarcomas. The most common liver metastases originate from colon, pancreas, breast, lung, and stomach carcinomas [1]. The highest prevalence of metastasis occurs with gallbladder, pancreas, colon, and breast carcinoma; the lowest with prostate carcinoma. In children, most common primary sites for metastatic lesions to the liver are neuroblastoma, Wilms tumor, and leukemia.

53.1 Liver Metastases from Colorectal Cancer

About 25 % of patients with colorectal cancer present synchronous liver metastases and approximately 50 % of patients develop liver metastases during the course of the disease. Metastasis to the liver is the leading cause of death in at least two-thirds of these patients. At present, the only accepted potentially curative standard treatment in patients with liver

G. P. Fragulidis (✉)
2nd Department of Surgery, Aretaieio Hospital, University of Athens Medical School, 76, Vas. Sophias Street, 11528 Athens, Attica, Greece
e-mail: gfragulidis@aretaieio.uoa.gr

A. D. Gouliamos et al. (eds.), *Imaging in Clinical Oncology*,
DOI: 10.1007/978-88-470-5385-4_53,

metastases of colorectal cancer is liver resection. Thus, all patients with resectable colorectal disease should be offered hepatic resection. In recent series, the 5-year overall survival rate after resection in selected patients is 37–58 %. Without any treatment, the survival rate is less than 1 %. Currently, only 10–20 % of patients with hepatic colorectal metastases are eligible for resection. Nevertheless, the absolute number of patients amenable to resection is increasing by means of improvements in systemic therapies for downstaging, in preoperative imaging and surgical techniques [2]. However, despite these very encouraging results, five-year recurrence rates following resection may be as high as 50 %. In 60–70 % of patients the recurrence will be extra-hepatic, often in combination with recurrent intrahepatic disease, and approximately 30 % will be isolated intrahepatic recurrence. For patients with extra-hepatic recurrence, regardless of whether there is an associated intrahepatic recurrence or not, surgery is usually contraindicated. Feasibly, it is patients with isolated intra-hepatic recurrence who represent the real hepatic surgical failure and it is this group of patients who currently presents the real challenge for hepatic imaging [3].

53.2 Hepatocellular Carcinoma

Hepatocellular carcinoma (HCC) is the most frequent primary liver neoplasm, being the major cause of death in cirrhotic patients. In a majority of cases, HCC occurs in the setting of cirrhosis with underlying chronic viral hepatitis (B or C) or alcoholism and more recently with non-alcoholic steatohepatitis. The annual incidence of HCC in the cirrhotic population is 3–5 % compared with 0.4 % in patients without cirrhosis. The diagnosis after the onset of symptoms, when the tumor stage is already advanced, is associated to a poor prognosis presenting 5-year survival rate in less than 10 % of patients. However, successful treatments are possible when the HCC is diagnosed at an early stage, and the 5-year survival rates of patients undergoing curative therapies, including liver transplantation, hepatic resection, and percutaneous ablative techniques, range between 40 and 75 %. It is estimated that about 30 % of patients with HCC are candidates for such curative interventions [4]. HCC in noncirrhotic patients usually manifests as either a large solitary mass or a dominant mass with small satellite nodules that more frequently shows necrosis and central scar formation. In contrast, the diagnosis can be quite challenging in the setting of a nodular cirrhotic liver regarding the differentiation of very small neoplastic lesions from hyperplastic nodules. Moreover, difficulty also arises in the differentiation of several variant types of HCC such as, clear cell type, fibrolamellar, sarcomatoid, sclerosing HCC and combined HCC–cholangiocarcinoma, as they do not share imaging characteristics typical of HCC [5].

53.3 Intrahepatic Cholangiocarcinoma

Cholangiocarcinomas typically present in one of two ways: either as mass lesions within the liver [intrahepatic cholangiocarcinoma (ICC)] or with biliary tract obstruction attributable to large duct obstruction (ductal cholangiocarcinoma). Therefore, they are classified as intrahepatic tumors (8–13 %) or extrahepatic tumors (87–92 %). The ICC arise from intrahepatic ducts, which extend from the periphery of the liver to the second-order bile ducts within the liver. ICC is the most common etiology of primary, malignant intra-hepatic mass lesions in the absence of other primary solid malignancies or cirrhosis, and it is the second most common primary hepatic tumor after HCC. The incidence of ICC is reported about 10 % of primary liver cancers. Risk factors for ICC include chronic biliary tract diseases such as primary sclerosing cholangitis (PSC), hepatolithiasis, choledochal cysts and liver fluke infections.PSC is associated with a prevalence of cholangiocarcinoma of 5–15 %. Patients with ICC are typically at an advanced pathological stage at the time of diagnosis, and are therefore associated with very poor prognosis [6].

References

1. Udayasankar U, Abbas C, Pardeep M, William CS (2008) Diagnostic imaging and image-guided interventions of hepatobiliary malignancies. In: Blake MA, Kalra MK (eds) Imaging in oncology. Springer Science+Business Media, LLC, pp 199–228
2. Abdalla EK, Adam R, Bilchik AJ, Jaeck D et al (2006) Improving resectability of hepatic colorectal metastases: expert consensus statement. Ann Surg Oncol 13(10):1271–1280
3. Wong P (2009) Further defining liver imaging—physician and radiologist in dialogue. Eur Gastroenterol Hepatol Rev 4(2):14–18
4. Willatt JM, Hussain HK, Adusumilli S et al (2008) MR imaging of hepatocellular carcinoma in the cirrhotic liver: challenges and controversies. Radiology 247(2):311–330
5. Ayuso C, Rimola J, Garcia-Criado A (2011) Imaging of HCC. Abdom Imaging 37:215–230
6. Blechacz B, Komuta M, Roskams T, Gores GJ (2011) Clinical diagnosis and staging of cholangiocarcinoma. Nat Rev Gastroenterol Hepatol 8(9):512–522. doi: 10.1038/nrgastro.2011.131

54 Imaging Findings in Liver Malignancies

Christos N. Mourmouris

54.1 Introduction

The liver is an important organ in the era of oncology. Primary hepatic neoplasms have significantly increased during the last decades. The liver also is the most common site of metastasis from primary tumors such as colon, breast, lung, pancreas, and stomach. In both cases, the accurate detection of malignant liver disease is crucial to patient management. However, since benign liver lesions are also very common, it is important to use all the available imaging modalities for the characterization of a focal liver lesion. The goal of liver imaging in oncology is detection and characterization of a lesion, staging of a neoplasm, evaluation of treatment response, and assessment of vascular anatomy for surgical planning or chemotherapy.

For the purpose of this chapter, we will focus on the two most common primary tumors of liver, hepatocellular carcinoma (HCC) and cholangiocarcinoma, and also on metastatic tumors.

C. N. Mourmouris (✉)
Imaging Department Hygeia Hospital,
4 Erythrou Stavrou Str, 15124, Marousi, Greece
e-mail: cmourmouris@yahoo.gr

54.2 Hepatocellular Carcinoma

Hepatocellular carcinoma (HCC) is the most frequent primary liver tumor. HCC occurs in the setting of cirrhosis with underlying chronic viral hepatitis or alcoholism.

If the diagnosis established after the onset of symptoms, usually the tumor is already in advanced stage which is associated to a poor diagnosis (0–10 %, 5-year survival). As a result, early detection of HCC is crucial in order to achieve effective treatment and long-term survival (50–70 %, 5-year survival).

54.2.1 Diagnosis

To detect HCC at an early stage it is important that high-risk patients undergo periodic liver screening test in order to detect focal liver lesion. For this purpose, ultrasonography (US) is the essential screening test. It is not expensive, not invasive, well accepted by the patients, and can be repeated without risk, typically every 3–6 months. The sensitivity and specificity of US for the detection of HCC in cirrhotic patients are high (60–80 % and 45–94 % respectively) [1]. The goal of the examination is to detect tumors smaller than 2 cm, because they have low probability of vascular invasion and appropriate treatments can be applied. However, the presence of diffuse liver disease decreases the sensitivity of US for the detections of focal lesions. In addition, distinction of small HCCs from other

A. D. Gouliamos et al. (eds.), *Imaging in Clinical Oncology*,
DOI: 10.1007/978-88-470-5385-4_54, © Springer-Verlag Italia 2014

solid benign lesions such as, regenerative and dysplastic nodules, which are found very frequent in cirrhotic patients may be difficult and sometimes impossible. The radiological appearances of HCC on US are variable. Large lesions are often heterogeneous due to necrosis and fibrosis. In these cases, it may be easy to suggest the diagnosis of HCC. On the other hand, small HCCs have less specific findings. They are usually hypoechoic, but other appearances like mixed or hyperechoic nodules, especially if fatty infiltration is present, are possible. In conclusion, every new focal lesion >1 cm which is detected on US in a cirrhotic liver is suspicious and further investigation is recommended.

Contrast-enhanced US (CEUS) is using microbubbles in order to provide microflow imaging of nodules and depict the vascular features of HCC. The most common feature of HCC using CEUS is the presence of early, intense, and homogeneous intratumoral enhancement in the arterial phase. After the arterial enhancement, HCC shows rapid washout resulting in an isoechoic or hypoechoic appearance in the portal and delayed phase. Recent studies demonstrated that CEUS has sensitivity, specificity, and positive predictive value greater than 90 %. However, Vilana et al. [2] demonstrated that small intrahepatic cholangiocarcinoma may mimic the enhancement pattern of HCC and concluded that CEUS should not be used as the only imaging modality to characterize HCC.

CT is the most common imaging modality for the diagnosis of HCC. The two main reasons are their wide availability and short examination time. Recent technological advances in CT technology (from single slice to multislice scanners) have strongly enhanced the performance of CT in liver imaging concerning the speed of acquisition, spatial resolution, and the ability to scan the liver during multiple phases of contrast enhancement is more accurate than possible before. Additionally, the introduction of powerful workstations and the improvements in postprocessing methods results in the acquisition of detailed three-dimensional images of the liver including vascular anatomy.

The standard protocol for the examination of the liver consists of three phases: arterial, portal, and delayed phase. Iannaccone et al. [3] demonstrate the value of delayed phase for the detection of HCC (≤2 mm) due to its ability to depict HCC capsule a finding that can be detected only on delayed images.

HCC arising in a noncirrhotic liver typically presents as a hyperattenuated lesion in arterial phase following by rapid washout to iso or mostly hypoattenuatted in the portal or delayed phase. Although there are other morphologic features of HCC such as peripheral rim enhancement on delayed phase, suggesting the presence of a fibrous capsule, extension into the portal vein or hepatic veins, internal mosaic appearance that may help the diagnosis of HCC; however, the depiction of this typical enhancement pattern is the most reliable criteria to characterize a lesion as HCC [4]. Colli et al. [5] estimate that sensitivity and specificity were 68 and 93 %, respectively. Kim et al. [6] demonstrate that MDCT showed better sensitivity than spiral CT for detecting HCC (65–79 vs. 37–54 %).

However, the diagnosis can be quite challenging in the setting of a cirrhotic liver regarding the differentiation of very small neoplastic lesions from hyperplastic nodules. Additionally, a number of benign lesions hemangiomas, focal confluent fibrosis, benign regenerative nodules, and transient hepatic attenuation difference can stimulate small HCC on CT [7]. Brancatelli et al. [8] report an 8 % false-positive rate when CT studies prior to transplantation were compared with pathological examination of explanted livers but most of the lesions were small (<1.5 cm).

MRI has established as the best imaging modality for the liver lesion detection and characterization, because it provides higher lesion to liver contrast over CT and does not use radiation. Over the past few years, MR imaging of the liver has progressed substantially. Technical advances in hardware and software including parallel imaging, powerful gradient system with increased speed, new 3D gradient echo sequences with increased resolution and

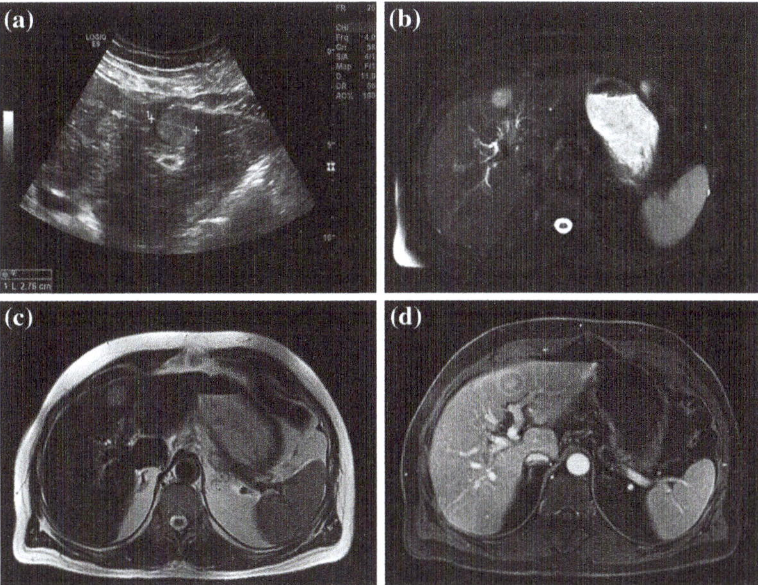

Fig. 54.1 Hepatocellular carcinoma. Appearances at different imaging modalities, **a** Ultasound: hyperechoic nodule, **b–d** MRI: Hyperintense nodule on T2W with and without fat suppression. On dynamic study after the administration of contrast media the lesion enhanced on delayed phase. The capsule of the lesion is also enhanced

volumetric imaging, and 3T MRI with increased SNR have strongly enhanced the ability to imaging the liver.

HCC imaging features on MRI are variable reflecting the variable characteristics of this malignancy. HCC may have variable appearance on T1W images and typically has increased signal intensity on T2W images. However, the most important sequence in the detection of HCC is the dynamic study of liver following the intravenous contrast media administration where the typical enhancement pattern of HCC (hyperenhancement during the arterial phase and rapid washout during the portal or the delayed phase) may well demonstrated (Fig. 54.1). In this case, the sensitivity and specificity are 90 and 95 %, respectively [9]. The sensitivity of MRI for the diagnosis of HCC is slightly better when compared with CT (81 vs. 68 % respectively). MR imaging is sensitive for the detection of lesions measuring 2 cm or larger but is insensitive for the diagnosis of small HCC (<1 cm). However, the sensitivity of MRI decreases significantly for the detection of small HCC nodules (>90 % when tumor is larger than 2 cm and 4–33 % when tumor is smaller than 1 cm) [10].

Several of liver-specific contrast agents have been used in order to increase the sensitivity and specificity of MRI concerning the diagnosis of HCC especially in a cirrhotic liver. Two hepatobiliary agents with extracellular properties Gd-BOPTA and Gd-EOB-DTPA were recently introduced. These agents are taken up to varying degrees by functioning hepatocytes and are excreted in the bile. Because of their properties, the agents cause T1 shortening of the liver and biliary tree resulting in an increased contrast to noise ratio for nonhepatocellular lesions compared with that of the background liver. Thereby, the lesion conspicuity on delayed T1W images is increased. Kim et al. [11] reported that gadoxetic acid–enhanced MRI and MDCT have similar accuracy in the preoperative detection of HCC, but MRI may be better than MDCT in the detection of HCC 1 cm in diameter or smaller. Ahn et al. [12] reported that adding hepatobiliary phase images in gadoxetic acid-enhanced MRI modest improvement in the diagnosis of HCC may be achieved.

Recently, diffusion-weighted imaging (DWI) has been introduced in protocol studies dedicated to the liver. DWI detects the random motion of water molecules within biological tissues which are not influenced by magnetic field strength or by perfusion or microcirculation and quantified as the apparent diffusion coefficient (ADC). Vandecaveye et al. [13] reported sensitivity 95 % for detection of malignant lesions compared to

80 % for conventional MRI and the improved accuracy was most beneficial for differentiating malignant lesions smaller than 2 cm.

The most challenging part in imaging cirrhosis is the characterization of nodules smaller than 2 cm which often have nonspecific imaging characteristics. Over 41–62 % of those lesions showed absence of arterial hypervascularity, venous washout or both. Due to the recent advances on CT and MR scanners, there is an increasing demand for detection smaller tumors as possible because curative therapies are most effective. As a result, the American Association for the study of the Liver disease (AASLD) updated the recommendations for noninvasive diagnostic criteria of HCC. The recommendations are discussed in the previous chapter.

54.2.2 Staging

Once the diagnosis of HCC is established the next crucial step is to define the staging of the disease. The goal of the staging is to provide a guide assess in order to choose the best treatment to every particular case.

Unlike with most cancers staging of HCC is not simply a process of measuring tumor extent, nodal involvement, and metastasis. The staging of HCC is complicated by the fact that HCC almost always is found on the background of cirrhosis and therefore liver function and the physical status of the patient has to be taken into account. For these reasons, the staging process is complicated. Several staging systems have been proposed. Although there is no consensus about which system is the best, many have preferred the Barcelona Clinic Liver Cancer (BCLC) system. The BCLC combines tumors borders, hepatic function, patient physical status, and treatment indications [14].

The goal of imaging techniques in the staging of HCC is: (1) to determine the size, number and location of the lesions, to detect major vascular invasions, nodal disease, and distant metastases; (2) to assess the extent of chronic liver disease and the presence of portal hypertension with its associated clinical manifestations.

Typically, patients with an established diagnosis of HCC should undergo staging with a contrast-enhanced CT of the chest, abdomen, and pelvis.

54.2.3 Assessment of Treatment Response

Surgical treatment in patients with HCC is standard for curative treatment; however, most of the patients are not candidates for resection due to advance liver disease especially in cirrhotic patients. As a result, patients with HCC in the early and intermediate stages undergo loco-regional therapies, such as percutaneous ablation, RFA, and embolization procedures.

Liver transplantation is theoretically the most radical treatment for HCC. However, the risk of recurrence is increased especially for the first 2 years. Therefore, a close follow-up of these patients is strongly recommended.

The evaluation of surgery is not subject to controversy. Due to the risk of recurrence during the first 2 years after surgery, follow-up of these patients is recommended.

On the other hand, assessment of tumor response after loco-regional treatment is important in order to evaluate the efficacy of the treatment. Therefore, the development of reliable and reproducible criteria is mandatory. Unfortunately, RECIST criteria cannot apply reliably in patients with HCC, because the aim of all effective loco-regional therapies is not tumor shrinkage of the lesion but the necrosis of the tumor. As a result in 2000, a panel of experts on HCC of the European Association for the Study of the Liver (EASL) agreed that estimating the reduction in viable tumor volume (recognized as nonenhanced areas using dynamic imaging techniques) should be considered the optimal method for assessing local response to treatment in patients with HCC [15]. Therefore, most authors reporting results of loco-regional therapy for HCC evaluate tumor response according to this recommendation. Complete response (CR) is defined as the absence of enhanced tumor areas, reflecting complete tissue necrosis, partial response (PR) was defined a decrease >50 % of enhanced areas inside the treated lesion and progressive disease (PD) was defined as an increase >25 % in the size of ≥1 measurable lesions or the appearance of new lesions [16].

Both dynamic CT and MRI may be applied in order to monitor treatment response after locoregional treatment demonstrating high accuracy.

54.2.4 Conclusion

Over the past few years, imaging techniques have progressed substantially. Recent technological advantages in the development of CEUS, MDCT, and MRI have improved significantly the ability for detection and characterization of nodules in patients with liver cirrhosis. However, it should be recognized that challenges remain in imaging evaluation of the cirrhotic liver particularly in the detection of small HCC (<1 cm) and their differentiation from a number of benign liver pathologies.

54.3 Cholangiocarcinoma

Cholangiocarcinoma is a primary tumor arising from the epithelium of the biliary ducts and is the second most common primary hepatobiliary cancer after HCC. Cholangiocarcinomas generally are classified as intrahepatic, hilar, and extrahepatic. Hilar cholangiocarcinoma is the most common accounting 40–60 % of cases. When the tumor is located at the confluence of the right and left hepatic ducts is called Klatskin tumor.

Because of their location, these tumors tend to become symptomatic late when patients are in advanced stage, and therefore are not usually resectable at the time of presentation. This is variable as, due to obstruction, jaundice may present early and force the patient to seek help. A multimodality imaging approach is used in patients with a suspected malignant cause for biliary obstruction.

Ultrasound is the initial screening imaging modality for evaluating biliary dilatation in patients with jaundice, because it is inexpensive and widely available. B-mode US is a highly sensitive method for confirming biliary duct dilatation, localization of the site of obstruction, and excluding gallstones. The tumor may not be seen on US and biliary dilatation might be the only indirect sign of a cholangiocarcinoma. The sensitivity and specificity of US are variable depending on tumor type, quality of equipment, and operator's experience.

CT is the initial imaging modality for the assessment of cholangiocarcinoma. However, with the development of multidetector CT scanners, the whole abdomen can be covered with slices <1 mm in less than 15 s. With these detailed datasets we can create high-quality multiplanar reformatted images in order to assess the biliary system and to depict the level and the cause of the biliary obstruction. Using advanced postprocessing techniques, we can provide detailed images of the liver vasculature (CT angiography) in order to depict the involvement of critical vessels, the relationship of the tumor to the vessels and the presence of any vascular anomalies or variants helping in surgical planning [17]. We also have the ability, at the same scan, to examine the whole abdomen for potential metastatic disease.

The standard protocol for the assessment of cholangiocarcinoma includes arterial and portal phase. A delayed scan (3–5 min after the intravenous administration of contrast media) is recommended.

The CT findings of cholangiocarcinoma vary depending on its anatomic position within the biliary system. Many of the tumors may not directly visualize and the isolated dilatation of the intrahepatic bile ducts may be the only sign. Typically, cholangiocarcinomas are hypoattenuatting masses that do not show significant enhancement during the arterial and portal phase, while they enhanced during the delayed phase due to the fibrous stroma they contain. Nonunion of the dilated right and left hepatic ducts is a typical finding of infiltrating hilar cholangiocarcinoma. This is very useful when a distinct mass cannot be seen. The overall accuracy of CT for assessing resectability varies between 60 and 75 % [18].

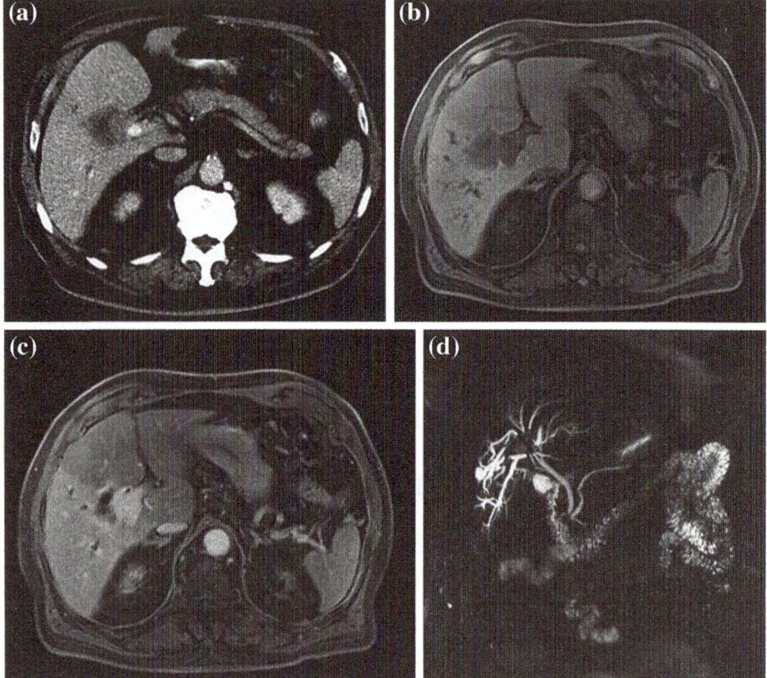

Fig. 54.2 Imaging study of a patient with hilar cholangiocarcinoma. Contrast-enhanced CT (**a**), MRI (**b**, **c**) and MRCP (**d**). An enhanced space—occupying at the hilum of the liver is observed. The lesion is in contact with portal vein. The ducts of the *right* hepatic lobe are dilated. On MRCP images, an abrupt cutoff at the confluence of the RHD and LHD is observed

MRI in combination with magnetic resonance cholangiopancreatography (MRCP) is the preferred imaging technique for the comprehensive evaluation of cholangiocarcinoma. Due to high contrast resolution, MRI is superior to CT in detecting small hillar lesions, intrahepatic, and periductal tumor infiltration. The appearance of intrahepatic cholangiocarcinoma is variable on T2W images depending on the amount of fibrous tissue they contain. After the administration of contrast media, most of them show a heterogeneous enhancement that gradually peaks on delayed phase (Fig. 54.2). More than 50 % of patients will have satellite nodules [19]. It is also important to note that small intrahepatic cholangiocarcinomas <2 cm with less fibrosis, may mimic HCC, since they show an intense enhancement during the arterial phase with prolonged enhancement during the delayed phase. However, they do show the wash-out pattern which is the key for differential diagnosis [20].

MRCP is a noninvasive imaging study of choice in depicting the level of biliary obstruction and associated upstream biliary dilatation. The accuracy of MRCP is comparable to ERCP [21].

54.3.1 Conclusion

The imaging characteristics of cholangiocarcinoma are extremely variable, since these tumors vary greatly in growth pattern and location. Imaging studies play a crucial role in order to define the location and the extension of the tumor and also to assess respectability.

54.4 Liver Metastases

Metastases are by far the most common malignant tumor of the liver. Mostly, 20–25 % of patients with known primary tumor have hepatic metastases at the time of diagnosis. The most common sites of primary malignancy that seeds to liver are colorectal cancer, pancreatic adenocarcinoma, gastric carcinoma, and breast and lung cancer. However, the incidence of solid benign liver lesion is approximately 20 %. The most frequent benign lesion is hemangioma with a prevalence rate of 7–21 %. Focal nodular hyperplasia (FNH) is by far less common (3 %). Additionally, pseudo liver tumors such as transient hepatic attenuation differences (THAD), focal fatty sparing may also be cause of confusion.

Therefore, imaging of the liver in patients with known primary malignancy not only requires high sensitivity, but the ability to reliable differentiates malignant from benign tumors.

Ultrasound is currently the first screening method to be used in the search for hepatic metastases. It is inexpensive and easily available. It is highly accurate to differentiate a cyst from a solid lesion. However, the sensitivity to detect a focal solid lesion is decreased in comparison to CT and MRI especially if fatty infiltration is present. Although the reported sensitivity of US for the detection of liver metastases varies from 40 to 70 % [22], there are many limitations such as high operator dependency, pure acoustic window, and obesity.

CEUS improves the sensitivity of US in the detection of solid lesions by about 20 %. The reported sensitivity varies from 80 to 86 % [23] and it is comparable to contrast-enhanced CT and MRI. The key to establish the diagnosis is the enhancement pattern. Metastatic lesions demonstrate contrast washout during the delayed phase, while benign lesions demonstrate prolonged enhancement in the portal and late phases.

Contrast-enhanced CT is the most widely used imaging modality for detection of liver metastases. It has high sensitivity and specificity (93 and 100 % respectively) [24]. Other advantages of the method is the wide availability and the short examination time which allow a chest—abdomen—pelvis CT scan in less than 15 s breath hold using modern MDCT scanners. Main limitations of the method include radiation dose and the decreased sensitivity for the detection and characterization of lesions smaller than 1 cm.

Typically, the examination should perform during the portal venous phase after the intravenous administration of the contrast media. However, the protocol should modified by adding an arterial phase when patients with known vascular tumors such as melanoma and renal cell carcinoma are examined.

Contrast-enhanced CT is contraindicated in patients with a previous history of allergic reaction to iodine contrast media. Renal failure is also another major contraindication. In these cases, accuracy of unenhanced CT is poor and an MRI scan should be performed to evaluate the liver. Similarly, MRI scan should be performed if liver is fatty infiltrated.

Typically, hypovascular liver metastases appeared as rounded, well-defined, or ill-defined hypoattenuatting lesions on portal phase imaging. Some lesion may show peripheral wash-out sign. On the other hand, hypervascular metastases demonstrate homogeneous late arterial enhancement on CT scan, although inhomogeneous enhancement may be seen due to areas of necrosis or hemorrhage.

MRI is the best imaging test for accurate detection of liver metastases, especially if liver resection is being considered. The main advantages of MRI include high spatial resolution, better lesion-to-liver contrast than CT, and lack of radiation. MRI can be safely used in patients with renal failure or with a history of previous iodine allergy. The main disadvantages of MRI include high cost, long procedure time, and the need for the patient to hold his breath for longer periods than CT.

On MRI, metastases typically appeared as hypointense lesions on T1W images and hyperintense on T2W images. After the intravenous administration of contrast media, the enhancement pattern is similar to those on CT images. Most liver metastases show restricted water diffusion on DW images, and therefore appear as hyperintense lesions (Fig. 54.3).

The accurate detection of liver metastases is a major concern, especially when a patient is being evaluated for curative liver resection. Although there is some debate on which contrast agent to use, MRI using liver-specific contrast media (hepatobiliary and reticuloendothelial) is more sensitive than CT in detecting liver metastases. Several studies have consistently shown that superiority. In a metaanalysis comparing CT, MRI, and FDG/PET for the detection of liver metastases from colorectal cancer, Niekel et al. found that sensitivity on a per-lesion

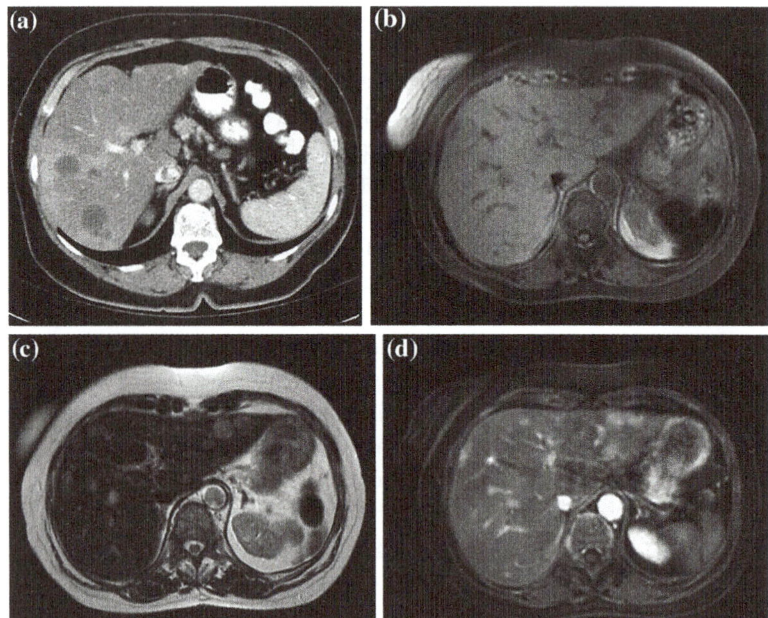

Fig. 54.3 Imaging study of a patient with a history of breast cancer. **a** Contrast-enhanced CT shows multiple hypodense lesions with peripheral enhancement. **b–d** Multiple liver metastases on MRI. The lesions are hypointensed on T1W images (**b**) and hyperintenced on T2W (**c**). After the administration of the contrast media the lesions show peripheral enhancement

basis were 74.4, 80.3, and 81.4 %, respectively and on per-patient basis were 83.6, 88.2, and 94.1 %, respectively. Especially for lesions smaller than 1 cm, the sensitivity for MRI was higher than those for CT [25, 26].

54.4.1 Conclusion

Optimal detection of liver metastases can alter patient management. Contrast-enhanced MDCT is an accurate technique to evaluate liver and extra-hepatic disease in patients with a known extra-hepatic malignancy. Contrast-enhanced MRI with gadolinium chelates offers an accurate nonradiation imaging technique for the detection of liver metastases especially for lesions <1 cm. However, when a patient is candidate for surgical therapy MR imaging enhanced with liver-specific contrast agents is strongly recommended.

References

1. Bolondi J (2003) Screening for hepatocellular carcinoma in cirrhosis. J Hepatol 39:1076–1084
2. Vilana R, Forner A, Bianchi L et al (2010) Intrahepatic peripheral cholangiocarcinoma in cirrhotic patients may display a vascular pattern similar to hepatocellular on contrats enhanced ultrasound. Hepatology 51:2020–2029
3. Iannaccone R, Laghi A, Catalano C et al (2005) Hepatocellular carcinoma: role of unenhanced and delayed phase multi-detector row helical CT in patients with cirrhosis. Radiology 234:460–467
4. Choi B, Lee J (2010) Advancement in HCC imaging: diagnosis, staging and treatment efficacy assessments. J Hepatobilliary Pancreat Sci 17:369–373
5. Colli A, Fraquelli M, Casazza G et al (2006) Accuracy of ultrasonography, spiral CT, magnetic resonance and alpha-fetoprotein in diagnosing hepatocellular carcinoma: a systematic review. Am J Gastroenterol 101:513–523
6. Kim SH, Choi BI, Lee JY et al (2008) Diagnostic accuracy of MDCT and contrast-enhanced MRI in the detection of hepatocellular carcinomas meeting the Milan Criteria before liver transplantation. Intervirology 51(suppl 1):52–60
7. Ariff B, Lloyd C, Khan S et al (2009) Imaging of liver cancer. World J Gastroenterol 15(11):1289–1300
8. Brancatelli G, Federle MP, Grazioli L et al (2002) Hepatocellular carcinoma in non-cirrhotic liver: CT clinical and pathological findings in 39 US residents. Radiology 222:89–94
9. Marrero JA, Hussain HK, Nghiem HV et al (2005) Improving the prediction of hepatocellular carcinoma in cirrhotic patients with arterial enhancing liver mass. Liver Transpl 11:281–289
10. Willatt JM, Hussain HK, Adusumilli S et al (2008) MR imaging of hepatocellular carcinoma in the cirrhotic liver: challenges and controversies. Radiology 247:311–330

11. Kim SH, Kim CS, Chung GH et al (2009) Gadoxetic-acid enhanced MRI versus triple-phase MDCT for the preoperative detection of hepatocellular carcinoma. AJR 192:1675–1681
12. Ahn S, Kim M, Lim J et al (2010) Added value of gadoxetic acid—enhanced hepatobilliary phase MR imaging in the diagnosis of hepatocellular carcinoma. Radiology 255:459466
13. Vandecaveye V, De Keyzer F, Verslype Ch et al (2009) DWI provides additional value to conventional dynamic contrast enhanced MRI for detection of hepatocellular carcinoma. Eur Radiol 19:2456–2466
14. Bruix J, Sherman M (2005) Management of hepatocellular carcinoma. Practice guidelines committee, American association for the study of liver diseases. Hepatology 42:1208–1236
15. Bruix J, Sherman M, Llovet JM et al (2001) Clinical management of hepatocellular carcinoma. Conclusions of The Barcelona 2000 EASL conference. European association for the study of the liver. J Hepatol 35: 421–430
16. Forner A, Ayuso C, Varela M et al (2009) Evaluation of tumor response after locoregional therapies in hepatocellular carcinoma. Cancer 115:616–623
17. Sainani N, Catalano O, Holalkere N et al (2008) Cholangiocarcinoma: current and novel imaging techniques. Radiographics 28:1263–1287
18. Slattery J, Sahani D (2006) What is the current state of the art imaging for detection and staging of cholangiocarcinoma. Oncologist 11:913–922
19. Baron R, Ferris J (2004) Primary tumors of the liver and the biliary tract. In: Husband J, Reznek R (eds) Imaging in oncology. Taylor and Francis, London, pp 245–272
20. Ayuso C, Rimola J, Garcia-Criado A (2011) Imaging of HCC. Abdom Imaging 37:215–230
21. Rosch T, Meining A, Fruhmorgen S et al (2002) A prospective comparison of the diagnostic accuracy of ERCP, MRCP, CT and EUS in biliary strictures. Gatsrointest Endosc 55:870–876
22. Paulson EK (2001) Evaluation of the liver metastatic disease. Semin Liver Dis 21:225–236
23. Konopke R, Kersting S, Saeger HD et al (2005) Detection of liver lesions by contrast enhanced ultrasound—comparison to intraoperative findings. Ultraschall Med 26:107–113
24. Ward J, Naik KS, Guthrie JA et al (1999) Hepatic lesion detection: comparison of MR imaging after the administration of superparamagnetic iron oxide with dual-phase CT using alternative free response receiver operating characteristic analysis. Radiology 210:459–466
25. Oliva M, Saini S (2004) Liver cancer imaging: role of CT, MRI, US and PET. Cancer Imaging 4:S42–S46. doi:10.1102/1470-7330.2004.0011
26. Niekel M, Bipat S, Stoker J et al (2010) Diagnostic Imaging of colorectal liver metastases with CT, MR imaging FDG PET and/or FDG PET/CT: a meta analysis of prospective studies including patients who have not previously undergone treatment. Radiology 257:674–684

Clinical Implications of Liver Malignancies

55

Georgios P. Fragulidis

55.1 Colorectal Liver Metastases

To determine the performance of preoperative imaging in patients with liver metastases, two methods are used as standard of reference. First, intraoperative clinical, US, and pathology findings, to evaluate how many lesions are missed by preoperative imaging but detected intraoperatively. Second, postoperative follow-up to detect lesions missed by both the pre- and intraoperative examinations and to determine how many lesions originally thought to be benign, turned out to be malignant. Although all of the imaging modalities perform relatively well in terms of sensitivity per patient, when the data were analyzed with respect to sensitivity per lesion there was a greater difference between the modalities. This difference was mainly due to variance in the ability to detect lesions <1 cm in size.Therefore, one of the biggest tasks of imaging techniques is the detection and sensitivity for metastatic lesions <1 cm in size [1].

MRI is a more sensitive modality than CT for lesions <1 cm with better also sensitivity both in per patient (81.1 vs. 74.8 %) and in per lesion (86.3 vs. 82.6 %) analyses. Moreover, MRI can currently detect small remnant metastases that are not detectable with other imaging modalities because of the fatty liver development in patients who receive chemotherapy. Indeed, surveillance of pathological response of liver metastases to chemotherapy can be assessed by imaging from the change in tumor size, the morphological changes unrelated to size, and the metabolic activity. In addition to the tumor size, MRI can evaluate the morphological changes that are nonsize-based, progressed from a complex, heterogeneous solid mass to a pseudocystic mass, which is classified as optimal, incomplete, or absent response to chemotherapy. Metabolic activity is currently evaluated primarily with FDG-PET–CT. Preliminary studies suggest that the degree of chemotherapy-induced change in tumor glucose metabolism is predictive of patient outcome, and that the use of FDG-PET for therapy monitoring is clinically feasible. However, the role of PET in monitoring the response to treatment in liver metastases from CRC remains to be further defined since the lack of FDG uptake or complete response using PET does not imply complete pathological response.Thus, it is apparent that MRI is one of the most sensitive imaging modality for evaluating the liver in the initial staging and follow-up of colorectal cancer patients [2].

Concerning the ultimate preoperative imaging modality, this should combine high sensitivity and high specificity rate for the accurate anatomic information of the tumor location in relation to the major anatomic structures to further define resectability. The current definition of resectability includes the potential for

G. P. Fragulidis (✉)
2nd Department of Surgery, Aretaieio Hospital, University of Athens Medical School, 76, Vas. Sophias str, Athens, Attica 11528, Greece
e-mail: gfragulidis@aretaieio.uoa.gr

A. D. Gouliamos et al. (eds.), *Imaging in Clinical Oncology*,
DOI: 10.1007/978-88-470-5385-4_55, © Springer-Verlag Italia 2014

complete tumor resection with tumor-free margins (R0 resection), with preservation of at least two disease-free liver segments with viable vascular inflow, outflow, and biliary drainage and a future liver remnant (FLR) volume > 20–30 %, depending on hepatic *reserve*. A tumor-free resection margin is associated with a lower local recurrence rate and improved long-term survival [3].

Tumor margins for resection can be difficult to define, since half of the patients have tumor regrowth at the periphery of the metastasis when chemotherapy is interrupted, increasing the risk for disease recurrence. Although surgical resection margins are currently selected using preoperative imaging, intraoperative ultrasound (IOUS), and palpation, none of which take into account the possibility of this "dangerous halo", the proliferating tumor cells infiltrating the parenchyma surrounding the metastasis. Tumor-specific DNA has also been detected up to 4 mm beyond the visible tumor margin. Therefore, a negative margin should be attainable for a patient to be deemed resectable and aiming for 1 cm margins should be encouraged when possible. Intraoperative assessment of resectability is performed with IOUS and several studies have shown that it reveals important information not seen during preoperative imaging and thus, it was significantly more sensitive than CT and/or MRI. These additional unsuspected findings may change surgical planning in up to 51 % of patients. As a result, IOUS is now used routinely to assist in planning for liver resection, mainly to enable detection of additional tumors and evaluation of the relationship of tumors to major vascular structures [2, 4].

Currently, liver failure is the main cause of postoperative mortality and it is primarily the result of inaccurate prediction of remnant post-operative liver function.

Therefore, determining technical resectability should focus on preserved structures and FLR, rather than those which require resection. Regarding the minimum amount of remnant liver following resection, most agree that 20–30 % and 40 % of the preoperative volume should be preserved for those with normal and abnormal parenchyma (i.e., fibrosis, cirrhosis, steatosis due to preoperative chemotherapy, etc.), respectively. In certain cases, the use of parenchymal sparing resection techniques such as segmental and subsegmental resections and intraoperative thermal ablation (RFA) can often avoid an unnecessary large volume resection. Multiple studies have demonstrated that CT and MRI-based volumetric measurement results in a reliable estimation of FLR with very little variability [3, 5].

55.1.1 Conclusions

The goals of preoperative imaging of liver metastases from CRC should be the identification of intra- and extrahepatic disease, relevant liver anatomy, and remnant liver volume. MRI may be used to better characterize indeterminate lesions and relevant anatomy, rule out the presence of occult disease and assessing lesions in the presence of steatosis, a common finding after extensive chemotherapy treatment. Surgery remains the best treatment option for these patients when R0 resection can be achieved with preservation of a functioning liver remnant of 20–30 %. IOUS is useful for intraoperative staging and planning liver resection. PET scan is often performed to identify marginal liver lesions and mainly in patients scheduled for metastasectomy with a high risk for extrahepatic disease.

55.2 Hepatocellular Carcinoma

Studies in explanted and preoperative livers show that MRI has an advantage over CT in terms of characterization and diagnosis of Hepatocellular carcinoma (HCC). However, the diagnostic performance of HCC on dynamic contrast-enhanced CT and MR imaging depends on the tumor size, with sensitivity and specificity values significantly higher for lesions larger than 2 cm in diameter compared with those smaller than 2 cm. The detection of small tumors remains the most challenging area in imaging the cirrhotic liver. In lesions > 2 cm, a single investigation with typical vascular pattern suffices. Diagnosis of HCC can also be established without biopsy in patients with cirrhosis with lesions 1–2 cm in diameter if the typical vascular pattern is present in two imaging modalities. In a different setting, a nodule biopsy should be performed. If the biopsy is negative, the lesion should be followed-up by imaging techniques every 3–6 months until it disappears, or it enlarges or changes its vascular profile to a typical HCC pattern [1].

In addition, lesions smaller than 2 cm in size and better differentiated histologically, do not imitate to the classical imaging features. This is revealed by their atypical imaging appearances, where 87 % of well-differentiated lesions and 41–62 % of lesions smaller than 2 cm showed either absence of arterial hypervascularity, venous washout, or both. Moreover, recent data demonstrated that washout can be observed in contrast-enhanced US (CEUS) in hypervascular liver lesions different from HCC, for instance in cirrhotic patients with intrahepatic cholangiocarcinoma with a median nodule size of 3.2 cm. Thus, the authors stayed that CEUS should not be used as the sole imaging technique to confidently characterize HCC [6]. As a concern, the American Association for the Study of the Liver diseases (AASLD) updated the recommendation for non-invasive diagnostic criteria of HCC [7] (Fig. 55.1). Contrast-enhanced US has been eliminated as a diagnostic technique suitable for the characterization of HCC lesions because it may produce false positive findings for HCC in patients with intrahepatic cholangiocarcinoma. US should be reserved for detection purposes along the screening programs, for guiding the fine needle biopsy (FNB) when it is required, to apply an ablative percutaneous treatment if indicated and to evaluate the local therapeutic response after these local therapies.

Nodules less than 1 cm in size are considered not feasible to be confidently diagnosed and in some cases they may not even correspond to premalignant or malignant foci. Instead of

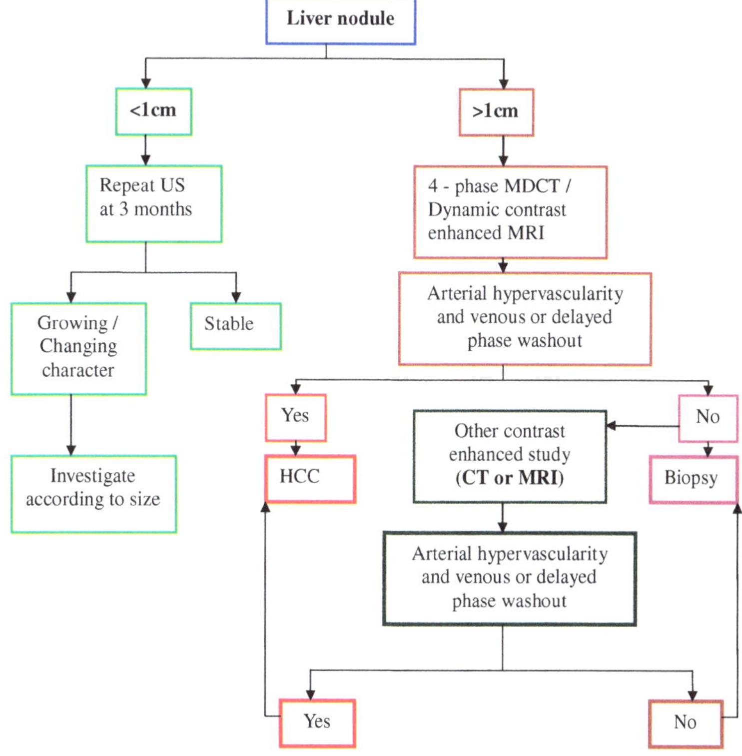

Fig. 55.1 Diagnostic algorithm for suspected HCC (CT, computed tomography; MDCT, multidetector CT; MRI, magnetic resonance imaging; US, ultrasound). From the AASLD Guidelines for the management of HCC. (http://www.aasld.org/practiceguidelines).

aggressively chasing the diagnosis through biopsy which can be technically challenging due to size, in a suspicious nodule for HCC closer imaging follow-up at 3 monthly intervals should be performed. Typically, nodules are declared benign only if they regress or remain stable for 2 years, since HCC nodules can grow very slowly. If the lesion shows no changes in the follow-up US after this period of time, the patient can revert to standard surveillance.

FDG-PET is generally accepted to have low sensitivity (50–68 %) for intrahepatic HCC and is therefore not considered to be useful for diagnosis of HCC. However, in the setting of extrahepatic disease FDG-PET seems to be an effective accurate method for HCC staging with sensitivity of 13–84 %, depending on the size of the lesions [8].

From the clinical perspective, the use of imaging in HCC diagnosis can be divided into two main categories. The first regards the surveillance and prospective screening of patients at high-risk of developing HCC and the second is in the diagnosis of HCC based on an abnormal screening test and determination of the stage. A screening strategy focus on those patients with chronic HBV or HCV virus infection that has progressed to cirrhosis since more than 40 % of these patients will develop HCC. A 6 month surveillance interval is recommended in both measurements of serum alpha-fetoprotein (AFP) levels combined with US of the liver for HBV-HCV carriers and patients with chronic hepatitis. The presence of elevated AFP > 200 ng/mL is no longer required, as it is recognized that there are inherent false-positives (in cirrhotic patients) and false negatives. Combined AFP and US further increases the detection rate and it has been found to reduce mortality, having yielded sensitivities of 50–60 % in cohort or case-control studies [9]. In the event of abnormal results at surveillance US or AFP-level testing > 20 ng/mL, contrast-enhanced MR imaging or CT are the best imaging techniques currently available [10]. Concerning liver biopsy, several limitations due to location of the tumor, clotting disorders and ascites exist. In addition, biopsy is not free of risks such as bleeding or seeding and some groups may contraindicate liver biopsy prior to surgery or transplantation. The risk of tumor cells seeding following liver biopsy is reported as 2.92 % and the time over which seeding occurred was 1–58 months. In a recent study, a positive diagnosis was obtained in only 70 % of cases and the false negative rate for a second biopsy was 38.9 %. This raises the need of well-defined noninvasive criteria that, while avoiding the demand for a positive biopsy, would allow a confident diagnosis based on the imaging characterization [11].

Management and staging process of HCC is not predominantly based on biology of the tumor, but also depends on underlying liver function and the patient's general physical status. For this reason the staging process is complicated and several staging systems have been proposed to predict the prognosis of HCC. These include the modified TNM, the Barcelona Clinic Liver Cancer (BCLC), the Okuda, the Cancer of the Liver Italian Program, and other classifications. They use different variables related to the severity of liver disease, number and size of tumor nodules and cancer spread. For patients with cirrhosis, the Child-Pugh classification is used most widely to stratify patients according to their underlying liver disease, although other measures are increasingly used. Patients with HCC should undergo staging with a contrast-enhanced CT of the chest, abdomen, and pelvis. An MRI may alternatively be used to stage the abdominal cavity. Adjunctive studies such as bone scan or PET imaging should be used more selectively. Thus, the role of imaging in the staging of HCC is: (a) to definitively diagnose HCC without the need for biopsy; (b) to evaluate tumor burden by determining the size, number and location of hepatic lesions, the presence of major vascular invasion, nodal disease, and distant metastases; (c) to evaluate the extent of chronic liver disease and portal hypertension [9].

Although surgical treatment in patients with HCC is the standard for curative care, most are not candidates for resection due to advance liver disease especially in cirrhotic patients. Therefore, most patients with HCC in the early and intermediate stages undergo loco-regional therapies, including percutaneous ablation, RFA, and embolization procedures (TACE). Liver transplantation is theoretically the most radical treatment for HCC. Transplantation could simultaneously cure the tumor and underlying cirrhosis, and effectiveness of the procedure is not affected by the degree of liver function impairment. Mazzaferro and colleagues showed that selection of patients with one HCC of 5 cm or smaller, or up to three nodules of 3 cm or smaller, without vascular invasion or extrahepatic spread (known as the Milano criteria) offered 4 year survival of 75 %, with recurrence rates below 15 %. Due to the risk of recurrence, especially during the first 2 years after surgery (up to 65 %) mainly due to dissemination rather than metachronous tumor, follow-up of these patients is strongly recommended [12, 13].

55.2.1 Conclusions

Patients with cirrhosis are at highest risk of developing HCC, and early detection by surveillance is the only way to diagnose HCC when curative treatments are feasible. HCC screening is centered on ultrasonography combined with tumor marker measurements at intervals of 3–6 months. CT/MRI performed concurrently in the very high-risk group, increases the possibility of detection of HCC in the single nodule stage. Histologic diagnosis by biopsy is indicated when imaging findings are atypical. For determining whether surgery is indicated, evaluations of the extent of the HCC and liver function are essential. Surveillance allows diagnosis at early stages when the tumor might be curable by resection, liver transplantation, or ablation.

55.3 Intrahepatic Cholangiocarcinoma

Intrahepatic Cholangiocarcinoma (ICC) arising from small ducts is often diffuse and multicentric and may present with imaging features of both HCC and cholangiocarcinoma. Up to 81 % of ICC's are characterized by a progressive contrast uptake throughout the arterial and venous phase, and especially in the delayed venous phase images. Satellite nodules are seen at imaging in 65 % usually when they are larger than 1 or 2 cm, while 37 % of the patients who are diagnosed preoperatively with a solitary tumor have multiple satellite lesions in the resected specimen. MRI and CT are comparable in the detection of satellite lesions but CT is preferable for the depiction of vascular encasement. Vascular involvement is depicted in approximately 50 % of cases and more often concerns the portal branch than the hepatic veins. Therefore, the presence of segmental or lobar atrophy is strongly associated with ipsilateral portal vein encasement. Lymph nodes around the cardiac portion of the stomach and along the lesser gastric curvature should be also examined in addition to nodes in the hepatoduodenal ligament in ICC of the left lobe. The overall accuracy of detecting metastatic lymph node at imaging is 77 % and the most common error on preoperative imaging is underestimation of nodal involvement. The sensitivity of PET for the detection of mass-forming ICC of >1 cm diameter has been reported as 85–95 %, with a sensitivity of 100 %. PET imaging may be helpful in demonstrating extrahepatic metastases and its sensitivity and specificity for detection of nodal and distant metastatic disease is 100 and 94 %, respectively [14].

The characteristic presentation of ICC is an incidental hepatic mass lesion and the diagnosis is often made during evaluation of solitary masses within the liver. Levels of tumor markers, such as carbohydrate antigen 19–9 (CA19-9) or carcinoembryonic antigen (CEA), might be raised, but these markers lack sensitivity for diagnostic use. Besides, concomitant increases of the levels of CA19-9 and α-fetoprotein should suggest a mixed hepatocellular-cholangiocarcinoma. *It is important to be emphasized that imaging is not always reliable for the diagnosis of ICC's < 2 cm in size, since they can mimic HCC because of the absence of the progressive enhancement pattern.* Thus, the need for a liver biopsy and a histopathology diagnosis depends upon the clinical setting and preoperative imaging. In patients with cirrhosis and an uncategorized lesion, a biopsy is justified because the distinction between HCC and ICC changes management and could thus have an important effect on outcome. In noncirrhotic patients who qualify for surgery, a liver biopsy may not be required if a decision has been made to proceed with surgical resection. However, in patients who are not candidates for surgical treatment, a liver biopsy is usually performed before initiation of systemic therapy [14].

Contrary to extrahepatic cholangiocarcinoma the staging in ICC by imaging is poor. Multivariate analyses have shown that tumor size of 2 or 3 cm or more, lymph node metastasis, satellite lesions or intrahepatic metastasis at presentation, symptomatic tumors, and vascular invasion are independent factors associated with poor postoperative outcome. Therefore, the goal of imaging is to get the best accuracy in assessing these findings for the decision making process to determine resectability. For ICC three staging systems exist, though none fulfills the criteria of an ideal staging system. The major difference between these staging systems lies in the T-staging approach. The 7th edition American Joint Committee on Cancer (AJCC)/International Union against Cancer (UICC) TNM staging system requires histologic evaluation for the T*is* (carcinoma in situ) and for the T4 stages and is therefore not reliable for preoperative staging. The Liver Cancer Study Group of Japan (LCSGJ) staging system is inadequate owing to the lack of correlation between the T stages and survival. The National Cancer Center of Japan (NCCJ) includes all established independent prognostic factors and enables preoperative staging, however has only a suboptimal correlation with survival after hepatic resection [14].

Surgical resection should be considered for patients with localized disease, as this is the only strategy with the potential for cure in the absence of primary sclerosing cholangitis (PSC). Resection in patients with PSC is discouraged, as ICC in often multifocal in this setting with recurrence of the disease following resection occurring in >90 % of patients. Hence, in PSC patients with early ICC liver transplantation is the preferred definitive therapy. Liver transplantation is generally not recommended for patients with intrahepatic cholangiocarcinoma unless in the context of an approved trial protocol due to the poor outcomes. For nonresectable but localized tumors, potential options include locoregional approaches such as transarterial chemoembolization (TACE) or systemic chemotherapy. Untreated, survival of patients with advanced intrahepatic cancers is short (3.0 ± 5.3 mo). After surgical resection with curative intent, 1 and 5 year survival of 68 and 32 %, respectively, have been reported [15].

55.3.1 Conclusions

The typical presentation of an intrahepatic cholangiocarcinoma is an incidental hepatic mass lesion. Contrast-enhanced CT or MRI imaging will be necessary to determine the size, number and location of the lesions, vascular invasion, and the extent to which the tumor has spread. Distinguishing ICC from HCC is important as they respond differently to therapy. The resectability rate of ICC is low because this disease is frequently beyond the limits of surgical therapy at the time of diagnosis. Tumors that are medically fit for hepatic resection must be completely resected with negative histological margins, no evidence of metastases, disseminated disease, and extensive lymphadenopathy. Curative resection (R0) is the most effective treatment and the only therapy associated with prolonged disease-free survival.

References

1. Wong P (2009) Further defining liver imaging—physician and radiologist in dialogue. Eur Gastroenterol Hepatol Rev 4(2):14–18
2. Adam R, De Gramont A, Figueras J et al (2012) The oncosurgery approach to managing liver metastases from colorectal cancer: a multidisciplinary international consensus. Oncologist 17:1225–1239
3. Weiss MJ, D'Angelica MI (2012) Patient selection for hepatic resection for metastatic colorectal cancer. J Gastrointest Oncol 3(1):3–10

4. Sahani DV, Kalva SP, Tanabe KK et al (2004) Intraoperative US in patients undergoing surgery for liver neoplasms: comparison with MR imaging. Radiology 232:810–814
5. Frankel TL, Kinh Gian Do R, Jarnagin WR (2012) Preoperative imaging for hepatic resection of colorectal cancer metastasis. J Gastrointest Oncol 3:11–18
6. Ayuso C, Rimola J, Garcia-Criado A (2011) Imaging of HCC. Abdom Imaging 37:215–230
7. Bruix J, Sherman M (2011) AASLD practice guideline management of hepatocellular carcinoma: an update DOI 10.1002/hep.24199
8. Tan CH, Albert Low SC, Thng CH (2011) APASL and AASLD consensus guidelines on imaging diagnosis of hepatocellular carcinoma: a review. Int J Hepatol 519783:11. doi:10.4061/2011/519783
9. Choi BI, Lee JM (2010) Advancement in HCC imaging: diagnosis, staging and treatment efficacy assessments Imaging diagnosis and staging of hepatocellular carcinoma. J Hepatobiliary Pancreat Sci 17:369–373
10. Willatt JM, Hussain HK, Adusumilli S et al (2008) MR imaging of hepatocellular carcinoma in the cirrhotic liver: challenges and controversies. Radiology 247(2):311–330
11. Williams R (2012) Looking after the liver as well as the tumour. In: Williams R, Taylor-Robinson SD (eds) Clinical dilemmas in primary liver cancer. Wiley-Blackwell, UK, pp 67–72
12. Mazzaferro V, Regalia E, Doci R et al (1996) Liver transplantation for the treatment of small hepatocellular carcinomas in patients with cirrhosis. N Engl J Med 334:693–699
13. Llovet JM, Schwartz M, Mazzaferro V (2005) Resection and liver transplantation for hepatocellular carcinoma. Semin Liver Dis 25(2):181–200
14. Blechacz B, Komuta M, Roskams T, Gores GJ (2011) Clinical diagnosis and staging of cholangiocarcinoma. Nat Rev Gastroenterol Hepatol 8(9):512–522. doi:10.1038/nrgastro.2011.131
15. Cho SY et al (2010) Survival analysis of intrahepatic cholangiocarcinoma after resection. Ann Surg Oncol 17:1823–1830

56 Introduction to Pancreatic Cancer

Georgios P. Fragulidis

Pancreatic cancer (PC) (pancreatic ductal adenocarcinoma) constitutes 90 % of all primary malignant tumors arising from the pancreatic gland. In up to 60–70 % the tumor is located in the head and the remaining is equally distributed in the body and in the tail. Due to aggressiveness of the tumor, the diagnosis of PC is rarely made at an early stage. More than 90 % of PCs appear in the late stage of disease and only 10 % of patients have resectable tumors at the time of diagnosis. This is one of the main reasons for failing to achieve a cure in most patients [1]. The goal of pancreatic imaging is the early detection and characterization of clinically relevant pancreatic lesions. Incidental pancreatic lesions are increasingly common and can range from benign incidental lesions to malignant. Consequently, the detection of a mass on imaging is nonspecific and 5–15 % of pancreatic resections show benign pathology given the significant overlap of patient symptoms in benign and malignant pancreatic disorders. In addition, no pancreatic mass is visualized on imaging evaluation in 10 % of cases since the tumor may be isoattenuating. Thus, the presence and location of a mass may be assumed from secondary signs such as mass effect, an abnormal convex contour of the pancreas, ductal obstruction, and vascular invasion. Therefore, the use of a multimodality approach combines the strengths of individual imaging modalities and has a synergistic effect in improving diagnostic yield. Imaging techniques currently used for diagnosis and preoperative staging of PC include transabdominal ultrasound (US), contrast-enhanced multisection computed tomography (CT), magnetic resonance imaging (MRI), MR cholangiopancreatography (MRCP), and PET scan and invasive imaging modalities like endoscopic ultrasound (EUS), endoscopic retrograde cholangiopancreatography (ERCP), and intraductal ultrasound (IDUS).

Reference

1. Sharma C, Eltawil KM, Renfrew PD, Walsh MJ, Molinari M (2011) Advances in diagnosis, treatment and palliation of pancreatic carcinoma: 1990–2010. World J Gastroenterol 17(7): 867–897. doi: 10.3748/wjg.v17.i7.867

G. P. Fragulidis (✉)
2nd Department of Surgery, Aretaieio Hospital, University of Athens Medical School, 76, Vas. Sophias str, 11528 Athens, Attica, Greece
e-mail: gfragulidis@aretaieio.uoa.gr

A. D. Gouliamos et al. (eds.), *Imaging in Clinical Oncology*,
DOI: 10.1007/978-88-470-5385-4_56, © Springer-Verlag Italia 2014

57 Imaging in Pancreatic Cancer

Christos N. Mourmouris

57.1 Introduction

Pancreatic ductal adenocarcinoma is the fifth leading cause of cancer deaths in the Western hemisphere. It represents 90 % of all malignant tumors arising from the pancreatic gland. Early pancreatic cancer often does not cause symptoms and the later symptoms are usually non-specific and varied. Therefore, pancreatic cancer is often not diagnosed until it is advanced. And despite all the advances in oncological treatments, the overall 5-year-survival rates remain poor (<5 %). On the other hand surgery is still the only curative option but only a minority of cancers is resectable.

Therefore the role of the imaging modalities should be to: (a) detect early the pancreatic cancer and (b) stage the tumor and determine if it is locally resectable.

57.2 Diagnosis

The diagnostic approach usually begins with abdominal ultrasound because it is widely available and noninvasive. Ultrasound (US) may detect pancreatic cancer as an ill-defined hypoechoic mass but usually is performed in order to exclude gallstones, choledocholithiasis, and signs of common bile duct obstruction in patients who are present with abdominal pain and jaundice. The accuracy of US for detection of pancreatic cancer is 50–70 % [1]. However the body habitus, the overlying bowel gas, and the variable operator dependency decrease the sensitivity of the method.

CT is the standard imaging modality for accurate diagnosis and staging of pancreatic cancer. The standard protocol for the evaluation of the pancreas consists of two phases after the intravenous administration of contrast media (pancreatic and portal venous phase). During the pancreatic phase or late arterial phase (approximately 30–40 s after the injection of the contrast media) the contrast between the normal parenchyma and the lesion is maximal and also there is sufficient enhancement of the arteries in order to evaluate possible vascular tumor involvement. Portal venous phase is optimal for detecting potential metastatic disease and for the assessing of the peripancreatic veins [2].

State–of-the-art protocol with MDCT scanners includes acquisitions with very thin slices (<1 mm) which is crucial for optimizing lesion detection. These isotropic or nearly isotropic data sets are used with postprocessing techniques (MPR, MIP VRT) in order to depict high quality reformatted images. Recent reports have demonstrated the role of reformatted images in the preoperative evaluation of pancreatic cancer regarding the invasion of the peripancreatic vessels and the potential resectability of the pancreatic tumor [3].

C. N. Mourmouris (✉)
Imaging Department Hygeia Hospital,
4 Erythrou Stavrou Str, 15124, Marousi, Greece
e-mail: cmourmouris@yahoo.gr

A. D. Gouliamos et al. (eds.), *Imaging in Clinical Oncology*,
DOI: 10.1007/978-88-470-5385-4_57, © Springer-Verlag Italia 2014

Typically, pancreatic cancer present as a hypoattenuated mass but in 10 % of cases may be isoattenuating to the pancreatic parenchyma thereby leading to misdiagnosis. However, the presence and the location of a tumor may be indicated from secondary signs. Prokesh et al., demonstrated that secondary signs are important and should be considered as indicators of a tumor when a mass cannot be seen [4]. The "double duct sign" which refers to simultaneous dilatation of the common bile and pancreatic ducts is a reliable sign of an obstructing lesion, however, pancreatic adenocarcinoma is not the only cause of the sign [5]. The reported sensitivity of CT ranges between 76 and 92 % for tumor detection [1].

MRI can be used in imaging for pancreatic cancer in patients with equivocal findings on MDCT. Pancreatic adenocarcinoma typically demonstrated as low signal intensity mass on T1W and T2W and contrast enhanced T1 images mass. MRI has better soft tissue contrast resolution than CT and thus is superior in detecting small tumors and metastases. The accuracy of MR imaging in the detection and staging adenocarcinoma ranges between 90 and 100 % [6]. MRCP is a useful technique which in collaboration with MRI helps for detection of pancreatic cancer. MRCP is better than CT for depicting the anatomy of the biliary tree and pancreatic duct. It is also reported that it is as sensitive as ERCP and thus may help to avoid unnecessary interventional procedures (Fig. 57.1).

One of the main challenges in the diagnosis of pancreatic cancer is the differentiation between pancreatic adenocarcinoma and chronic pancreatitis. Patients with chronic pancreatitis show an increased incidence for pancreatic cancer. Also chronic pancreatitis and pancreatic cancer coexist in up to 5 % of cases. Both of these lesions are associated with fibrosis thereby imaging appearances are quite similar. As a result chronic pancreatitis is a significant factor that leads to misdiagnosis due to its tumor like appearance. Secondary signs such as duct contour, calcification, enhancement, lymph nodes, and metastases may be useful to rule out a diagnosis. MRCP may also help in the differentiation between these two processes. A positive duct penetrating sign refers to a smoothly stenotic or normal main pancreatic duct penetrating through the apparent tumor which may be useful in the distinction from

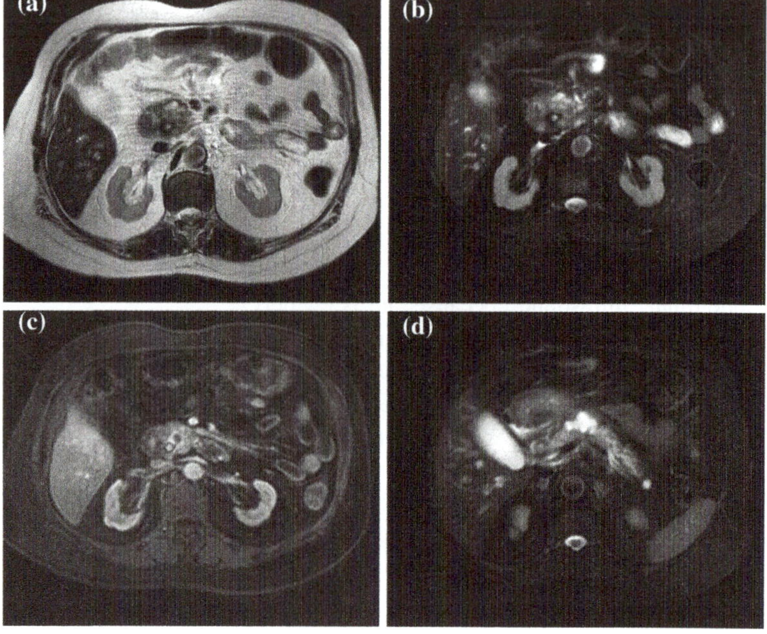

Fig. 57.1 Space occupying lesion at the head of the pancreas. The lesion appeared slightly hypointense on T1W images (**a**) hypeintense on T2W (**b**) and after the administration of the contrast media the lesion enhanced inhomogeneously (**c**). A stent is placed in the CBD. The distal part of the pancreatic duct is dilated (**d**)

pancreatic cancer [7]. Nevertheless in equivocal cases biopsy may still be necessary.

Endoscopic US has an important role in the detection of small tumors. It can help detect masses as small as 0.2–0.3 cm that may be undetectable by CT or MRI. It has high sensitivity and specificity (93 and 100 %, respectively) [8].

57.3 Staging

The staging of pancreatic cancers is performed according to the TNM system.

Ninety percent of pancreatic adenocarcinomas are demonstrated as focal mass. CT and MRI are very accurate for the assessment of T stage. While T1 and T2 stage are distinguished on the basis of size, T3 stage is defined as an extension into the peripancreatic soft tissues such as duodenum, common bile duct, or peripancreatic fat and T4 stage is defined as an extension into the stomach, colon, and large vessels which is unresectable. Attention should be given for detection of potential local infiltrative disease which may be demonstrated as subtle infiltration of peripancreatic tissue. Local invasion may lead to underestimation of the extent and stage of the tumor.

An important step during the staging process of pancreatic cancer is to define the relationship of the tumor to critical arterial and venous structures, since their involvement may exclude surgical resection.

The most widely used grading system for the assessment of vascular invasion is one that proposed by Raptopoulos et al. [3, 9]. Grade 0: normal, with a fat plane or normal pancreas between the tumor and the vessel. Grade 1: loss of the fat plane between the tumor and the vessel, with or without displacement of the vessel. Grade 2: flattening or slight irregularity of one side of the vessel (i.e., <180° of the perimeter). Grade 3: tumor around two sides of vessel, narrowing of the vessel lumen (i.e., >180° of the perimeter). Grade 4: one major vessel is occluded.

It should be noted that splenic artery and vein are not always critical because pancreatic tail tumors can be resected en bloc with the spleen as long as the tumor can be removed from the superior mesenteric—portal vein confluence and celiac axis.

The accuracy of CT and MRI for predicting vascular invasion is quite similar (90 and 87 % respectively) [10].

In regard to the N-stage although the identification of enlarged peripancreatic lymph nodes is important, however, CT and MRI are not accurate for determination of malignant adenopathy.

Unfortunately 60 % of patients who are present with pancreatic adenocarcinoma have advanced disease. CT and MRI have high sensitivity for the detection of liver metastasis. However, the ability of these modalities to detect small liver metastases and peritoneal deposits are limited.

57.4 Conclusion

Pancreatic ductal adenocarcinoma is the fifth leading cause of cancer deaths in the Western hemisphere. Despite all the advances in oncological treatments, the overall 5-year-survival rates remain poor (<5 %). However, recent technological advantages in CT and MRI technology improved the ability for early detection of pancreatic cancer and proper staging. As a result more patients can benefit from the surgery.

References

1. Tummala P, Junaidi O, Agarwal B (2011) Imaging of pancreatic cancer: an overview. J Gastrointest Oncol 2:168–174
2. Low G, Panu A, Millo N et al (2011) Multimodality imaging of neoplastic and non-neoplastic solid lesions of the pancreas. Radiographics 31:993–1015
3. Brennan D, Zamboni G, Raptopoulos V et al (2007) Comprehensive pre-operative assessment of pancreatic adenocarcinoma with 64-section volumetric CT. Radiographics. 27:1653–1666
4. Prokesch RW, Chow LC, Beaulieu CF et al (2002) Isoattenuating pancreatic adenocarcinoma at MDCT: secondary signs. Radiology 224:764–768
5. Menges M, Lerch MM, Zeitz M (2000) The double duct sign in patients with malignant and benign pancreatic lesions. Gastrointest Endosc 52:74–77

6. Hanbidge AE (2002) Cancer of the pancreas: the best image for early detection—CT, MRI, PET or US? Can J Gastroenterol 16(2):101–105
7. Kalra M, Maher M, Mueller P et al (2003) State of the art imaging of pancreatic neoplasms. BJR 76:857–865
8. Wiersema MJ (2002) Identifying contraindications to resection in patients with pancreatic carcinoma: the role of endoscopic ultrasound. Can J Gastroenterol 16:109–11
9. Raptopoulos V, Steer ML, Sheiman RG et al (1997) The use of helical CT and CT angiography to predict vascular involvement from pancreatic cancer: correlation with findings at surgery. AJR 168: 971–977
10. Arslan A, Buanes T, Geitung JT (2001) Pancreatic carcinoma: MR, MR angiography and dynamic helical CT in the evaluation of vascular invasion. Eur Radiol 38:151–159

Clinical Implications of Pancreatic Cancer

58

Georgios P. Fragulidis

Ultrasound (US) is used for diagnosis of a pancreatic tumor rather than staging, although liver metastasis and ascites may be seen. US coupled with Doppler gives a reasonable measure of vascular patency and can improve accuracy in assessing vascular invasion. Because the results of US are highly operator dependent with relatively poor sensitivity and the accuracy for diagnosing pancreatic tumors is 50–70 %, the utility of the transabdominal US in the diagnosis of PC is limited. Thus, multisection CT should be used first in the detection of pancreatic adenocarcinoma and distant metastases. Currently, pancreatic section thickness of 1 mm is obtained allowing true volume acquisition with vascular details better than angiography when assessing vascular invasion, providing diagnostic and staging information with an approximate rate of 99 %. The presence of circumferential vessel involvement of more than 180 degrees, radiological absence of a fat plane between tumor and vessel, vascular occlusion with collaterals, and teardrop sign, allow remarkable degree of accuracy in diagnosing vascular invasion [1].

MRI is performed when other imaging modalities provide insufficient data for the clinical staging of the tumor, or when treatment planning cannot be based on the images obtained by other techniques. MRI with cholangiopancreatography gives much information for the evaluation of primary tumor and metastatic dissemination. Nevertheless, with the improvement in CT scan technology, recent studies have shown that MRI might have lower sensitivity in comparison to multisection CT (82–94 % vs. 100 %) [2]. The accuracy of MRI for vascular visualization and resectability of the tumor is quite similar to that of CT. However, MRCP is better than CT for defining the anatomy of the biliary tree and pancreatic duct, to evaluate the bile ducts both above and below a stricture and to identify intrahepatic mass lesions. It is also reportedly sensitive as ERCP in detecting pancreatic cancers and does not require contrast material to be administered into the ductal system. In certain cases, MRCP is routinely used in patients with high grade stenosis of the gastric outlet or proximal duodenum or in those with specific postsurgical anatomy (e.g., Billroth II, Roux-en Y biliary bypass), which make the biliary ductal system difficult to access by ERCP [1]. Regarding the use of MRI in an "all-in-one" staging method (MRI, coupled with angiography and MRCP) is a subject under debate.

Endoscopic US (EUS) has a recognized role in the detection of small tumors and it has been shown to be accurate in diagnosing and staging pancreatic cancer. Fine needle aspiration (FNA) biopsy guided by endoscopic ultrasonography may provide tissue diagnosis in patients who are not surgical candidates. Due to its ability to

G. P. Fragulidis (✉)
2nd Department of Surgery, Aretaieio Hospital, University of Athens Medical School, 76, Vas. Sophias str, 11528 Athens, Attica, Greece
e-mail: gfragulidis@aretaieio.uoa.gr

A. D. Gouliamos et al. (eds.), *Imaging in Clinical Oncology*,
DOI: 10.1007/978-88-470-5385-4_58, © Springer-Verlag Italia 2014

reliably identify lymph nodal metastasis in celiac and mediastinal lymph nodes, EUS-FNA can prove to be beneficial in preoperative assessment of resectability. From the point of view of the detection of vascular invasion, EUS has shown good accuracy, especially for venous invasion. Although EUS is invasive, highly operator-dependent, it is appropriate to incorporate EUS in the preoperative assessment when there is suspicion of pancreatic cancer.

PET differentiates malignant and benign pancreatic pathologies with a sensitivity of 85–100 % and a specificity of 67–99 % often higher than that of CT, although false negatives results exist in the case of strongly differentiated tumors, small periampullary tumors or in cases of hyperglycemia. False-positive results may also occur when focal pancreatitis is associated with early pancreatic carcinoma. Interestingly, the clinical management of patients undergoing PET can be changed in 16 % of cases because of distant metastases. Another very important characteristic of PET-CT is its ability to provide useful information on tumor viability, and this technique also allows monitoring of tumor response to treatment [1, 2].

Endoscopic Retrograde Cholangiopancreatography (ERCP) has high sensitivity and specificity for cancer, and is useful in detecting tumors if there is main pancreatic ductal involvement as in Intraductal Papillary Mucinous Neoplasm (IPMN). In contrast to other imaging modalities, tissue diagnosis of the involved ducts may be achieved using needle aspiration, brush cytology, and forceps biopsy (triple sampling), improving the sensitivity for diagnosing cancer to 77 %. In addition, new technology may allow the ERCP and EUS scope to be combined into one instrument to provide both diagnostic and therapeutic techniques in the same setting. The use of a 2 mm probe fed into the pancreatic duct during ERCP (Intraductal Ultrasound, IDUS) can help to detect focal ductal lesions <1 mm in height. In a study comparing IDUS to standard ERCP, EUS and, CT, the authors showed that IDUS is more sensitive and specific in identifying the cause of strictures than either of the other techniques (100 % sensitivity, 93 % specificity for cancer). The role of ERCP in stent placement to relieve biliary obstruction prior to surgery for potentially resectable pancreatic cancers is currently debated and should be individualized based on specific clinical situation. However, stent placement can performed in cases presented an unresectable or borderline resectable tumor requiring chemotherapy ± radiation and thus would benefit from an ERCP for biliary drainage [3].

The role of diagnostic imaging in PC is to demonstrate the tumor and its relationship to surrounding vessels to determine the possibility of curative resection and plan the operative intervention. The size of pancreatic tumor is a major determinant of resectability and up to 83 % of tumors ≤2 cm are resectable compared to only 7 % of tumors >3 cm in size. Surgery is the only chance of cure and the presence of negative resection margins of the primary tumor represent the strongest prognostic factor. The 5-year-survival rate in patients with resectable tumors can be as high as 20–25 % and compares favorably with patients with unresectable tumor, very few of whom survive 5 years after diagnosis [4].

In the absence of metastatic disease which precludes resection, assessment of vascular invasion is an important parameter for determining resectability for pancreatic cancer. This is a relatively frequent discovery in pancreatic cancer found in 21–64 % of patients and current imaging modalities have improved and allowed detection of vascular invasion with more accuracy. The superior mesenteric vessels are the most frequently involved vessels due to their intimate relationship with the head, the uncinate process and body of the pancreas. This depiction is crucial for preoperative planning, because the posterior and lateral surfaces of the portal and superior mesenteric vein can be evaluated only after the surgical procedure is well advanced. It has to be mentioned though that limited venous invasion does not represent an absolute contraindication for surgery. Evidently, surgical exploration remains the "gold standard" in terms of evaluation of resectability, especially from the point of view of vascular involvement which is one of the most important challenges in pancreatic surgery [1].

Although that, the tumor, node, and metastasis system may be used for pancreatic cancer staging, in clinical decision making pancreatic cancers can be categorized as *resectable*, *locally advanced*, or *metastatic*. Patients with distant metastases (liver, lungs, and peritoneum) or local invasion of the surrounding organs (stomach, colon, small bowel) are usually not surgical candidates. The initial imaging with multisection CT of the abdomen and pelvis is the best way to assess most tumors and identify distant metastases and arterial involvement. If the patient has high surgical risk or if CT shows unresectable disease, FNA can confirm the diagnosis, and no further staging work-up is necessary. If the CT scan is indeterminate, endoscopic ultrasonography can identify smaller lesions and further delineate vascular involvement. Multisection CT is the most accurate in assessing the stage of the tumor (73 %), locoregional invasion (74 %), vascular involvement (83 %), distant metastases (88 %), final TNM stage (46 %), and overall tumor resectability (83 %). A decision analysis demonstrated that the best strategy to assess tumor resectability was based on CT as an initial test and the use of EUS to confirm the results of resectability CT. Staging laparoscopy is generally reserved for patients whose physicians highly suspect metastasis but have not yet identified it [5].

Multisection CT is the preferred initial imaging modality in patients with clinical suspicion for pancreatic cancer, and should be considered as the initial imaging study regardless of suspected tumor type. MRI is performed for further lesion characterization and to increase specificity in the setting of cystic pancreatic lesions and small liver lesions. EUS is the most accurate examination and can be a useful adjunct to CT/MRI in determining resectability of pancreatic cancer. EUS/EUS-FNA can also provide a definite determination about the presence of pancreatic cancer in patients with nonspecific findings suggestive of cancer on conventional imaging, with ERCP utilized for palliative stent placement as necessary. Patients with resectable disease who are surgical candidates can undergo definitive surgery without preoperative histologic confirmation. MRCP seems favorable in differentiating pancreatic cancer from chronic pancreatitis. PET scans can provide information on occult metastasis but its clinical benefit is not established.

References

1. Buchs NC, Chilcott M, Poletti PA, Buhler LH, Morel P (2010) Vascular invasion in pancreatic cancer: imaging modalities, preoperative diagnosis and surgical management. World J Gastroenterol 16(7):818–831. doi:10.3748/wjg.v16.i7.818
2. Sharma C, Eltawil KM, Renfrew PD, Walsh MJ, Molinari M (2011) Advances in diagnosis, treatment and palliation of pancreatic carcinoma: 1990–2010. world J gastroenterol 17(7):867–897, doi: 10.3748/wjg.v17.i7.867
3. Rabinowitz CB, Prabhakar HB, Sahani DV (2008) Recent advances in imaging of pancreatic neoplasms In: Blake MA, Kalra MK (eds) imaging in oncology. Springer, LLC, NY, pp 229–254
4. Tummala P, Junaidi O, Agarwal B (2011) Imaging of pancreatic cancer: an overview. J Gastrointest Oncol 2:168–174. doi: 10.3978/j.issn.2078-6891.2011.036
5. Freelove R, Walling AD (2006) Pancreatic cancer diagnosis and management. Am Fam Physician 73(3):485–493

Introduction to Peritoneal Cavity Carcinoma

59

Paris A. Kosmidis

The most frequent tumors in the peritoneal cavity are the metastatic. Ovarian, gastric, and colon cancers are the commonest which spread through intraperitoneal seeding. Other primary cancers, such as melanoma, lung, and breast cancers can spread through mesenteric arteries to peritoneum. Lymphoma may disseminate to the peritoneal cavity through lymphatic pathways [1].

CT and MRI are the most frequently used imaging methods for detecting peritoneal implants. These methods are also useful for response evaluation and follow-up. In case of increased accuracy, PET and diffuse-weighted images may be used effectively. This is particularly important for ovarian and colon cancers in which surgical interventions in cases of exclusive peritoneal disease are promising.

Pseudomyxoma peritonei is a special type of neoplasia which spread throughout the peritoneal cavity following rupture of a mucin-producing tumor of the appendix or ovary.

Primary peritoneal malignant tumors are rare and include mesothelioma, peritoneal serous carcinoma, leiomyosarcoma, and desmoplastic small round cell tumors [2].

References

1. Meyers MA (2000) Intraperitoneal spread of malignancies. In: Meyers MA (ed) Dynamic radiology of the abdomen: normal and pathologic anatomy, 5th edn. Springer, New York, 131–263
2. Levy A, Arnaiz J, Shaw J et al (2008) Primary peritoneal tumors: imaging features with pathologic correlation. Radio Graphics 28:583–607

P. A. Kosmidis (✉)
2nd Medical Oncology Department, Hygeia Hospital, 4, Er.Stavrou and Vas Sofias Ave, 15123, Marousi, Athens, Greece
e-mail: parkosmi@otenet.gr

A. D. Gouliamos et al. (eds.), *Imaging in Clinical Oncology*,
DOI: 10.1007/978-88-470-5385-4_59, © Springer-Verlag Italia 2014

Imaging of Peritoneal Cavity Carcinoma 60

Panos K. Prassopoulos, Nikolaos A. Courcoutsakis
and Apostolos K. Tentes

60.1 Introduction

The malignant peritoneal neoplasms are much more common than the benign. The secondary tumors are more frequently encountered than the primary ones. Imaging evaluation is important for the diagnosis, estimation of disease extent, and preoperative planning. A thorough analysis of imaging examinations is required, since imaging findings are nonspecific in a considerable number of cases and additionaly, there is an overlapping of imaging findings between primary and secondary malignant peritoneal neoplasms.

The primary peritoneal tumors arise from the mesothelial or submesothelial layers of the peritoneum affecting diverse age group of patients. Clinical manifestation of these tumors independently of their histologic origin is usually nonspecific; symptoms include gastrointestinal complaints, nausea, abdominal discomfort and/or abdominal distention, symptoms from small bowel (SB) obstruction, and presence of a palpable mass in a number of cases. The majority of secondary peritoneal tumors results from intraperitoneal spread of intra-abdominal malignancies.

60.2 Primary Peritoneal Malignant Tumors

The *primary peritoneal malignant tumors* (*PPMT*) are rare lesions with poor prognosis that are classified according to their histogenesis as *mesothelial* [peritoneal malignant mesothelioma (PMM), well-differentiated papillary mesothelioma], *epithelial* (primary peritoneal serous carcinoma), *smooth muscle tumor* (leiomyosarcoma). There are also peritoneal tumors from *uncertain origin* (solitary fibrous tumor, desmoplastic small round cell tumor) [1, 2].

PMM is derived from peritoneal mesothelium, it may be associated with asbestos exposure and is most often seen in middle-aged men. Peritoneal involvement may occur, either alone (in only 30 % of the cases) or in association with pleural involvement. PMM may be classified as diffused that is highly aggressive and practically incurable, or localized with better prognosis after complete surgical excision [2, 3]. On CT, PMMs have a wide range of appearances varying from the "dry" form (large confluent peritoneal masses with no or minimal ascites) to "wet" form (nodular or diffuse peritoneal thickening and ascites). Enhancement of the peritoneal nodules or masses is typically seen on

P. K. Prassopoulos (✉) · N. A. Courcoutsakis
Department of Radiology and Medical Imaging, University Hospital of Alexandroupolis, Democritus University of Thrace, Greece
e-mail: pprasopo@med.duth.gr

N. A. Courcoutsakis
e-mail: ncourcou@med.duth.gr

A. K. Tentes
Department of Surgery, General Hospital of Didimotichon, Thrace, Greece
e-mail: atentes@did-hosp.gr

A. D. Gouliamos et al. (eds.), *Imaging in Clinical Oncology*,
DOI: 10.1007/978-88-470-5385-4_60, © Springer-Verlag Italia 2014

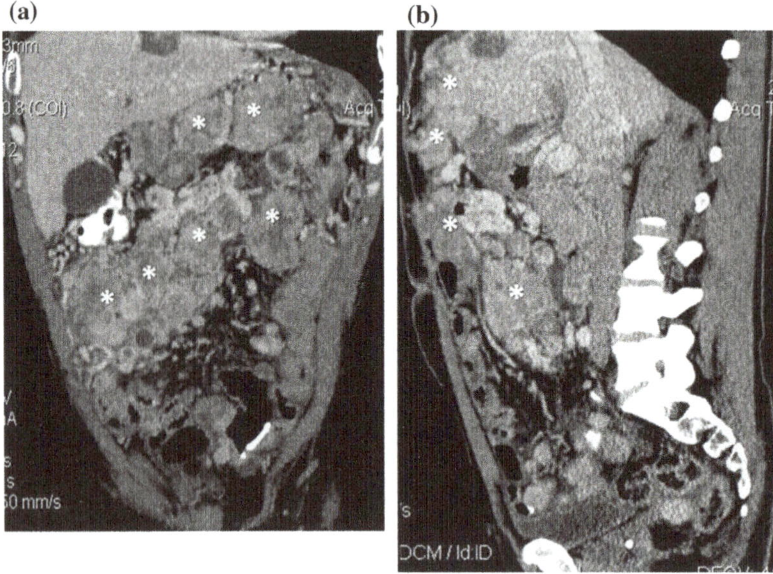

Fig. 60.1 Peritoneal mesothelioma, "dry" form. Coronal (*left*) and sagittal (*right*) CT reformatted images of a patient with peritoneal mesothelioma. There are multiple, confluent, soft tissue masses (*asterisks*) throughout the peritoneal cavity exhibiting peripheral enhancement

CT, while omental thickening or mass and a stellate mesenteric appearance may also be seen [2, 3] (Fig. 60.1). In contrary to pleural mesothelioma PMM is not calcified. Stellate or pleated mesenteric infiltration is common. Based on CT findings, PMMs should be differentiated from peritoneal carcinomatosis (PC) or tuberculosis. If asbestos related lung or pleura disease coexist the diagnosis of PMM is strongly suggested [1, 3].

Primary papillary serous carcinoma (*PSC*) is a rare malignant tumor predominately seen in postmenopausal women. Histologically, PSC is identical to serous papillary carcinoma of the ovary. On CT, multiple areas of involvement are depicted and omental caking is usually present. The extensively calcified omentum is a characteristic sign of the disease. The ovaries are normal. PSC should be differentiated from PC [2, 3].

Desmoplastic small round cell tumor(*DSRCT*) is a highly aggressive malignant tumor, most often seen in adolescents and young adults. On CT, the typical findings are multiple round peritoneal soft-tissue masses with heterogeneous enhancement with central low-attenuation (due to necrosis) and omental involvement [1–3]. Lymphadenopathy, hepatic metastases, hydronephrosis, and bowel obstruction may be seen. In some cases ascites is present.

Liposarcomas arise more frequently from the retroperitoneum than from the mesentery or peritoneum. They may have a variable CT and MR imaging appearance which merely reflects their tissue composition, ranging from predominantly fat, fluid, and soft-tissue elements to entirely soft-tissue density masses [1, 2]. Fat attenuation is less likely to be found in higher grade liposarcomas (Fig. 60.2).

The less infrequent sarcoma in the peritoneal cavity is *malignant fibrous histiocytoma* which is manifested at CT as a large, solitary mass often loculated with distinctive margins that exhibits heterogeneous enhancement. *Leiomyosarcomas* found in the mesenteries are rarely primary and most often represent peritoneal extension from leiomyosarcomas arising from the stomach or the SB. The intraperitoneal spread of leiomyosarcomas is believed to occur by invasion of the serosa or by embolic metastases. Peritoneal leiomyosarcomatosis is defined as the peritoneal dissemination of leiomyosarcomas and manifests peritoneal nodules, omental infiltration, and large peritoneal masses [1, 4].

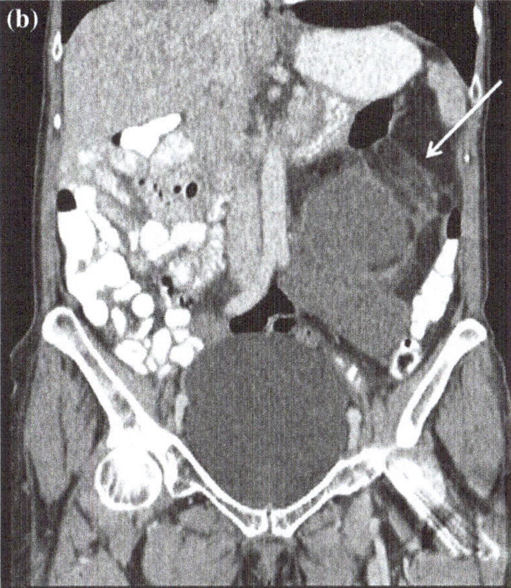

Fig. 60.2 62-year-old female with a history of abdominal pain. **a** Axial and coronal, **b** contrast-enhanced CT images show a large inhomogeneous mass in the left upper quadricept of the abdomen (*arrow*), with soft tissue and fatty areas. The mass is surgically proven liposarcoma

60.3 Secondary Peritoneal Tumors

Secondary neoplasms are the most common malignancies involving the peritoneal cavity. They can disseminate through the peritoneum by four distinctive pathways: direct invasion along peritoneal folds, intraperitoneal seeding, lymphatic permeation, and embolic hematogenous spread. These types of malignant dissemination are manifested by specific imaging patterns of disease spread. Although the imaging patterns of metastatic disease may coexist, many neoplasms metastasize predominantly by one particular route that may indicate the primary site (Fig. 60.1).

60.3.1 Direct Spread Along Peritoneal Reflections

Primary neoplasms of the stomach, colon, pancreas, and ovary that have penetrated beyond the borders of these organs can spread directly along the adjacent visceral peritoneal attachments (mesenteries, ligaments, omenta) to involve other intra-abdominal organs or anatomic areas. Invasion occurs through the areolar tissue that is enclosed by the mesothelial peritoneal membranes on the surface of the mesenteries, ligaments, and omenta. Early peritoneal invasion is manifested as linear strands in the fat adjacent to primary tumor, local thickening of the peritoneal folds, and changes in the CT density or the MRI-signal intensity of the peritoneal fat. A mass contiguous with the primary neoplasm reflects a more advanced form of dissemination. Involvement of the peritoneal folds may occupy the total length of the corresponding peritoneal reflection to reach and invade other intra-abdominal structures. Under this concept the peritoneal reflections act as bridges between abdominal organs allowing involvement from one organ to another and constitute a common route for malignant dissemination [5]. In this way, gastric malignancy from the greater curvature may extend to the spleen via the gastrosplenic ligament; from the anterior-inferior gastric wall to invade the superior margin of the transverse colon along the gastrocolic ligament (and vice versa); from the lesser curvature of the stomach invasion of the left liver lobe or the porta hepatis may occur along the gastrohepatic or the hepatoduodenal ligament, respectively. Biliary or even hepatic tumors may also spread along the gastrohepatic and hepatoduodenal ligaments. A carcinoma at the head of the pancreas may directly invade the porta hepatis and

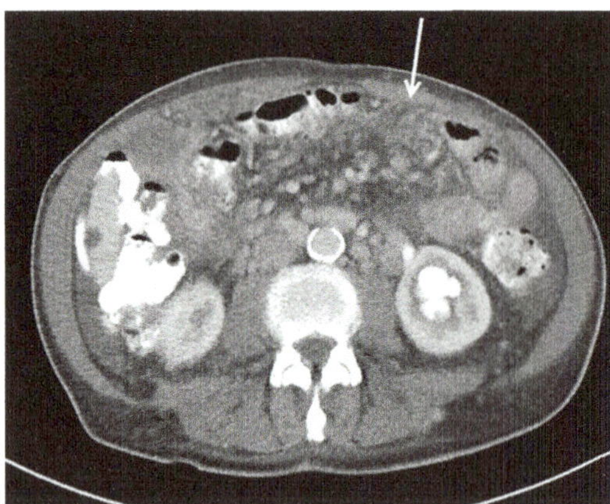

Fig. 60.3 65-year-old female with a history of ovarian cancer. Axial contrast-enhanced CT image demonstrates soft tissue masses (nodular pattern) along the great omentum (*arrow*). Stranding of the mesenteric fat and a small amount of ascites are also present

neighboring liver parenchyma via the hepatoduodenal ligament; a neoplasm of the body of the pancreas may spread along the transverse mesocolon to the inferior border of the transverse colon (and vice versa); a tumor of the pancreatic tail may migrate to the spleen through the splenopancreatic ligament (connecting the pancreatic tail with the splenic hilum and containing the splenic vessels) or to the splenic flexure of the colon through the phrenicocolic ligament. Ovarian carcinoma may spread diffusely through all adjacent peritoneal surfaces (Fig. 60.3).

60.3.2 Intraperitoneal Seeding

Intraperitoneal seeding is a common mechanism of spread in advanced intra-abdominal malignancies with most common primaries the ovarian (71 %), gastric (17 %), and colorectal (10 %) cancers. When cancer cells from a growing primary neoplasm reach the peritoneal surface, they are carried out by the peritoneal fluid and disseminated throughout the peritoneal cavity.

Distribution of disease in PC is promoted by peritoneal fluid circulation which is governed by body habitus, gravity, peristaltic motion of the intestine, intra-abdominal pressure gradients, adhesions, and predetermined anatomic routes formed by peritoneal reflections and attachments [5]. Normally present peritoneal fluid (about 100 cc) or ascites tend to accumulate in the most depended portion of the peritoneal cavity, namely the pouch of Douglas and then, symmetrically, to the lateral paravesical spaces. From there fluid can migrate to the upper abdomen due to the lower hydrostatic pressure at the subdiaphragmatic area than the pelvis, produced by respiratory movements. Fluid migration occurs along both the paracolic gutters and especially the right one that is wider and deeper than the left. In addition, fluid movement along the left paracolic gutter is obstructed at the level of the splenic flexure by the phrenicocolic ligament. Peritoneal fluid in the paracolic gutters is distinguished from retroperitoneal fluid by the preservation of the retroperitoneal fat posteriorly to the ascending or descending colon, provided there is not a complete ascending or descending mesocolon.

Ascites in the upper abdomen usually accumulates in the pouch of Morison (or hepatorenal space, the most depended portion of the peritoneal cavity in the upper abdomen), the subdiaphragmatic spaces, and the perihepatic and perisplenic spaces. Any amount of fluid that may be found in the inframesocolic compartment of the abdomen tends to move toward the lower pelvis; in the right inframesocolic compartment ascites flows along the surface of the SB mesentery to a pouch at the ileocecal conjunction and in continuation to the pelvis, while in the left inframesocolic compartment the fluid is directed to the surface of the sigmoid mesocolon and, thereafter, to the pelvis. Pooling of ascites along with cancer cells is followed by their adhesion to the mesothelial surface and the invasion of the subperitoneal space for proliferation and vascular neogenesis [6]. PC is the term given to malignant tumor seeding of the peritoneum. The most common seeding sites include the pouch of Douglas, the distal SB mesentery near the ileocecal junction, the sigmoid mesocolon, the right paracolic gutter, the pouch of Morison, and the right subdiaphragmatic area. More aggressive

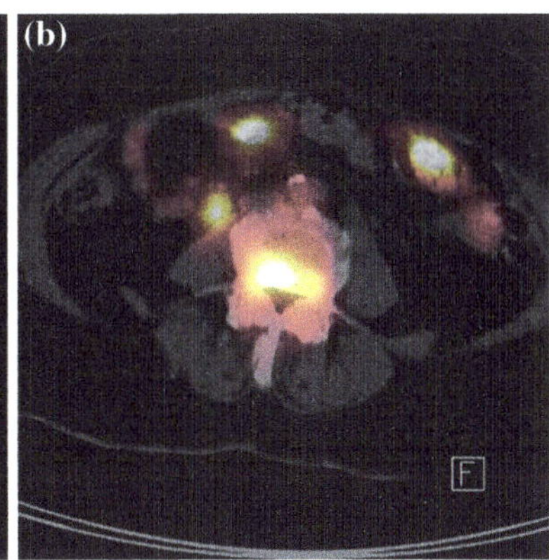

Fig. 60.4 70-year-old female with a history of ovarian cancer. **a** Axial CT image demonstrates two soft tissue lesions at the anterior surface of the peritoneum (*arrows*). **b** In fusion axial PET/CT image these lesions show increased metabolic activity and are considered as peritoneal implants. The *right ureter* (*arrowhead*) is dilated by another peritoneal implant (not shown)

neoplasms tend to exhibit malignant peritoneal deposits closer to the primary tumor, as opposed to less aggressive neoplasms that usually manifest deposits in remote areas in the abdominal cavity. Variable amounts of ascites may accompany peritoneal seeding, but ascites is not always present. Ascitic fluid is sometimes loculated and/or septated, due to malignant adhesions and may appear as a cystic lesion with mass effect.

Cross-sectional imaging examinations demonstrate a variety of types of peritoneal implants that may be demonstrated as thickening and enhancement of the peritoneum, nodules, or plaques on the peritoneal surfaces, masses, or stranding of the mesenteric fat [7] (Fig. 60.4). Implantation of tumor deposits along the peritoneal surfaces of the diaphragm, liver, and spleen, results in smooth, nodular, or plaque-like thickening and contrast enhancement of the parietal peritoneal lining. Some implants (usually from mucinous primary tumors of the colon or the ovary) may exhibit low attenuation values on CT, enhance after contrast material injection, and may mimic loculated fluid. Calcifications within peritoneal implants prior to chemotherapy suggest that the primary site is either serous papillary cystadenocarcinoma of the ovary or rarely gastric carcinoma. In the subcapsular liver area or in the spleen nodules and/or masses may indent parenchyma creating a "scalloping"-called pattern [8]. The gastrohepatic, the gastrosplenic, and the falciform ligaments when involved became thicker and fat-stranding may appear. The SB mesentery is frequently involved by intraperitoneally disseminated tumor. Common, although nonspecific, imaging findings include scattered nodules, rounded, ill-defined soft-tissue or cystic masses, and mesenteric fixation and thickening of the mesentery. The latter may demonstrate either a stellate or a pleated form [9]. In the stellate appearance, a radiating configuration of the mesenteric folds with thickened rigid perivascular bundles and encased, straightened vascular structures is observed. In the pleated appearance, sheets of soft tissue produce thickening of the mesenteric folds. Extensive involvement of the mesentery may be associated by fixation of the mesenteric folds, which is more evident on repeated CT or MRI in the lateral or prone position. Peritoneal seeding may result in metastatic tumor nodules in the visceral peritoneal surfaces adherent to the serosa of SB loops. A specific pattern of SB involvement named "layered-type" of involvement has been described, referring to extensive coating of intestinal loops by thin cancerous plaques [10].

Larger metastatic mesenteric lesions maintain their relationship with the distal SB mesentery and they may cause inferior and medial displacement of ileal loops. In cases of severe desmoplastic response to the seeded metastases, the marked fixation and angulation of SB loops may lead to obstruction. The greater omentum is also usually involved by PC, since it is the site for reabsorption of the peritoneal fluid that carries cancer cells in those patients. Early omental involvement is manifested on CT as omental thickening with increased attenuation values of the fat, fat stranding, nodules or irregular soft-tissue permeation of the omental fat. In advanced seeding spread, the deposits range from discrete nodules to thick, confluent solid omental masses, the so-called "omental-cake". On postcontrast CT, the metastatic implants may enhance and be more readily seen within the low attenuation omentum. On MRI, implants present with low-signal intensity within the high signal omental fat on T1-weighted images and exhibit enhancement. Extensive involvement of the omentum is manifested by a crescent-shaped mass, intermediate in signal intensity, exhibiting diffuse enhancement after administration of gadolinium. Fat suppression postgadolinium T1-weighted MR images facilitate the depiction of omental involvement.

Mutli-detector CT (MDCT) with thin collimation and coronal and sagittal reformations is considered as the preferable modality for detecting the presence, location, and extent of PC. Furthermore, the Peritoneal Surface Malignancy Group has accepted CT as the fundamental imaging modality in the preoperative selection process [11]. Overall diagnostic accuracy of 94 %, specificity of 92 % and sensitivities between 75 and 81 % have been reported for MDCT; however, sensitivity for the identification of smaller lesions by MDCT is significantly lower [12]. CT accuracy for the detection of peritoneal lesions varies with their location within the abdomen, being highest in the gutters, over the free surface of spleen and liver, and less sensitive in the pelvis and mid-abdomen. Also, a wide interobserver variability among radiologists in the interpretation of CT scans of patients with PC of colorectal or appendiceal origin has been reported; this variability is more remarkable in the detection rate of lesions smaller than 1 cm, and of lesions on the SB and its mesentery [13]. MRI was considered to have a complementary role in PC. However, contrast-enhanced T1-weighted MR images with fat saturation can improve the detection of smaller or equivocal implants or of numerous very small implants that may be manifested as a contiguous "sheet-like" enhancement along the peritoneal surfaces. Peritoneal tumors often enhance slowly and are best seen on images obtained 5 min after injection of gadolinium. In addition, Diffusion-weighted (DW) MRI has been described to improve sensitivity for small hypercellular implants of peritoneal malignant tissue due to increased contrast between the hyperintense spot of malignant tissue and the surrounding hypointense normal tissue [14]. Consequently, the combination of diffuse-weighted images (DWI) and conventional MRI improves the accuracy of MRI for depicting peritoneal implants; therefore DWI is suggested as an indispensable part of any MRI evaluation in patients suspected for PC [15]. FDG PET-CT adds to conventional imaging in the detection and staging of PC and is a useful diagnostic tool in monitoring response to therapy and in long-term follow-up. PET/CT imaging findings considering as positive for peritoneal tumor include (a) areas with increased FDG uptake corresponding to a CT abnormality and not related to physiologic uptake, (b) CT abnormalities with strong suspicion of tumor even in absence of a corresponding FDG uptake, (c) abnormal FDG uptake with strong suspicion of tumor even in absence of a corresponding CT abnormality [16]. At present, DW-MRI and FDG-PET/CT are equally promising methods for the evaluation of PC [15, 17] and could be suggested especially for monitoring therapeutic response and disease recurrence.

PC was regarded as a lethal disease with disappointing prognosis up to few years ago; the majority of the patients died within 6 months after diagnosis and only palliative treatment was applied. The innovations in peritoneal surface malignancy therapeutics and the application of more aggressive methods, namely cytoreductive surgery (CRS) in combination with hyperthermic intraperitoneal chemotherapy (HIPEC), have significantly improved the long-term survival rate in these patients [18]. The evolution of CRS has not only revolutionized the treatment of PC but it is also a challenge for imaging. CRS aims in complete resection of tumor-bearing peritoneal surfaces and abdominal organs. Optimal CRS requires excision of any visible malignant peritoneal deposit. Complete CRS is followed by HIPEC to eliminate minimal residual PC. CRS with HIPEC is associated with significantly improved progression-free and overall survival. However, the method carries a significant morbidity, it is time- and resource consuming and it is considered efficacious if it is performed in selected patients with peritoneal surface malignancy. Imaging techniques have an important role in the preoperative evaluation of PC and in the selection of candidates for CRS-HIPEC. Analysis of imaging findings should be performed on a site-by-site basis and the presence, type and size of peritoneal seeding should be reported in every region of the peritoneal cavity. Preoperative assessment of the overall disease burden and the extent of involvement in specific peritoneal areas are of decisive significance in the selection of patients that could benefit from CRS and in surgical planning [19]. For example, extensive involvement of the hepatoduodenal ligament, the SB and/or mesenteric root, hepatic metastases, pelvic side wall invasion, involved lymph node beyond to celiac axis or of the ligament of Treitz may preclude a complete CRS [20]. On the other hand, infiltration of the ligaments suspending the stomach by PC may indicate the need for gastrectomy. The role of imaging is emphasized by recent evidence that residual disease larger than 1 cm was present on early postoperative CT in almost half of the patients deemed to have optimally debulked disease at primary cytoreduction [21] (Fig. 60.2).

Involvement of the SB and its mesentery is considered as an independent prognostic factor of survival in patients with PC. The extent of SB/SB mesentery involvement by peritoneal seeding is crucial in the selection process of candidates for CRS and it is also important for surgical planning. Furthermore, SB mesentery is a common location of suboptimally debulked disease after CRS. As opposed to the clinical significance of an accurate preoperative evaluation of peritoneal seeding affecting the SB/SB mesentery, cross-sectional imaging presents the lowest sensitivity and diagnostic accuracy in this specific area. CT-enteroclysis with SB distention by negative contrast medium results in increased sensitivity and specificity in the diagnosis of the extent of SB/SB mesentery involvement by PC and it has been proposed in the preoperative work-up in candidates for CRS [10] (Fig. 60.5).

(a)

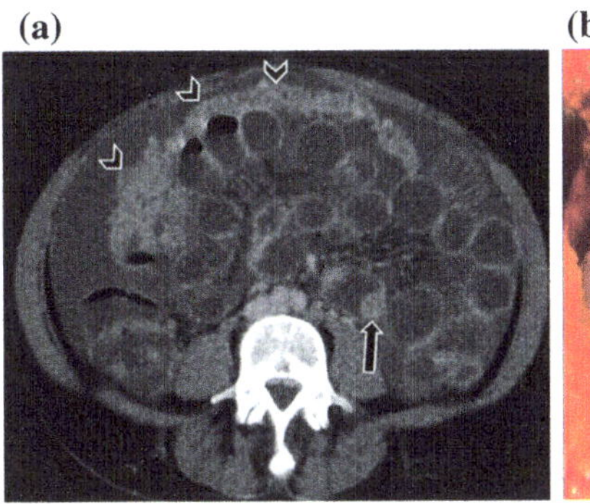

(b)

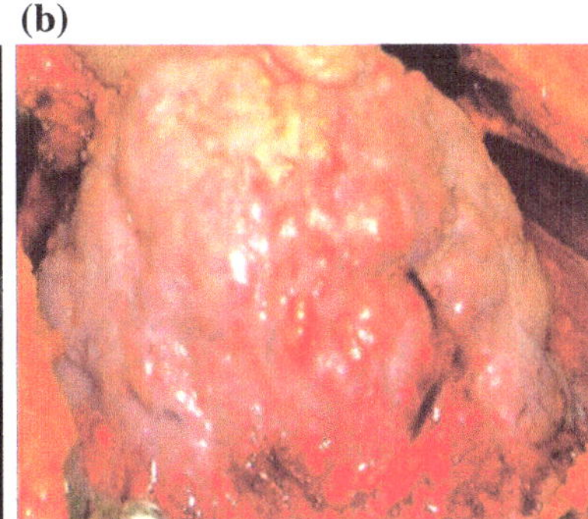

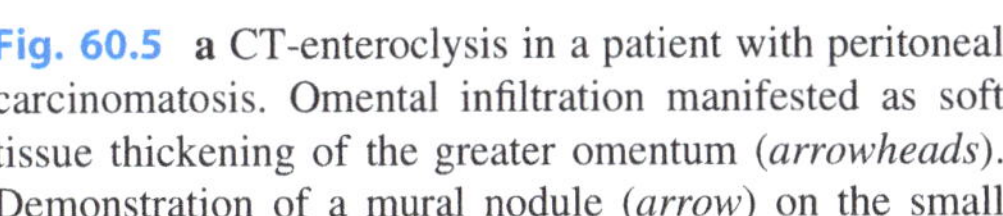

Fig. 60.5 **a** CT-enteroclysis in a patient with peritoneal carcinomatosis. Omental infiltration manifested as soft tissue thickening of the greater omentum (*arrowheads*). Demonstration of a mural nodule (*arrow*) on the small bowel wall is facilitated by the distention of the intestinal loops after CT-enteroclysis (**b**). Extensive omental infiltration in the same patient seen at surgery

Pseudomyxoma peritonei is a peculiar type of neoplasia spread throughout the abdominal cavity after rupture of a benign or malignant mucin-producing tumor of the appendix or ovary. Imaging manifestations include masses of low attenuation on CT and moderately high signal intensity on MRI, accompanied by ascites with septations representing the margins of mucinous nodules. Additional cross-sectional imaging findings include scalloping of visceral surfaces of the liver and spleen by adjacent mucinous peritoneal implants as well as soft-tissue thickening of the peritoneal surfaces, reflecting the more solid components of the tumor.

There are two nonmalignant great mimickers of PC: *tuberculosis* (TBC) and *eosinophilic peritonitis* (EP). Peritoneal tuberculosis may exhibit free or loculated ascites, thickened strands with crowded vascular bundles within mesentery, smooth uniform thickening of the peritoneum, and a smudged pattern of omental involvement infiltrated by small ill-defined soft-tissue [22]. Imaging findings of TBC and EP are similar to these seen in PC. However, high-attenuation ascites (20–45 HU) and mesenteric lymphadenopathy with peripheral enhancement and central low attenuation on CT, when present, indicate TBC. EP is a benign disease of unknown etiology, although allergic diathesis is present in most of the patients. It affects young to middle age individuals and responds to corticosteroids. EP is characterized by peripheral eosinophilia, eosinophilic infiltration of GI tract, and eosinophilic ascites. Diffuse peritoneal thickening and enhancement and "soft-tissue" omental infiltration are common manifestations of EP on imaging [23].

60.3.3 Embolic Metastases

Embolic metastases to the mesentery are usually arising from melanoma and lung or breast carcinoma and they can spread via mesenteric arteries to locate along the antimesenteric border of the SB. CT manifestations include focal bowel wall thickening and thickening of the mesenteric folds [9]. Melanoma deposits may become large and ulcerated. Breast cancer deposits may cause multiple areas of SB luminal narrowing with prestenotic dilatations.

60.3.4 Lymphatic Dissemination

Lymphatic permeation to mesenteric lymph nodes plays a minor role in the spread of metastatic carcinoma, but it is the main pathway of dissemination of lymphoma. Enlarged mesenteric lymph nodes occur at presentation in approximately 50 % of patients with gastrointestinal non-Hodgkin's lymphoma. Confluent lymphomatous nodes may surround the superior mesenteric vessels, producing a "sandwich-like" appearance. Coexisted lymphomatous mural involvement and thickening of the small-bowel loops affects predominantly their mesenteric border (Fig. 60.5).

References

1. Levy A, Arnaiz J, Shaw J et al (2008) Primary peritoneal tumors: imaging features with pathologic correlation. Radiographics 28:583–607
2. Pickhardt P, Bhalla S (2005) Primary neoplasms of peritoneal and subperitoneal origin: CT findings. Radiographics 25:983–995
3. Jeong Y, Kim S, Wook Kwak S et al (2008) Neoplastic and non-neoplastic conditions of serosal membrane origin: CT findings. Radiographics 28: 801–818
4. Rha S, Ha H, Kim A et al (2003) Peritoneal leiomyosarcomatosis originating from gastrointestinal leiomyosarcomas: CT features. Radiology 227: 385–390
5. Meyers MA (2000) Intraperitoneal spread of malignancies. In: Meyers MA (ed) Dynamic radiology of the abdomen: normal and pathologic anatomy, 5th edn. Springer, New York, pp 131–263
6. Confuorto G, Giuliano ME, Grimaldi A et al (2007) Peritoneal carcinomatosis from colorectal cancer: HIPEC? Surg Oncol 16(Suppl 1):S149–S152
7. Raptopoulos V, Gourtsoyiannis N (2001) Peritoneal carcinomatosis. Eur Radiol 11:2195–2206
8. Pannu H, Bristow R, Montz F et al (2003) Multidetector CT of peritoneal carcinomatosis from ovarian cancer. Radiographics 23:687–701
9. Sheth S, Horton KM, Garland MR et al (2003) Mesenteric neoplasms: CT appearances of primary

and secondary tumors and differential diagnosis. Radiographics 23:457–473
10. Courcoutsakis N, Tentes AA, Astrinakis E et al (2012) CT-Enteroclysis in the preoperative assessment of the small-bowel involvement in patients with peritoneal carcinomatosis, candidates for cytoreductive surgery and hyperthermic intraperitoneal chemotherapy abdom Imaging. doi: 10.1007/s00261-012-9869-3
11. Yan TD, Morris DL, Shigeki K et al (2008) Preoperative investigations in the management of peritoneal surface malignancy with cytoreductive surgery and perioperative intraperitoneal chemotherapy: expert consensus statement. J Surg Oncol 98:224–227
12. Marin D, Catalano C, Baski M et al (2010) 64-section multi-detector row CT in the preoperative diagnosis of peritoneal carcinomatosis: correlation with histopathological findings. Abdom Imaging 35:694–700
13. De Bree E, Koops W, Kröger R et al (2004) Peritoneal carcinomatosis from colorectal or appendiceal origin: correlation of preoperative CT with intraoperative findings and evaluation of interobserver agreement. J Surg Oncol 86:64–73
14. Koh DM, Collins DJ (2007) Diffusion-weighted MRI in the body: applications and challenges in oncology. AJR 188(6):1622–1635
15. Iafrate F, Ciolina M, Sammartino P et al (2012) Peritoneal carcinomatosis: Imaging with 64-MDCT and 3T MRI with diffusion-weighted imaging. Abdom Imaging 37:616–627
16. DeGaetano AM, Calcagni ML, Rufini V et al (2009) Imaging of peritoneal carcinomatosis with FDG PET-CT: diagnostic patterns, case examples and pitfalls. Abdom Imaging 34:391–402
17. Soussan M, Des Guetz G, Barrau V et al (2012) Comparison of FDG-PET/CT and MR with diffusion-weighted imaging for assessing peritoneal carcinomatosis from gastrointestinal malignancy. Eur Radiol 22:1479–1487
18. Sugarbaker P (2009) From the guest editors: introduction: progress in the management of carcinomatosis. Cancer J 15:182–183
19. Tentes KA, Courcoutsakis N, Prassopoulos P (2012) Combined cytoreductive surgery and perioperative intraperitoneal chemotherapy for the treatment of advanced ovarian cancer, ovarian cancer—clinical and therapeutic perspectives. In: Samir F (ed) Ovarian cancer—clinical and therapeutic perspectives. In Tech - Publishers pp 143–167. [ISBN 978-953-307-810-6]
20. Nougaret S, Addley H, Colombo PE et al (2012) Ovarian carcinomatosis: how the radiologist can help plan the surgical approach. Radiographics 32:1775–1800
21. Lakhman Y, Akin O, Sohn JM et al (2012) Early postoperative CT as a prognostic biomarker in patients with advanced ovarian, tubal, and primary peritoneal cancer deemed optimally debulked at primary cytoreductive surgery. AJR 198:1453–1459
22. Gourtsoyiannis N, Daskalogiannaki M, Prassopoulos P (2001) Imaging of the peritoneum, mesentery and omentum. In: Grainger RG, Allison DJ (eds) Diagnostic radiology. Churchill Livingstone, London, pp 1141–1163
23. Pickhardt PJ, Bhalla S (2005) Unusual nonneoplastic peritoneal and subperitoneal conditions: CT findings. Radiographics 25:719–730

61 Introduction to the Large Bowel

Paris A. Kosmidis and Christos A. Pissiotis

Colorectal cancer is the third most common cancer in the world. In the USA, 150,000 new cases are diagnosed annually whereas in Europe the respective incidence is 400,000 [1]. The ratio of colonic to rectal cancer is 2:1. Colorectal cancer is more common in males than females [2].

Colorectal cancer is highly a preventable disease. Screening and removal of premalignant polyps have contributed to the decline of the incidence during the past three decades.

Early diagnosis is extremely important which result a 5-year survival of 90 %. The 5-year survival of patients with this disease has improved significantly during the past 10 years due to the improved surgical techniques and novel molecular agents.

However, the contribution of new imaging technology is of paramount importance. The early detection of polyps, the accurate staging and restaging, the assessment of response to treatment as well the surveillance are issues directly related to imaging techniques. In particular, imaging contribution for residual liver metastatic lesions, evaluation of response following radio-chemotherapy for rectal cancer are important information to the oncologist for decision making process. CT, CT colonography, MRI, PET-CT, and endorectal ultrasound are useful and necessary techniques which make the radiologist's role great and his cooperation with the oncologist mandatory.

References

1. World Health Organization. Global burden of disease. http://www.who.int/entity/healthinfo/global_burden_disease
2. Parkin DM, Bray F, Ferlay J et al (2005) Global cancer statistics, 2002. CA Cancer J Clin 55:74–108

P. A. Kosmidis (✉)
2nd Medical Oncology Department,
Hygeia Hospital, 4, Er.Stavrou and Vas Sofias Ave, 15123, Marousi, Athens, Greece
e-mail: parkosmi@otenet.gr

C. A. Pissiotis
Professor of Surgery, Hygeia Hospital, 4, Er. Stavrou and Vas Sofias Ave, 15123, Marousi, Athens, Greece
e-mail: c.pissiotis@hygeia.gr

A. D. Gouliamos et al. (eds.), *Imaging in Clinical Oncology*,
DOI: 10.1007/978-88-470-5385-4_61, © Springer-Verlag Italia 2014

62 CT and CT-Colonography

Dimitrios T. Kechagias

62.1 Computed Tomography

Preoperative CT is indicated in suspicion of hematogenous or distal nodal metastatic disease or invasion into adjacent organs or formation of abscess and presence of atypical symptoms.

Abdominal CT must be performed with an intravenous contrast agent. The portal phase must be used either as a single phase or combined with arterial and late phases.

At CT colorectal cancer appears as a soft tissue mass or wall thickening with luminal narrowing. Colonic obstruction, perforation, and fistula are complications that can be visualized with CT. Local spread is seen by loss of fat planes between colon and adjacent organs, extracolic mass, thickening and infiltration of pericolic fat, and involvement of adjacent organs (Fig. 62.1). The sensitivity, specificity, positive predictive value, and negative predictive value of CT in identifying tumor extension in pericolic fat ranges from 74 to 79 %, 33–67 %, 91, and 15 %, respectively. In one series the sensitivity and specificity of CT in indentifying T3 and T4 tumors were 87 and 49 %, respectively. Sensitivity and specificity for tumor infiltration beyond the muscularis propria were 95 and 50 %, respectively [1].

The specificity of CT for N staging based on size criteria is high (96 %) but the sensitivity is low. The accuracy ranges from 62 to 75 % [2]. Small or normal-sized nodes may have micrometastatic disease whereas large nodes (larger than 1–1.5 cm in short axis diameter) may be reactive. Radiological T and N categories using CT staging are independent prognostic factors for both overall survival and free survival in patients who underwent curative resection.

Hepatic metastases are seen as hypoattenuating lesions in portal phase of contrast-enhanced CT with a sensitivity of more than 90 % for lesions larger than 1 cm of diameter. The accuracy, specificity, and sensitivity are 85, 97, and 74.4 %, respectively. Cystic or calcified hepatic metastases can be seen in mucinous cancer. Lungs, adrenal glands, bones, and peritoneum are other common sites of metastatic disease.

CT can be used to find lung metastases preoperatively but not as a routine procedure.

CT is useful for the treatment planning especially for postoperative comparison. The accuracy of preoperative CT in staging ranges from 48 to 77 %. Poor prognostic features like T-stage, N-stage, extramural extension, and involvement of retroperitoneal surgical margin can be predicted using CT with accuracy of 82–94.1 %. In this way, patients with a poor prognosis can be indentified and may be suitable for neoadjuvant chemotherapy [1].

Recurrent tumor after surgery looks like as a soft-tissue mass in the surgical site which enlarges over time, enlarged regional lymph

D. T. Kechagias (✉)
CT, MRI and PET/CT Departments, Hygeia Hospital, 4 Erythrou Stavrou Str, 15124 Marousi, Greece
e-mail: dikechagias@hotmail.com

A. D. Gouliamos et al. (eds.), *Imaging in Clinical Oncology*,
DOI: 10.1007/978-88-470-5385-4_62, © Springer-Verlag Italia 2014

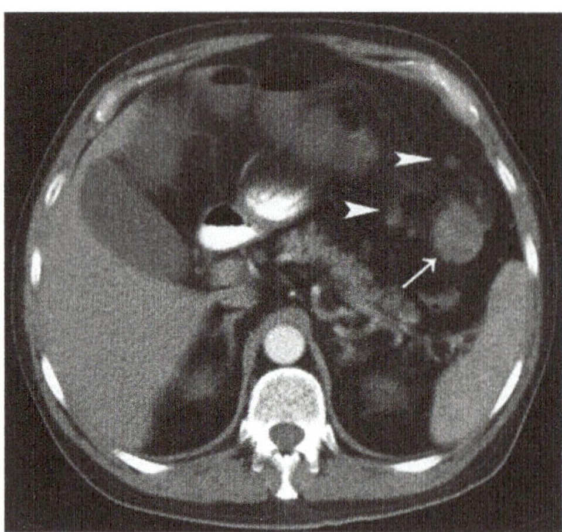

Fig. 62.1 Enhanced CT of the abdomen shows a mass in the left colic flexure (*arrow*), infiltration of the pericolic fat, and small lymph nodes (*arrowheads*)

nodes, and invasion of adjacent structures. CT is helpful to diagnose recurrent metastases in liver or extra abdominal sites.

62.2 CT Colonography

62.2.1 Introduction

The first description of Computed tomographic colonography (CT colonography) or virtual colonoscopy was reported in 1994. It is a minimally invasive examination for the colon and rectum.

62.2.2 Indications-Contraindications

CT colonography is useful in patients with incomplete colonoscopy due to colonic tortuosity or stenosis, diverticulosis, obstructive cancer, or in those with contraindication for optical colonoscopy (anticoagulant drugs or diseases with increased risk from anesthesia). CT colonography can also be used for colon cancer screening. The examination is contraindicated in colon perforation, toxic megacolon, recent rectal operation, proctitis and polyp excision, or biopsy into the last 6 days period.

62.2.3 Technique

The day before the study, a clear liquid diet along with cathartics for adequate bowel preparation is required, because polyps cannot be differentiated from retained stools. Barium and/or iodine oral contrast agents can be used for tagging of residual fluid and solid stool.

CT colonography with cathartic—free faecal tagging yields high positive predictive values (92.8 %) and is well accepted by the patients [3].

The colon is distended with carbon dioxide or room air through a small-caliber rectal catheter by automated or manual insufflation. No sedation is needed.

The abdomen is scanned with the patient in prone and supine positions in less than 2 min. Approximately 10 min is the duration of the CT table procedure. Intravenous contrast is helpful for differentiation of colonic fluid from polyps and for patients with more advanced symptoms. 2-D images in axial coronal and sagittal planes and 3-D image display techniques for interpretation are used. Evaluation of extracolonic structures is feasible with 2-D images (Fig. 62.2).

62.2.4 Efficacy and Test Performance Characteristics

Measurements of polyp size at CT colonography are 1–2 mm smaller than colonoscopic and 1–2 mm larger than pathologic measurements.

The reference standard for the CT colonography performance characteristics for detection of polyps is optical colonoscopy. In one series, the sensitivity and specificity for large polyps is 90 and 86 %, respectively [4] whereas in another one, sensitivity of 85 % and specificity of 87 % for large polyps was achieved [5]. Detection rates for advanced neoplasia are similar in CT colonography and colonoscopy.

CT colonography compared with colonoscopy has a negative predictive value (NPV) of 96.3 % overall. The positive predictive value (PPV) is 90 %. When limited to fecal occult blood tests, the positive persons NPV is 84.9 %.

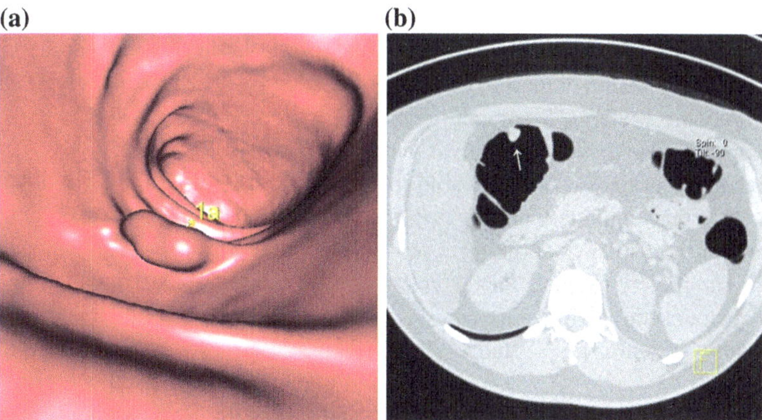

Fig. 62.2 Colonic adenoma with pathological confirmation in a patient who underwent CT colonography as a screening test. **a** 3-D image shows a polypoid lesion (1a). **b** 2-D axial CT image shows a soft tissue polypoid lesion (*arrow*) located at the right colic flexure

The per-patient and per-lesion PPVs of CT colonography after incomplete colonoscopy for masses (≥20 mm), large polyps (10–19 mm), and medium polyps (6–9 mm) are 90.9 and 91.7 %, 64.7 and 70 %, and 33.3 and 30.4 %, respectively [6].

In a post–hoc analysis of data from the US National CT Colonography trial no statistically significant differences have been found in the diagnostic performance of CT colonography between patients older than 65-years of age and younger participants for the detection of intermediate-size and large adenomas. Some meta-analyses have been published to summarize the available data. In one, 47 studies providing data of 10,546 patients were included. Overall per-polyp and per patient sensitivity of CT colonography was 66 and 69 %, respectively. Overall CT colonography specificity was 83 % [7].

A recent meta-analysis included 49 studies (compromising a total of 11,151 patients) and calculated sensitivity of CT colonography 96.1 % [8]. Another one included five studies (compromising 4,086 asymptomatic patients) and estimated sensitivity for patients with polyps or adenomas ≥6 mm 75.9 % and corresponding specificity 94.6 %, whereas for patients with polyps or adenomas ≥10 mm sensitivity 83.3 % and specificity 98.7 % [9].

62.2.5 Safety

Complications from CT colonography are rare. The incidence of symptomatic colonic perforation is small but definite. Rates at between 0.06 and 0.08 % have been reported, which approaches the complication rates reported for colonoscopy. This comparison may be biased because CT colonography is performed in many patients after colonoscopy failed. Risk factors are age, diverticular disease, colonic obstruction, and recent colonoscopy, especially with recent biopsy.

Low—pressure delivery of carbon dioxide for colonic distention may be safer than insufflation of room air. Pneumatosis of the right colon, a rare asymptomatic condition which is self-limited is associated with delivery of carbon dioxide at CT colonography.

Another issue is the radiation exposure. The effective dose for CT colonography is approximately 7–10 mSv for dual positioning, both supine and prone. Median effective dose for CT colonography is significantly lower for screening than for daily practice protocols (4.4 and 7.6 mSv respectively). Although low radiation dose protocols are used, these do not appear to reduce overall radiation exposure. The benefits from CT colonography screening every 5 years from the age of 50–80 years outweigh the radiation risks [10].

62.2.6 Patient Acceptance

For CT colonography sedation or recovery time is not required. Patients prefer CT colonography over colonoscopy because the test is noninvasive, they avoid sedation/anesthesia, they are able to drive after the test, they avoid colonoscopy risks and the test is able to identify abnormalities outside the colon. The preference rates for CT colonography and colonoscopy in patients who had experienced both procedures are 77 and 13.8 %, respectively [11].

The worst part of the procedure is bowel preparation. Limited bowel preparation for CT colonography with faecal tagging only without laxatives does not prevent high diagnostic accuracy.

62.2.7 Follow-Up

Diminutives polyps ($\leq$5 mm in size) detected at CT colonography screening, must be ignored according to American College of Radiology because the risk cancer is extremely low. Referral of patients with diminutive polyps for colonoscopy would dramatically increase the cost of screening.

CT colonography follow-up of the patients would be expensive with increased risk of radiation exposure.

In normal CT colonography follow up in 5 years with CT colonography is recommended. When one or more polyps $\geq$10 mm in size or three or more polyps 6–9 mm in size found in CT colonography, polypectomy is recommended. One or two lesions with size between 6 and 9 mm should be followed-up with CT colonography every 3 years.

In patients without recurrence of the disease in laboratory or clinical tests, contrast-enhanced CT colonography is accurate for surveillance in colorectal cancer postoperatively. The per-patient and per-lesion sensitivity is 81.8 and 80.8 %, respectively for advanced neoplasia and 80 and 78.5 %, respectively for all adenomatous lesions. The specificity is 93.1 %. The negative predictive values for adenocarcinoma, advanced neoplasia and all adenomatous lesions are 100, 99.1, and 97 %, respectively [12].

62.2.8 Extracolonic Findings

Incidental extracolonic findings are observed with reported rates from 15 to 69 %. Clinically significant findings are found 4.5 to 11 % [13]. Many patients may benefit from detection of previously unsuspected pathology; others may suffer needless anxiety, testing. and cost for clinically insignificant lesions.

62.2.9 Role for Colon Rectal Cancer Screening

Screening using CT colonography as a primary method is feasible. Similar yields for advanced neoplasia are seen in CT colonography, colonoscopy and sigmoidoscopy screening. Crucial factors for the viability of a primary screening test like CT colonography are the impact of extracolonic findings and cost-effectiveness. Good quality data regarding the impact of extracolonic findings and good quality information regarding the cost-effectiveness are lacking. In first round g guaiac Faecal Occult Blood Test/Faecal Immuno chemical Test (FOBT/FIT) positives CT colonography triage is not clinically effective [14].

If widely available, CT colonography may increase adherence to screening as a result of its general acceptance by patients. CT colonography may be the primary screening modality for all patients followed by colonoscopy in the same day if lesions are found. Alternatively colonoscopy may be used for high-risk patients and CT colonography for low-risk patients.

62.2.10 Conclusion

Abdominal CT can accurately indentify liver metastases and locally advanced colon cancer. CT can be used to find lung metastases but not as a routine procedure preoperatively. CT can identify high risk (T3/T4) tumors with more than 5 mm extramural depth which would be considered as candidates for neoadjuvant therapy.

Recent data show similar detection rates of advanced neoplasia for CT colonography screening and colonoscopic screening. Based on data, CT colonography is an acceptable examination for colon cancer screening which increases the overall prevalence of colon cancer screening. In case of negative for polyps ≥6 mm or cancer initial CT colonography, follow up in 5 years with CT colonography is recommended. Patients with three or more polyps 6–9 mm in size or polyps ≥10 mm in size should be referred for colonoscopy.

Technological advances in multi-detector row CT scanners and computer—aided detection software in addition to stool-tagging low-preparation techniques will allow increase adherence to population-based CT colonography screening.

References

1. Dighe S, Swift I, Magill L, Handley K, Gray R, Quirke P, Morton D, Seymour M, Warren B, Brown G (2012) Accuracy of radiological staging in identifying high-risk colon cancer patients suitable for neoadjuvant chemotherapy: a multicentre experience. Colorectal Dis 14(1):438–444
2. Burton S, Brown G, Bees N, Norman A, Biedrzycki O, Arnaout A, Abulafi AM, Swift RI (2008) Accuracy of CT prediction of poor prognostic features in colonic cancer. Br J Radiol 81(961):10–193
3. Zueco Zueco C, Sobrido Sampedro C, Corroto JD, Rodriguez Fernández P, Fontanillo Fontanillo M (2012) CT colonography without cathartic preparation: positive predictive value and patient experience in clinical practice. Eur Radiol 22(6):1195–1204
4. Johnson CD, Chen MH, Toledano AY, Heiken JP (2008) Accuracy of CT colonography for detection of large adenomas and cancers. N Engl J Med 359:1207–1217
5. Regge D, Laudi C, Galatola G, Della Monica P, Bonelli L, Angelelli G, Asnaghi R, Barbaro B, Bartolozzi C, Bielen D, Boni L, Borghi C, Bruzzi P, Cassinis MC, Galia M, Gallo TM, Grasso A, Hassan C, Laghi A, Martina MC, Neri E, Senore C, Simonetti G, Venturini S, Gandini G (2009) Diagnostic accuracy of computed tomographic colonography for the detection of advanced neoplasia in individuals at increase risk of colorectal cancer. JAMA 301:2453–2461
6. Copel L, Sosna J, Kruskal JB, Raptopoulos V, Farrell RJ, Morrin MM (2007) CT colonography in 546 patients with incomplete colonoscopy. Radiology 244(2):471–478
7. Chaparro M, Gisbert JP, Del Campo L, Cantero J, Maté J (2009) Accuracy of computed tomographic colonography for the detection of polyps and colorectal tumors : a systemic review and meta-analysis. Digestion 80:1–17
8. Pickhardt P, Hassan C, Halligan S, Marmo R (2011) Colorectal cancer: CT colonography and colonoscopy for detection-systemic review and meta-analysis. Radiology 259(2):393–405
9. de Haan MC, van Gelder RE, Graser A, Bipat S, Stoker J (2011) Diagnostic value of CT-colonography as compared to colonoscopy in an asymptomatic screening population: a meta-analysis. Eur Radiol 21:1747–1763
10. Berrington de González A, Kim KP, Knudsen AB, Lansdorp-Vogelaar I, Rutter CM, Smith-Bindman R, Yee J, Kuntz KM, van Ballegooijen M, Zauber AG, Berg CD (2011) Radiation-related cancer risks from CT colonography screening: a risk-benefit analysis. AJR Am J Roentgenol 196(4):816–823
11. Pooler BD, Baumel MJ, Cash BD, Moawad FJ, Riddle MS, Patrick AM, Damiano M, Lee MH, Kim DH, Muñoz del Rio A, Pickhardt PJ (2012) Screening CT colonography: multicenter survey of patient experience, preference, and potential impact of adherence. AJR 198:1361–1366
12. Kim HJ, Park SH, Pickhardt PJ, Yoon SN, Lee SS, Yee J, Kim DH, Kim AY, Kim JC, Yu CS, Ha HK (2010) CT colonography for combined colonic and extracolonic surveillance after curative resection of colorectal cancer. Radiology 257(8):697–704
13. Levin B, Lieberman DA, McFarland B, Smith RA, Brooks D, Andrews KS, Dash C, Giardiello FM, Glick S, Levin TR, Pickhardt P, Rex DK, Thorson A, Winawer SJ; American Cancer Society Colorectal Cancer Advisory Group; US Multi-Society Task Force; American College of Radiology Colon Cancer Committee (2008) Screening and surveillance for the early detection of colorectal cancer and adenomatous polyps, 2008: a joint guideline from the American Cancer Society, the US Multi-Society Task Force on Colorectal Cancer, and the American College of Radiology CA Cancer J Clin 58(3):130–160
14. de Haan M, Halligan S, Stoker J (2012) Does CT colonography have a role for population-base colorectal cancer screening? Eur Radiol 22:1495–1503

63 MR Findings of Rectal Carcinoma

Sofia N. Gourtsoyianni

63.1 Role of MRI in Rectal Cancer

Magnetic Resonance Imaging (MRI) has a central role in current rectal cancer treatment. MRI-based preoperative local staging directs neoadjuvant treatment strategies aimed primarily at the reduction of local recurrence (LR). Short course preoperative radiotherapy and long course of chemoradiotherapy (CRT) are used in patients presenting with $\geq$ T3 stage rectal cancer based on their LR risk category as staged by endorectal ultrasound (ERUS) and MRI.

ERUS remains the most accurate modality for assessment of tumor ingrowth into rectal wall layers and as such is highly specific for superficial tumors [1]. However, due to its inherent low contrast resolution, ERUS cannot clearly depict mesorectal fascia (MF) and thus cannot stratify patients presenting with locally advanced rectal cancers(LARC) according to their risk for LR. As a consequence of neoadjuvant treatment, MRI also has a role in assessment of treatment response preoperatively, especially in cases in which potential downstaging will alter the surgical plan.

MRI allows an accurate prediction of T and N stage as well as being the best method of assessing the relation of the tumor to the potential circumferential resection margin (CRM)—the MF—with a reported 92 % concordance between MRI using phased array coils and histopathology report [2]. In rectal cancer, the presence or absence of tumor within 1 mm of the surgical CRMs strongly influences outcome and is an independent predictor of survival and LR.

S. N. Gourtsoyianni (✉)
Division of Imaging Sciences, King's College London, Imaging 2, Level 1, Lambeth wing, St. Thomas' Hospital, Lambeth Palace Road, London, SE1 7EH, UK
e-mail: sgty76@gmail.com

63.2 Identification of Poor Rectal Cancer Prognostic Factors by Imaging

A major concern after surgery with curative intent is the high rate of LR, ranging from <10 to 50 %, with an average recurrence rate of 29 % [3]. LR is caused by incomplete resection of the primary tumor. It has been shown to directly correlate with the shortest distance between the primary tumor or involved lymph node and the MF (Fig. 63.1), previously referred to as the CRM. The shorter this distance is, the higher the rate of a LR [4, 5]. Although LR has a small impact on patient's survival rate it has a profound influence on patient's quality of life. Introduction of total mesorectal excision (TME), that is removal of rectum and mesorectal fat along MF, as a surgical approach for rectal cancer has significantly reduced the chance for LR to less than 10 % in certain centers even without neoadjuvant therapy [6].

LR rate varies among different stages of rectal cancer. According to the Dutch TME trial [7] Stage III (T × N + M0) disease benefited

A. D. Gouliamos et al. (eds.), *Imaging in Clinical Oncology*,
DOI: 10.1007/978-88-470-5385-4_63, © Springer-Verlag Italia 2014

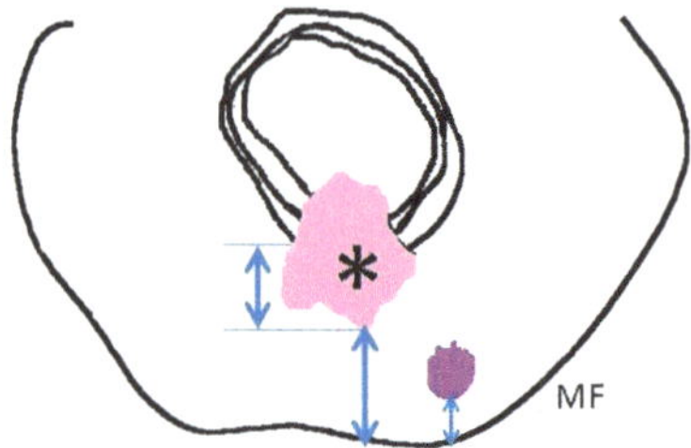

Fig. 63.1 Schematic drawing demonstrating distance to MF from either primary tumor (*) or separate tumor deposited in the mesorectal fat (lymph node, purple color structure). Whichever is closest to the MF in each case should be used for distance measurement for accurate stratification of patient according to personalized local recurrence risk

the most from short course of preoperative radiation but LR rate was still 11 % despite the addition of preoperative RT. The latter group is often being referred to as locally advanced rectal cancer (LARC) and a long course of radiotherapy combined with chemotherapy (CRT) has been known to be effective for downstaging of bulky T3 and T4 stage tumors, improving R0 resections as well as increasing the number of sphincter preservation surgeries in low lying tumors.

Three different patient categories can be stratified according to their risk for LR by MR Imaging: (a) *the GOOD*, patients with early or superficial rectal cancer that can be treated exclusively by surgery, (b) the *BAD*, patients presenting with operable tumor with wide CRM, who would benefit from short radiotherapy scheme, and (c) the UGLY, the patients with locally advanced cancer and narrow or involved CRM (CRM ≤2 mm) who would benefit from a long scheme of chemoradiation prior to surgery (Fig. 63.2) [8]. In addition MR imaging is able to identify rectal cancer poor prognostic factors. These include: (a) large T3 stage tumors with extramuscular extension >5 mm as well as T4 stage tumors, (b) narrow or involved CRM, (c) presence of metastatic lymph nodes (N+), and (d) extramural venous invasion (EMVI) as well as (e) peritoneal involvement/perforation.

63.2.1 The T Stage

Radiologists should determine whether tumor is resectable T1–T3 stage or non-resectable T4 stage. T3 stage disease can be subdivided into T3a, T3b, T3c, and T3d disease according to the radial outgrowth of tumor distance from the breached muscularis propria. This is not a TNM staging classification but uses pragmatic MRI-based categories. T3a = <1 mm, T3b = 1–5 mm, T3c = >5–15 mm, and T3d = >15 mm. Hermanek et al. [9] showed that tumor penetration of >4 mm was an important risk factor for the subsequent development of metastases. For T3 tumors penetration into the muscularis propria >5 mm is associated with poorer survival [10–13]. In the latter study, patients

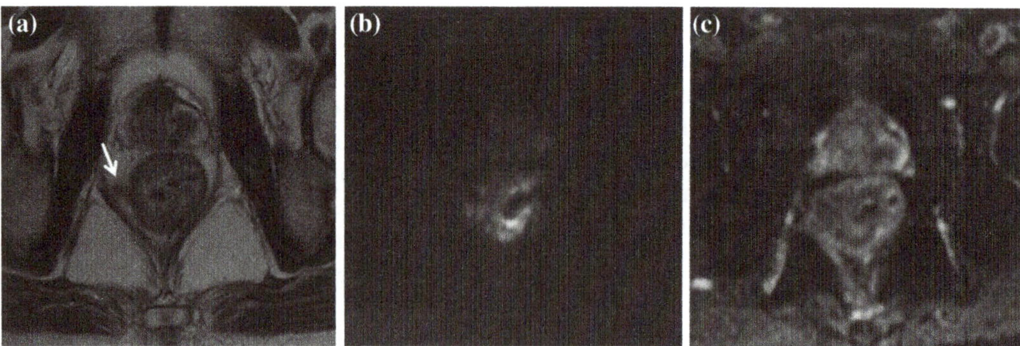

Fig. 63.2 T2-weighted axial rectal MRI image showing low-lying LARC extending beyond muscularis propria, at 9 o' clock (*arrow*), and almost abutting the right levator ani muscle. Tumor demonstrates moderate signal intensity on T2-weighted MRI image (**a**) high signal intensity on b-value 1000 SE EPI diffusion image (**b**) while ADC map at the same anatomical level reveals restriction of diffusion (low signal area) (**c**)

with >5 mm penetration had a 5-year survival of only 54 % [13].

T staging of rectal adenocarcinoma in the area of the sphincters is more difficult. Anatomical extent of tumor spread both above the sphincters, in the area of the mesorectum, and at the height of the levator/sphincters should be described. Replacement of the muscle coat of the internal sphincter by tumor, extension to the intersphincteric plane or invasion into it, and the external anal sphincter as well as infiltration or extension beyond the levators can be identified by high resolution MR imaging. On T2-weighted images, the muscularis propria layer is identified as a fine low signal intensity line, while the submucosal layer beneath it presents with high signal intensity. The mesorectal fat appears as high signal intensity area surrounding the low signal intensity line of the muscularis propria, while the MF is depicted as a thin intermediate signal intensity band surrounding the mesorectal fat (Fig. 63.3).

In T2-weighted images rectal adenocarcinoma is visualized as an intermediate signal intensity space occupying lesion that extends in the majority of cases intraluminally. In T1 weighted images it presents with isointense signal intensity to the rest of the rectum. Mucin containing type of rectal tumor presents with high signal intensity on T2-weighted images, pathognomonic of mucin (Fig. 63.4). Stage T4 can be easily recognized with high resolution MRI when there is invasion of adjacent pelvic organs (uterus, cervix, bladder, seminal vesicles, prostate, or sacrum) or structures (pelvic side wall, anal sphincter) or invasion to the peritoneum. Local tumor perforation through the peritoneal membrane is common and also indicates an unfavorable prognosis, not only due to associated peritonitis, but also because of the risk of dissemination of malignant cells within the abdominal cavity resulting in transcoelomic spread and peritoneal involvement [14].

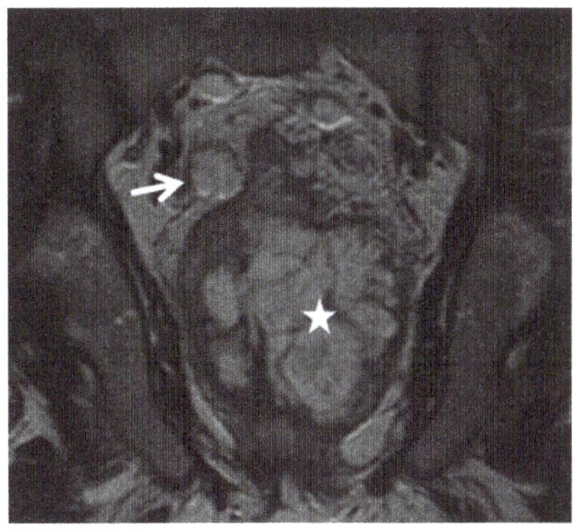

Fig. 63.4 T2-weighted coronal MRI image: a bulky, space occupying lesion is noted in the mid rectum. The high signal intensity of the mass is pathognomonic of a mucinous type of adenocarcinoma (*). Note the mesorectal lymph nodes on the right side also appear with same signal intensity as the primary tumor suggestive of involvement (*arrow*)

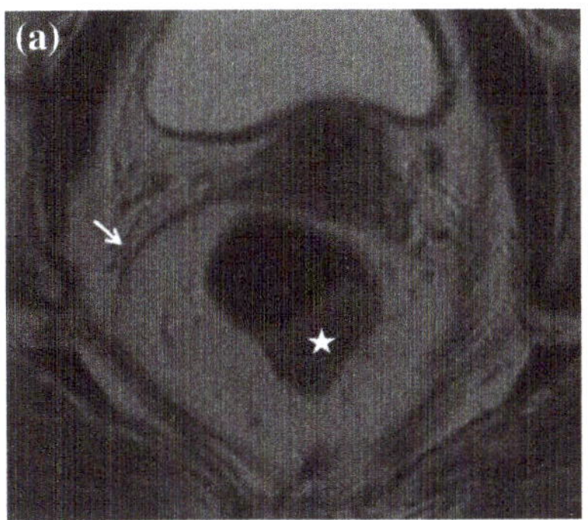

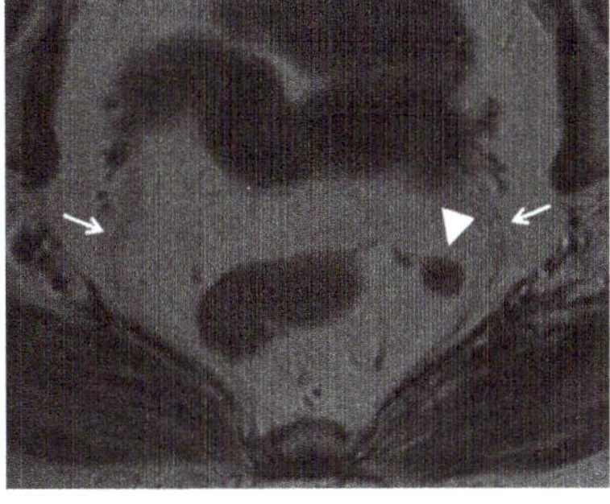

Fig. 63.3 T2-weighted axial rectal MRI in a 58-year-old female showing tumor inside the rectal lumen with minimal extension beyond muscularis propria, in keeping with a stage T3a (*) (**a**). A mesorectal lymph node is noted cranially (**b**) which contains heterogeneous intermediate signal intensity and has irregular borders (*arrowhead*) indicating features of malignancy. MF (*arrows*), however, is not threatened by tumor or involved lymph node

63.2.2 Involved CRM

MRI has so far been proven to be the most precise imaging modality for depiction and prediction of MF invasion and for measurement of the distance from the tumor [15]. The level two evidence has been given by a European multicenter study, the MERCURY study, in which MRI was proven to be 88 % accurate for prediction of an involved CRM with a sensitivity of 59 %, specificity of 92 %, PPV of 54 %, and NPV of 94 % [2]. The CRM is at risk not only from direct tumor spread but also metastatic deposits in lymph nodes that lie close to or against the MF, and through extension along lymphatics, blood vessels, and nerves. If the CRM is involved by tumor then the mode of involvement should be stated (e.g., primary spread, lymph node, tumor deposit, vascular, lymphatic, or perineural), as well as the minimum distance between the closest tumor site and the MF (Fig. 63.1).

63.2.3 Nodal Disease

According to the TNM staging system, N1 corresponds to involvement of 1–3 nodes and N2 to involvement of 4 or more nodes. Lymphatic spread of upper part of rectum is along the superior rectal vessels to the inferior mesenteric vessels while the lower part of the rectum presents with an additional lateral lymphatic spread along the middle rectal vessels to the internal iliac vessels. Early anatomical studies have shown that metastatic lymph nodes are found within 3 cm of primary tumor and can be less than 5 mm in diameter in 15–42 % of the patients. In addition involved nodes are located mostly in the laterodorsal part of the mesorectum, at tumor height or above [16]. Positive nodes distal to the tumor are rare, and occur in patients with more proximal nodal metastases. Positive extramesorectal nodes mainly occur in patients with distal rectal cancer with nodal metastases in the mesorectum. With standard TME lymph nodes within the mesorectum are removed but presence of lymph nodes outside the mesorectum, for example in the hypogastric region and external iliac as well as obturator region have to be reported in order to be included in the radiation portal fields and for the surgeon to remove if considered to be involved. Although high resolution MR images allow identification of lymph nodes with a diameter of 2 mm, reliable detection of nodal metastasis is not possible so far. A meta-analysis has shown [17] that only lymph node specific contrast-enhanced MRI with ultrasmall particles of iron oxide (USPIO) can achieve sensitivities and specificities high enough for clinical decision making for prediction of malignant nodes. However, at the time of writing, USPIO is no longer commercially available.

Lymph node characterization is based on morphologic criteria, such as size, shape, border contour, and signal intensity (Fig. 63.4). When applying them at MRI an 85 % sensitivity and 97 % specificity have been reported [18]. Mesorectal lymph nodes regardless of size present in most of the cases with a homogeneous intermediate T2 weighted signal intensity except in case of mucinous adenocarcinoma in which they are significantly larger in size and present with high signal intensity like the primary tumor (Fig. 63.3). Mixed MR signal intensity within lymph nodes corresponds to tumor deposit.

63.2.4 EMVI

Extramural vascular invasion (EMVI) can frequently be seen as serpiginous extension of tumor signal extending from the muscularis propria into mesorectal fat (Fig. 63.5) and is defined as involvement of a vascular structure. EMVI apart from poor prognostic factor of survival has been acknowledged as an independent predictor of metastatic disease [19]. High resolution MRI has 80 % accuracy of predicting EMVI when compared to histopathology. EMVI is present in 40 % of rectal cancers and MRI-EMVI positive tumor patients have a worse outcome and a 50 % risk of developing metastases compared with

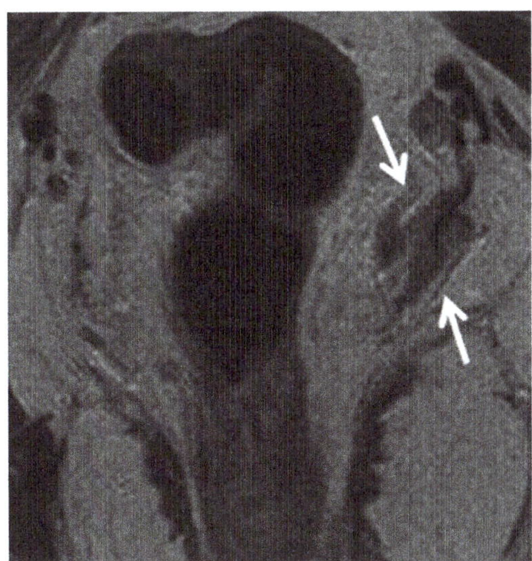

Fig. 63.5 Coronal T2-weighted MRI image shows low lying rectal tumor and nodular intermediate signal intensity tumor tissue extending along into a left perirectal vein within the mesorectal fat (*arrows*) which itself is expanded and irregular in contour, imaging findings suggestive of presence of EMVI

12 % in for EMVI negative patients [19, 20]. This feature is also readily identified on preoperative MRI, and predicts for systemic failure with good concordance between MRI-EMVI and eventual pathology EMVI prognostic outcome, suggesting that patients with macroscopic EMVI have a 30 %, 3 year survival.

63.3 MRI Restaging After Chemoradiation Therapy

LARC patients undergo neoadjuvant chemoradiation therapy (CRT) for their tumor to be downsized and downstaged, especially patients presenting with low rectal cancers so that sphincter sparing surgery may be performed. 50 % of the patients achieve partial response while in 15–30 % of patients complete pathological response is achieved and this has led to the question whether a more conservative surgery can be applied in the good responders or even a wait and see policy in the very selected patients with complete clinical response (yT0) following treatment may be adopted [21]. If this is the case it is imperative to image the patients following completion of neoadjuvant therapy.

Imaging has to take place at least 6 weeks after completion of CRT scheme to allow for tumor shrinkage and recovery from side effects. Huh et al. [22] performed a comparison study between ERUS and computed tomography (CT) regarding restaging of the depth of invasion after neoadjuvant treatment and showed an overall accuracy of 38.3 % for ERUS and 46.3 % for CT. Overstaging was more common than understaging with both imaging modalities, while complete pathology-proved remission was not correctly predicted by any imaging modalities.

Most striking feature of response after neoadjuvant treatment is the development of fibrosis around the tumor area, which has characteristic low T2-weighted signal intensity (Fig. 63.6). Conventional MRI has a reported moderate accuracy for prediction of MF involvement after CRT therapy, mainly due to its inability to differentiate between diffuse fibrosis with/without presence of small tumor foci. Another common change post neoadjuvant treatment is replacement of tumor by mucin pools, which have characteristic high T2 weighted signal intensity.

Morphological MR imaging criteria that correspond to free of disease/involved MF have been reported, as well as criteria indicating disease being confined to the rectal wall (ypT0-T2). Vliegen et al. [23] tried to assess the sensitivity and specificity of MRI after CRT for predicting tumor invasion of the MF and to determine morphologic MR imaging criteria for MF invasion.

Four types of MRI morphologic tissue patterns were associated with whether or not MF invasion was present at histology examination: (a) development of fat pad larger than 2 mm, (b) development or persistence of spiculations, (c) development of diffuse hypointense “fibrotic” tissue, and (d) persistence of diffuse iso- or hyperintense tissue. High resolution MR images combined with radiologists’ rising level of familiarity regarding the assessment of reactive

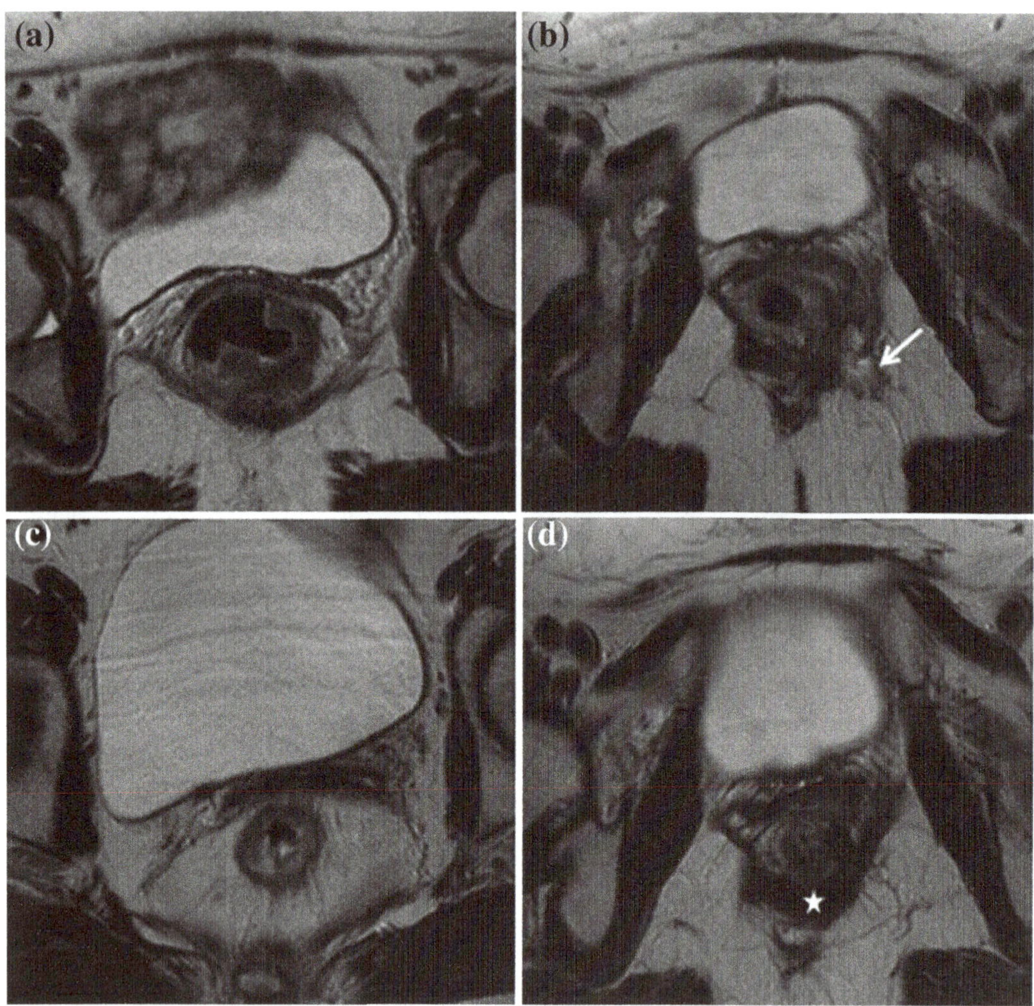

Fig. 63.6 T2-weighted axial rectal MRI of a patient presenting with a semi-annular locally advanced low lying rectal tumor, stage T4 at baseline MRI, with involvement of left sphincteric complex and extension to the left ischiorectal fossa (*arrow*) (**a**, **b**). Patient underwent long scheme of CRT and tumor showed regression, same anatomical levels are demonstrated (**c**, **d**). Downsizing and downstaging was achieved with development of dense fibrotic tissue (*) around the tumor area (**d**)

changes post CRT have increased local staging accuracy of MRI, including both T and N stage reporting.

A modified imaging grading system for CRT response assessment based on percentage of tumor and fibrosis identified respectively on preoperative MRI that has been proposed according to the criteria published by Dworak et al. [24] which are used at histopathology reporting [25]. Introduction of imaging techniques such as Diffusion weighted imaging, especially when combined with morphological T2w sequences for tumor assessment response have shown promising results. Addition of DWI to T2w imaging has been reported to improve prediction of tumor clearance from MF and provide a higher inter-observer agreement [26]. Neoadjuvant chemoradiation treatment results in a decrease in size and number of malignant- and benign-appearing mesorectal nodes on MRI [27] rendering MRI a useful tool for assessing nodal response to neoadjuvant treatment.

63.4 Conclusion

MRI allows for an accurate depiction of high risk for LR rectal cancer patients, as it is an excellent tool for accurate measurement of tumor to MF distance. Nodal involvement remains a difficult radiological diagnosis although nodes as small as 2 mm can be depicted with high resolution MR images. MRI will detect accurately yp T0–T2 stage post-treatment as well as ypN0 patients. However, precise cellular composition of scar, low SI area, in close proximity of MF cannot be assessed by single MRI, but functional MRI sequences, such as DWI show promise for decreasing overstaging and aiding in accurate diagnosis of complete response.

References

1. Bipat S, Glas AS, Slors FJ et al (2004) Rectal cancer: local staging and assessment of lymph node involvement with endoluminal US, CT, and MR imaging-a meta-analysis. Radiology 232(3): 773–783
2. MERCURY Study Group (2006) Diagnostic accuracy of preoperative magnetic resonance imaging in predicting curative resection of rectal cancer: prospective observational study. BMJ 333:779
3. Pahlman L (2000) Neoadjuvant and adjuvant radio- and radio-chemotherapy of rectal carcinomas. Int J Colorectal Dis 15:1–8
4. Wibe A, Rendedal P, Svensson E et al (2002) Prognostic significance of the circumferential resection margin following total mesorectal excision for rectal cancer. BJS 89:327–334
5. Quirke P, Durdey P, Dixon MF et al (1986) Local recurrence of rectal adenocarcinoma due to inadequate surgical resection: histopathological study of lateral tumor spread and surgical excision. Lancet 2:996–999
6. Heald RJ, Ryall RD et al (1986) Recurrence and survival after total mesorectal excision for rectal cancer. Lancet 1:1479–1482
7. Kapiteijn E, Marijnen C, Nagtegaal I et al (2001) Preoperative radiotherapy combined with totalmesorectal excision for resectable rectal cancer. N Engl J Med 345:638–646
8. Beets-Tan RG, Beets GL (2004) Rectal cancer: review with emphasis on MR imaging. Radiology 232(2):335–346
9. Hermanek P, Guggenmoos-Holzmann I, Gall FP (1989) Prognostic factors in rectal carcinoma. A contribution to the further development of tumor classification. Dis Colon Rectum 32(7):593–599
10. Gunderson LL, Sargent DJ, Tepper JE et al (2004) Impact of T and N stage and treatment on survival and relapse in adjuvant rectal cancer: a pooled analysis. J Clin Oncol 22(10): 1785–1796
11. Lindmark G, Gerdin B, Påhlman L et al (1994) Prognostic predictors in colorectal cancer. Dis Colon Rectum 37(12):1219–1227
12. Cawthorn SJ, Parums DV, Gibbs NM et al (1990) Extent of mesorectal spread and involvement of lateral resection margin as prognostic factors after surgery for rectal cancer. Lancet 335(8697): 1055–1059
13. Merkel S, Mansmann U, Siassi M et al (2001) The prognostic inhomogeneity in pT3 rectal carcinomas. Int J Colorectal Dis 16(5):298–304
14. Shepherd NA, Baxter KJ, Love SB (1997) The prognostic importance of peritoneal involvement in colonic cancer: a prospective evaluation. Gastroenterology 112(4):1096–1102
15. Beets-Tan RG, Beets GL, Vliegen RF et al (2001) Accuracy of magnetic resonance imaging in prediction of tumor free resection margin in rectal cancer surgery. Lancet 357(9255):497–504
16. Engelen SM, Beets-Tan RG, Lahaye MJ et al (2008) Location of involved mesorectal and extramesorectal lymph nodes in patients with primary rectal cancer: preoperative assessment with MR imaging. Eur J Surg Oncol 34(7):776–781
17. Will O, Purkayasthas S, Chan C et al (2005) Diagnostic precision of nanoparticle–enhanced MRI for lymph-node metastases: a meta-analysis. Lancet Oncol 7:52–60
18. Brown G, Richards CJ, Bourne MW et al (2003) Morphologic predictors of lymph node status in rectal cancer with use of high-spatial-resolution MR imaging with histopathologic comparison. Radiology 227(2):371–377
19. Brown G (2008) Staging rectal cancer: endoscopic ultrasound and pelvic MRI. cancer imag; 4(8 SupplA):S43–A45
20. Smith NJ, Barbachano Y, Norman AR et al (2008) Prognostic significance of magnetic resonance imaging-detected extramural vascular invasion in rectal cancer. Br J Surg 95(2):229–236
21. Habr-Gama A (2006) Assessment and management of the complete clinical response of rectal cancer to chemoradiotherapy. Colorectal Dis 8(Suppl 3):21–24
22. Huh JW, Park YA, Jung EJ et al (2008) Accuracy of endorectal ultrasonography and computed tomography for restaging rectal cancer after preoperative chemoradiation. J Am Coll Surg 207(1):7–12
23. Vliegen RF, Beets GL, Lammering G et al (2008) Mesorectal fascia invasion after neoadjuvant chemotherapy and radiation therapy for locally advanced rectal cancer: accuracy of MR imaging for prediction. Radiology 246(2):454–462

24. Dworak O, Keilholz L, Hoffmann A (1997) Pathological features of rectal cancer after preoperative radiochemotherapy. Int J Colorectal Dis 12(1):19–23
25. Taylor FG, Swift RI, Blomqvist L et al (2008) A systematic approach to the interpretation of preoperative staging MRI for rectal cancer. AJR 191(6):1827–1835
26. Park MJ, Kim SH, Lee SJ et al (2011) Locally advanced rectal cancer: added value of diffusion-weighted MR imaging for predicting tumor clearance of the mesorectal fascia after neoadjuvant chemotherapy and radiation therapy. Radiology 260(3):771–780
27. Koh DM, Chau I, Tait D et al (2008) Evaluating mesorectal lymph nodes in rectal cancer before and after neoadjuvant chemoradiation using thin-section T2-weighted magnetic resonance imaging. Int J Radiat Oncol Biol Phys 71(2):456–461

64 PET-CT Staging of Rectal Carcinoma

Maria G. Skilakaki

64.1 Introduction

Rectal cancer is one of the most frequent causes of cancer related mortality in Western countries. The expectation of cure strongly depends on the local extent of initial tumor, infiltration of lymph nodes, and presence of distant metastatic disease. Accurate initial staging, early recognition of recurrence, and assessment of residual masses after treatment are mandatory for optimal management of patients with rectal cancer. Fusion imaging with combined Positron emission tomography (PET) and Computed tomography (CT) has been introduced in clinical practice since 2001. The glucose analogue, 18F-fluorodeoxyglucose (18F FDG), due to its ability to accumulate in highly metabolic lesions, is the most widely used radiotracer for PET tumor imaging. As a noninvasive whole-body imaging modality able to provide metabolic and anatomic information, 18F FDG-PET/CT has been extensively used in the evaluation of patients with rectal carcinoma [1].

64.2 Diagnosis and Initial Staging

Although rectal tumors (with the exception of mucinous adenocarcinomas) are FDG avid, PET/CT is not generally recommended for the initial diagnosis and staging of rectal cancer because it has a low sensitivity for locoregional staging due to its limited spatial resolution combined with the intense FDG uptake by the primary tumor and its inability to detect microscopic lymph nodal disease. However, several studies in the literature that have investigated the specific impact of PET/CT on management of patients with locally advanced and low rectal tumors reported a change in management in 12–27 % of cases. This is mainly due to more accurate tumor volume delineation for preoperative radiation treatment planning, discrimination of responders from nonresponders to chemoradiotherapy, and detection of abnormal metabolic activity in inguinal lymph nodes, a common place of metastasis in patients with low rectal cancer (Fig. 64.1).

Moreover, an intense FDG uptake before therapy seems to be bad prognostic factor related to reduced overall survival. It is therefore currently widely acceptable the use of FDG-PET/CT in the initial staging of patients with locally advanced rectal carcinomas who will receive chemoradiation preoperatively [2–4].

M. G. Skilakaki (✉)
Evangelismos General Hospital, 45–47 Ipsilantou street, 10676, Athens, Greece
e-mail: skmaria@otenet.gr

A. D. Gouliamos et al. (eds.), *Imaging in Clinical Oncology*,
DOI: 10.1007/978-88-470-5385-4_64, © Springer-Verlag Italia 2014

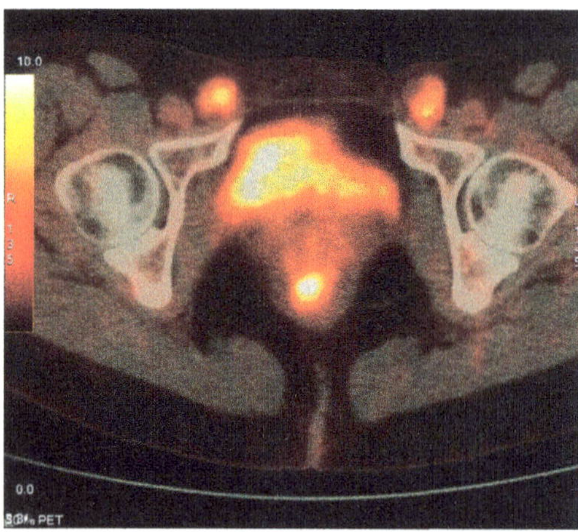

Fig. 64.1 58-year-old male with low rectal cancer. Axial fused PET/CT at the level of the pelvis shows abnormal metabolic activity in the primary tumor and in inguinal lymph nodes

64.3 Detection and Staging of Recurrent Disease

Locoregional recurrence and hepatic metastatic disease are the most common sites of relapse in patients with rectal carcinoma and usually occur in the first two years after resection of the primary tumor. Early diagnosis of local recurrence at the level of the anastomosis and identification of liver metastases are very important for patient care because surgery is the only curable option. One of the most challenging matters in post-therapy patients with locally advanced primary tumors is differentiation of surgical scarring and radiation fibrosis from viable tumor. PET/CT performed 3–6 months after radiotherapy is able to diagnose tumor recurrence by detecting abnormal metabolic activity in the presacral surgical bed and has been noted to have a sensitivity of 84–100 %, specificity of 80–100 %, positive predictive value of 76–88 %, and negative predictive value of 92–100 %. Thus, on this aspect PET/CT is superior to multi-detector CT and MRI [3, 5–7] (Fig. 64.2). Moreover, FDG-PET/CT with its whole-body imaging capabilities has a significantly higher sensitivity (92 %) for detection of extra-hepatic metastatic disease than does CT or MRI and can play a crucial role on determining whether patients are suitable candidates for curative surgery. It seems that incorporation of PET/CT into the preoperative investigation of patients with recurrent disease and potential resectable local or hepatic lesions leads to reduced morbidity due to futile surgery and probably also to a considerable cost saving [5, 6, 8].

Another situation in which PET/CT is very helpful is the evaluation of patients with progressively elevated carcinoembryonic antigen (CEA) and no identifiable lesions on conventional imaging modalities (Fig. 64.3). In this patient population FDG-PET and PET/CT have reported sensitivity, specificity, positive and negative predictive values for detection of recurrence 79–100, 50–83, 89–95 and 85–100 %, respectively, [6–8].

64.4 Monitoring Treatment Response and Planning of Radiation Therapy

Traditionally, cancer response to therapy is based on comparison of tumor sizes visualized on conventional imaging modalities (most commonly CT) before and after treatment. According to response evaluation criteria in solid tumors (RECIST) a tumor is considered responding when there is at least a 30 % decrease of its largest diameter. Although the RECIST criteria are widely accepted in current clinical practice, there is a weak correlation between changes in tumor size and patient outcome. Moreover, biologic response to therapy may precede morphologic changes and residual masses may lack any malignant activity. Several recent studies show that the combined functional and anatomical information provided by FDG-PET/CT seem to be very helpful in monitoring therapeutic activity [1, 5, 6].

Preoperative chemoradiotherapy in locally advanced rectal tumors has been noted to downstage the disease and allow sphincter preserving surgery in selected cases. Furthermore, it has been reported to increase the rate of complete surgical resection and reduce the risk of local recurrence,

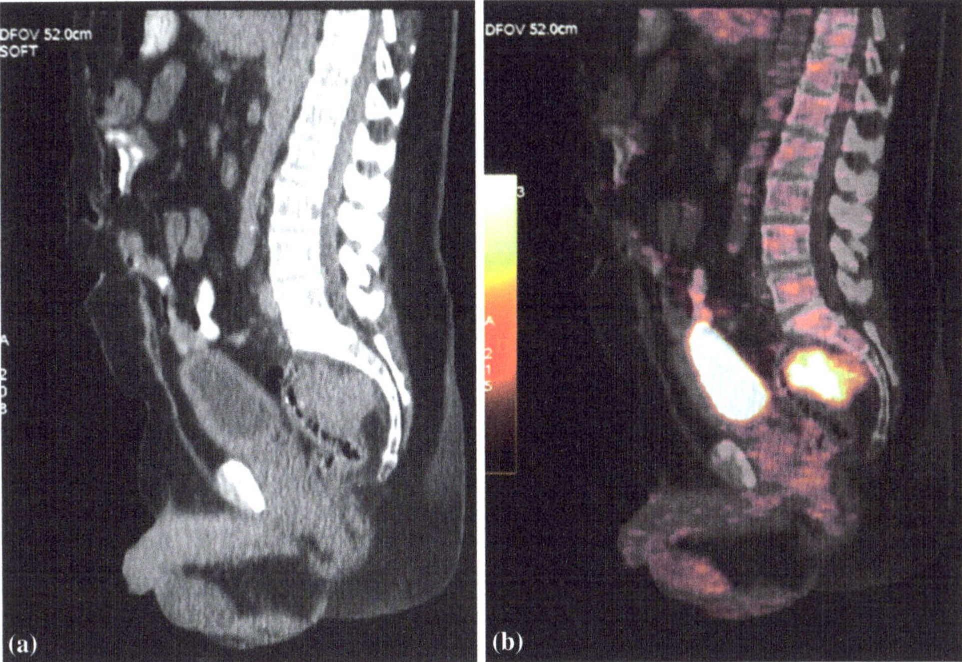

Fig. 64.2 **a**, **b** 62-year-old patient with rectal carcinoma, status post surgery, and chemoradiotherapy. Sagittal CT and fused PET/CT images reveal increased FDG uptake in a presacral mass representing local recurrence

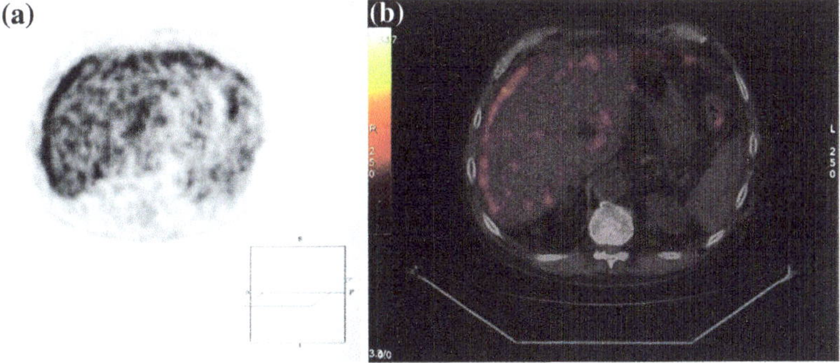

Fig. 64.3 **a**, **b** 68-year-old-man status post-treatment for rectal cancer presenting with rising CEA serum levels and negative results on CT imaging. Axial PET and corresponding fused PET/CT image of the abdomen show diffuse infiltration of the anterolateral peritoneum

compared with postoperative treatment [1, 6, 9, 10]. Discrimination of responders from nonresponders with FDG-PET/CT has based on reduction in post-treatment tumor standardized uptake value (SUV), a semiquantitative estimation of FDG activity within a selected lesion. However, there is a substantial variability among different studies in selecting optimal time for imaging and defining a minimum post-therapeutic SUV reduction indicative of response. In addition, hypermetabolic inflammatory changes, that may be present after radiation therapy, can cause issues with image interpretation and limit the accuracy of FDG-PET/CT in assessing tumor response [3]. Thus, the role of FDG-PET/CT imaging for monitoring neoadjuvant therapy response in patients with rectal cancer has not been yet fully investigated.

Another field, in which FDG-PET/CT can provide additional information, is the early detection of residual tumor after local ablation of liver metastases. Identification of increased focal metabolic activity in the area of a treated lesion is considered as persistent disease. The reported negative predictive value of PET/CT scans performed at 1–4 weeks and at 3–11 months after the ablative procedure is 100 %, whereas the positive predictive value ranges from 80 to 88 % [3, 6].

Finally, limited data in the literature support the use of FDG-PET/CT in radiotherapy planning for rectal cancer. PET/CT is reported to provide useful information for identification of more aggressive tumor subvolumes that should receive higher doses of radiation leading to accurate delineation of tumor volume, more effective local tumor control, and decreased toxicity [4].

64.5 Conclusions

FDG-PET/CT can be reliably used in the evaluation of patients with rectal carcinoma, particularly for the assessment of residual presacral masses after treatment, the localization and staging of recurrent disease before surgery, and the investigation of cases with progressive elevation of serum CEA and negative findings on conventional imaging techniques. Preliminary data reveal a potential role of PET/CT in the evaluation of response to chemoradiotherapy and planning of radiation therapy.

References

1. De Geus-Oei LF, Vriens D, van Laarhoven HWM et al (2009) Monitoring and predicting response to therapy with 18F-FDG PET in colorectal cancer: a systematic review. J Nucl Med 50:43S–54S
2. Lonneux M (2008) FDG-PET and PET/CT in colorectal cancer. PET Clin 3:147–153
3. O'Connor OJ, McDermott S, Slattery J et al (2011) The use of PET-CT in the assessment of patients with colorectal carcinoma. Intern J Surg Oncol, p 14, Article ID 846512
4. Patel DA, Chang ST, Goodman KA et al (2007) Impact of integrated PET/CT on variability of target volume delineation in rectal cancer. Technol Cancer Res Treat 6(1):31–36
5. Hebertson RA, Lee ST, Tebbutt N et al (2007) The expanding role of PET technology in the management of patients with colorectal cancer. Ann Oncol 18:1774–1781
6. De Geus-Oei LF, Ruers TJM, Punt CJA et al (2006) FDG-PET in colorectal cancer. Cancer Imaging 6:S71–S81
7. Delbeke D, Martin WH (2011) FDG PET and PET/CT for colorectal cancer. Methods Mol Biol 727:77–103
8. Mosley CK, Schuster DM (2007) Practical PET/CT of the abdomen. In: Wani RL (ed) RSNA categorical course in diagnostic radiology—clinical PET and PET/CT imaging, pp 71–81
9. Guerra L, Niespolo R, Di Pisa G et al (2011) Change in glucose metabolism measured by 18F-FDG PET/CT as a predictor of histopathologic response to neoadjuvant treatment in rectal cancer. Abdom Imaging 36:38–45
10. Cascini GL, Avallone A, Delrio P et al (2006) 18F-FDG PET is an early predictor of pathologic tumor response to preoperative radiochemotherapy in locally advanced rectal cancer. J Nucl Med 47:1241–1248

65 Clinical Implications of Large Bowel Carcinoma

Paris A. Kosmidis and Christos A. Pissiotis

65.1 Screening

The colorectal cancer is a slow growing process which makes prevention very effective. The preference for the immunochemical fecal occult blood test over the classical hemoccult based on recent studies is a fact [1]. Barium enema was the usual screening imaging test in the past. However, its usage has been declined mainly due to the published study in which only 39 % of polyps found at colonoscopy, were detected by this imaging technique [2]. CT colonography (virtual colonoscopy) has a sensitivity of 90 % for polyps larger than 9 mm. However, there is a controversy over the potential radiation risk of this method. Certainly, it can be preferred for older high risk individuals [3].

P. A. Kosmidis
Department of 2nd Medical Oncology, Hygeia Hospital, 4, Er. Stavrou & Vas Sofias Ave, 15123, Marousi, Athens, Greece
e-mail: parkosmi@otenet.gr

C. A. Pissiotis (✉)
Department of Surgery, Hygeia Hospital, 4, Er. Stavrou & Vas Sofias Ave, 15123, Marousi, Athens, Greece
e-mail: c.pissiotis@hygeia.gr

65.2 Diagnosis and Staging

Colonoscopy with biopsy is the most often used method for diagnosis. Cross-sectional imaging follows colonoscopy for staging purposes in an effort to detect metastatic disease. CT and MRI are not recommended for detection of the colonic primary lesion, however, as always used for identification of extracolonic pelvic disease and/or metastatic lesions throught the body. A key point for staging is the liver lesion. NCCN guidelines indicate contrast-enhanced CT or MRI [4]. Detection of smaller lesions and those in liver with fat infiltration may be difficult. In such cases, MRI is more sensitive [5]. Newer techniques like DW-MRI may be proven more helpful in the near future. In these small liver lesions, PET Scan is not useful due to low resolution. However, PET-CT scan is extremely useful for whole-body imaging especially in restaging where lung or liver metastasectomy is the preferred mode of treatment.

Specifically for rectal cancer, staging is of major importance for treatment planning. Endorectal ultrasound (ERUS) and MRI visualize the extenth of the tumor as well as the circumferential resection margin which is significant for total mesorectal excision. As a matter of fact MRI has an advantage over ERUS in this visualization. MRI is almost equivalent to histopathology for identification of this margin [6]. Regarding T and N stage, MRI and ERUS have similar accuracy [7]. Restaging of rectal cancer following treatment with chemoradiotherapy is

A. D. Gouliamos et al. (eds.), *Imaging in Clinical Oncology*,
DOI: 10.1007/978-88-470-5385-4_65, © Springer-Verlag Italia 2014

difficult and probably inaccurate due to local edema and fibrosis. ERUS has a 35 % positive predictive value for residual cancer [8] whereas MRI has 43 % accuracy [9] and PET is limited. It is also difficult to identify by imaging a 25 % of patients who achieve a pathological complete response, and therefore omit surgery [10]. However, the identification of decreasing tumor is extremely important because these patients may preserve their sphincter. There are indications that decreasing the mass my >75 %, as it is shown by MRI, is a prediction of preserving the sphincter. Similar, a reduction of the volume of the mass by 45 % is an independent prognostic factor for longer disease-free and overall survival [11, 12].

65.2.1 Evaluation of Treatment Response

Assessing the response to any treatment in hepatic and extra-hepatic metastatic lesions is critical for decision-making process. Systemic and occasionally local treatment of initially nonresectable lesions are often very effective and this leads to resection with prolonged survival. Typically, this response is detected by imaging technique with decrease in the size and enhancement of the heterogenous or ring enhanced lesions. MRI has more sensitivity for lesions less than 1 cm due to superior soft tissue contrast. Therefore, MRI is the preferred modality compared to CT [13]. It is interesting to mention that certain local therapies may initialy induce increase the size of the lesions, although these lesions are responding. There are new criteria which assess the response of the remaining tumor using morphological and functional imaging. PET-CT and enhancing residual volume by MRI are preferred in this setting [14]. This field is rapidly changing and new studies are awaited.

PET-CT scan as a routine test at baseline staging is not recommended. During restaging in patients who are candidates for liver metastasectomy PET-CT play an important role for identification of those with extra-hepatic disease. The percentage of these patients is 27 % and their treatment is changed [15]. Regarding response evaluation by PET-CT, no definitive conclusion has been made. The early metabolic and functional changes induced by the treatment and especially by the new molecular agents can be captured by the PET. However, the changes in the size and the glycolysis induced by the treatment are at the present time responsible for the inaccurate evaluation of response by the PET [16]. PET-CT is also useful in those patients with an unexplained elevation of CEA.

65.3 Surveillance

The ideal surveillance strategy for colorectal cancer has not been defined. NCCN guidelines recommend CT scans of upper and lower abdomen as well as chest every year for 5 years [4]. Colonoscopy is recommended one year following surgery and then at 3 years and then every 5 years. Certainly, large studies will define exactly the optimal surveillance strategy.

References

1. Smith A, Young GP, Cole SR et al (2006) Comparison of a brush-sampling fecal immunochemical test for hemoglobin with a geniac-based fecal occult blood test in detection of colorectal neoplasia. Cancer 107:2152–2159
2. Ninawer SJ, Stewart ET, Zamber AG et al (2000) A comparison of colonoscopy and double-contrast barium enema for surveillance after polypectomy. National polyp study work group. N Engl J Med 342:1766–1772
3. McHigh M, Osei-Anto A, Klabunde CN et al (2011) Adoption of CT colonography by US hospitals. J Am Coll Radiol 8:169–174
4. National Comprehensive Cancer Network (NCCN) (2012) NCCN clinical practice guidelines in oncology. Colon cancer, Version 3, 2012. Accessed April 23
5. Khalil HI, Patterson SA, Panicek DM (2005) Hepatic lesions deemed too small to characterize at CT: prevalence and importance in women with breast cancer. Radiology 235:872–878
6. Phang PT, Gollup MJ, Loh BD et al (2012) Accuracy of endorectal ultrasound for measurement of the closest predicted radial mesorectal margins for rectal cancer. Dis Colon Rectum 55:59–64

7. Lahaye MJ, Engelen SM, Nelemans PJ et al (2005) Imaging for predicting the risk factors—the circumferential resection margin and nodal disease—of—local recurrence in rectal cancer: a meta-analysis. Semin Ultrasound CT-MRI 26:259–268
8. Maretto I, Pomerri F, Pucciarelli S et al (2007) The potential of restaging in the prediction of pathologic response after preoperative chemoradiotherapy for rectal cancer. Ann Surg Oncol 14:455–461
9. Suppiah A, Maslekar S, Alabi A et al (2008) Transanal endoscopic microsurgery in early rectal cancer time for a trial? Colorectal Dis 10:314–327
10. Mehta VK, Cho C, Ford JM et al (2003) Phase II trial of preoperative 3D conformal radiotherapy, protracted venous infusion 5-fluorouracil and weekly CPT-11 followed by surgery for ultrasound-staged T3 rectal cancer. Int J Radiat Oncol Biol Phys 55:132–137
11. Yeo SG, Kim DY, Park JW et al (2012) Tumor volume reduction rate after preoperative chemoradiotherapy as a prognostic factor in locally advanced rectal cancer. Int J Radiat Oncol Biol Phys 82:e193–e199
12. Barbaro B, Fiorucci C, Tebala C et al (2009) Locally advanced rectal cancer: MR imaging in prediction of response after preoperative chemotherapy and radiation therapy. Radiiology 250:730–739
13. Floriani I, Torri V, Rulli E et al (2010) Performance of imaging modalities in diagnosis of liver metastases from colorectal cancer: a systematic review and metaanalysis. J Magn Reson Imaging 31:19–31
14. Kuehl H, Antoch G, Stergar H et al (2008) Comparison of FDG-PET, PET-CT and MRI for follow-up of colorectal liver metastases treated with radiofrequency ablation: initial results. Eur J Radiol 67:362–371
15. Park IJ, Kim HC, Yu CS et al (2006) Efficacy of PET/CY in the accurate evaluation of primary colorectal carcinoma. Eur J Surg Oncol 32:941–947
16. Lin M, Wong K, Ng WL et al (2011) Positron emission tomography and colorectal cancer. Crit Rev Oncol Hematol 77:30–47

Part X
Neuroendocrine Tumors

Introduction to Neuroendocrine Tumors

66

George C. Nikou

Neuroendocrine cells are characterized by the production of a neurotransmitter, neuromodulator, or neuropeptide hormone, the presence of dense-core secretory granules from which the hormones are released by exocytosis in response to external stimulus and also, the absence of axons and synapses. They are derived from the diffuse endocrine system and can be found in the gastrointestinal and respiratory tract, in pancreas, pituitary gland, epiphysis, thyroid (C cells), parathyroid gland, adrenal gland (medulla), and paraganglia. Skin (Merkel cells), thymus, kidneys, ovary, prostate gland, and testis also contain these cells.

Neuroendocrine tumors (NETs) represent a very heterogeneous group of neoplasms arising from these specific cells and, comprise approximately 2 % of all malignant tumors of gastroenteropancreatic system [1]. Although they are characterized by a relatively slow tumor growth, they have a malignant potential and, in fact, most of them are diagnosed when liver metastases have been developed. Additionally, these tumors may be sporadic or may occur as part of the Multiple Endocrine Neoplasia I (MEN-1) syndrome, Von Hippel–Lindau (VHL) syndrome, neurofibromatosis (NF-1), or tuberous sclerosis.

Gastoenteropancreatic neuroendocrine tumors (GEP-NETs) include those of the gastrointestinal tract (GI-NETs), classically known as "carcinoids", and also the pancreatic neuroendocrine tumors (pNETs) , formerly known as "islet cell tumors". Although the term "carcinoid" is no longer acceptable to pathologists, most clinicians still find it of practical use, in describing NETs of the GI tract and the "carcinoid syndrome".

Carcinoid tumors are derived predominantly from enterochromaffin or Kultchisky cells. They have been found in almost every organ of the human body, but are traditionally subdivided according to their embryological origin into foregut carcinoids (bronchus, stomach, pancreas), midgut (small bowel, appendix and caecum), and hindgut carcinoids (colon, rectum).

pNETs are derived from the endocrine cells of the pancreatic islet of Langerhans and may be functioning or nonfunctioning. Functioning tumors are associated with a clinical syndrome which is caused by hormone release, and are named according to the hormone that they secrete, whereas nonfunctioning, include those that have all the histological characteristics of such a tumor, but no specific clinical syndrome related to hormone hypersecretion [2].

pNETs may be functioning or nonfunctioning. In the former group, the predominant symptoms are those of the hormonal hypersecretion. These tumors get their name from the predominant peptide that they secrete. The most common

G. C. Nikou (✉)
Section of Gastrointestinal Neuroendocrinology,
1st Department of Propaedeutic Internal Medicine,
Laikon Hospital, Medical School of Athens
University, 68, Plateon Street,
15235 Vrilissia-Athens, Greece
e-mail: gcnikou@yahoo.gr

A. D. Gouliamos et al. (eds.), *Imaging in Clinical Oncology*,
DOI: 10.1007/978-88-470-5385-4_66, © Springer-Verlag Italia 2014

ones include gastrinomas, insulinomas, VIPomas, glucagonomas, somatostatinomas, growth-hormone releasing factor secreting tumors (GRFomas), and ACTH secreting tumors of the pancreas (ACTHomas). In nonfunctioning tumors symptoms are due to the tumor itself. These tumors often produce hormones, but remain clinically silent for the following reasons: (a) the hormones produced may not develop a known specific clinical syndrome (PPomas), (b) the tumor may produce a known peptide, but fails to release it, or (c) the tumor produces biologically inactive precursor forms of hormones. Other rarer pNETs have recently been considered as causing syndromes, including pNETs causing hypercalcemia (producing parathormone and parathormone-related protein), pNETs secreting calcitonin, and pNETs with histopathological characteristics of GI carcinoids .

Although GEP-NETs are rare entities, it is thought that recently, these tumors have had an increase in their reported incidence. Earlier studies had found an incidence of 0.8–2.1 cases per 100,000 per year, while recent data estimate their incidence approaching 3 per 100,000 (some studies even higher), with a continuing slight predominance in women. This may be due to increased awareness of the clinicians and improvement of diagnostic studies. Autopsy series have found an incidence of 8.4 cases of gastrointestinal carcinoids per 100,000 people.

Carcinoid tumors represent more than 50 % of all neuroendocrine tumors of the gastroenteropancreatic system and they occur most frequently in the small intestine (25 %), appendix (14 %), and rectum (12 %). Nonfunctioning tumors comprise the 30–40 % of the whole group of pNETs, while among the functioning pNETs, insulinoma is the most common (17 %), followed by gastrinoma (15 %) [3].

The histopathological examination of neuroendocrine tumors aims at classifying the tumors according to their tissue origin, biochemical behavior, and prognosis. The histological diagnosis of these tumors relies first on the identification of general markers of neuroendocrine differentiation, and then on cell-specific characterization. Neuroendocrine differentiation is evaluated by immunohistochemistry, using antibodies against secretory granule proteins (chromogranin-A, synaptophysin) and cytosolic proteins (neuron-specific enolase, protein gene product 9.5). The cell-specific characterization of neuroendocrine tumors requires hormone immunohistochemistry.

According to the recently revised classification of the World Health Organization (WHO), the following types of GEP-NETs have been recognized: (1) well-differentiated neuroendocrine tumors and (2) poorly differentiated neuendocrine carcinomas (small or large cell type) [4]. Criteria for categorization of these tumors include general morphologic description, mitotic rate (2 or more mitoses/mm^2), proliferative index (as assessed by nuclear Ki67 expression), tumor size, and evidence of invasion of blood vessels/nerves/adjacent organs. Most NETs are well-differentiated tumors (those of the gastrointestinal tract were formerly called "carcinoids" by the pathologists) with absent or low cytological atypia, and a low-mitotic (<2 mitoses/mm^2) and proliferation index (<2 % Ki67 positive cells). Poorly differentiated NET carcinomas (formerly called "atypical carcinoids") exhibit a high-grade malignant behavior with cellular atypia, high mitotic index (>10 mitoses/mm^2), and >20 % Ki67 positive cells. These tumors do not express chromogranin-A, but retain cytosolic markers together with synaptophysin.

A number of genetic syndromes including Multiple Endocrine Neoplasia syndrome type-1 (MEN-1), von Hippel–Lindau syndrome (VHL), neurofibromatosis type-1 (NF1), and tuberous sclerosis may be associated with GEP-NETs. In the normal cells, the genes associated with these disorders play a role in tumor suppression, while aberrations in these regulatory genes can lead to the development of neoplasms, including NETs.

MEN-1 syndrome is an autosomal dominant inherited disorder, associated mainly with primary hyperparathyroidism (>95 %), neuroendocrine pancreatic tumors (50–75 %), and pituitary tumors (20–40 %). Apart from those three classical manifestations of the syndrome, several other endocrinopathies are overrepresented in carriers of the MEN-1 gene, including different types of adrenocortical proliferation (hyperplasia, adenoma, and rarely carcinoma), NETs of thymus, lung and stomach, and also lipomas and ependymomas.

The MEN-1 gene is located at chromosome 11q13 (Menin gene) and is a suppressor gene. Genetic mapping studies show somatic loss of heterozygosity (LOH) suggesting the two-hit hypothesis. Initially, a germline mutation affect the MEN-1 gene, making the carrier of the inherited defective gene heterozygous and predisposed to tumor development (first hit), and then a somatic inactivation of the unaffected allele by LOH occurs (second hit).

The diagnosis of MEN-1 requires the presence of at least two of the three classical lesions. Hyperparathyroidism (HPT) is the initial manifestation of MEN-1, usually presenting in the third decade of life, followed by the development of an pNET between the ages of 35 and 50 years. Overall, approximately 10 % of pNETs are associated with MEN-1. However, nonfunctioning pNETs (20–30 %) and gastrinomas (25 %) have a strong association, whereas it is rare for insulinomas (<5 %) to be associated with MEN-1. Early recognition of MEN-1 syndrome is an important first step in the management of pNETs, because patients with and without MEN-1 differ in clinical presentation, management, and also prognosis [5].

A common feature of most GEP-NETs is the high expression of somatostatin receptors, which was proved to be very important for their management [6]. Five somatostatin receptor subtypes (SSTR 1–5) have been cloned and pharmacologically characterized. SSTR-2 is expressed in 90 % of carcinoids and in 80 % of pNETs. An exception is insulin-producing pancreatic tumors, where less than 50 % express the SSTR-2. Other SSTRs may be expressed but to a much lesser extent.

References

1. Warner R (2005) Enteroendocrine tumors other than carcinoid : a review of clinically significant advances. Gastroenterology 128:1668–1684
2. Nikou GC, Marinou K, Thomakos P et al (2008) Chromogranin A levels in diagnosis, treatment and follow-up of 42 patients with non-functioning pancreatic endocrine tumours. Pancreatology 8:510–519
3. Hemminki K, Li X (2001) Incidence trands and risk factors of carcinoid tumors : a nationwide epidemiologic study from Sweden. Cancer 92:2204–2210
4. Rindi G, Arnold R, Bosman FT, Capella C, Klimstra DS, Kloppel G et al (2010) Nomenclature and classification of neuroendocrine neoplasms the digestive system. In: Bosman FT, Carneiro F, Hruban RH, Theise ND (eds): WHO classification of tumours in the digestive system, 4th edn. IARC, Lyon, pp 13–14
5. Toumpanakis CG, Caplin ME (2008) Molecular genetics of gastroenteropancreatic neuroendocrine tumors. Am J Gastroenterol 103(3):729–732
6. Reubi JC (1995) Neuropeptide receptors in health and disease : the molecular basis for in vivo imaging. J Nucl Med 36:1825–1835

67 Neuroendocrine Tumors

Dimitra N. Nikolaou, Dimitrios A. Fotopoulos and Eugenia I. Gialakidi

Neuroendocrine tumor (NET) imaging encompasses a large heterogeneous host of lesions. Thorough knowledge of their characteristics and the clinical implications and underlying associations is mandatory, as they can occur sporadically, or can be associated with various syndromes. The constellation of specific findings could aid in tumor detection and possibly characterization.

Hyperfunctioning tumors are related to the specific symptoms associated with the specific substance they secrete, hence their detection is a targeted process. They usually tend to be detected when they are smaller.

Nonhyperfunctioning tumors are either detected in patients who seek medical advice for nonspecific symptoms related to impingement upon nearby structures by the tumor itself, or are detected completely incidentally. They can be of any size, but usually they tend to be diagnosed at a later stage with relatively larger tumor size. Therefore, careful scrutiny should be exercised so as not to miss incidentally detected tiny lesions that have not yet produced any symptoms, as their nonhyperfunctioning condition does not entail any substance-specific syndrome.

NET's are universally hypervascular structures which enhance rapidly in the early arterial phase of scanning, yet to a lesser extent a tiny minority of them enhances mainly in the portal phase. Multidetector CT has increased detection rate, rendering bowel wall layers visible, something that facilitates tumor detection, especially when located within intestinal wall. Double scanning, both in the arterial phase and the portal phase with thin collimation is strongly advocated [1, 2].

MRI has spatial resolution lower than that of CT, and therefore lags behind in ability to depict as accurately bowel wall stratification, being of limited value in detection of primary gastrointestinal wall tumors. Its role is mainly to detect hepatic metastases and to further characterize lesions in solid organs in equivocal cases (Fig. 67.1).

In the case of suspected hyperfunctioning tumors (where a hypervascular mass is to be specifically spotted) bowel should be filled with nonionic oral contrast material (water, milk) so that enhancing tumor may not be rendered inconspicuous by adjacent dense orally administered material [1].

Hyperfunctioning tumors tend to be homogeneous and solid, whereas with size increase there is an increased probability for development of calcifications, necrosis, and cystic areas. Non-hyperfunctioning tumors are also more

D. N. Nikolaou (✉) · D. A. Fotopoulos · E. I. Gialakidi
Kyanous Stavros Hospital, 102 Vasilissis Sofias, 11528, Athens, Greece
e-mail: dimnik1970@yahoo.gr

D. A. Fotopoulos
e-mail: radiolog@hol.gr

E. I. Gialakidi
e-mail: e.gialakidi@gmail.com

A. D. Gouliamos et al. (eds.), *Imaging in Clinical Oncology*,
DOI: 10.1007/978-88-470-5385-4_67, © Springer-Verlag Italia 2014

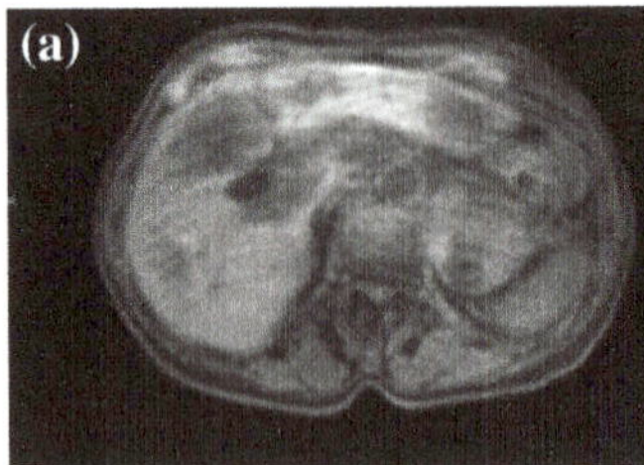

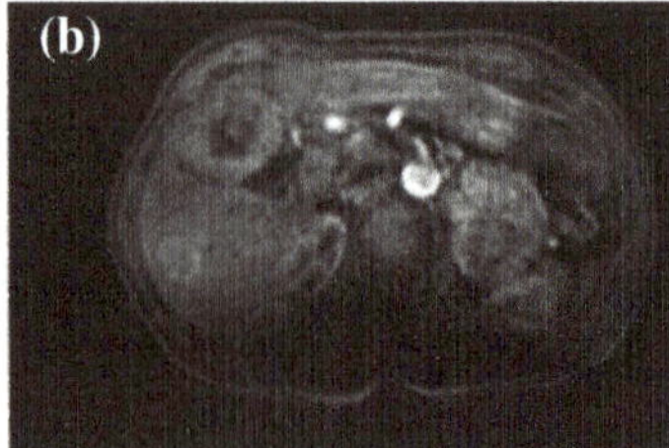

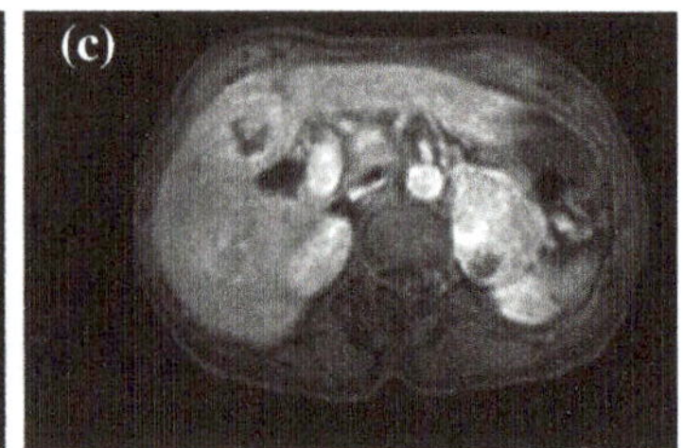

Fig. 67.1 Transaxial T1-weighted MR images (**a**), gadolinium-enhanced axial T1-weighted images arterial (**b**) and portal venous phase (**c**). *Right* lobe lesion rendered significantly less conspicuous in the portal venous phase compared to the arterial phase

frequently homogeneous and solid, but they tend to manifest additional necrosis, calcification, or cystic areas to a greater extent than their hyperfunctioning counterparts.

67.1 Pancreatic Neuroendocrine Tumors

Pancreatic non-hyperfunctioning tumors and insulinomas are located throughout the pancreas without specific predilection for a specific area. Most frequent location of gastrinomas is the pancreatic head. Somatostatinomas and Vipomas are more frequently encountered at the pancreatic tail.

Pancreatic gastrinomas are larger than their duodenal counterparts (3–4 vs. 1 cm on average, respectively), yet duodenal carcinomas are by far more frequent (four times as common) [1]. Therefore, it goes without saying that duodenal gastrinomas could be easily missed, unless the duodenal lumen is adequately distended with negative oral contrast medium. One additional clue that could increase conspicuity of these tumors is specific inspection of the so-called gastrinoma triangle, defined as the area bounded by the common bile duct, second and third part of duodenum and pancreatic head [1].

An indirect sign is thickened gastric folds caused by increased gastrin levels secreted by the tumor. Evidence of MEN 1 syndrome could coexist, as there is documented association with this entity.

In case of cystic neuroendocrine tumors confusion with other entities could arise, so that they might be mistaken for other cystic pancreatic lesions, including intraductal papillary mucinous neoplasm (IPMN), serous and mucinous cystadenomas, and pseudocyst. Nevertheless, there is a specific sign that favors the diagnosis of cystic neuroendocrine tumor, which is an enhancing rim separating the tumor from the adjacent pancreatic parenchyma. This finding is absent from the rest of the tumors listed above (Fig. 67.2).

Adjacent structures could pose diagnostic pitfalls for inadvertent diagnosis of pancreatic neuroendocrine tumor. These are most commonly aneurysms of the hepatic and gastroduodenal artery (near pancreatic head) and splenic artery (near pancreatic tail) [2].

67.2 Specific Features in Favor of p-NETs

Calcification within a pancreatic tumor should favor diagnosis of a neuroendocrine tumor, as calcification within a pancreatic adenocarcinoma coexists only with preexisting chronic pancreatitis (in that case specific signs should be sought for, like pancreatic atrophy, widespread calcification throughout parenchyma, and pancreatic duct dilatation).

A recently described feature of pancreatic neuroendocrine tumors is their tendency to be accompanied by pancreatic duct stenosis with a transition point of upstream dilatation, unaccounted for by tumor proximity or tumor size. This study documented that ductal dilatation was not the result of any mass effects, as even small tumors could elicit the same effect, and therefore

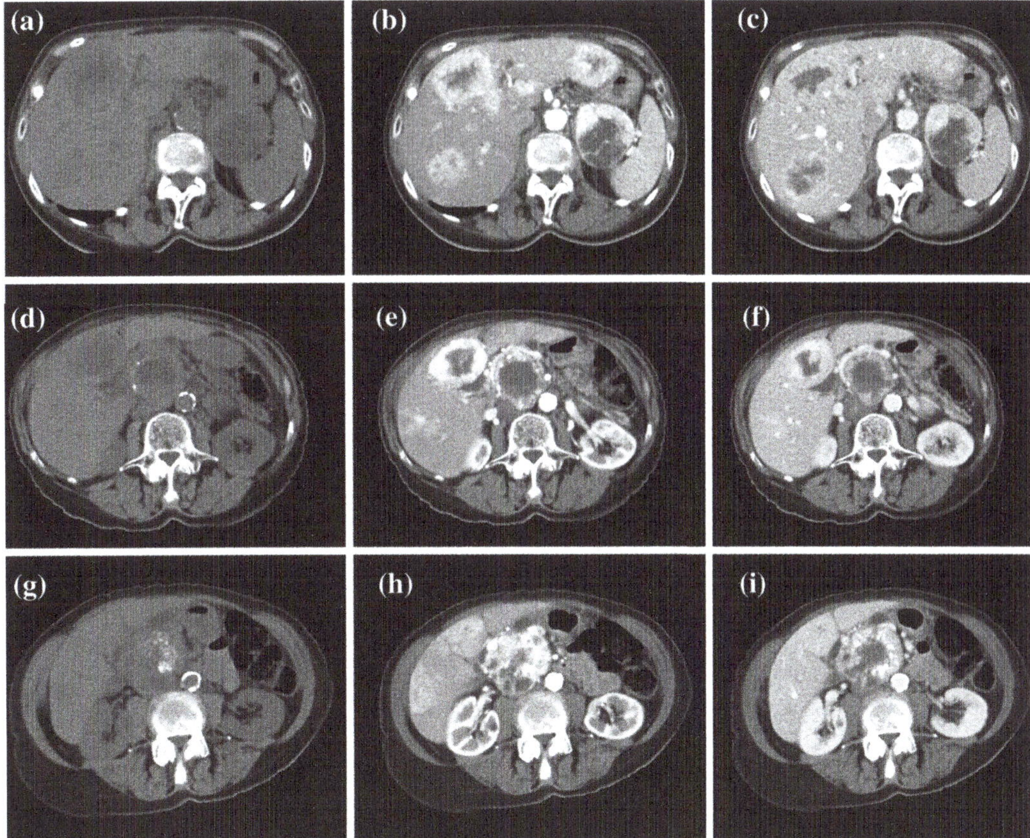

Fig. 67.2 CT images non contrast enhanced (**a**, **d**, **g**), arterial phase (**b**, **e**, **h**), and portal phase (**c**, **f**, **i**). Cystic lesion within head of pancreas. Central area of necrosis (fluid–fluid level with debris). Peripheral calcification and early enhancement (rim sign) is seen. The presence of calcification within lesion favors diagnosis of NET over adenocarcinoma. Rim enhancement favors NET over IPMN. Hepatic adrenal metastases display identical enhancement with primary tumor

the proposed mechanism could rather be fibrotic changes produced by serotonin secreted by the tumor itself. The authors of the same study also suggested that whenever pancreatic ductal dilatation is noted, search should be made for even subtle evidence of enhancing mass that could qualify for pancreatic NET [3].

An important part of the radiology report is the presence of venous invasion, a feature that is common for the nonhyperfunctioning tumors, rarely encountered among the hyperfunctioning tumors, which nevertheless according to a recent study is missed up to two-thirds of cases studied. This could have potential implications upon the surgical technique applied, if not known preoperatively with subsequent inadequate tumor excision regarding the unreported part of venous invasion, which will lead to tumor recurrence. This only holds true for macroscopic invasion as CT cannot detect microscopic venous invasion. Pancreatic adenocarcinomas typically displace adjacent vessels without invasion [4].

67.3 p-NETs Identification Pearls and Pitfalls

Pearls:

- thickened gastric folds (gastrinoma?)
- rim enhancement (discriminator for cystic lesions)
- tumor calcification

- early arterial enhancement (solid part of solid and cystic lesions)
- pancreatic duct dilatation in the absence of mass effects

Pitfalls: to avoid overdiagnosis

- adjacent vascular structures (identical enhancement to vascular structures)
- splenule (identical enhancement to spleen an all phases)
- metastases to the pancreas (front-runner: renal cell carcinoma) [5, 6].

67.4 NETs of the Gastrointestinal Tract (GI-NETs)

When neuroendocrine tumors are located within the gastrointestinal tract they manifest as subepithelial masses that enhance in the early arterial phase. It should be remembered though that detection of an enhancing subepithelial mass within the gastrointestinal wall should encompass a host of other much commoner entities, including gastrointestinal stromal tumors (GIST) and hypervascular metastases [2].

They are unusual in the foregut (hypopharynx and esophagus).

When located in the gastric wall they have been divided into three categories (enterochromaffin cell tumors, or ECLomas), of which types I and II are associated, respectively, with atrophic gastritis and Zollinger–Ellison syndrome, and type III, that carries the worst prognosis, which is not associated with any underlying condition. They can assume configurations similar to primary gastric adenocarcinomas with ulceration and can be solitary tumors or multiple tumors of varying sizes, ranging from small nodules to large masses [7, 8].

Neuroendocrine tumors in the small intestine are commonly accompanied by bowel wall kinking and bowel loop convergence, owing to desmoplastic reaction elicited by vasoactive amines like serotonin secreted by the tumor (Fig. 67.3). The same factor could also involve intestinal wall perfusion due to fibrosis encasing vessels with subsequent evidence of ischemia (manifest as decreased intestinal wall enhancement) [2]. Punctate calcifications are encountered up to 70 %. Their tendency to metastasize increases with tumor growth from 1 to 2 cm more than 80-fold.

Among neuroendocrine tumors of the colon their commonest location is in the rectum, followed by those of the right colon and then by those of the appendix [7]. Appendiceal tumors can also display evidence of calcification and can be indistinguishable from appendicoliths. They can manifest as appendicitis, in which case the accompanying findings are identical to that of appendicolith-induced appendicitis. Sometimes the appearance of tumors located in the cecum assumes a circumferential configuration identical to that of primary adenocarcinoma of the colon. Contribution of Computed Tomography is to stage, not to detect those tumors.

Neuroendocrine tumors of the colon tend to be detected earlier than those of the small intestine, that is to say they are of smaller size (less than 1 cm, as opposed to those of the small intestine, which exceed 2 cm at time of diagnosis), have not traversed the muscularis propria, and consequently have not reached regional lymph nodes [7, 8].

Neuroendocrine tumor metastases have identical appearance with the primary tumors. Metastases of G-NETS tend to be to a greater extent located in the peritoneum and lymph-nodes, as opposed to liver and lung metastases, which tend to be of rather extra-gastrointestinal origin. This assumption could possibly aid in the detection of the primary tumor, as this affects survival [9].

67.5 Nuclear Medicine/Molecular Imaging

γ-camera-SPECT, as well as PET offers functional as well as metabolic imaging. Ideal solution so far is provided by hybrid imaging systems SPECT/CT and PET/CT which combine functional and anatomic information.

The radionuclides most frequently used for detection fall within two categories.

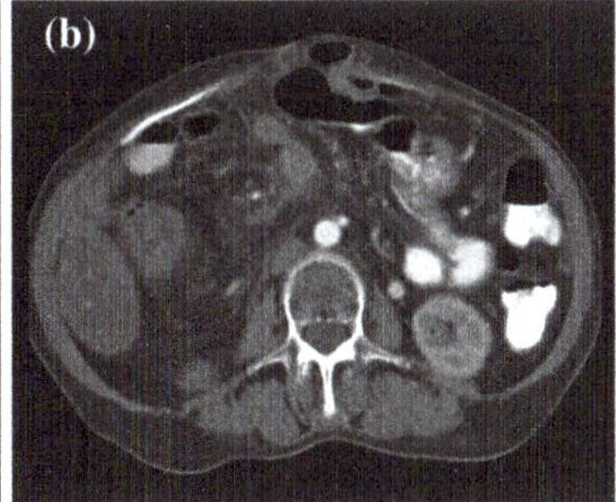

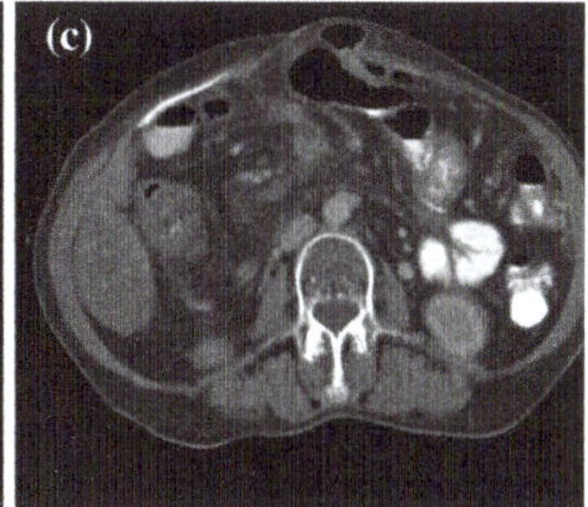

Fig. 67.3 CT images **a** non contrast enhanced, **b** Arterial phase, **c** Portal phase. Metastatic lymph node with sunburst appearance, tethering of surrounding structures is seen

- radionuclides for single photon emission MIBG-metaiodobenzyl guanidine tagged with I-131 or I-123, octreoscan (In-111-pentetreotide/DTPA-D-Pheoctreotide)
- radionuclides for positron emission (PET)
  - F-18-FDG, F-18-fluorodesoxyglucoze
  - F-18/C-11-DOPA, F-18/C-11-dihydroxyfenylalanine
  - F-18-FDA, F-18-fluodopamine
  - C-11-HTP, C-11hydroxytryptophan
  - GA-68 DOTADATE, DOTADOC, or DOTANOC

SPECT imaging

MIBG: I-123—tagged is the preferred radionuclide due to lower energy of I-123 at 159 keV compared to 364 keV of I-131, and also due to absence of β-radiation, shorter imaging time, and better image quality.

I-123-MIBG has high sensitivity and specificity (90 %). It is indicated for detection, localization, staging, and follow-up of neuroendocrine tumors and their metastases, as well as for evaluation of response to treatment. Tumor uptake of I-131 is the prerequisite for possible I-131-MIBG treatment.

Cessation of certain medications is mandatory for 2–3 weeks prior to radionuclide administration (antihypertensives, tricyclic antidepressants, sympathomimetic agents). It is taken up normally at sites of increased sympathetic innervation (heart, liver, spleen, intestine, salivary glands, lungs at 2 h) and is secreted by the kidneys. Normal adrenal medulla visualization is possible, mainly with I-123.

Positive uptake evaluation is made by comparison to background at 24 h and by radionuclide hepatic uptake.

67.6 Octreoscan

Somatostatin receptor scan (Five subtypes of SSTR1-5 receptors)

SSTRs are overexpressed in a large number of neoplasias (neuroendocrine tumors, other tumors), as well as nonneoplastic conditions (e.g., granulomatous). Endogenous somatostatin has a very short half life (T1/2 = 1–2 min), rendered therefore inadequate means for diagnosis and therapy of neuroendocrine tumors, synthetic somatostatin analogs, peptidase-resistant have been created: octreotide, lantreotide, vapreotide).

Tagging is achieved with radionuclides suitable either for γ-camera imaging (Tc-99 m, In-111) or for PET (F-18, C-11, Ga-68).

Endogenous somatostatin has high affinity for all five SSTR subtypes, whereas synthetic analogs manifest variable degree of affinity for each subtype. The somatostatin analog most widely used is In-111-tagged octreotide. It is bound mainly to SSTR subtype 2, to a lesser extent to subtype 5, and even less so to subtype 3. It is mainly indicated for detection and localization of tumors that express SSTRs, detection of metastases, staging, restaging, and follow-up of patients with known disease, and is an indispensable tool for targeted radiotherapy [10].

It is normally distributed at sites where SSTRs exist (mainly 2 and 5) like spleen, liver, pituitary, nasal mucosa, salivary glands, and thyroid. It is secreted by the urinary system and gastrointestinal tract.

Currently, attempts are made for somatostatin analogs tagging with Tc-99 m (Neospect, tektrotyd) owing to high cost of In-111.

(see Chap. 65.1)

PET radionuclides are divided into four categories:

- Glucose metabolism (F-18-FDG)
- Catecholamine carrying and storage (mainly C-11/F-18-L-DOPA)
- Serotonin analogs
- 68-Ga-tagged somatostatin analogs.

18-F FDG contrary to rest of oncology cases is not a radionuclide of choice for the study of well-differentiated, low malignancy neuroendocrine tumors. It plays a complementary role in negative octreoscan study [11].

Of greater help are the Ga-68 tagged somatostatin analogs, which are advantageous over octreoscan for the following reasons:

a. cause less radiation exposure with a more rapid imaging protocol.
b. PET has greater spatial resolution than γ-camera
c. offer greater affinity with β-radiation emitting peptides (tagged with Y-90, Lu-177)and are therefore, more suitable for charting before choice of treatment.

(see Chap. 65.2)

References

1. Horton KM, Hruban RH, Yeo C et al (2006) Multi–detector row CT of pancreatic islet cell tumors. Radiographics 26:453–464
2. Lee NK, Kim S, Kim GH et al (2010) Hypervascular subepithelial gastrointestinal masses: CT-pathologic correlation. Radiographics 30(7):1915–1934
3. Kawamoto S, Shi C, Hruban RH, Choti MA et al (2011) Small serotonin-producing neuroendocrine tumor of the pancreas associated with pancreatic duct obstruction. AJR Am J Roentgenol 197(3): W482–W488
4. Balachandran A, Tamm EP, Bhosale PR et al (2012) Original research:venous tumor thrombus in nonfunctional pancreatic neuroendocrine tumors. AJR 199(3):602–608
5. Palmowski M, Hacke N, Satzl S et al (2008) Metastasis to the pancreas: characterization by morphology and contrast enhancement, features on CT and MRI. Pancreatology 8:199–203
6. Raman SP, Hruban RH, Cameron JL et al (2012) Pancreatic imaging mimics: part 2, pancreatic neuroendocrine tumors and their mimics AJR 199:309–318
7. Chang S, Choi D, Lee SJ et al (2007) Neuroendocrine tumors of the gastrointestinal tract: classification, pathologic basis and imaging features. Radiographics 27(6):1667–1679
8. Scarsbrook AF, Ganeshan A, Statham J, Thakker RV, Weaver A, Talbot D, Boardman P, Bradley KM, Gleeson FV, Phillips RR (2007) Anatomic and functional imaging of metastatic carcinoid tumors. Radiographics 27(2):455–477
9. Bhosale P, Shah A, Wei W et al (2013) Carcinoid tumours: predicting the location of the primary neoplasm based on the sites of metastases. Eur Radiol 23:400–407
10. Niederer M, Seidl S, Buck A et al (2009) Correlation of immunohistopathological expression of somatostatin receptor 2 with standardized uptake values in 68 Ga-DOTATOC PET/CT. Eur J Med Imaging 36:48–52
11. Rufini V, Calcagni ML, Baum RP (2006) Imaging of neuroendocrine tumors. Semin Nucl Med 36(3): 228–247

68 Clinical Implications of Neuroendocrine Tumors

George C. Nikou

A particular feature of carcinoids and especially those of midgut origin, is the abnormal metabolism of tryptophan. In healthy people, about 99 % of tryptophan is used to make nicotinic acid and 1 % is made into 5-hydroxytryptamine (serotonin). However, in patients with carcinoids, the production of 5-hydroxytryptamine and subsequently 5-hydroxindoleacetic acid predominates, and the latter can be measured in the urine of most patients. A deficiency in nicotinic acid can develop and the patients may have features of pellagra. Apart from 5-hydroxytryptamine, these tumors may produce several other hormones, like kinins, prostaglandins, substance P, histamine, gastrin, somatostatin, corticotrophin, and chromogranin-A. Unless these hormone products are directly secreted into the systemic circulation (intestinal drainage is into the portal system), they do not usually cause any systemic signs or symptoms. Usually only when liver metastases are present, the systemic features of midgut carcinoids associated the hormonal hypersecretion ("carcinoid syndrome" including flushing and diarrhoea) become apparent. However, diarrhoea in midgut carcinoids may be also due to paracrine secretion of the intestine, gut lymphangiectasia, or bacterial overgrowth.

Apart from metabolic abnormalities, midgut carcinoids may cause pronounced fibrosis locally in the peritumoral tissues and the peritoneal cavity, and distantly in the heart or lungs.

Carcinoid heart disease is associated with midgut carcinoids which metastasize to the liver. The cardiac manifestations are caused by the paraneoplastic effects of vasoactive substances such as 5-hydroxytryptamine, histamine, and tachykinins released by the malignant cells rather than any direct metastatic involvement of the heart. The vasoactive tumor products are inactivated by the liver, lungs, and brain, but the presence of hepatic metastases may allow large quantities of these substances to reach the right side of the heart, without being activated by the liver. The preferential right heart involvement (tricuspid valve, pulmonary valve) is most likely related to inactivation of vasoactive substances by the lungs (by the monoamine oxidase system). In the 5–10 % of cases with left-sided valvular pathology (affecting mainly the mitral valve), one should suspect either extensive liver metastases, bronchial NET, or a patent foramen ovale [1].

Most carcinoids have no specific symptoms and usually they are discovered incidentally at the time of endoscopy or surgery for other abdominal disorders. For example, appendiceal carcinoids are revealed during appendicectomy for acute appendicitis, gastric carcinoids are detected during upper GI endoscopy for investigation of dyspepsia, etc. Thus, the presence of these tumors

G. C. Nikou (✉)
Section of Gastrointestinal Neuroendocrinology,
1st Department of Propaedeutic Internal Medicine,
Laikon Hospital, Medical School of Athens
University, 68, Plateon Street, 152 35
Vrilissia-Athens, Greece
e-mail: gcnikou@yahoo.gr

A. D. Gouliamos et al. (eds.), *Imaging in Clinical Oncology*,
DOI: 10.1007/978-88-470-5385-4_68, © Springer-Verlag Italia 2014

may be undetectable for years without obvious signs or symptoms. When symptoms do occur they are associated with: (a) local tumor mass effects, including vague abdominal pain, which often leads to false diagnoses (i.e., irritable bowel syndrome) (b) mesenteric or retroperitoneal fibrosis caused usually by small bowel NETs. Patients with mesenteric fibrosis often present with symptoms indicating intestinal obstruction or ischemia, while patients with retroperitoneal fibrosis may develop hydronephrosis and renal failure secondary to stenosis of the ureters, and (c) the systemic effects of the hormonal products of the tumor. A typical example is the classical "carcinoid syndrome", which results from the synergistic interaction between 5-hydroxytryptamine metabolites, kinins, and prostaglandins released by the tumor to the systemic circulation, circumventing metabolism in the portal vein or pulmonary arterial circulation. Thus, it can occur in patients with midgut carcinoids metastasized to the liver, or with bronchial NETs. Paroxysmal flushing (90 %) triggered by foods, alcohol or exercise, and diarrhea (70 %) are the most common symptoms, followed by abdominal pain (40 %), valvular heart disease (40–45 %), telangiectasia (25 %), wheezing (15 %), and pellagra (5 %) [2, 3]. "Carcinoid crisis" is a life-threatening complication of this syndrome, including hypotension (occasionally hypertension), tachycardia predisposing to arrhythmias, bronchial wheezing, flushing, and central-nervous system abnormalities. It can be precipitated by an anaesthetic or interventional procedure in these patients. "Atypical carcinoid syndrome" is much less common and may occur in patients with gastric metastatic NETs, and excess production of histamine. It includes a generalized flushing, lacrimation, hypotension, cutaneous oedema, and bronchoconstriction.

When tumor-associated fibrosis affects the cardiac valves (usually those of the right side of the heart), symptoms and signs of right-heart failure may develop, while when valves of the left-side of the heart are also involved, the patient may complain of increasing dyspnoea and weakness [1].

Similarly, symptoms of pNETs may be caused by the mechanical effects of the tumor itself or by the systemic effects of tumor hormonal products. For example, patients with gastrinomas often present with recurrent peptic ulcers, resistant to treatment, erosive esophagitis, and chronic diarrhea, associated to hypergastrinaemia [4]; patients with insulinomas develop symptoms (e.g., faintness, perspiration) as a result of hypoglycemia, secondary to insulin hypersecretion; VIPomas patients have a severe secretory diarrhoea, which causes dehydration and hypokalemia, due to VIP (Vasoactive Intestinal Polypeptide) hypersecretion [5]. Additionally, in patients with glucagonomas, a characteristic necrolytic migratory erythema, in combination with weight loss and diabetes mellitus may occur, as systemic effects of glucagon hypersecretion.

In patients with nonfunctioning pNETs the presenting symptoms are not specific and include dyspepsia, abdominal pain, weight loss, jaundice, etc., associated with the tumor growth or the development of metastases.

GEP-NETs represent a very heterogenous group of neoplasms. The majority of them exhibit rather long periods of tumor stabilization or even tumor shrinkage, whereas others may have an aggressive behavior, resulting in patient's poor survival. The natural history of GEP-NETs is still not entirely clear. This is probably due to the fact that, these tumors are rather rare, often with slow evolution and many times are diagnosed once they have already metastases. Additionally, most of the previous studies include only a fraction of the total number of these tumors and also, they do not distinguish the different types of GEP-NETs.

The overall 5 year survival in GEP-NETs, regardless of site and presence of metastases, has estimated to be 67.2 % in the largest series. Among the group of carcinoids, those of the appendix and rectum seem to carry better prognosis, compared with those of colon, small intestine, and stomach. It is also recognized that almost all pNETs with the exception of 90 % of insulinomas, have a long-term malignant potential. Most of them (more than 60 %) have already developed hepatic metastases at the time of diagnosis. At the same time, nonfunctioning pNETs tend to be more advanced because their lack of a clinical hormone-produced syndrome leads to a greater delay in diagnosis.

According to the larger studies, survival of patients with GEP-NETs depends on several clinical, histopathological and biochemical factors. However, most of them are not definitive reliable markers for prognosis.

The presence of metastases is the most important clinical factor and has been associated with a reduced 5-year survival (<50 %). Distant metastases, most commonly to the liver, confer a poorer outcome than do regional metastases (lymph nodes). That is the reason for early screening of the relatives of patients with MEN-1 syndrome. When the pancreatic lesion in these patients is revealed and treated surgically before the development of distal metastases, the prognosis will be definitively better. Also tumor size, especially in carcinoid tumors is associated with the development of metastases, and therefore poorer survival. Other clinical factors that may affect GEP-NETs prognosis are the patients' age over 50 years and the co-existence of other malignant lesions (GI adenocarcinomas). In patients with midgut carcinoids particularly, the presence of the "carcinoid syndrome" and especially the carcinoid heart disease are associated with poorer prognosis [1, 6].

Certain histological features are generally considered as indicators of a higher degree of malignancy and a poorer prognosis. Major criteria are the depth of tumor invasion to the muscularis propria, angioinvasion, and lymphatic invasion, the presence of necroses and especially the mitotic index. The presence of necroses and more than 2 mitoses/50 high-power fields classify the tumor as of intermediate grade of malignancy. Additionally, potential histochemical indicators of malignant behavior of GEP-NETs include the antigen Ki67, and in some cases the tumor suppressor protein p53. Ki67, which has also been adopted by the recent WHO classification for GEP-NETs is considered as a good prognostic indicator for GEP-NETs.

The diagnosis of NETs is based upon: (I) the clinical features, especially in functioning tumors, (II) the levels of several peptides and amines, that represent tumor products, in blood and urine (biomarkers), (III) the localization of primary and/or metastatic lesions by imaging studies, and (IV) the histopathological confirmation (through a biopsy or a surgical specimen) which represents the "gold standard" and should be obtained whenever possible.

Several endoscopic, radiological and molecular/nuclear medicine studies have been used for detection and demonstration of primary and metastatic NET lesions. Precise assessment of tumor load, at diagnosis, is important to determine, whether a patient is a candidate for curative or cytoreductive surgery, while appropriate imaging studies at follow-up will evaluate the disease course and the response to treatment.

In terms of radiological studies, *Transabdominal ultrasound* is of limited value in revealing the primary lesion of GEP-NETs, although the use of ultrasound "microbubble" contrast medium may increase the sensitivity of US, for the detection of liver metastases. *Computed Tomography* (*CT*). Multidetector CT is the most widely used cross-sectional imaging study for assessment of tumor load and follow-up of the disease in GEP-NETs. When combined with EUS, the sensitivity for detection of small pNETs, such as insulinomas, is approaching 100 %. Moreover, the detection of an occult small bowel NET can be facilitated with *CT enteroclysis,* with reported sensitivity and specificity of 85 and 97 %, respectively. *Magnetic Resonance Imaging* (*MRI*). The use of T1 weighted and T1 fat-saturated sequence can detect the primary pancreatic lesion in 94 % of pNETs, but with lower sensitivity for extrapancreatic lesions. MRI is usually used over CT in younger patients, in patients with iodine allergy and in those with renal impairment. MRI is also considered as the imaging of choice for spinal NET metastases, while it seems also to be more sensitive than CT for small hepatic metastases. In the era of marked improvements in CT and MRI techniques, Interventional radiological procedures, such as *Selective angiography with Calcium (as secretagogue) injection* is rarely used. This procedure has more than 90 % sensitivity in revealing small pancreatic insulinomas and also duodenal gastrinomas, while its sensitivity is further increased when it is combined with *Intraoperative ultrasound (IOUS)*. The latter, in combination with the surgical palpation of the pancreas and duodenal wall has revealed the vast majority of pancreatic insulinomas and gastrinomas (97 and 100 %), and also most of the small duodenal gastrinomas in MEN-1 patients. Additionally, *IOUS* can provide a precise examination of the liver parenchyma for the detection of small metastases [7].

Nuclear medicine/Molecular imaging studies have a central role in patients' diagnosis. *Indium-111-diethylentriamine penta-acetic acid (DTPA)-octreotide (Octreoscan)* is recognized as the gold standard modality for GEP-NETs' imaging, with an overall sensitivity of approximately 80–90 %. The simultaneous performance of single photon emission computed tomography (SPECT), using a triple-head camera, increases its sensitivity and specificity. Octreoscan may detect unsuspected lesions, not shown by the previous conventional studies, which is crucial when surgery is planned. Furthermore, it may predict the response to treatment with somatostatin analogues. However, its sensitivity is lower in small volume disease, in high-grade NETs and also in insulinomas (<50 %) [8]. *Meta-iodobenzylguanidine scintigraphy (^{123}I-MIBG)* scintigraphy is considered as the imaging modality of choice for pheocromocytomas (with a sensitivity and specificity of 87 and 99 %, respectively) and also paragangliomas and neuroblastomas. Additionally, it has a complementary role in medullary thyroid carcinomas and in metastatic midgut NETs, especially to assess whether treatment with ^{131}I-MIBG can be considered.

Positron Emission Tomography (PET) molecular imaging studies have been increasingly used in NETs. The first and widely used *FDG-PET,* that is utilizing [^{18}F]Fluoro-2-deoxy-D-glucose as a tracer, can be beneficial in poorly differentiated GEP-NETs. According to recent data, FDG-PET is more sensitive than Octreoscan, in NETs with higher proliferation index.

Recently, labeling of PET isotopes, such as ^{68}Ga, to somatostatin analogues has led to the development of *^{68}Ga-DOTATOC and ^{68}Ga-DOTATATE PET* scans. These new imaging modalities can be completed within a few hours compared to 24–48 h for Octreoscan and also, seem to identify additional tumor lesions. Moreover, new tracers, such as 5-hydroxytryptophan (5-HTP) labeled with ^{11}C, and L-dihydroxy-fluoro-phenylalanine labeled with ^{18}F, have led to the development of *^{11}C-5-HTP-PET* and *^{18}F-DOPA-PET*, respectively. These PETs seem to be valuable diagnostic tools as the can detect small lesions, not revealed by other methods. However all these, specific for NETs, PET studies are not yet widely available [9].

The optimal management of patients with GEP-NETs involves the coordination of several specialities. A multidisciplinary approach by gastroenterologists, oncologists, endocrinologists, radiologists, nuclear medicine physicians, histopathologists, and surgeons is required in order to achieve a more individualized therapeutic approach for each patient [10].

References

1. Bhattacharyya S, Toumpanakis C, Chilkunda D (2011) Risk factors for the development and progression of carcinoid heart disease. Am J Cardiol, vol 15,107(8):1221–6
2. Nikou GC, Lygidakis NJ, Toubanakis C et al (2005) Current diagnosis and treatment of gastrointestinal carcinoids in a series of 101 patients: the significance of serum chromogranin-A, somatostatin receptor scintigraphy and somatostatin analogues. Hepatogastroenterology 52(63):731–741
3. Nikou GC, Toubanakis C, Moulakakis C et al (2011) Carcinoid tumors of the duodenum and the ampulla of vater: current diagnostic and therapeutic approach in a series of 8 patients. Int J Surg 9:248–253
4. Nikou GC, Toubanakis C, Nikolaou P et al (2005) Gastrinomas associated with MEN-1 syndrome: new insights for the diagnosis and management in a series of 11 patients. Hepatogastroenterology 52(66):1668–1676
5. Nikou GC, Toubanakis C, Nikolaou P (2005) VIPomas: an update in diagnosis and management

in a series of 11 patients. Hepatogastroenterology 52(64):1259–1265

6. Hemminki K, Li X (2001) Incidence trands and risk factors of carcinoid tumors : a nationwide epidemiologic study from Sweden. Cancer 92:2204–2210
7. Bushnell DL, Baum RP.(2011) Standard imaging techniques for neuroendocrine tumors. Endocr Met Clin North Am 40(1):153–62 Mar 2011
8. Kwekkeboom DJ, Krenning EP, Scheidhauer K et al (2009) ENETS consensus guidelines for the standards of care in neuroendocrine tumors: somatostatin receptor imaging with (111)In-pentetreotide. Neuroendocrinology 90(2):184–189
9. Miederer M, Weber MM, Fottner C (2010) Molecular imaging of gastroenteropancreatic neuroendocrine tumors. Gastroenterol Clin North Am 39(4):923–935
10. Nikou GC, Marinou K, Thomakos P et al (2008) Chromogranin A levels in diagnosis, treatment and follow-up of 42 patients with non-functioning pancreatic endocrine tumours. Pancreatology 8:510–519

Part XI
Urogenital Cancer

Introduction to Adrenal Cancer

69

Dionysios N. Mitropoulos

69.1 Incidentally Found Adrenal Lesions ("Incidentalomas")

The more frequent and widespread use of cross-sectional imaging has resulted in an increase of the detection of adrenal lesions in patients with no suspicion of adrenal disease. Imaging along with clinical evaluation is critical for the characterization of an incidentaloma as benign or malignant. Clinical criteria are an earlier cancer diagnosis (malignancy in even 50 % of cases), the size of the lesion (direct relationship to malignancy), and symptoms at presentation. The decision for a surgical or non-surgical management of patients with incidentalomas in nowadays influenced by their imaging characterization [1].

69.2 Malignant Adrenal Tumors

In contrast to incidentalomas, malignant adrenal tumors are very rare and comprise adrenocortical carcinomas, pheochromocytomas/paragangliomas, and metastatic lesions.

D. N. Mitropoulos (✉)
1st Department of Urology, University of Athens Medical School, 75 Mikras Asias, 11517 Athens, Greece
e-mail: dmp@otenet.gr

69.3 Adrenocortical Carcinomas (ACCs)

ACCs account for <5 % of incidentalomas, may appear at any age and show a bimodal distribution in children <5 year of age and in adults in their fourth and fifth decades of life. The clinical signs are those of autonomous adrenocortical steroid excess (mostly Cushing's syndrome or rapidly worsening androgenisation in women). In men, androgen excess is usually asymptomatic while feminization with gynecomastia and testicular atrophy is rare. In a small percentage of cases, symptoms are related to isolated mineralocorticoid excess (severe hypertension and profound hypokalemia). Patients with hormonally inactive ACCs have symptoms related to the local effects of a large (at least 10 cm in diameter) tumor such as abdominal discomfort, back pain, indigestion, nausea, and vomiting [2]. The surgical approach (open or laparoscopic) is equivocal as far as the postoperative benefits and the oncological outcomes [3].

69.4 Pheochromocytomas (PCCs) and Paragangliomas (PGLs)

The malignancy of PCCs and PGLs is defined, according to the WHO classification, by the presence of metastases at nonchromaffin sites distant from that of the primary tumor and not by local invasion. Clinically, malignant cases may lack the typical signs of hypertension,

A. D. Gouliamos et al. (eds.), *Imaging in Clinical Oncology*,
DOI: 10.1007/978-88-470-5385-4_69, © Springer-Verlag Italia 2014

palpitations, headache, and diaphoresis. Imaging and nuclear medicine techniques are used for the localization of the primary tumor and in the evaluation of the extent of the disease, staging, and treatment decision making, respectively [3].

69.5 Metastatic Lesions

The presence of a primary tumor elsewhere and a synchronous or metachronous detection of an adrenal lesion raise the question of a potential adrenal metastasis that has to be thoroughly evaluated. An adrenal biopsy can be proposed in indeterminate cases [3].

References

1. Sundin A (2012) Imaging of adrenal masses with emphasis on adrenocortical tumors. Theranostics 2:516–522
2. Zini L, Porpiglia F, Fassnacht M (2011) Contemporary management of adrenocortical carcinoma. Eur Urol 60:1055–1065
3. Henry J-F, Peix J-L, Kraimps J-L (2012) Positional statement of the European society of endocrine surgeons (ESES) on malignant adrenal tumors. Langenbecks Arch Surg 397:145–146

70 Ultrasound Findings in Adrenal Cancer

Ioannis A. Tsitouridis and Georgios E. Glataganas

The ultrasound (US) evaluation of normal adrenal glands is difficult. This is because bowel gas on the left side can often produce acoustic shadowing which obscures the gland, the adrenal glands reveal an echotexture very close to that of surrounding tissues, and also because of the small size of the glands.

The normal adrenal gland on US has a typical Y or inverted V shape and the central medulla is hyperechoic with a hypoechoic cortex.

The right adrenal gland is visible using optimized techniques but the left adrenal gland is visible in about 40–50 % of the cases [1].

70.1 Malignant Tumors

70.1.1 Metastasis

Metastasis to adrenal glands are the second more common solid tumor after adenoma. These lesions have heterogeneity on ultrasound because they are less homogeneous, in contrast to adenomas, although both of them are circumscribed lesions. In rare cases metastasis has irregular margins.

70.1.2 Adrenal Carcinoma

The tumor is not usually detected until it becomes very large (often >8 cm) and in the majority of cases reveals inhomogeneous hypoechoic pattern with irregular margins (Fig. 70.1).

Besides this hypoechoic appearance, intratumoral hemorrhage, necrotic foci with or without liquefaction and calcification may occur, changing the echopoor pattern.

70.1.3 Pheochromocytoma

Pheochromocytoma is a neoplasm which has its origin in adrenal medulla and is always detected when it reaches several centimeters in diameter.

These tumors have a round shape with smooth margins and mixed echogenicity (Fig. 70.2).

With color Doppler imaging pheochromocytoma and lymphoma are usually hypervascularized, in contrast to metastasis and adrenal carcinoma which are hypovascularized tumors.

I. A. Tsitouridis (✉) · G. E. Glataganas
Department of Radiology, General Hospital Papageorgiou, Thessaloniki, Ring Road Thessaloniki Efkarpia, 685111 Thessaloniki, Greece
e-mail: tsitouridis.1@gmail.com

G. E. Glataganas
e-mail: gialim@hol.gr

A. D. Gouliamos et al. (eds.), *Imaging in Clinical Oncology*,
DOI: 10.1007/978-88-470-5385-4_70, © Springer-Verlag Italia 2014

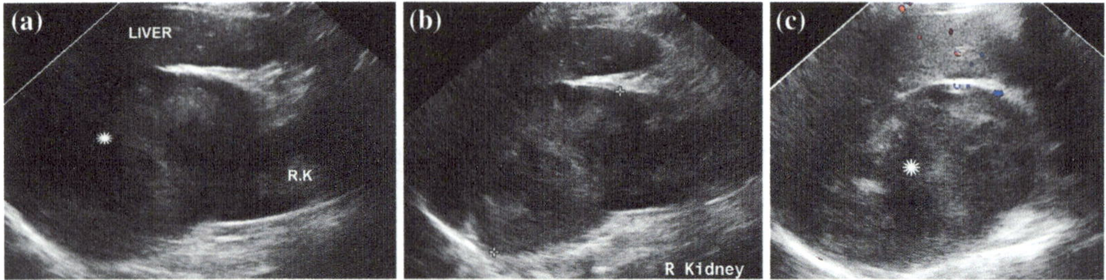

Fig. 70.1 **a**, **b**, **c** Oblique sagittal sonograms which reveal a large adrenal carcinoma with mixed echogenicity and poor vascularity (*asterisk*). There is no clear cleavage plane between the lesion and liver parenchyma

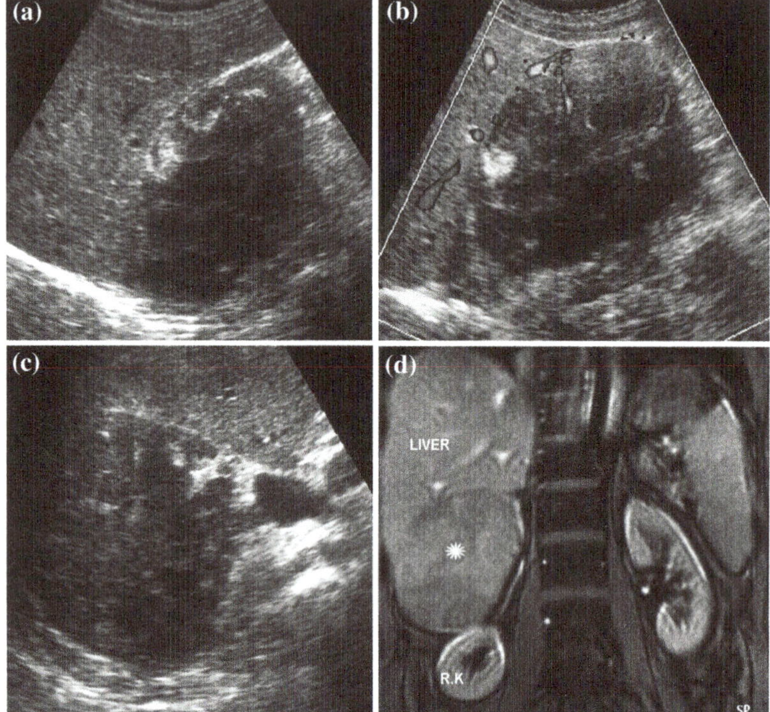

Fig. 70.2 **a**, **b** Oblique sagittal grayscale and color Doppler sonograms which reveal a large pheochromocytoma of the right adrenal gland. **c** Axial grayscale sonogram and **d** coronal T1-FLASH post contrast MRI scan which shows the location of the lesion between the liver and the dislocated right kidney

Bibliography

1. Dietrich CF, Wehrmann T, Hoffmann C, Hermann G, Caspary WF, Seifert H (1999) Detection of the adrenal glands by endoscopic or transabdominal ultrasound. Endoscopy 29(9):859–864

CT and MRI Findings in Adrenal Cancer 71

Fotios D. Laspas

71.1 Introduction

The incidental detection of adrenal lesions ("incidentalomas") has increased with the widespread and frequent use of cross-sectional imaging. Accurate characterization of an incidentaloma is important, particularly in patients with a known primary carcinoma. CT and MRI are the most common methods used for characterization and follow-up of the incidentaloma. Although cross-sectional imaging findings can suggest or confirm a diagnosis for most adrenal masses, in a small minority they will not yield a definitive diagnosis and functional methods (such as positron emission tomography) or percutaneous biopsy procedures may be necessary.

When an adrenal lesion is encountered, the major clinical problem is to differentiate benign lesion (such as adenoma and myelolipoma) from malignant disease (including adrenocortical carcinoma-ACC, pheochromocytoma-PCC and metastasis) [1]. The vast majority of these lesions will prove to be benign (the most common lesion incidentally detected is the benign adrenal adenoma); however, the probability of metastasis significantly increases if the patient has a diagnosis of an extra-adrenal malignancy [2]. The imaging characterization of adrenal lesions with CT and MRI is mainly based on the conventional morphologic features of the lesion, the intracellular lipid concentration of the mass and the contrast washout differences between benign and malignant masses [2].

71.2 Conventional Morphologic Features

Adenomas are generally small, homogeneous, well-defined lesions with uniform enhancement [3]. Although the presence of these structural features is nonspecific for adenoma, the absence strongly suggests another diagnosis. Lesions larger than 4 cm in diameter are much more likely to be malignant [2]. Myelolipoma can be sometimes large but the existence of areas of macroscopic fat indicates the diagnosis [4]. Both benign and malignant lesions can be of inhomogeneous attenuation particularly after the administration of intravenous contrast medium. However, large necrotic areas in an adrenal lesion usually suggest malignancy. Rarely, an adenoma can hemorrhage and has heterogeneous appearance [3]. Moreover, metastases are often homogeneous, especially when small.

The typical appearance of ACC is of a large, inhomogeneous (owing to the presence of necrosis or hemorrhage) mass that enhances heterogeneously after intravenous administration of contrast agent (Fig. 71.1). Sometimes the tumor becomes so large that it can be difficult to determine its origin. Calcification may be

F. D. Laspas (✉)
CT&MRI Department, Hygeia Hospital,
4, Erythrou Stavrou Str. & Kifisias Av, Attica
15123 Marousi, Athens, Greece
e-mail: fotisdimi@yahoo.gr

A. D. Gouliamos et al. (eds.), *Imaging in Clinical Oncology*,
DOI: 10.1007/978-88-470-5385-4_71, © Springer-Verlag Italia 2014

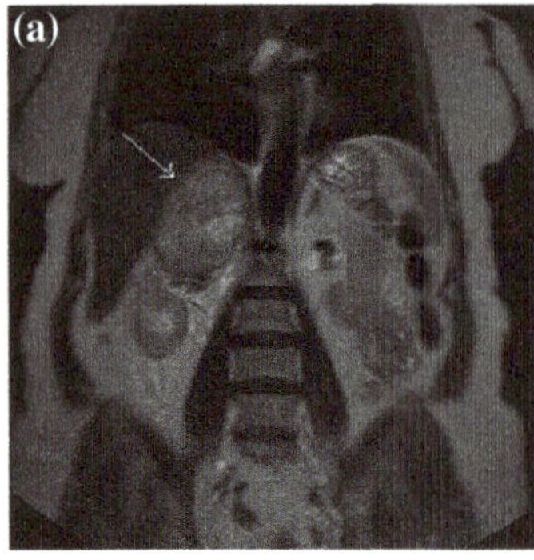

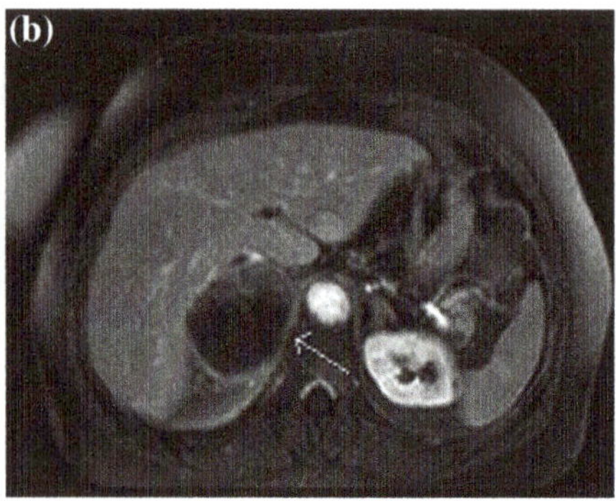

Fig. 71.1 Coronal T2-weighted MR image (**a**) and axial T1-weighted contrast-enhanced MR image (**b**) of a large adrenocortical carcinoma (*arrow*). The mass exhibits heterogeneous signal intensity on the T2-weighted image and heterogeneous pattern of contrast enhancement

identified on CT, more commonly centrally located. However, small lesions are often homogeneous and well-defined, and difficult to distinguish from benign adenomas. Staging of ACC is based on tumor size and invasion of adjacent organs (T), nodal involvement (N), and distant metastases (M) [5]. CT is the most common method used in ACC staging showing the local and distal spread of the tumor. Invasion of adjacent vascular structures (such as the renal vein and inferior vena cava), which is important information for the surgical planning, is not rare. Preservation of fat planes between the tumor and neighboring organs indicates no local invasion. Hematogenous metastases most commonly occur to the lungs, liver, and bones [5].

Pheochromocytoma is a rare catecholamine-secreting tumor, which is usually benign but in percentage of 10 % is malignant. Pheochromocytoma usually manifests clinically, but up to 10 % of patients are asymptomatic (hormonally inactive). A non-functioning pheochromocytoma often poses an imaging dilemma. Another 10 % are also bilateral or extra-adrenal in location or familial. Pheochromocytoma also is associated with various syndromes. The appearances of pheochromocytoma are nonspecific on CT and MRI and frequently overlap with other adrenal masses [6]. Small pheochromocytomas are usually homogeneous, whereas larger pheochromocytomas are usually heterogeneous with areas of hemorrhage and necrosis (even when they are benign). Metastatic spread is the only reliable criterion for malignant disease [6]. Most pheochromocytomas show avid enhancement after the administration of contrast agent. Although it has been thought that the use of intravenous iodinate contrast agent at CT can provoke an adrenergic crisis in patients with pheochromocytoma, more recent experience indicates that the use of nonionic contrast media is safe [4].

The adrenal gland is a common site of metastatic disease, particularly from lung cancer [4]. Metastases are the most common malignant tumor of the adrenal glands. Not infrequently, metastases are bilateral but may also be unilateral. The diagnosis of adrenal metastasis should be considered when there is a primary malignancy elsewhere or there is evidence of other metastases. Similar to most adenomas, metastases tend to be homogeneous and well-defined, especially when small.

71.3 Intracellular Lipid Concentration

About 70 % of adenomas contain significant intracellular fat (lipid-rich adenomas), whereas almost all malignant lesions do not [2]. These adenomas are of low attenuation on unenhanced CT. Conversely, almost all nonadenomatous lesions contain little or no intracellular fat and

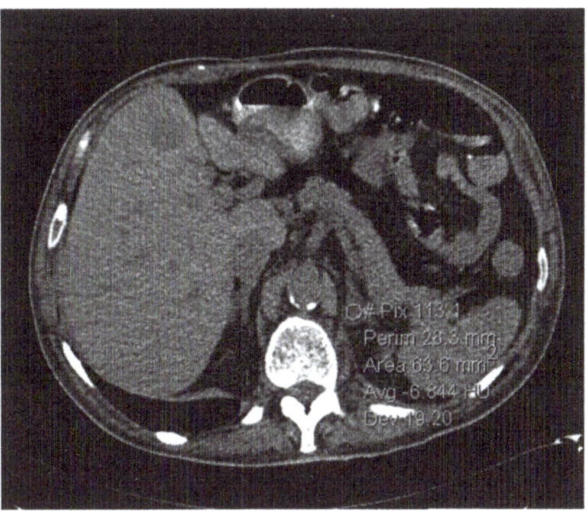

Fig. 71.2 Adenoma in a patient with colorectal cancer (stable for 24 months). Axial unenhanced CT scan shows a small (<2 cm) left adrenal nodule with attenuation of −6.8 HU

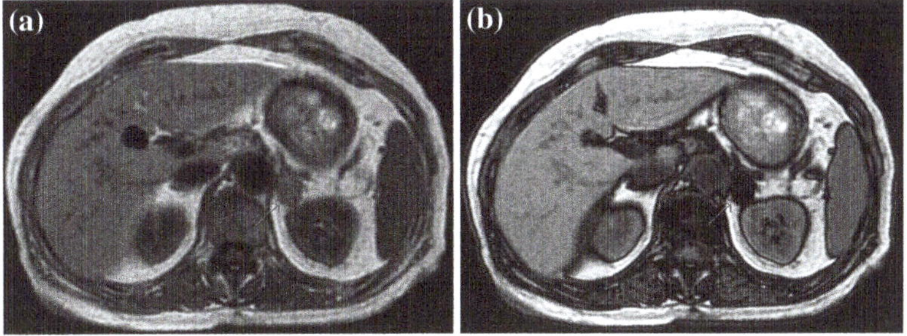

Fig. 71.3 Axial MR in-phase (**a**) and out-of-phase (**b**) images of a 2 cm left adrenal lesion (*arrow*) in a 62-year-old woman. The lesion shows marked signal intensity loss consistent with adenoma

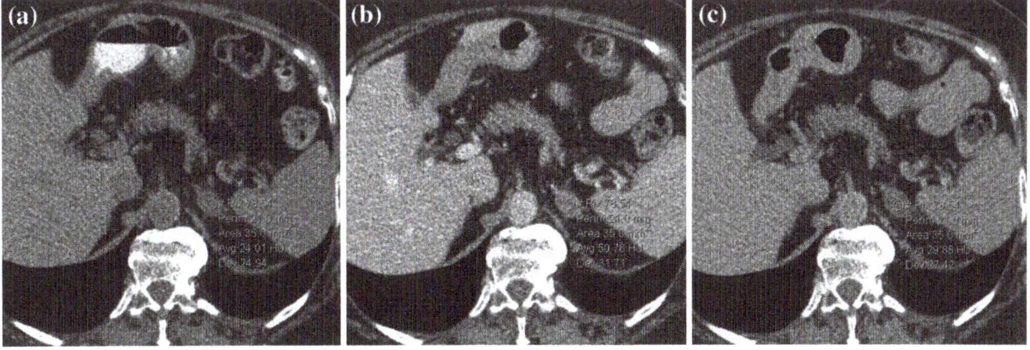

Fig. 71.4 Incidental left adrenal mass in a 54-year-old woman. The lesion measures 24 HU on precontrast CT (**a**) 51 HU on early enhanced scan (**b**), and 30 HU in the delayed phase (**c**). The absolute washout of this lesion is 78 %, consistent with an adenoma

their attenuation values at unenhanced CT are consequently higher. A density equal to or below 10 HU at unenhanced CT is generally used to diagnose an adenoma (Fig. 71.2). The 10 HU threshold results in a high specificity of 98 % for the diagnosis of an adenoma [1].

Table 71.1 Adrenal adenoma contrast washout characteristics

APW	(enhanced CT-delayed CT)/(enhanced CT-unenhanced CT) × 100	>60 %
RPW	(enhanced CT-delayed CT)/enhanced CT × 100	>40 %

Chemical shift imaging is the most accurate and commonly performed MRI technique for distinguishing between adenomas and malignancies [7]. This MRI method is also dependent on the detection of intracellular lipid in solid adrenal lesion. Lipid-rich adenomas have signal loss on out-of-phase imaging compared with in-phase images (Fig. 71.3). Chemical shift imaging shows similar sensitivity and specificity for the characterization of adrenal masses to those of unenhanced CT [1, 7].

However, up to 30 % of adrenal adenomas do not contain enough intracellular lipid (lipid-poor adenomas) and remain indeterminate and indistinguishable from malignant lesions on unenhanced CT scan or chemical shift imaging. Therefore, lesions above 10 HU on an unenhanced CT require further investigation.

71.4 Contrast Washout

As unenhanced CT and chemical shift MRI are both based on detection of intracellular lipid, they are limited in evaluation of lipid-poor adenomas. Fortunately, several authors showed that quantitative evaluation of delayed CT enhancement parameters of adrenal masses has been shown to be highly accurate for differentiating adenomas from malignant lesions [1]. Adenomas (lipid-rich and lipid-poor) commonly enhance rapidly and demonstrate rapid washout, while malignant lesions enhance also vigorously but have typically prolonged washout.

Attenuation values are measured on precontrast CT, early (at 60 s) and 15 min delayed enhanced images. Two methods are available to calculate percent washout: absolute percentage washout (APW), which requires a precontrast attenuation value, and relative percentage washout (RPW), which represents the percentage of the initial wash-in of enhancement that is washed-out at the time of delayed scanning (Fig. 71.4). Most investigators use an APW threshold of 60 % on a 15 min delayed scan or 40 % for RPW with reported sensitivity and specificity nearly 100 % [4]. Therefore, any lesion that demonstrates APW > 60 % or RPW > 40 % probably represents an adenoma (Table 71.1).

71.5 Conclusion

Noninvasive imaging methods can overcome the challenges of characterizing an adrenal mass with a high level of accuracy. The combination of conventional morphologic features, unenhanced CT, and washout values correctly differentiates nearly all adrenal adenomas from malignant lesions.

References

1. Taffel M, Haji-Momenian S, Nikolaidis P et al (2012) Adrenal imaging: a comprehensive review. Radiol Clin North Am 50(2):219–243
2. Blake MA, Cronin CG, Boland GW (2010) Adrenal imaging. AJR 194(6):1450–14560
3. Johnson PT, Horton KM, Fishman EK (2009) Adrenal mass imaging with multidetector CT: pathologic conditions, pearls, and pitfalls. Radiographics 29(5):1333–1351
4. Boland GW, Blake MA, Hahn PF et al (2008) Incidental adrenal lesions: principles, techniques, and algorithms for imaging characterization. Radiology 249(3):756–775
5. Bharwani N, Rockall AG, Sahdev A et al (2011) Adrenocortical carcinoma: the range of appearances on CT and MRI. AJR 196(6):706–714
6. Blake MA, Kalra MK, Maher MM et al (2004) Pheochromocytoma: an imaging chameleon. Radiographics 24:87–99
7. Elsayes KM, Mukundan G, Narra VR et al (2004) Adrenal masses: mr imaging features with pathologic correlation. Radiographics 24:73–86

SPECT in Adrenal Glands

72

Fani J. Vlachou

Adrenal glands are divided morphologically and functionally in two parts:

1. The adrenal cortex, which consists of three layers: the glomerulosa zone, responsible for the production of mineralocorticoids (aldosterone), the fasciculata zone, which generates glucocorticoides (cortisol), and the reticulata zone, which generates sex hormones (androgen).
2. The adrenal medulla, which generates catecholamines (epinephrine, norepinephrine, and dopamine).

Adrenal tumors are 2.1 % of tumors on average, 3 % during middle age, and 10 % in elderly people, with 60 % of adrenal tumors being detected in people aged between 60 and 80 years.

Increase in use of imaging methods, CT, and MRI, led to a significant rise in random discoveries of adrenal gland tumors, the so-called incidentalomas where no symptoms of the adrenal gland disease are detected and where inactive adenoma constitutes 80 % of cases, metastases 25 %, aldosteronism 1 %, whereas pheochromocytoma, adrenal carcinoma, and subclinical syndrome Cushing constitute 5 % of cases each.

Kloos [1] conducted a meta-analysis regarding incidentalomas, during which 36–94 % of non-oncologic patients and 7–68 % of oncologic patients were diagnosed with adrenal cortex adenoma. Moreover, 0–21 % of non-oncologic patients and 32–73 % of oncologic patients were diagnosed with adrenal metastasis. Cysts were found in 4–22 % of cases, myelolipoma in 7–15 % of cases, and pheochromocytoma in 0–11 % of cases. Despite most cases of incidentalomas (80 %) are considered benign tumors, the possibility of malignant tumors to occur should not be excluded. The conventional imaging methods, CT and MRI, play an important role toward that direction.

Fine needle biopsy (FNA) provides great accuracy in discrimination between benign and metastatic lesions of the adrenal gland (80–100 %); however this differentiation cannot be easily applied in many cases.

In the event of adrenal gland tumor three questions are posed: Is it a hormonally active tumor? Is it a malignant tumor, or is it a metastatic tumor? Diagnosis is performed taking into consideration the medical record, clinical examination as well as laboratory and especially hormonal control. It is completed with tumor imaging using anatomic imaging methods (CT, MRI) which are supplemented with functional scintigraphy.

Adrenal cortex tumors may imply adenoma, hyperplasia, or carcinoma while medulla tumors may imply pheochromocytoma, ganglioneuroma, or neuroblastoma. Other tumor cases may include myelolipoma, hamartoma, or metastases.

F. J. Vlachou (✉)
Department of Nuclear Medicine, Hygeia Hospital, Kifissias Avenue & 4 Erythou Stavrou Street, 15123, Maroussi, Athens, Greece
e-mail: fanivlachou@yahoo.com

A. D. Gouliamos et al. (eds.), *Imaging in Clinical Oncology*,
DOI: 10.1007/978-88-470-5385-4_72, © Springer-Verlag Italia 2014

Primary aldosteronism (PA) is a syndrome related to increased production of aldosterone generated by adrenal glands and attributed either to aldosterone producing adenoma (APA) or to bilateral adrenal hyperplasia (BAH).

In most cases, hypertension occurs due to PA. A proportion of 5–20 % of hypertensive patients is found with PA, which is characterized by increased aldosterone secretion and reduced renin secretion because of the fact that the renin-angiotension-aldosterone axis remains inert.

Several imaging modalities have been employed to discriminate between BAH and APA. In addition to CT, MRI, and adrenal venous sampling (AVS), which is the gold standard examination, adrenal scintigraphy using cholesterol-based radiopharmaceutical such as iodine-131-6-B-iodomethyl norcholesterol (NP59) and selenium 75-6-β-selenomethyl norcholesterol is a commonly used method.

CT cannot detect any possible Conn's adenoma in PA patients. Therefore, NP59 scintigraphy is selected as the most suitable method, since unilateral adrenal visualization implies solitary adrenal adenoma, while bilateral visualization implies bilateral hyperplasia. Treatment of PA patients is performed surgically, in the occurrence of APA, whereas pharmaceutical therapy is recommended in a bilateral hyperplasia case. This is the reason why differential diagnosis between these two pathological conditions is critical. Several multimodality diagnostic algorithms have been suggested to distinguish BAH from APA. Each modality carries an important role. CT and MRI published sensitivities vary from 40 to 100 % and from 70 to 100 %, respectively [2]. Dexamethasone suppression of normal adrenal cortex enhances the accuracy of NP59-based adrenal scintigraphy which ranges from 47 to 94 % in various studies [3].

Adenomas smaller than 1.5 cm are possibly not visible due to low spacial resolution of planar imaging. The establishment of SPECT/CT images appears as a solution to this problem, offering better resolution as well as functional and anatomic information, ameliorating the accuracy of this modality.

Adrenocortical scintigraphy based on radiolabeled cholesterol analogue is acknowledged as the most accurate imaging technique in discrimination between benign and malignant adrenal lesions and involves three patterns: [1]

(a) The concordant pattern: increased uptake of radiopharmaceutical in the adrenal mass demonstrated by CT or MRI represents benign adenoma providing an accuracy of 100 %.
(b) The discordant pattern: decreased or no uptake in the adrenal mass demonstrated by CT or MRI represents space-occupying lesions (metastasis, tumor, etc.)
(c) The non-lateralizing pattern: normal, symmetrical adrenal uptake in the masses >2 cm represents pseudoadrenal mass, providing 100 % accuracy.

Adrenal medulla is part of the sympathetic nervous system that produces catecholamines (epinephrine, norepinephrine, and dopamine) which function as hormones or as neurotransmitters.

Pheochomocytomas (PCC's) and paragangliomas (PGL's) are both tumors: the former group originates from the chromaffin cells of the adrenal medulla and the latter from extra adrenal chromaffin cells of nervous ganglia.

Five percentage of incidentaloma cases are related to PCC, which are also responsible for hypertension in 0.5 % of hypertensive patients. Tumors of this kind may be malignant (10 % of cases), bilateral (10 % of cases), outside the adrenal gland (20 % of cases), or linked to hereditary causes (10 % of cases) such as multiple endocrine neoplasia 2 syndrome (MEN 2A, MEN 2B), von Hippel-Lindau syndrome, etc.

PCC diagnosis includes measurements of plasma-free metanephrines and/or catecholamines found in 24 h urine and/or in plasma. If values are high, anatomic as well as functional imaging modalities appear to be of great help in detection of PCC and possible metastases.

CT sensitivity diagnosis reaches 93–100 % for intraadrenal PCCs and approximately 90 % for extra adrenal tumors with 1 cm diameter, while MRI sensitivity is even higher; however, specificity of both of these anatomic imaging modalities varies from 50 to 90 % [4].

During functional imaging of tumors originating from adrenal medulla and nervous ganglia, various radiopharmaceuticals are used such as radiolabeled catecholamines (14C-dopamine, 11C-epinephrine), radiolabeled inhibitors of catecholamines (tyrosin derivates), neuroblockers (guanethidine analogs), and somatostatin receptors.

MIBG scintigraphy is considered the gold standard functional imaging modality for PCCs and PGLs. Sensitivity of I-131 MIBG ranges from 77 to 90 % and specificity ranges from 95 to 100 %, while the sensitivity of I-123 MIBG is 83–100 % and the specificity is about 95–100 % (I-123 MIBG has the advantage of SPECT/CT images improving the modality's sensitivity) [4].

Despite the fact that FDG-PET/CT seems to have greater sensitivity which rises to 100 % with use of new radiopharmaceuticals such as 18F-Fluorodopamine, MIBG scintigraphy emerges as a valuable method in cases of malignant PCC and neuroblastoma not only for staging, but also for monitoring treatment response. Moreover, it proves to be useful in selecting patients suitable for I-131 MIBG treatment.

Neuroblastoma is the most common pediatric malignancy, representing about 30 % of pediatric cancers. 70–80 % of patients present metastatic disease, usually in the bone marrow, cortical bone, lymph nodes, and liver.

I-123 MIBG is the radiopharmaceutical of choice for imaging neuroblastoma, having a reported sensitivity of about 70 % and high specificity of about 100 % (SPECT/CT improve anatomic localization) (Figs. 72.1a, b, c and 72.2a, b, c).

I-123 MIBG scintigraphy is considered superior to FDG-PET/CT in higher stage disease (stage IV), as it allows better detection of bone marrow and bone metastases, nevertheless FGD-PET/CT is superior in early stage of the disease (stages I and II), in patients whose tumors have low uptake of MIBG, as well as in patients whose scintigraphic findings are not consistent with the clinical symptoms [5].

Pheochromocytomas, paragangliomas, and neuroblastomas are classified as neuroendocrine tumors since they originate from the sympathoadrenal system. Radiolabeled somatostatin analogs are of great importance in their imaging.

As far as somatostatin analogs are concerned, the most commonly applied radiopharmaceutical in clinical practice is In-111 pentetreotide, used for scintigraphic imaging of neuroendocrine tumors such as [6]:

- Sympathoadrenal system tumors (pheochromocytoma, neuroblastoma, ganglioneuroma, and paraganglioma)
- Gastroenteropancreatic (GEP) tumors (carcinoid, gastrinoma, insulinoma, glucagonoma, VIPoma, etc.)
- Medullary thyroid carcinoma
- Pituitary adenoma
- Merkel cell carcinoma
- Small-cell lung cancer (SCLC).

Radiolabeled somatostatin analogs contribute significantly to imaging neuroendocrine tumors due to the tumoral overexpression of somatostatin receptors (sst). In-111 pentetreotide links to somatostatin receptors and is strongly associated with subtypes 2 and 5.

In-111 pentetreotide is less sensitive than MIBG in benign PCC imaging, whereas its sensitivity is higher for malignant and metastatic PCC imaging and similar to FDG-PET/CT (87 %).

As far as paragangliomas' imaging is concerned, In-111 pentetreotide is the radiopharmaceutical of choice having a sensitivity of 94 % [7].

As in malignant PCC, In-111 pentetreotide has a high sensitivity of about 88 % which is similar to FDG-PET/CT and in any case excels that of MIBG.

An excessive quantity of vasoactive peptides and neuropeptides is generated by carcinoid tumors. The gastrointestinal tract is acknowledged as the origin of carcinoid tumors site in 73–85 % of cases; bronchopulmonary system is the origin in 10–20 % and rarely are other organs. These tumors are slow growing; nevertheless 40 % of the patients at the time of the diagnosis are found with metastasis. In addition

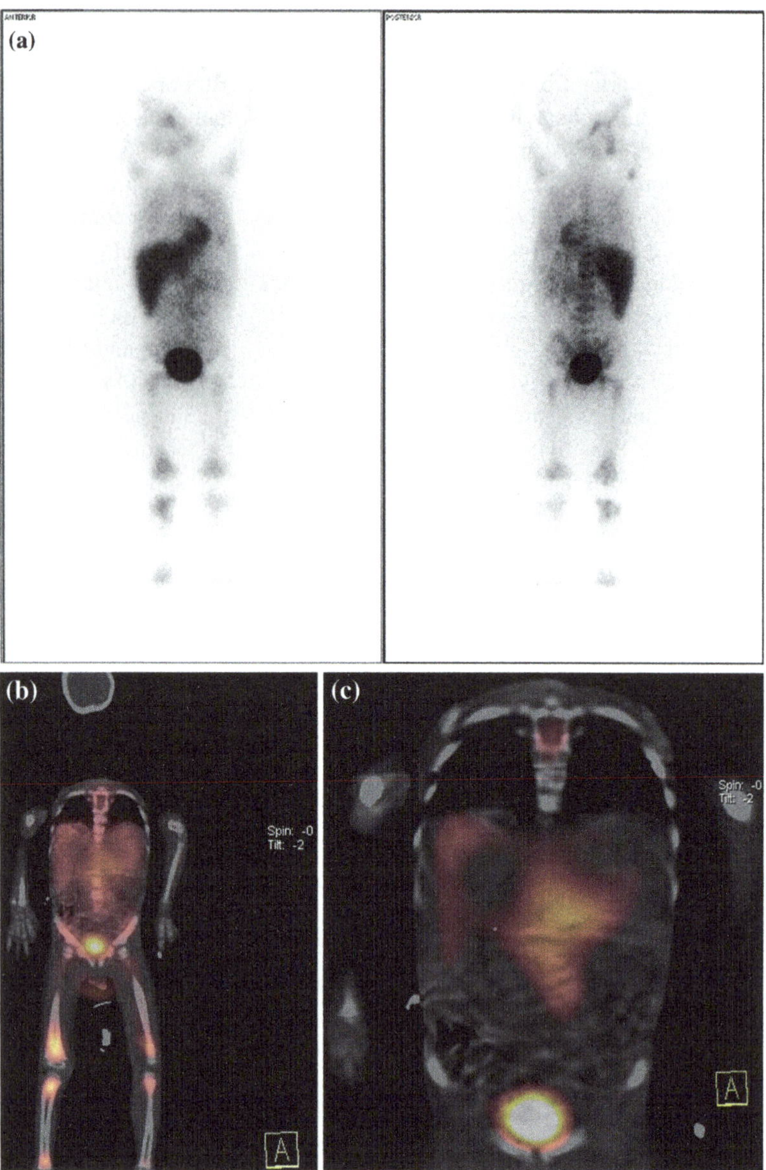

Fig. 72.1 Initial staging. **a** I-123 MIBG whole body. **b**, **c** I-123 MIBG SPECT/CT images reveal abdominal mass with increased uptake of the radiopharmaceutical, as well as bone marrow involvement at lower limbs

to this, it is important to mention that only about one-third of the patients share the symptoms of typical carcinoid syndrome (flushing, diarrhea, abdominal pain, etc.).

Diagnosis of carcinoid tumor is performed with measurements of serum chromogranin-A and of urinary 5-HIAA (5 Hydroxyindoleacetic acid). In-111 pentetreotide imaging provides higher sensitivity results than conventional imaging modalities (CT or MRI) rising to 80–90 % [7] explaining why this is the most appropriate method for carcinoid tumors localization and staging.

Gastrinoma generates an excessive amount of gastrine leading to overproduction of gastric acid and peptic ulcer (Zollinger-Ellison syndrome). Gastrinomas are characterized malignant in 50–60 % of cases, while they are associated with MEN1 syndrome in 25 % of cases. The majority of gastrinomas is identified in the pancreas and concerns slow growing tumors. In-111 pentetreotide is recommended as

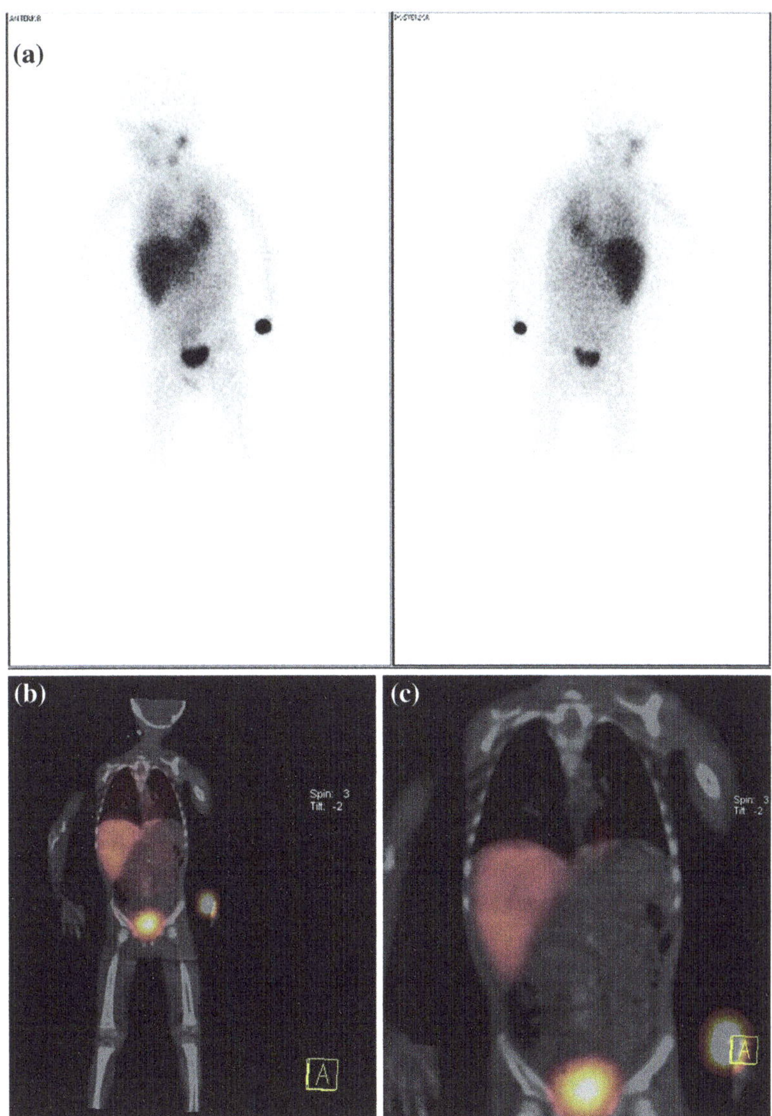

Fig. 72.2 Restaging-favorable response to treatment (chemotherapy). **a** I-123 MIBG whole body. **b**, **c** I-123 MIBG SPECT/CT images: no abnormal uptake is observed

the most appropriate radiopharmaceutical for imaging gastrinomas, providing sensitivity of 75–93 % [7].

Glucagonomas involve tumors that emanate from pancreas and overproduced glucagon, a peptide of significance in glucose metabolism. The symptoms of diabetes, dermatitis, deep venous thrombosis, and depression constitute the clinical syndrome of glucagonoma.

Tumors called VIPomas emanate from the pancreas and over produced VIP, a neuropeptide that leads to vasodilatation. The clinical syndrome known as Verner-Morrison syndrome includes watery diarrhea, hypokalemia and achlorhydria. In-111 pentetreotide for imaging VIPomas generated sensitivity results of 88 % [7].

The efforts made to discover new somatostatin analogs that demonstrate higher affinity for subtypes somatostatin receptors has enriched the nuclear medicine presenting new somatostatin analogs such as DOTA-TOC, DOTA-TATE, DOTANOC as well as new radiopharmaceuticals particularly for PET/CT imaging such as 18F-DOPA, 11C-5-HTP, 68 Ga-DOTATOC/DOTANOC, 68 Ga DOTATATE/DOTATOC, Gluc-Lys([18F]FP)TOCA, 64Cu-TETA OCTREOTIDE.

Apart from the great contribution to diagnosis of neuroendocrine tumors, radiolabeled somatostatin analogs with betta-emitting isotopes such as 90-Y and 177-Lu seem to be encouraging for treatment of patients with inoperable or metastatic neuroendocrine tumors.

References

1. Rubello D, Bui C, Csara D et al (2002) Functional scintigraphy of the adrenal gland. Eur J Endocrinol 147:13–28
2. Patel SM, Lingam RK, Beaconsfield TL et al (2007) Role of radiology in the management of primary aldosteronism. RadioGraphics 27:1145–1157
3. Yen RF, Wu VC, Liu KL et al (2009) 131-I-6β-Iodomathyl-19-Norcholesterol SPECT/CT for primary aldosteronism patients with inconclusive adrenal venous sampling and CT results. J Nucl Med 50:1631–1637
4. Ilias I, Divgi C, Pacak K (2011) Current role of metaiodobenzylguanidine in the diagnosis of pheochromocytoma and medullary thyroid cancer. Semin Nucl Med 41(5):364–367
5. Sharp SE, Shulkin BL, Gelfand MJ et al (2009) 123I-MIBG scintigraphy and 18F-FDG PET in neuroblastoma. J Nucl Med 50:1237–1243
6. Bombardieri E, Aktolun C, Baum RP et al (2003) In-pentetreodite scintigraphy procedure guidelines for tumour imaging. Guidelines Oncol Committee Eur Assoc Nucl Med 1–10
7. Intezo CM, Jabbour S, Lin HC et al (2007) Scintigraphic imaging of body neuroendocrine tumors. Radiographics 27:1355–1369

73 PET/CT Findings in Adrenal Cancer

Alexandra V. Nikaki

73.1 Introduction

Adrenal glands serve as potential sites for secondary infiltration of various cancers. Moreover, primary tumors can arise, either from the cortex or from the medulla of the glands. Single photon emitters with g-camera procedures have long been used for evaluation of primary tumors with high sensitivity and specificity. 18F-FDG-PET/CT has mostly been evaluated as a diagnostic tool in detection of adrenal metastasis, while other positron radiopharmaceutical has been used for the identification and evaluation of disease extend in primary adrenal tumors.

73.2 PET/CT in Evaluation of Adrenal Masses in Cancer and Non-Cancer Patients

Although adrenal masses incidentally discovered in general population are usually benign and diagnosis is usually achieved by CT and MRI, they are common cause of differential diagnostic problems when conventional imaging is indeterminate in non- cancer patients, or when they consist the only site of potential metastasis in cancer patients, usually from non-small cell lung cancer, gastrointestinal tract cancer, and melanoma [1–5]. In the first case scenario, with sensitivity and negative predictive value of up to 100 % [1] PET/CT may be helpful and should be considered [6].

As far as identification and characterization of adrenal masses in cancer patients is concerned, sensitivity, specificity, and accuracy of FDG-PET/CT have been demonstrated to be high (Figs. 73.1, 73.2). Qualitative analyses, using liver [2] or aorta uptake [7], quantitative measurements, using SUVmax cutoff values [2] or target to adjacent tissues and organs ratios, and a variety of interpretive criteria and scanning protocols have been used in order to augment the method's diagnostic capabilities. According to Jana et al. [2] visual interpretation is enough in discriminating benign and malignancy in cancer patients, SUVmax 3.4 was reported to yield 95 % sensitivity and 86 % specificity, while the utility of PET is invaluable for CT indeterminate adrenal lesions . Tumor-to-liver SUV ratio of 1.68, according to Kara et al. [4] corresponds to 90, 91.1, and 90.4 % sensitivity, specificity, and accuracy, respectively. In a meta-analysis of 21 eligible studies, including 1,391 lesions, about the utility of FDG-PET and PET/CT in characterizing adrenal masses as malignant or benign, reported sensitivity, specificity, accuracy, positive, and negative likelihood ratio are 0.97, 0.91, 0.98, 11.1, 0.04, thus demonstrating the unnecessary further exploration of adrenal masses with other imaging techniques [3]. The high negative and positive predictive value, of ~93 %, is, also,

A. V. Nikaki (✉)
Nuclear Medicine Department, Hygeia Hospital, Kallistratous 86, 15771, Zografou Athens, Greece
e-mail: anikaki@gmail.com

A. D. Gouliamos et al. (eds.), *Imaging in Clinical Oncology*,
DOI: 10.1007/978-88-470-5385-4_73, © Springer-Verlag Italia 2014

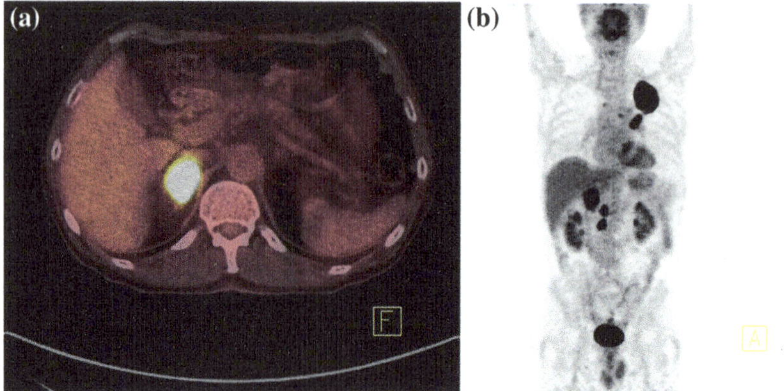

Fig. 73.1 **a**, **b** Adrenal metastasis in a patient with non-small-cell lung cancer- high FDG uptake

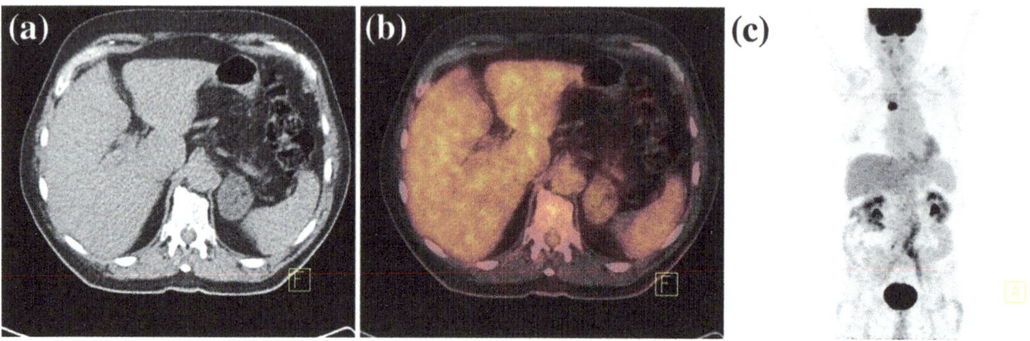

Fig. 73.2 **a**, **b**, **c** Adrenal myelolipoma in a patient with non-small-cell lung cancer—FDG uptake lower than liver uptake

confirmed in a later prospective study [8]. However, it is still questionable whether qualitative or quantitative (using SUVmax and/or SU ratios) is more suitable to be used for the identification of adrenal lesions and although visual analysis is considered adequate [9] perhaps in certain cases, exploitation of all the scanning and interpretation capabilities result in the highest possible diagnostic accuracy. Moreover, mild uptake, equally increased metabolic activity in both adrenal glands and size of less than 1 cm should be dealt with caution, as they might provoke false interpreting results [3, 7]. Lipid- poor and generally benign adrenal adenomas, as well as pheochromocytomas (PCCs) also constitute causes of false positive results [2, 7]. Addition of CT histogram analysis from PET/CT derived data, without the use of any kind of contrast material, in cancer patients, can even improve the, anyway high, diagnostic accuracy of FDG-PET/CT in characterization of adrenal masses [7].

73.3 PET/CT in Primary Tumors' Evaluation

Primary tumors of the adrenal glands arise either from the cortex, called adrenocortical carcinomas (ACC), or from the medulla, the most common being PCC.

PCCs are paragangliomas (PGs) that arise from adrenal medulla and are usually diagnosed by their biochemical- functional profile in addition to a CT scan or MRI that reveal an adrenal mass. I-131 or I-123- MIBG complements further diagnostic approach, while somatostatin receptor scintigraphy has also been used [10]. Apart from the above, current approaching strategies if PCC is suspected may include gene profile expression and specific radiopharmaceutical utilization, according to the mutations detected. Although studies are scattered and patient sample is small in most, several positron emitting radiopharmaceuticals have been used in PCC investigation, summarized in a review of Havekes et al. [10] with F-18-FDOPA, normally not concentrated at the adrenal glands, to present higher diagnostic accuracy in detection of PCCs as compared to I-123-MIBG, although VHL PGs are likely better detected with F-18-FDA. In addition, the above-mentioned PET radiopharmaceuticals can be used for multifocal and metastatic disease detection or exclusion and recurrence assessing [10]. In a small sample of 12 patients with suspected or known relapse of PG, FDOPA-PET was reported superior to I-123-MIBG in assessing the burden of disease and changed therapeutic management in one patient [11]. Positive and negative predictive values of FDOPA-PET for the detection of PCCs-PGs are reported 94 and 85 %, respectively, yielding an accuracy of 91 %, with false results arising one in VHL and one in SDHB, although uptake is not significantly different among the various genotypic tumor mutations [12]. Somatostatin analogues, such as DOTATOC, DOTATATE, and DOTANOC, labeled with positron emitting radionuclides- Ga-68- have also been used for evaluation of metastatic disease [10]. In a prospective study, Naswa et al. [13] demonstrated the superiority of Ga-68-DOTANOC over I-131-MIBG in evaluation of PCCs- PGs, concluding in alteration of therapeutic management of six patients. Evaluating the role of Ga-68-DOTATATE in PCCs- PGs at initial staging and follow-up, the authors proposed the utilization of this radiopharmaceutical in high-risk patients and patients with mutations correlated with familial syndromes [14]. However, during the process of dedifferentiation, tumors may lose their primary molecular characteristics and therefore less specific radiopharmaceutical, such as F18-FDG may be more suitable for usage. In metastatic SDHB associated PGs, FDG was reported to yield the highest sensitivity, up to 100 %, of the modalities used [15]. FDG-PET was also demonstrated to have higher sensitivity, as compared to I-123-MIBG and CT in evaluation of metastatic disease in biochemically established PCCs and PGs, with a specificity of 90.2 % [16].

Adrenocortical carcinoma is a rare tumor, with poor prognosis and high rates of recurrence. Metomidate (MTO), the methyl-ester of etomidate, with its high and specific adrenocortical binding, labeled with the positron emitting radionuclide C-11, has been evaluated in adrenal glands' pathology. Although C-11-MTO-PET could not differentiate between malignancy and benign pathology, reported sensitivity and specificity reach 89 and 96 % compared to histopathologic findings for distinguishing adrenocortical versus non-adrenocortical pathology, while a cutoff ratio of 1.4 of tumor-to-normal gland uptake is associated with a risk of 99.5 % for adrenocortical tumor [17]. Higher SUV values were reported for aldosterone secreting tumors, compared to nonfunctional adenomas and to adrenocortical carcinoma [17, 18]. False negative results were reported for lesions <1 cm and large necrosis [17]. C-11-MTO can serve as complementary to CT and MRI for evaluation of adrenal pathology [18, 19]. Razifar et al. [20] reported improvement of image quality, reduction of image noise, and increase of structure contrast by using principal component analysis – masked volume wise (MVW). Medication, such as adrenal steroid inhibitors and chemotherapeutic agents, may reduce C-11-MTO uptake both in adrenocortical carcinoma lesions and in normal tissues [21]. While C-11-MTO-PET is specific to adrenocortical versus non- adrenocortical pathology evaluation, F-18-FDG-PET has been proposed in discriminating benign versus malignancy in adrenal glands. FDG-PET, with a sensitivity of $\sim$90 %, equal to that of CT, is proposed to be used complementary to CT for detection of recurrent and metastatic adrenocortical carcinoma. High mitotic rate is significantly related to FDG uptake, while FDG-avidity and FDG uptake volume are significantly correlated with overall survival in the same group of patients [22]. However, such correlation of FDG uptake with overall survival in metastatic cancer and with disease-free survival in non-metastatic cancer is not demonstrated in initial staging of adrenocortical carcinoma [23]. The two described radiopharmaceutical may be utilized supplementary, since they answer specific and different clinical questions. Further studies are required until both find their exact position in adrenocortical pathology evaluation.

Imaging modalities used for detection and investigation of neuroblastoma, the most frequent solid extracranial tumor in children, include ultrasound, CT, MRI, bone, and MIBG scintigraphy. Although neuroblastoma tumors usually concentrate FDG, FDG-PET could likely be reserved for non-MIBG avid neuroblastoma and perhaps for early response assessment if baseline FDG-PET showed at least moderate FDG uptake and follow-up [24, 25]. As compared to I-123-MIBG scintigraphy, FDG-PET appears less effective in evaluation of neuroblastoma disease burden, thus cannot replace I-123-MIBG scintigraphy; however, it bears significant prognostic value, since (a) FDG uptake higher than the according MIBG uptake, (b) high tumoral SUVmax, and (c) identification of bone disease in PET is all correlated with lower survival interval in refractory or recurrent neuroblastoma patients going to receive I-131 therapy [26]. F-18-FDOPA has also been evaluated in advanced stage neuroblastoma at initial staging and during follow-up in suspicion of recurrence; the authors reported sensitivity and accuracy of 90 % in a lesion-based analysis, higher than the according of I-123-MIBG, thus proposing FDOPA as potential radiopharmaceutical for neuroblastoma exploration either at initial staging, or at restaging of the disease, as well as in inconclusive MIBG results [27].

73.4 Conclusion

F-18-FDG-PET/CT in evaluation of adrenal glands' tumors is currently widely applied in cancer patients, in search of metastatic adrenal lesions, particularly in non-small cell lung cancer patients; it can, also, be used in non-cancer patients as a complementary tool in cases of inconclusive CT and MRI. Other radiopharmaceuticals, such as FDOPA, Ga-68- somatostatin receptors' analogues have been explored in primary tumors of medulla. C-11-MTO is specific for distinguishing of adrenocortical versus non-adrenocortical pathology. Further research is required so as the above-described positron emitting radiopharmaceutical reach their definite applications.

References

1. Tessonnier L, Sebag F, Palazzo FF et al (2008) Does 18F-FDG PET/CT add diagnostic accuracy in incidentally identified non-secreting adrenal tumours? Eur J Nucl Med Mol Imaging 35(11): 2018–2025
2. Jana S, Zhang T, Milstein DM et al (2006) FDG-PET and CT characterization of adrenal lesions in cancer patients. Eur J Nucl Med Mol Imaging 33(1):29–35
3. Boland GW, Dwamena BA, Jagtiani Sangwaiya M et al (2011) Characterization of adrenal masses by using FDG PET: a systematic review and meta-analysis of diagnostic test performance. Radiology 259(1):117–126
4. Ozcan Kara P, Kara T, Kara Gedik G et al (2011) The role of fluorodeoxyglucose-positron emission tomography/computed tomography in differentiating between benign and malignant adrenal lesions. Nucl Med Commun 32(2):106–112
5. Xu B, Gao J, Cui L et al (2012) Characterization of adrenal metastatic cancer using FDG PET/CT. Neoplasma 59(1):92–99
6. Terzolo M, Stigliano A, Chiodini I et al (2011) AME position statement on adrenal incidentaloma. Eur J Endocrinol 164:851–870
7. Perri M, Erba P, Volterrani D et al (2011) Adrenal masses in patients with cancer: PET/CT characterization with combined CT histogram and standardized uptake value PET analysis. AJR Am J Roentgenol 197(1):209–216
8. Ansquer C, Scigliano S, Mirallié E et al (2010) 18F-FDG PET/CT in the characterization and surgical decision concerning adrenal masses: a prospective multicentre evaluation. Eur J Nucl Med Mol Imaging 37(9):1669–1678
9. Boland GW, Blake MA, Holalkere NS, Hahn PF (2009) PET/CT for the characterization of adrenal masses in patients with cancer: qualitative versus quantitative accuracy in 150 consecutive patients. AJR Am J Roentgenol 192(4):956–962
10. Havekes B, Kathryn King K, Edwin W, Lai EW et al (2010) New imaging approaches to pheochro-

mocytomas and paragangliomas. Clin Endocrinol (Oxf) 72(2):137–145
11. Rufini V, Treglia G, Castaldi P et al (2011) Comparison of 123I-MIBG SPECT-CT and 18F-DOPA PET-CT in the evaluation of patients with known or suspected recurrent paraganglioma. Nucl Med Commun 32(7):575–582
12. Rischke HC, Benz MR, Wild D et al (2012) Correlation of the genotype of paragangliomas and pheochromocytomas with their metabolic phenotype on 3,4-dihydroxy-6-18F-fluoro-L-phenylalanin PET. J Nucl Med 53(9):1352–1358
13. Naswa N, Sharma P, Nazar AH et al (2012) Prospective evaluation of ^{68}Ga-DOTA-NOC PET-CT in phaeochromocytoma and paraganglioma: preliminary results from a single centre study. Eur Radiol 22(3):710–719
14. Maurice JB, Troke R, Win Z et al (2012) A comparison of the performance of ^{68}Ga-DOTATATE PET/CT and ^{123}I-MIBG SPECT in the diagnosis and follow-up of phaeochromocytoma and paraganglioma. Eur J Nucl Med Mol Imaging 39(8):1266–1270
15. Timmers HJ, Kozupa A, Chen CC et al (2007) Superiority of fluorodeoxyglucose positron emission tomography to other functional imaging techniques in the evaluation of metastatic SDHB-associated pheochromocytoma and paraganglioma. J Clin Oncol 25(16):2262–2269
16. Timmers HJ, Chen CC, Carrasquillo JA et al (2012) Staging and functional characterization of pheochromocytoma and paraganglioma by 18F-fluorodeoxyglucose (18F-FDG) positron emission tomography. J Natl Cancer Inst 104(9):700–708
17. Hennings J, Lindhe O, Bergström M et al (2006) [11C]metomidate positron emission tomography of adrenocortical tumors in correlation with histopathological findings. J Clin Endocrinol Metab 91(4):1410–1414
18. Hennings J, Sundin A, Hägg A, Hellman P (2010) 11C-metomidate positron emission tomography after dexamethasone suppression for detection of small adrenocortical adenomas in primary aldosteronism. Langenbecks Arch Surg 395(7):963–967
19. Hennings J, Hellman P, Ahlström H, Sundin A (2009) Computed tomography, magnetic resonance imaging and 11C-metomidate positron emission tomography for evaluation of adrenal incidentalomas. Eur J Radiol 69(2):314–323
20. Razifar P, Hennings J, Monazzam A et al (2009) Masked volume wise principal component analysis of small adrenocortical tumours in dynamic [11C]-metomidate positron emission tomography. BMC Med Imaging 22(9):6
21. Khan TS, Sundin A, Juhlin C et al (2003) 11C-metomidate PET imaging of adrenocortical cancer. Eur J Nucl Med Mol Imaging 30(3):403–410
22. Leboulleux S, Dromain C, Bonniaud G et al (2006) Diagnostic and prognostic value of 18-fluorodeoxyglucose positron emission tomography in adrenocortical carcinoma: a prospective comparison with computed tomography. J Clin Endocrinol Metab 91(3):920–925
23. Tessonnier L, Ansquer C, Bournaud C et al (2013) ^{18}F-FDG uptake at initial staging of the adrenocortical cancers: a diagnostic tool but not of prognostic value. World J Surg 37(1):107–112
24. Boubaker A, Bischof Delaloye A (2003) Nuclear medicine procedures and neuroblastoma in childhood. Their value in the diagnosis, staging and assessment of response to therapy. Q J Nucl Med 47(1):31–40
25. Chawla M, Kumar R, Agarwala Sandeep et al (2010) Role of positron emission tomography-computed tomography in staging and early chemotherapy response evaluation in children with neuroblastoma. Indian J Nucl Med 25(4):147–155
26. Papathanasiou ND, Gaze MN, Sullivan K et al (2011) 18F-FDG PET/CT and 123I-metaiodobenzylguanidine imaging in high-risk neuroblastoma: diagnostic comparison and survival analysis. J Nucl Med 52(4): 519–525
27. Piccardo A, Lopci E, Conte M et al (2012) Comparison of 18F-dopa PET/CT and 123I-MIBG scintigraphy in stage 3 and 4 neuroblastoma: a pilot study. Eur J Nucl Med Mol Imaging 39(1):57–71

Clinical Implications of Adrenal Cancer 74

Paris A. Kosmidis

Metastases are the commonest malignant tumors of the adrenal gland. Metastases can be unilateral or bilateral. Primary adrenal gland malignant tumors are rare and comprise adrenocortical carcinomas (ACCs), pheochromocytomas (PCCs), and paragangliomas (PGs).

74.1 Metastatic Tumors

Adrenal gland is a significant target organ for metastasis in patients known to have cancer i.e., lung. CT is mostly done for initial diagnosis and staging of cancer in different organs and has contributed to the increased incidental finding of an adrenal mass [1, 2]. This is an important finding for the decision-making process. It upgrades the stage of the disease and may change the decision for operation of the primary site. Lately, single metastatic lesion in the adrenal gland from cancers such as lung cancers may be removed with reasonable survival benefit for the patients.

PET-CT scan has facilitated the most accurate diagnosis of malignancy and it is a desirable imaging test to be done prior to surgery. Certainly, in equivocal cases a biopsy in mandatory.

P. A. Kosmidis (✉)
2nd Medical Oncology Department, Hygeia Hospital, 4, Er.Stavrou and Vas Sofias Ave Marousi, 15123, Athens, Greece
e-mail: parkosmi@otenet.gr

CT and/or MRI are very helpful imagine tests for response evaluation following treatment either surgery or chemotherapy and targeted treatment. Reappearance of a mass or progressively increasing mass declares progressive disease.

On the contrary, elimination of the size of the tumor means responsive disease. Unchanged mass declares stable disease. Careful evaluation of the tumor mass density is necessary to identify areas of necrotic tissue within the mass following treatment which is usually compatible with good response.

Ultrasound, CT, and MRI are very accurate and commonly used imagine tests for the follow-up of these patients [1, 2].

74.2 Primary Tumors

CT is the commonest used imagine test for diagnosis, staging, and follow-up of patients with primary adrenal gland tumors. MIBG scanning is a complementary test for staging pheochromocytoma [1, 2].

References

1. Blake MA, Cronin CG, Boland GW (2010) Adrenal Imaging. AJR 194(6): 1450–1460
2. Taffel M, Haji-Manenian S, Nikolaidis P et al (2012) Adrenal imaging: a comprehensive review. Radiol Clin North Am 50(2):219–243

A. D. Gouliamos et al. (eds.), *Imaging in Clinical Oncology*,
DOI: 10.1007/978-88-470-5385-4_74, © Springer-Verlag Italia 2014

75 Introduction to Renal Cancer

Dionysios N. Mitropoulos

Renal cell carcinoma (RCC) is the 3rd most common genitourinary cancer and its rate has increased 2 % per year for the past 65 years. RCCs are usually solitary but may also be multifocal or even bilateral. Many renal tumors are asymptomatic until the late stages of the disease; the classic triad of flank pain, gross haematuria, and palpable abdominal mass is now rare. Paraneoplastic syndromes (hypertension, cachexia, weight loss, pyrexia, neuromyopathy, amyloidosis, elevated sedimentation rate, anaemia, abnormal liver function, hypercalcemia, polycythemia) are found in almost 30 % of symptomatic patients, while a few present with symptoms due to metastatic disease (bone pain or persistent cough) [1, 2]. The rate of incidentally detected tumors has been steadily increasing with the dissemination of imaging, and nowadays exceeds 50 % of all RCCs [1, 2]. The incidentally found tumors are more often smaller and of lower stage [1]. Small renal masses (defined as enhancing tumors <4 cm in diameter) may be indolent, even if malignant; however, not all small renal cancers are biologically less aggressive, and size at presentation does not predict their growth rate if left untreated [1–3].

Following detection, the diagnostic work-up of renal masses has to characterize their cystic or solid nature, to differentiate benign from malignant lesions, and to provide information about the clinical stage of the disease (Table 75.1) [1, 2] in case malignancy is suspected. Cystic renal masses should be classified according to Bosniak [1] and treated accordingly (Table 75.2). For the characterization of solid renal masses the most important criterion is the presence of enhancement on CT or MRI using iodinated or gadolinium contrast media, respectively, depending on renal insufficiency and history of allergies [4]. Criteria for using MRI as a primary or secondary to CT diagnostic tool have to be provided. Reliable characterization of benign renal lesions (i.e., oncocytoma, angiomyolipoma, complex cyst) is of outmost importance since patients could avoid invasive treatment. Percutaneous renal mass core biopsy is being increasingly used in diagnosis, follow-up surveillance, ablative treatments, and in cases of metastatic disease before systemic treatment. Although, in most series, a core biopsy demonstrates high specificity and high sensitivity for the presence of malignancy, it should be noted that 10–20 % of biopsies are nonconclusive [1]. Clinical staging (Table 75.1) should include local extension (size, location, and invasion), evaluation of locoregional lymph nodes, lung and abdominal visceral metastases, and evaluation of venous thrombosis along with delineation of vascular anatomy (the latter is especially helpful when nephron-sparing surgery or

D. N. Mitropoulos (✉)
1st Department of Urology, University of Athens Medical School, 75 Mikras Asias, 115 17, Athens, Greece
e-mail: dmp@otenet.gr

A. D. Gouliamos et al. (eds.), *Imaging in Clinical Oncology*,
DOI: 10.1007/978-88-470-5385-4_75, © Springer-Verlag Italia 2014

Table 75.1 The 2010 TNM classification system of RCC [1, 2]

T—primary tumor	
Tx	Primary tumor cannot be assessed
T_0	No evidence of primary tumor
T_1	Tumor ≤7 cm in greatest dimension, limited to the kidney
T_{1a}	Tumor ≤4 cm in greatest dimension
T_{1b}	Tumor >4 cm but ≤7 cm in greatest dimension
T_2	Tumor >7 cm in greatest dimension, limited to the kidney
T_{2a}	Tumor >7 cm but ≤10 cm in greatest dimension
T_{2b}	Tumor >10 cm in greatest dimension
T_3	Tumor extends into major veins or directly invades adrenal gland or perinephric tissues but not into the ipsilateral adrenal gland and not beyond Gerota's fascia
T_{3a}	Tumor grossly extends into the renal vein or its segmental (muscle-containing) branches or tumor invades perirenal and/or renal sinus (peripelvic) fat but not beyond Gerota's fascia
T_{3b}	Tumor grossly extends into the vena cava below the diaphragm
T_{3c}	Tumor grossly extends into vena cava above the diaphragm or invades the wall of the vena cava
T_4	Tumor invades beyond Gerota's fascia (including contiguous extension into the ipsilateral adrenal gland)
N—Regional lymph nodes	
N_x	Regional lymph nodes cannot be assessed
N_0	No regional lymph node metastasis
N_1	Metastasis in a single regional lymph node
N_2	Metastasis in more than one regional lymph node
M—Distant metastasis	
M_0	No distant metastasis
M_1	Distant metastasis

Table 75.2 The Bosniak classification of renal cysts [1]

Category	Features	Work-up
I	A simple benign cyst with a hairline-thin wall that does not contain septa, calcification, or solid components. It measures water density and does not enhance with contrast material	Benign
II	A benign cyst that may contain a few hairline-thin septa. Fine calcification may be present in the wall or septa. Uniformly high-attenuation lesions of <3 cm, which are sharply marginated and do not enhance	Benign
IIIF	These cysts might contain more hairline-thin septa. Minimal enhancement of a hairline-thin septum or wall can be seen. There may be minimal thickening of the septa or wall. The cyst may contain calcification that might be nodular and thick, but there is no contrast enhancement. There are no enhancing soft-tissue elements. This category also includes totally intrarenal, nonenhancing, high-attenuation renal lesions of >3 cm. These lesions are generally well-marginated	Follow-up. A small proportion are malignant
III	These lesions are indeterminate cystic masses that have thickened irregular walls or septa in which enhancement can be seen	Surgery or follow-up. Malignant in >50 % lesions
IV	These lesions are clearly malignant cystic lesions that contain enhancing soft-tissue components	Surgical therapy recommended. Mostly malignant tumor

ablative treatments are considered). Correct identification of T_4 and further subclassification of T_3 tumors is essential for prognosis and surgical treatment planning. A plain chest X-ray can be sufficient for assessment of the lung in low-risk patients, but chest CT is most sensitive. Brain imaging and bone scanning are recommended only in the presence of symptoms, while PET is rarely recommended [1, 2].

Treatment options for RCC include radical or partial nephrectomy , ablation, and active surveillance. Ipsilateral adrenalectomy is not performed routinely anymore, especially when the preoperative staging shows a normal gland, no suspicious nodule is found intraoperatively, and when there is no direct involvement of the upper pole. Lymph node dissection does not affect survival and can be limited, for staging purposes, to the hilar region or to those which are palpable or have been identified by preoperative imaging. Radical nephrectomy includes en block removal of all the contents of Gerota's fascia. Partial (nephron-sparing) nephrectomy is currently recommended for management of T_1 renal masses when technically feasible [1, 2], and typically includes clamping of the renal artery, although, there have been reports of successful attempts with zero ischemia that have been facilitated by three-dimensional reconstruction of renovascular-tumor anatomy [5]. Recent studies indicate that nephron-sparing surgery confers a survival advantage and a lower risk of severe chronic kidney disease [6]. However, in some patients with localized RCC, nephron-sparing surgery is not suitable because of locally advanced tumor growth, unfavorable location, and significant deterioration of a patient's general health [1, 2]. The anatomic characteristics of organ-confined tumors are used in three preoperative scoring systems (RENAL, PADUA, and C-INDEX) to predict the risk of prolonged warm ischemia or surgical complications after partial nephrectomy [7]. Old (ultrasonography) or novel (near infrared fluorescence imaging after intravenous indocyanine green) technologies can be also used intra-operatively to distinguish renal cortical tumors from normal tissue and to highlight the renal vasculature. Image-guided or not guided ablative treatments (radiofrequency ablation, cryoablation, high-intensity focused ultrasound, microwave, and laser) are used either percutaneously (image-guided) or during laparoscopy [1]. Radiofrequency ablation (RFA) using a needle probe with temperatures up to 105 °C applied in either monopolar or bipolar configuration causes cell death and coagulation necrosis. Hypothermic ablation decreases tissue temperature to −40 °C and results in cell damage attributed to freezing, apoptosis, coagulation necrosis, and immunologic reaction. Microwave, laser, and high-intensity focused ultrasound ablation are still considered experimental. Active surveillance involves careful monitoring for progression and is crucially based on imaging. There are no reports of a correlation between local tumor progression and an increased risk of metastatic disease. It is particularly indicated for elderly or patients unfit for invasive treatments [1].

The intensity of the follow-up program for an individual patient is based on the risk of tumor recurrence and includes evaluation of the chest and the abdomen. Local or distant recurrences may occur in approximately 20–40 % of patients within 5 years after radical nephrectomy, while isolated recurrences in the nephrectomy bed are uncommon. Local recurrences after partial nephrectomy may occur either early (within 6–24 months in patients with locally advanced disease) or late (later than 48 months in patients with localized disease) and are most likely the result of previously undetected multifocal RCC. Assessment of tumor viability could be particularly difficult following application of ablation techniques and imaging changes have to be further studied and characterized [3].

RCC is resistant to conventional chemotherapy and radiotherapy. The evolvement of targeted treatments following the recent advances in cytogenetics and molecular biology of RCC has displaced immunotherapy. Evaluation of the response to systemic therapies is typically on the response evaluation criteria in solid tumors (RECIST) that define the minimum size of measurable lesions, the number of lesions that should be followed, and the use of a one-dimensional measure of disease burden to classify response into complete or partial, stable disease, and progression. However, these criteria may not apply for measuring tumor responses in RCC where shrinkage is probably less important than a decrease in attenuation and other morphology and structure criteria. Moreover, when targeted treatments are given in a neo-adjuvant mode, imaging is essential for the presurgical evaluation of tumor thrombus progression and regression and of structural changes (necrosis, intratumoral nodules) [7].

References

1. Ljungberg B, Cowan NC, Hanbury DC et al (2010) EAU Guidelines on renal cell carcinoma: the 2010 update. Eur Urol 58:398–406
2. Motzer RJ, Agarwal N, Beard C et al (2009) Kidney cancer. J Natl Compr Cancer Netw 7:618–630
3. Stakhovskyi O, Yap SA, Leveridge M et al (2011) Small renal mass: what the urologist needs to know for treatment planning and assessment of treatment results. AJR 196:1267–1273
4. Israel GM, Bosniak MA (2005) How I do it: evaluating renal masses. Radiology 236:441–450
5. Gill IS, Patil MB, Abreu AL et al (2012) Zero ischemia anatomical partial nephrectomy: a novel approach. J Urol 187:807–814
6. Kim SP, Thompson RH, Boorjian SA et al (2012) Comparative effectiveness for survival and renal function of partial and radical nephrectomy for localized renal tumors: a systematic review and meta-analysis. J Urol 188:51–57
7. Chapin BF, Delacoix SE Jr, Wood CG (2011) Renal cell carcinoma: what the surgeon and treating physician need to know. AJR 196:1255–1262

76 US Findings in Renal Cancer

Ioannis A. Tsitouridis and Georgios E. Glataganas

Although ultrasound (US) is not the method of choice for evaluation of the renal cell cancer, it is still the initial and the most frequently used imaging method performed. The majority of asymptomatically diagnosed renal tumors are detected by US. Renal cell carcinoma is found incidentally in 0.18–0.80 % of asymptomatic patients undergoing abdominal US exam [1]. Early detection has led to an improved prognosis for the patients with renal cell carcinoma. Nevertheless, to date the standard method for detection, characterization and staging is the contrast-enhanced computed tomography.

Renal cell carcinoma is a de novo solid tumor but could appear into a cystic lesion or it could be initially cystic [2]. US exam is only occasionally necessary for characterization of the small renal masses, the cystic renal lesions, and venous renal tumor extension. Not infrequently US provides valuable information about the renal cell tumor.

In comparison with the normal renal parenchyma, renal cell tumor may be isoechoic, hypoechoic, and slightly or markedly hyperechoic (Figs. 76.1, 76.2, 76.3, 76.4). Tumors 3 cm or less in diameter were markedly hyperechoic like angiomyolipomas in 32 % of cases and tumor larger than 3 cm were markedly hyperechoic only in 2 % of cases [3].

Areas of necrosis, hemorrhage, fibrosis abscess, or calcification within the mass may alter the sonographic appearance of renal cell carcinoma.

The specific indications for the sonographic study include:

(a) the evaluation of the small renal masses,
(b) the detection of the pseudocapsule in renal cell carcinoma,
(c) the characterization of complex cystic renal masses,
(d) Venous renal tumor extension.

76.1 Small Renal Masses

Approximately 30 % of all renal cell tumors detected on US are 3 cm or less in diameter [4].

Although the majority of renal cell carcinomas attain large size before they are detected, small renal cell tumors, (smaller than 3 cm) are also under consideration, because many of them reveal an aggressive behavior.

Lesions 3 cm or smaller reveal extension of the tumor beyond the renal capsule (T3/T4) in 38 % of cases and a high nuclear grade (Fuhrman grade 3 or 4) in 28 % of cases [5].

Comparison studies of CT and US show that CT depicts more and smaller masses (75 % of masses 10–15 mm in size and 100 % of masses

I. A. Tsitouridis (✉) · G. E. Glataganas
Department of Radiology, General Hospital Papageorgiou, Thessaloniki, Ring Road Thessaloniki Efkarpia, 685111 Thessaloniki, Greece
e-mail: tsitouridis.1@gmail.com

G. E. Glataganas
e-mail: gialim@hol.gr

A. D. Gouliamos et al. (eds.), *Imaging in Clinical Oncology*,
DOI: 10.1007/978-88-470-5385-4_76, © Springer-Verlag Italia 2014

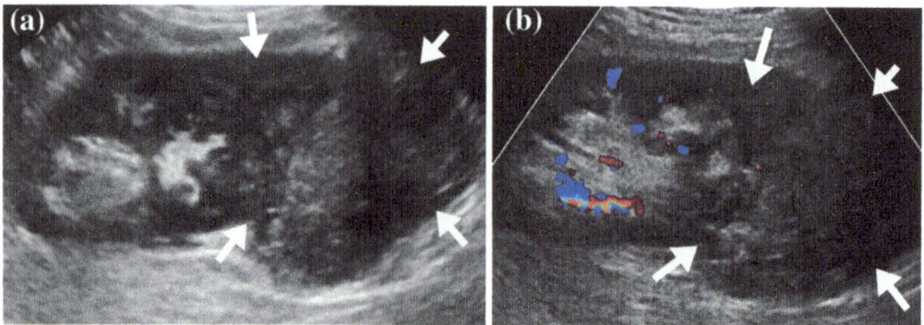

Fig. 76.1 **a**, **b** Sagittal sonograms of the left kidney. In the lower renal pole there is a large renal cancer with mixed echogenicity (*arrows*)

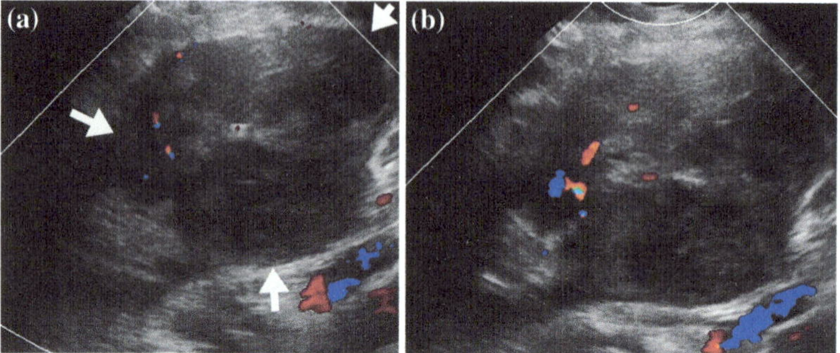

Fig. 76.2 **a**, **b** Sagittal sonograms of the left kidney. In the lower renal pole there is a large renal cancer with mixed echogenicity (*arrows*)

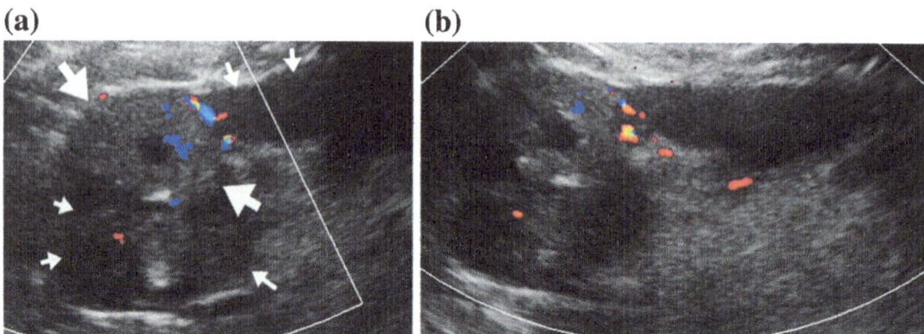

Fig. 76.3 **a**, **b** Sagittal sonograms of the left kidney (*small arrows*). In the periphery of the upper renal pole there is a slightly echogenic renal tumor with echopoor central area due to hemorrhage (*large arrows*)

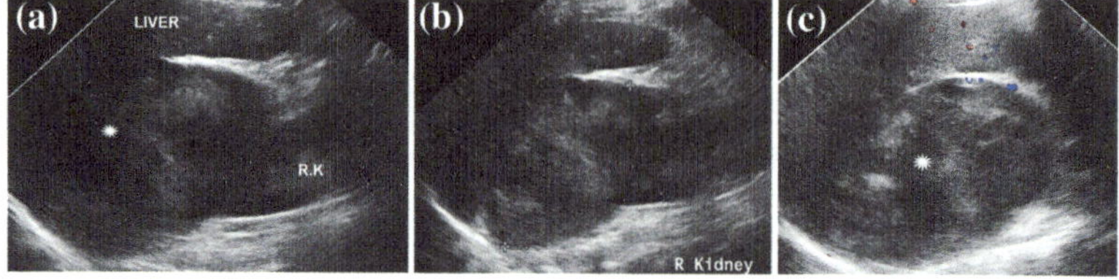

Fig. 76.4 **a**, **b** Oblique sagittal gray scale sonograms and **c** oblique axial color Doppler sonogram of the right kidney, which reveals in the upper pole a slightly echogenic tumor (*arrows*), with subcapsular hemorrhage (*asterisk*)

Fig. 76.5 **a**, **b** Axial and **c** sagittal color Doppler sonograms which reveal a small partially exophytic tumor (*arrows*), in the upper pole of the right kidney

15–20 mm) than US (28 % of tumors 10–15 mm in size and 58 % of masses 15–20 mm), [6].

The advantage of US includes its ability to distinguish cystic from solid lesion with limitation to the detection of small noncontour-deforming masses, small isoechoic intraparenchymal tumors, and tumors of polar origin with extrarenal growth.

This is quite useful for the very small renal carcinomas—smaller than 8–10 mm, because CT has limitation to the characterization of hypoattenuation in these masses in which pseudoenhancement may also be a problem.

Color Doppler US exam and US contrast agents provide subtle increase in the detection rate of small renal tumors. Renal blood vessels outside an isoechoic small tumor give rise to a vascular rim around the tumor which becomes more obvious (Figs. 76.5, 76.6, 76.7).

76.2 Detection of Pseudocapsule in Renal Cell Carcinoma

When such a pseudocapsule in a renal cell carcinoma exists, nephron sparing surgery is possible. The pseudocapsule is composed of fibrous tissue and compressed renal parenchyma [7].

High resolution sonography or older US machines using contrast-specific agents which improve sonographic visualization can detect this pseudocapsule as echogenic peripheral zone or line in 85.7 % of cases (Fig. 76.8) [7].

76.3 Characterization of Complex Cystic Renal Masses

In comparison to CT and MRI a major advantage of US is its ability in the evaluation of cystic lesions, because blood and fluid with high protein content may change the density in CT or the MR signal in MRI or may obscure some small intracystic papillary projections.

Partial volume effect is also very common in CT and MRI imaging and because of this effect, very thin septa are not available for detection.

Renal cell carcinomas with cystic degeneration due to massive necrosis have internal degenerative tissue components. US usually shows inhomogeneous fluid content with internal echoes suggestive of malignancy [4].

Contrast-enhanced US might better visualize intratumoral septa (number, thickness) or solid components [8].

In the majority of cases the role of US is limited to the evaluation of minimally complicated cysts to rule out a cystic tumor, while all the other complex cystic masses require evaluation with contrast-enhanced CT or MRI (Fig. 76.9) [9].

76.4 Extension into the Renal Vein or Inferior Vena Cava

This is the main criterion to the corresponding stage T3b and T3c of TNM staging system. US is performed to evaluate stage T3b and T3c only

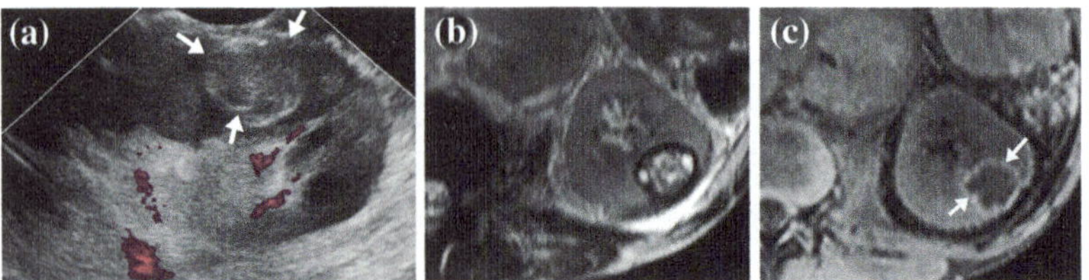

Fig. 76.6 **a** Sagittal color Doppler sonogram of the left kidney which reveals a small solid renal tumor in the lower renal pole (*arrows*). **b**, **c** Axial T2WI and T1WI post contrast MRI scans which shows the tumor with a peripheral capsule (*arrows*)

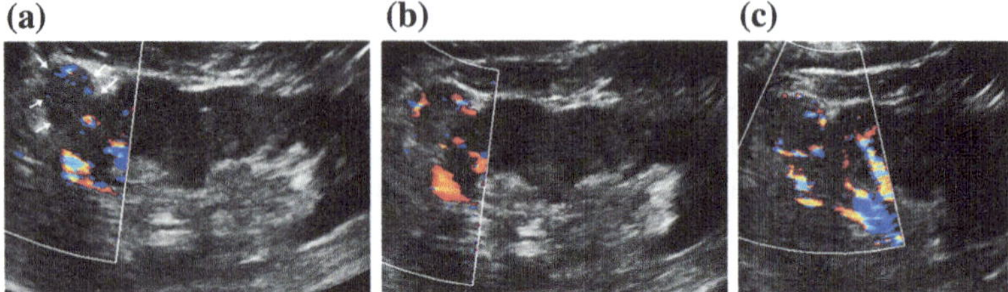

Fig. 76.7 **a**, **b** Sagittal and **c** oblique axial color Doppler sonograms of the left kidney. In the upper renal pole there is a small solid renal tumor (*arrows*) with rich vascularity

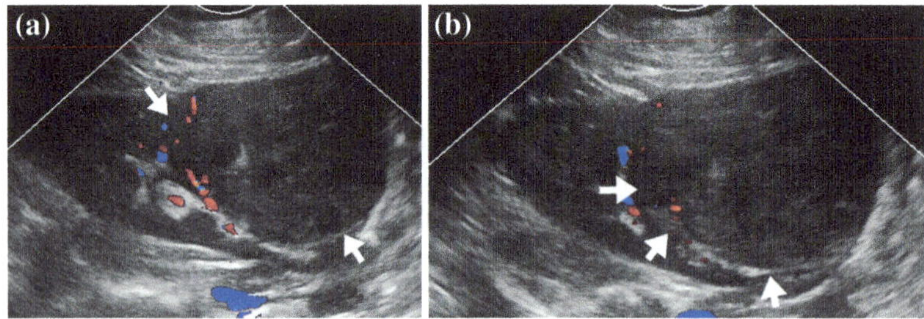

Fig. 76.8 **a**, **b** Sagittal color Doppler sonograms of the left kidney which reveals clearly a pseudocapsule in the periphery of a large sized tumor (*arrows*) in the lower renal pole

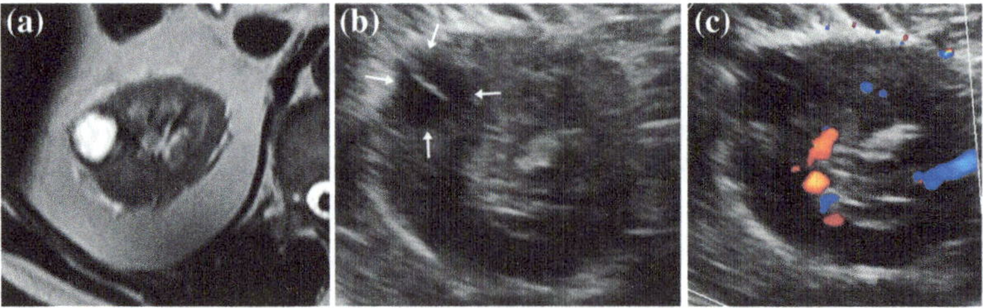

Fig. 76.9 **a** Axial T2WI MRI scan which reveals a complicated cyst with irregular internal margins, a peripheral capsule and internal inhomogeneous composition. **b**, **c** Axial gray scale and color Doppler sonograms which show the small cortical complicated cyst without any evidence of tumor behavior

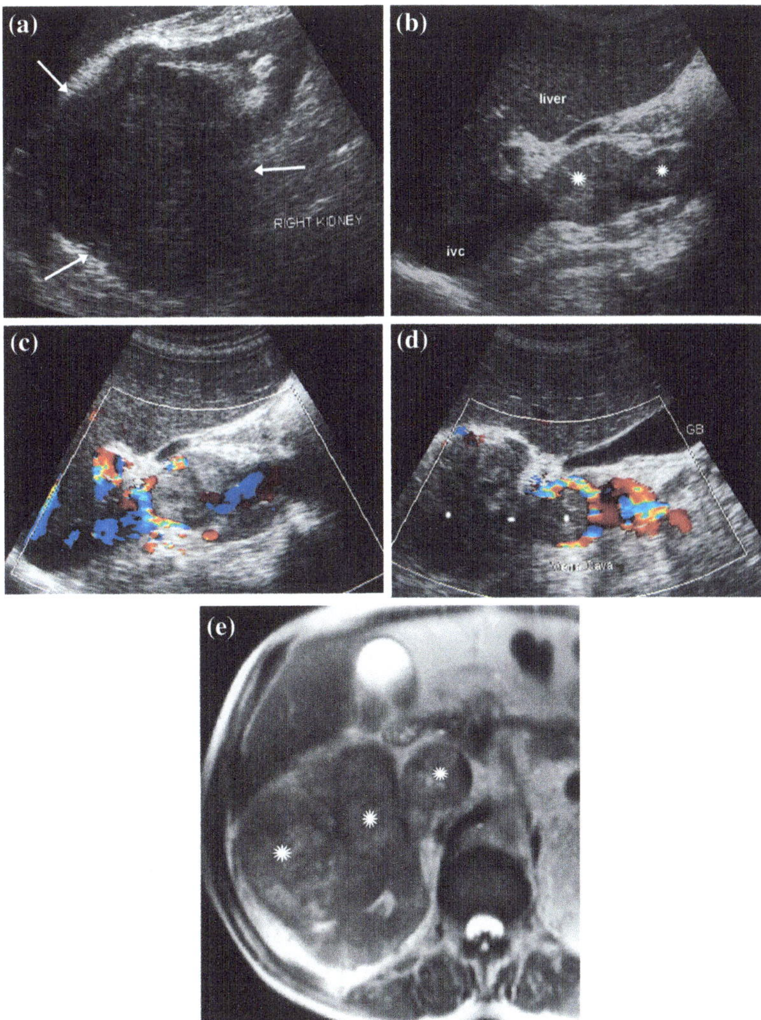

Fig. 76.10 **a** Oblique sagittal gray scale sonogram of the right kidney which reveals a large tumor in the upper renal pole (*arrows*). **b**, **c** Sagittal gray scale and color doppler sonograms of the inferior vena cava (*ivc*), which show the tumor invasion of ivc (*asterisk*), and **d**, **e** Axial color Doppler sonogram and axial T2WI MRI scan which show the tumor and the invasion of the ivc (*asterisk*)

when CT findings are equivocal, because overlying bowel gas precludes adequate visualization or obscure completely the renal vessels (especially the left renal vein), the retroperitoneum and the infrahepatic portion of inferior vena cava (Fig. 76.10).

A venous tumor extension was usually seen as an intravascular mass with echotexture similar to the corresponding renal cancer [10].

US is not the appropriate imaging method to stage renal cell carcinoma because is not accurate for the evaluation of:

- Tumor size of the large-sized tumors
- Perinephric tumor extension
- Local and regional lymph node enlargement
- Spread into contiguous organs
- Local or distant metastatic spread.

References

1. Levine E, King BF (2000) Adult malignant renal parenchymal neoplasms. In: Pollack HM, McClennan BL (eds) Clinical urography. Saunders, Philadelphia, pp 1440–1559
2. Feldberg MAM, Von Waes FGM (1982) Multilocular cystic renal cell carcinoma. AJR 138: 953–955
3. Forman HP, Middleton WD, Melson GL et al (1993) Hyperechoic renal cell carcinomas: increase in detection at US. Radiology 188:431–434

4. Helenon O, Correas JM (2006) Ultrasound and Doppler in kidney cancer. In: Gueimazi A (ed) Imaging of kidney cancer. Springer, Berlin Heidelberg, pp 15–28
5. Hsu RM, Chan DY, Siegelman SS (2004) Small renal cell carcinomas: correlation of size with tumor stage, nuclear grade and histologic subtype. AJR 182:551–557
6. Jamis-Dow CA, Choyke PL, Jennings SB et al (1996) Small ($\leq$3 cm) renal masses: detection with CT versus US and pathologic correlation. Radiology 198:785–788
7. Ascenti G, Gaeta M, Magno C et al (2004) Contrast-Enhanced second-harmonic sonography in the detection of pseudocapsule in renal cell carcinoma. AJR 182: 1525–1530
8. Park BK, Kim B, Kim SH et al (2007) Assessment of cystic renal masses based on Bosniak classification: comparison of CT and contrast-enhanced US. Eur J Radiol 61:310–314
9. Ascenti G, Mazzioti S, Zimbaro G et al (2007) Complex cystic renal masses: characterization with contrast-enhanced US. Radiology 243(1):158–165
10. Schwerk WB, Schwerk WN, Rodeck G (1985) Venous renal tumor extension: a prospective US evaluation. Radiology 156:491–495

CT and MRI Findings in Renal Cancer 77

Fotios D. Laspas

77.1 Introduction

Renal masses are very common and in some cases may represent a challenging diagnostic and clinical problem. With the expanding use of imaging methods in the abdomen, the vast majority of renal masses are discovered incidentally. Fortunately, most of these are cysts that do not require any further management. However, if a renal mass is not obviously a simple cyst, it becomes critical to differentiate between a complex but probably benign lesion, which can be observed, and a potentially malignant lesion, which require surgical intervention. Therefore, the proper evaluation of these masses is key to appropriate management.

77.2 Detecting and Characterization

With recent advances in imaging technology the diagnosis of most renal lesions is usually straightforward and renal cell carcinoma (RCC) can be diagnosed with high accuracy (better than 95 %) [1]. Multidetector CT remains the most widely available and primary imaging modality for detecting and characterization of renal lesions. The optimal scanning protocol should include unenhanced CT through the kidneys followed by imaging during the corticomedullary through the liver and kidneys and nephrographic phases of the entire abdomen. Excretory phase is occasionally helpful. The nephrographic phase is the most sensitive for detecting renal masses (almost all renal masses have lower attenuation than the homogeneously enhancing surrounding normal renal tissue) [2]. The role of MRI in the evaluation of renal masses is ever increasing. The use of advanced MRI techniques such as diffusion-weighted imaging and ADC measurements has increased the diagnostic capability of the method in assessing renal masses [3]. Therefore, MRI can be used when the CT findings are nondiagnostic. Furthermore, MRI can be used when optimal CT cannot be performed, as in the case of compromised renal function, severe iodinated contrast allergy or pregnancy where radiation exposure is a problem.

Renal masses can be broadly categorized into cystic or solid appearing lesions. The most important feature which differentiates a solid mass from a cystic lesion is the presence of enhancement after intravenous contrast agent (Fig. 77.1). A change of >20 HU is definite enhancement, while a difference of <10 HU between pre- and postcontrast CT scan is regarded as insignificant and a renal mass that enhances between 10 and 20 HU is indeterminate and needs further assessment for definitive characterization. The presence of enhancement

F. D. Laspas (✉)
CT&MRI Department, "Hygeia" Hospital,
4, Erythrou Stavrou Str. & Kifisias Av,
15123 Athens, Attica, Greece
e-mail: fotisdimi@yahoo.gr

A. D. Gouliamos et al. (eds.), *Imaging in Clinical Oncology*,
DOI: 10.1007/978-88-470-5385-4_77, © Springer-Verlag Italia 2014

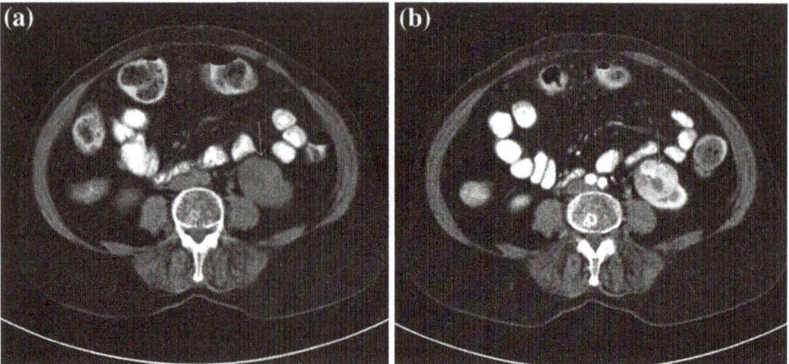

Fig. 77.1 Axial CT scans *before* (**a**) and *after* (**b**) intravenous contrast agent administration in a 54-year-old patient show a 2.8 cm enhancing mass in the left kidney. The lesion is found to be a renal cell carcinoma

at MRI cannot be measured easily and usually is assessed subjectively.

Cystic renal masses are composed predominantly of spaces filled with fluid. At imaging, these fluid-filled spaces have the characteristics of fluid (low-attenuation between 0 and 20 HU on CT and hyperintensity on T2W sequences similar to cerebral spinal fluid) and do not enhance after contrast agent administration. The Bosniak renal cyst classification is a worldwide and useful guide to the diagnosis and management of cystic renal masses (Fig. 77.2). This classification system was developed and based on only CT findings; nevertheless it is recently used in MRI interpretation (although cyst wall calcification is not well appreciated on MR images).

Solid renal masses consist predominantly of enhancing tissue. Although any solid mass in the kidney should be considered a RCC, benign lesions also may enhance. The presence of fat in a solid mass is of great importance, as its presence has long been considered diagnostic for angiomyolipoma (Fig. 77.3). Intralesional fat can be easily detected by CT using density measurement and by MRI using fat-suppression techniques. However, approximately 4.5 % of angiomyolipomas are fat-poor (no demonstrable fat on CT or MRI) and the imaging differentiation from RCC is impossible [2]. Moreover, there have been a few cases of fat-containing renal lesions that appeared to be RCC; most of them also contained calcifications [4]. Since angiomyolipomas rarely contain calcification, the presence of calcification in a lesion (even if macroscopic fat is seen on unenhanced images) indicates that RCC must be considered likely. In such cases, because the accuracy of MRI in detecting calcifications is relatively low, it is important always to assess CT examination of the patient (which will likely has been performed in most cases). Oncocytoma is the most common benign, solid, non-fat-containing renal

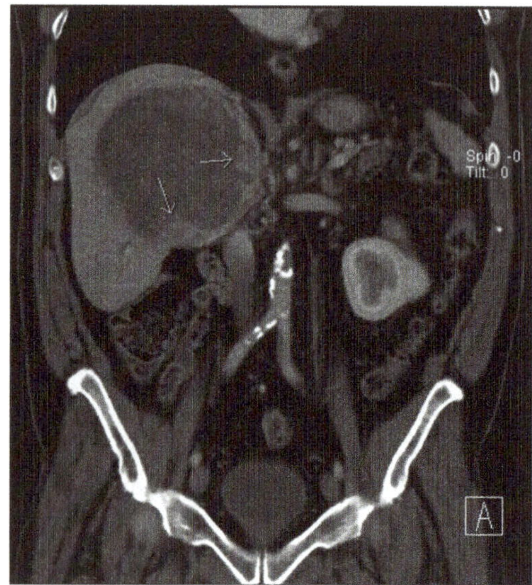

Fig. 77.2 Coronal multiplanar reconstruction (*MPR*) contrast-enhanced CT image shows a large cystic right renal lesion that contains distinct enhancing soft-tissue components (*arrows*), a finding consistent with a category IV cystic mass

mass. Although some imaging characteristics (homogeneous enhancement and central scar at CT or MR) are suggestive of oncocytoma, they may also be seen in RCC, and therefore the two entities are indistinguishable by imaging alone and a tissue diagnosis is needed. Silverman et al. [5] support that there is a direct relationship between malignancy and the size of the mass (the smaller the renal mass, the greater the incidence of benign lesions) and this must be taken into account when considering treatment options. Therefore, they support that it is reasonable to observe a solid mass less than 1 cm in diameter (which is usually difficult to be characterized) with CT or MR at 3–6 months and 12 months followed by yearly examinations.

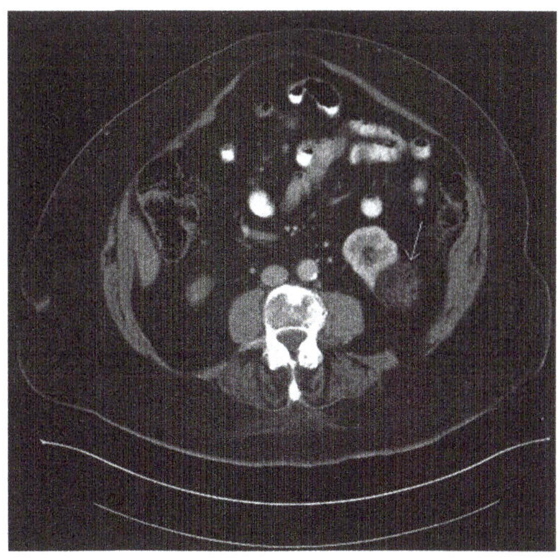

Fig. 77.3 Axial contrast-enhanced CT image shows fat attenuation within the renal lesion (*arrow*), a finding indicative of an angiomyolipoma

77.3 Staging

Since RCC is relatively resistant to both radiotherapy and chemotherapy and the only curative treatment remains complete surgical excision of the tumor, preoperative imaging is critical for appropriate treatment decisions providing important anatomic information to the surgeon. Staging is usually performed using multidetector CT, although MRI is equally accurate in staging of the primary tumor. MRI may be helpful when questions related to the staging of RCC are left unanswered at CT and also is used in patients who cannot undergo CT scanning with intravenous iodinated contrast agent.

Evaluation of perinephric tumor extension is the most common cause of imaging staging errors, as it is difficult to discriminate from nonspecific perinephric stranding from edema or previous inflammation. Moreover, both CT and MRI cannot reliably detect microscopic invasion of the perinephric fat. The reported sensitivity and specificity for predicting extension of tumor into the perinephric fat are 84 and 95 %, respectively [2]. Diagnosis of perinephric extension does not affect management, when the patient is candidate for radical nephrectomy (en block resection of all the contents of Gerota's fascia), but this is a key point if partial nephrectomy is considered (currently recommended for management of T1 renal masses). Moreover, due to increasing application of modern imaging modalities, the number of small incidentally detected renal tumors (at an earlier stage) is increasing and nephron-sparing surgical techniques have been advocated. Three-dimensional CT helps in preoperative evaluation of patients for partial nephrectomy defining the precise location of the renal mass, the depth of renal parenchymal invasion, and relationship of the tumor to the collecting system and the renal vessels.

Evaluation of the venous invasion, which is very important for the surgical approach, is well appreciated on cross-sectional imaging modalities (Fig. 77.4). For differentiation between clot and tumor thrombus, postcontrast images are required (the tumor thrombus enhances). Moreover, invasion of the inferior vena cava wall is important information for the surgeon. MRI is considered to be superior to CT in the assessment of the inferior vena cava wall invasion, although the accuracy of MRI has not yet been well documented [4].

Evaluation of ipsilateral adrenal gland invasion is important because the current trend is to spare the ipsilateral adrenal gland when it is assessed as normal at the preoperative imaging investigation. Direct RCC invasion outside the

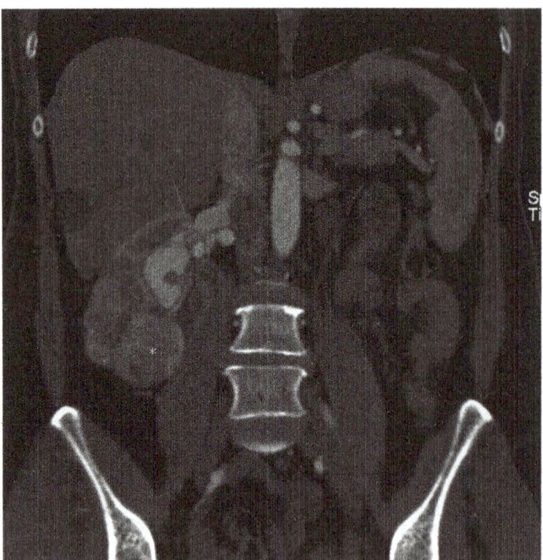

Fig. 77.4 Coronal multiplanar reconstruction (*MPR*) contrast-enhanced CT image in a 61-year-old woman shows a right renal lesion (asterisk). Moreover, a small filling defect (*arrow*) is seen within the right renal vein, a finding consistent with venous invasion

Gerota fascia into adjacent organs is well shown (focal change in attenuation or signal intensity within a neighboring organ), but it may not be possible to be proven (loss of fat planes between the tumor and surrounding organs raise the possibility of direct infiltration, but not always is confirmed surgically).

Both CT and MRI diagnosis of lymph node involvement is based on lymph node size (short-axis diameter larger than 1 cm). Although both methods are very effective in detection of lymph node enlargement, the limitation of using size criteria for detecting lymphatic metastases is well known. High false positive rates have been reported as malignant lymphadenopathy cannot be differentiated from nodal enlargement due to reactive hyperplasia [2]. Except from retroperitoneal lymph node involvement, mediastinal nodal involvement is also a frequent finding in patients with RCC as the lymphatic drainage of the kidneys is highly variable [6].

Distant RCC metastases are generally easy to identify with CT or MRI. Hematogenous metastases most commonly occur to the lungs, liver, bones, and brain, but essentially to any organ. CT is the ideal method for identifying hematogenous spread to lungs. Some authors still recommend that chest radiography can be sufficient for assessment of the lungs in low-risk groups (small tumors, T1) of metastatic disease, despite the fact it is far less sensitive than chest CT [6]. Both CT and MRI are sensitive techniques for the detection of liver metastases. Since RCC metastases are often hypervascular (like the primary tumor), hepatic metastases are most noticeable on scans obtained during the arterial phase. Brain imaging (CT or MRI) and bone scanning are generally performed only in the presence of symptoms and signs suggesting disease at these sites. Concerning cerebral metastases MRI is more sensitive for the detection of smaller lesions than CT. As bone metastases from RCC show variable uptake on bone scintigraphy, it may be limited in detecting the typical osteolytic bone metastases from RCC (the accuracy of bone scintigraphy in RCC varies from 10 to 60 %) [6]. Correlation with CT is helpful. MRI performs better for bone lesion characterization, but it is not used routinely [6].

77.4 Follow-up Evaluation-Response to Therapy

Multiple prognostic factors have been reported in the literature to predict RCC prognosis, however, the stage of the tumor at the time of presentation is the most important determinant of recurrent disease. The intensity of the follow-up program for an individual patient is primarily dependent on disease stage. More intensive surveillance is needed for patients who are at high risk for tumor recurrence. RCC recurrence may occur in the nephrectomy bed (local recurrence) or appears as distant metastases (most commonly in the lungs). CT offers the simplest way to assess RCC recurrence, while MRI is mainly used as a problem solving tool. Local recurrence manifests as an enhancing solid mass at the nephrectomy site (Fig. 77.5) with or without central necrosis. As during staging, brain imaging and bone scintigraphy are generally justified only in the presence of symptoms. The surveillance strategy after

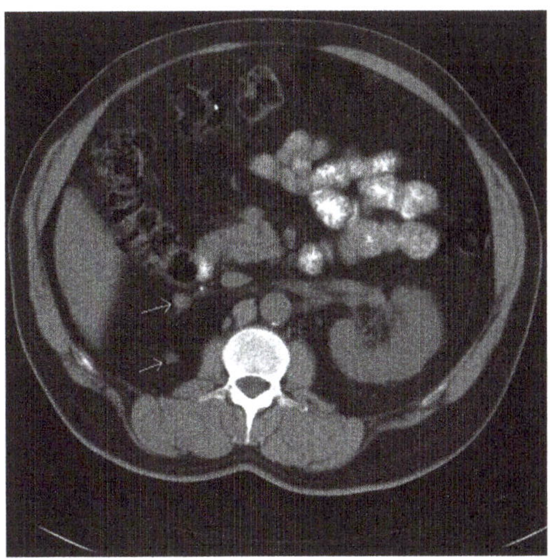

Fig. 77.5 68-year-old man who underwent right nephrectomy for renal carcinoma. Two years later, he developed two enhancing nodules (*arrows*) at the nephrectomy bed. Biopsy revealed recurrent tumor

nephron-sparing surgery is similar, except that greater consideration should particularly be given to the remnant kidney. Careful follow-up is also needed for patients who have undergone ablation treatment. After effective ablation, the tumor shows increased density on the unenhanced studies and does not enhance. The fat halo sign is a common postablation finding surrounding the ablated tumor. Any enhancement within the ablation zone on CT or MRI is a reliable sign of incomplete ablation or recurrence. A change in size is not an indicator of treatment efficacy [7].

Conventional disease response evaluation in patients with metastatic RCC was based on measurements of change in size. However, using size change in response criteria may be inadequate to new antiangiogenic agents, which show clinical benefit without tumor regression. To improve assessment of response to therapy in metastatic RCC, decrease in attenuation and reduced enhancement of target lesions should also be evaluated [7].

77.5 Conclusion

CT remains the mainstay of imaging in the detecting, characterizing, staging, and surveillance of renal lesions. MRI is increasingly used as a problem solving tool. Advanced MRI techniques such as diffusion-weighted imaging are being explored in investigating of renal lesions.

References

1. Barker DW, Zagoria RJ (2006) Renal cell carcinoma. In: Ali Guermazi (ed) Imaging of kidney cancer (medical radiology/diagnostic imaging). Springer, Berlin Heidelberg, pp 103–123
2. Leveridge MJ, Bostrom PJ, Koulouris G et al (2010) Imaging renal cell carcinoma with ultrasonography, CT and MRI. Nat Rev Urol 7(6):311–325
3. Wang H, Cheng L, Zhang X et al (2010) Renal cell carcinoma: diffusion-weighted MR imaging for subtype differentiation at 3.0 T. Radiology 257(1):135–143
4. Nikken JJ, Krestin GP (2007) MRI of the kidney-state of the art. Eur Radiol 17(11):2780–2793
5. Silverman SG, Israel GM, Herts BR et al (2008) Management of the incidental renal mass. Radiology 249(1):16–31
6. Patel U, Sokhi H (2012) Imaging in the follow-up of renal cell carcinoma. AJR 198(6):1266–1276
7. Murphy G, Jhaveri K (2011) The expanding role of imaging in the management of renal cell carcinoma. Expert Rev Anticancer The 11(12):1871–1888

78 PET/CT Findings in Renal Cancer

Alexandra V. Nikaki

78.1 Introduction

The incidence of renal carcinoma (RCC) at all stages is rising, with clear cell histologic type being the commonest [1]. However, it has been reported that 15 % of small renal masses are benign [2]. Partial or total nephrectomy is the current treatment for RCC. Contrast-enhanced computed tomography (CECT)-renal protocol [3] is the imaging modality of choice in detection and differentiation of solid renal masses versus cystic ones, even small ones of size <2 cm, however, it faces certain limitations consisting of its lower ability to differentiate between benign and malignant lesions, as well as indolent from aggressive phenotype [2, 3]. The role of magnetic resonance imaging (MRI) is currently mostly restricted to characterization of equivocal computed tomography (CT) findings, evaluation of perirenal fat and venous cava thrombosis. The urge of functional characterization of renal masses has brought the utilization of PET/CT at the foreground [2, 3].

A. V. Nikaki (✉)
Nuclear Medicine Department, Hygeia Hospital, Kallistratous 86, 15771 Zografou, Athens, Greece
e-mail: anikaki@gmail.com

78.2 18F-FDG-PET

78.2.1 Renal Mass Characterization and Initial Staging

Although FDG-PET has an established or promising role in initial staging and restaging of the majority of malignances, results are less optimal when renal masses are validated. Primarily, physiologic renal excretion of the radiopharmaceutical and secondary, inflammatory processes can provoke false positive results. Moreover, the variable degree of FDG uptake by the renal masses, as well as the spatial resolution of PET scanners can mislead to false negative diagnosis [2, 4].

Studies concerning the exploration of the value of FDG-PET imaging procedure in initial staging and restaging patients with renal cancer are only scattered, occupying a small sample of patients and the majority of them reveal no or little added information as compared to conventional imaging procedures. Reported sensitivity varies between 32 and 100 % and 47–75 % for renal cell carcinoma diagnosis and staging, respectively [2, 4].

First promising results for utilization of FDG-PET in exploration and characterization of RCC, with a reported sensitivity of 94 % [5], equal to that of CT, was not verified in more recent studies, although it should be mentioned that studies are subjected to referral bias, since most

A. D. Gouliamos et al. (eds.), *Imaging in Clinical Oncology*,
DOI: 10.1007/978-88-470-5385-4_78, © Springer-Verlag Italia 2014

patients were only referred to PET examination, if they were to be treated with surgical excision after CT and/or MRI indication [3, 5–7]. Aide et al. [6] demonstrated the high number of false negative PET examinations in evaluating suspicious renal masses, thus reporting a sensitivity of 47 %, however a high specificity (80 %), and the discordance between high FDG uptake by small low-grade renal malignances and low FDG uptake by large high- grade renal malignances, although the median size of visualized tumors was actually higher than that of nonvisualized ones. The last was also confirmed by Ozulker et al. [7] reporting an average 8.3 ± 4.3 cm of FDG-PET visualized tumors versus 3.5 ± 1.3 for nonvisualized ones; however, the authors also reported statistically significant higher Fuhrman grade in visualized tumors as compared to nonvisualized malignances. Reported accuracy was 50 %.

FDG-PET is reported to have a good sensitivity in characterizing the extent of disease, especially in detecting distant metastasis, thus showing higher accuracy than CT, concerning, more frequently, bone [6, 8, 9] and adrenal metastasis [6], renal vein and inferior vena cava infiltration, and tumor thrombus [7]. Advanced local disease, lymph node assessment, and predominantly distant metastasis are well identified by FDG-PET with higher sensitivity than CT and bone scintigraphy, thus concluding in alteration of patients' management in 9–13 % of cases, or even more according to more optimistic studies [5–9]. FDG avidity in metastatic lesions is demonstrated to be higher as compared to the primary site of the tumor, possibly indicating different biology and GLUT expression [3, 8]. Sensitivities in detecting metastatic disease range between 64 and 100 %, more closely to 100 % (for a review see Lawrentschuk et al. [4]). False results may occur in oncocytomas [5, 7]. Sensitivity could, likely, be improved by delayed imaging or with the use of diuretics, however, results are conflict and further investigation needs to be carried out.

High SUVmax either at the primary or at the metastatic foci, as well as increased number of FDG- avid lesions before treatment in metastatic or recurrent RCC patients has been reported to have prognostic significance and to be correlated with reduced overall survival [10, 11].

18F-FDG-PET has been investigated in small sample of pediatric population with Wilms tumor and was reported to correctly identify the primary site of the tumor and lymph node invasion and to rule out distant metastasis, and although it could be suitable for imaging Wilms tumor, it does not actually offer added information [12].

78.2.2 Relapse and Evaluation of Treatment Response

The role of FDG-PET is perhaps more decisive in the evaluation of possible renal bed recurrence or metastatic disease in restaging patients with renal cell carcinoma, especially considering the post-treatment changes that may influence CT interpretation. Regarding that FDG-PET is not subject to such alterations, it has been found accurate and useful in this portion of patients. Reported sensitivity is as high as 81–100 % [5, 13–16]. Specificity and accuracy according to Nakatani et al. [13] is 71 and 79 % respectively, while prognosis was better for PET negative patients. Lymph node invasion, local relapse, and adrenal metastasis were identified. During surveillance, Park et al. [14] demonstrated positive and negative predictive value of FDG-PET 77.3 and 92.6 %, respectively, with an overall accuracy of 85.7 in evaluating possible recurrence and metastatic disease; however, the reported results did not overweight those of other conventional modalities (Fig. 78.1a–e).

Apart from radical or partial nephrectomy, current therapeutic strategies for renal cancer, especially in advanced or recurrent cases, include tyrosine kinase inhibitors which target VEGF signaling and targeting mTOR. However, these approaches do not result, at least initially, in massive tumor shrinkage and size changes, since they act more as cytostatics rather than cytotoxics [3]. On the other hand it would be of great importance to determine which patients

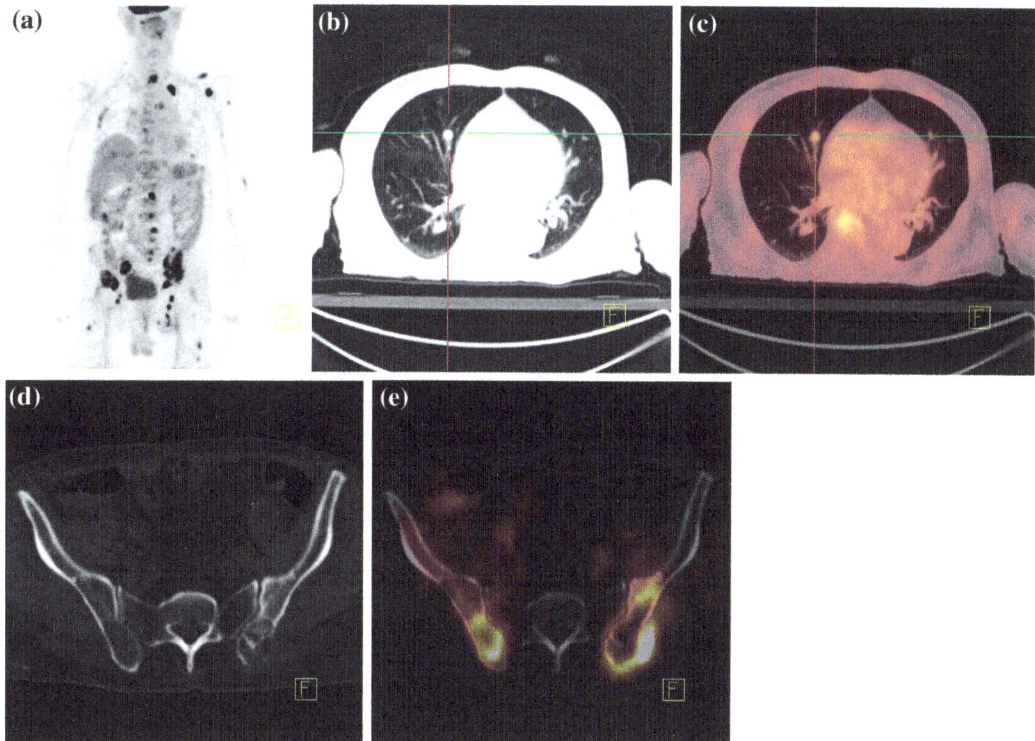

Fig. 78.1 **a** 18F-FDG-PET- MIP imaging reveals multiple metastatic lesions in a patient with renal carcinoma, who underwent surgical resection of the left kidney and had received multiple schemes of chemo and targeted therapy. **b**, **c** Nodule at the *right lung* (**b**) with 18F-FDG uptake (**c**), indicative of pulmonary metastasis. **d**, **e** Osseous distortion at CT imaging (**d**) with high 18F-FDG uptake at PET (**e**), compatible with osseous secondary invasion

mostly benefit from targeted therapies. FDG-PET has been evaluated in assessment of renal cell cancer response to tyrosine kinase inhibitors—sunitinib and sorafenib—and correlation with overall survival has been reported. Ueno et al. [17], in their prospective study, demonstrated that SUVmax reduction of >20 % early in the course of targeted treatment ($\sim$30 days after the initiation of treatment), was correlated with longer progression free interval. Moreover, when patients were categorized according to SUVmax reduction >20 or <20 % in not increasing masses according to CT criteria in good and intermediate responders, while mass size increase and/or new lesion apparent was indicative of poor response, both progression free and overall survival were statistically significantly different. Therefore, FDG-PET potentially could complement CT in evaluation of response to kinase inhibitors treatment and further discriminate patients with CT findings of stable disease [17]. However, Kayani et al. [10] reported prognostic significance of FDG-PET only 16 weeks after initiation of treatment with sunitinib, and not early in the course of therapy, although FDG-PET may provide information about tumors' biologic nature and sunitinib resistance according to the writers.

As for pediatric population with Wilms tumor, FDG-PET bears a potential role in post-treatment setting and in evaluating pretherapeutic relapse [12].

Conclusively, FDG-PET is likely not used in determining renal malignancy; however, it could play a role in selected cases of suspected distant metastasis, in providing functional prognostic information and evaluating response to treatment and recurrent disease.

78.3 Investigational Radiopharmaceutical for RCC Imaging

Considering the inadequate value of FDG-PET in characterizing and evaluating renal cell carcinoma and especially monitoring small renal masses, efforts have been made so as other imaging biomarkers to be manufactured. Carbonic anhydrase IX is a cell surface antigen, highly expressed in >95 % of clear cell renal cell carcinoma (ccRCC). Girentuximab (cG250), a chimeric antibody, labeled with I-124 (positron emitting radionuclide) binds with carbonic anhydrase IX and has been proposed for the evaluation of ccRCC [2]. After promising initial results in a small sample of patients [18], a multicenter open-label study was carried out, in which I-124-cG250-PET was performed in patients with renal masses, who were planned for surgical removal. With excellent interobserver agreement, reported average sensitivity and specificity are 86.2, 85.9 versus 75.5 and 46.8 %, respectively for CECT, while accuracy range between 85.6 and 86.9 % higher than the according reported for CECT and at least comparable to that of biopsy. Positive and negative predictive values are demonstrated 93.9–94.7 and 68.8–70.3 % respectively. Interestingly, I-124-cG250-PET could detect even small lesions of less than 2 cm with a sensitivity of 70.8 % and T1a and T1b lesions with a sensitivity of 82.8 and 95.7 %, respectively. Correlation with Fuhrman grade was not found and serious adverse effects attributed to girentuximab were not recorded. Moreover, I-124-cG250-PET can serve as a valuable tool in further stratification of patients, regarding that more indolent subtypes do not accumulate the radiopharmaceutical and patients can be put under close surveillance. I-124-cG250-PET has been characterized as the first molecular imaging procedure which bears specific prognostic information for a specific solid tumor [19].

Other radiopharmaceuticals have been proposed for evaluation of renal masses and RCC. 18F-Fluoromisonidazole, a marker of hypoxia has been evaluated to define possible oxygen-derivative alterations during sunitinib treatment and baseline 18F-Fluoromisonidazole was found to be linked to progression free survival in RCC patients treated with sunitinib, however not with overall survival [20]. 18F-Fluorothymidine, a proliferative marker, as well 18F-Fluoroethylcholine, a membrane synthesis marker, were also validated in RCC patients receiving tyrosine kinase inhibitor treatment, consisting a category of potential imaging agents in renal cell carcinoma [21, 22]. However, all these radiopharmaceutical are under investigation and further validation is required until they gain a role in daily imaging of renal cell carcinoma.

References

1. Cairns Paul (2011) Renal cell carcinoma. Cancer Biomark 9(1–6):461–473
2. Smaldone MC, Chen DY, Yu JQ, Plimack ER (2012) Potential role of (124)I-girentuximab in the presurgical diagnosis of clear-cell renal cell cancer. Biologics 6:395–407
3. Khandani AH, Rathmell WK (2012) Positron emission tomography in renal cell carcinoma: an imaging biomarker in development. Semin Nucl Med 42(4):221–230
4. Lawrentschuk N, Davis ID, Bolton DM, Scott AM (2010) Functional imaging of renal cell carcinoma. Nat Rev Urol 7(5):258–266
5. Ramdave S, Thomas GW, Berlangieri SU et al (2001) Clinical role of F-18 fluorodeoxyglucose positron emission tomography for detection and management of renal cell carcinoma. J Urol 166(3):825–830
6. Aide N, Cappele O, Bottet P et al (2003) Efficiency of [(18)F]FDG PET in characterising renal cancer and detecting distant metastases: a comparison with CT. Eur J Nucl Med Mol Imaging 30(9):1236–1245
7. Ozülker T, Ozülker F, Ozbek E, Ozpaçaci T (2011) A prospective diagnostic accuracy study of F-18 fluorodeoxyglucose-positron emission tomography/computed tomography in the evaluation of indeterminate renal masses. Nucl Med Commun 32(4):265–272
8. Kang DE, White RL Jr, Zuger JH et al (2004) Clinical use of fluorodeoxyglucose F 18 positron emission tomography for detection of renal cell carcinoma. J Urol 171(5):1806–1809
9. Wu HC, Yen RF, Shen YY et al (2002) Comparing whole body 18F–2-deoxyglucose positron emission tomography and technetium-99 m methylene

diphosphate bone scan to detect bone metastases in patients with renal cell carcinomas: a preliminary report. J Cancer Res Clin Oncol 128(9):503–506
10. Kayani I, Avril N, Bomanji J et al (2011) Sequential FDG-PET/CT as a biomarker of response to Sunitinib in metastatic clear cell renal cancer. Clin Cancer Res 17(18):6021–6028
11. Namura K, Minamimoto R, Yao M et al (2010) Impact of maximum standardized uptake value (SUVmax) evaluated by 18-Fluoro-2-deoxy-D-glucose positron emission tomography/computed tomography (18F-FDG-PET/CT) on survival for patients with advanced renal cell carcinoma: a preliminary report. BMC Cancer 10:667
12. Misch D, Steffen IG, Schönberger S et al (2008) Use of positron emission tomography for staging, preoperative response assessment and posttherapeutic evaluation in children with Wilms tumour. Eur J Nucl Med Mol Imaging 35(9):1642–1650
13. Nakatani K, Nakamoto Y, Saga T et al (2011) The potential clinical value of FDG-PET for recurrent renal cell carcinoma. Eur J Radiol 79(1):29–35
14. Park JW, Jo MK, Lee HM (2009) Significance of 18F-fluorodeoxyglucose positron-emission tomography/computed tomography for the postoperative surveillance of advanced renal cell carcinoma. BJU Int 103(5):615–619
15. Safaei A, Figlin R, Hoh CK et al (2002) The usefulness of F-18 deoxyglucose whole-body positron emission tomography (PET) for re-staging of renal cell cancer. Clin Nephrol 57(1):56–62
16. Kumar R, Shandal V, Shamim SA et al (2010) Role of FDG PET-CT in recurrent renal cell carcinoma. Nucl Med Commun 31(10):844–850
17. Ueno D, Yao M, Tateishi U et al (2012) Early assessment by FDG-PET/CT of patients with advanced renal cell carcinoma treated with tyrosine kinase inhibitors is predictive of disease course. BMC Cancer 12:162
18. Divgi CR, Pandit-Taskar N, Jungbluth AA et al (2007) Preoperative characterisation of clear-cell renal carcinoma using iodine-124-labelled antibody chimeric G250 (124I-cG250) and PET in patients with renal masses: a phase I trial. Lancet Oncol 8(4):304–310
19. Divgi CR, Uzzo RG, Gatsonis C et al (2013) Positron emission tomography/computed tomography identification of clear cell renal cell carcinoma: results from the REDECT trial. J Clin Oncol 31(2): 187–194
20. Hugonnet F, Fournier L, Medioni J et al (2011) Metastatic renal cell carcinoma: relationship between initial metastasis hypoxia, change after 1 month's sunitinib, and therapeutic response: an 18F-Fluoromisonidazole PET/CT study. J Nucl Med 52:1048–1055
21. Liu G, Jeraj R, Vanderhoek M et al (2011) Pharmacodynamic study using FLT PET/CT in patients with renal cell cancer and other solid malignancies treated with sunitinib malate. Clin Cancer Res 17(24):7634–7644
22. Middendorp M, Maute L, Sauter B et al (2010) Initial experience with 18F-fluoroethylcholine PET/CT in staging and monitoring therapy response of advanced renal cell carcinoma. Ann Nucl Med 24(6):441–446

79 Clinical Implications of Renal Cancer

Gerasimos J. Alivizatos

79.1 Diagnosis-Staging

Abdominal ultrasonography (US) and Multi detector CT (MDCT) scans are the common methods by which these tumors are identified today accidentally. The presence of enhancement is the criterion used to diagnose a kidney cancer and enhancement can be shown with CT scans, with MRI and ultrasounds. CT and MRI scans are the most appropriate imaging modalities for TNM classification. PET scans have been used in the diagnostic process and in the followup protocols, but its actual role in renal cell cancer cases has yet to be determined [1].

79.2 Follow up Strategies

The follow up investigations in patients with kidney tumors depend on the risk profiles (low, intermediate, and high risk profile) of each case. The imaging modalities used include chest X-ray, US, and CT scans.

CT remains the mainstay of imaging in the detecting, characterizing, staging, and surveillance of renal lesions. MRI is increasingly used as a problem solving tool. Advanced MRI technique such as diffusion-weighted imaging is being explored in the investigation of renal lesions [1].

Reference

1. Ljungberg B, Cowan NC, Hanbury DC et al (2010) EAU guidelines on renal cell carcinoma: the 2010 update. Eur Urol 58:398–406

G. J. Alivizatos (✉)
3rd Urological Department, Hygeia Hospital,
Erythrou Stavrou 4, 1523 Athens, Greece
e-mail: gali@hol.gr

A. D. Gouliamos et al. (eds.), *Imaging in Clinical Oncology*,
DOI: 10.1007/978-88-470-5385-4_79, © Springer-Verlag Italia 2014

80 Introduction to Urothelial Cancer

Andreas A. Skolarikos

The epithelium which covers the pyelocalyceal system, the ureter, and the urinary bladder constitutes a common source of human cancer development. Together with prostate, breast, lung, and colorectal cancers urothelial cancer constitutes the five most common human malignancies [1]. Among urothelial tumors, those originating from the urinary bladder are by far the most common, as they account for the 90–95 % of all locations [2]. Upper urinary tract urothelial cell carcinomas (UUT–UCCs)) originating from the pyelocalyceal system and ureteric epithelium account for the rest 5–10 % [1, 3–5]. It is estimated that approximately $10.1/10^5$ men and $2.5/10^5$ women are affected annually by bladder cancer. In comparison, the annual incidence of UUT–UCC is $1-2/10^5$ people, approximately [1–5]. Urothelial carcinoma is highly lethal as $4/10^5$ of men and $1.1/10^5$ of women with bladder cancer will annually die because of the disease [6].

The natural history of urothelial carcinoma varies depending on tumor location. Approximately 75–85 % of patients with bladder cancer present with nonmuscle invasive disease, while 60 % of patients with UUT-UCC are invasive at diagnosis [3–6]. Noninvasive lower tract tumors are most commonly treated with transurethral resection followed by chemotherapy or immunotherapy intravesical instillations. Multiple recurrences may usually occur, affecting patients' quality of life, increasing at the same time the risk of disease progression [7]. The standard treatment of noninvasive UUT–UCC is still radical nephroureterectomy. However, minimally invasive techniques which may spare the kidney are increasingly being used and are currently indicated under special circumstances. Muscle invasive bladder tumors as well as invasive UUT–UUC require accurate staging and when localized are treated with major extirpative surgical techniques. The later includes radical cystoprostatectomy and radical nephroureterectomy along with extensive lymphadenectomy on both occasions [8, 9]. Metastatic disease is still considered incurable as the response to chemotherapy is poor and major surgery is futile.

In this chapter, based on the importance of proper diagnosis, staging and follow-up of urothelial cancer, all contributors present the latest development in bladder and upper urinary tract cancer imaging. Whether, traditional and/or advanced imaging may result in earlier diagnosis, decrease the need for invasive diagnostic procedures such as cystoscopy or ureteroscopy, and increase accurate staging leading to enhancement of proper treatment selection remain to be seen.

A. A. Skolarikos (✉)
2nd Department of Urology, 47 Mitropoulou st
Xaidari, 12462 Athens, Greece
e-mail: andskol@yahoo.com

A. D. Gouliamos et al. (eds.), *Imaging in Clinical Oncology*,
DOI: 10.1007/978-88-470-5385-4_80, © Springer-Verlag Italia 2014

Table 80.1 Urothelial carcinoma classification

Transitional cell carcinoma
Urothelial carcinoma with mixed epithelial features (divergent differentiation)
Squamous cell carcinoma
Adenocarcinoma
Enteric type
Clear cell ("mesonephric") type
Signet ring cell type
Urachal carcinoma
Small cell-neuroendocrine carcinoma
Lymphoepithelioma-like carcinoma
Nested variant of urothelial carcinoma
Micropapillary carcinoma
Sarcomatoid carcinoma/carcinosarcoma
Microcystic carcinoma
Urothelial carcinoma with trophoblastic differentiation

80.1 Pathology, Classification, and Staging

Approximately 98 % of malignant tumors arising in the lower and/or upper urinary tract are of epithelial origin, and of those 90 % are transitional cell carcinomas. Table 80.1 shows the classification of urothelial carcinoma and its variants recognized by the World Health Organization (WHO) [10].

Table 80.2 shows the WHO/International society of urological pathology consensus classification of transitional cell neoplasms of the urinary bladder [10]. The system traditionally used for grading bladder tumors is also applied to UUT–UCC.

Bladder cancer is precisely staged through a combination of endoscopic inspection, histologic evaluation of endoscopically obtained material, physical examination under anesthesia, and radiographic imaging for evaluation of local, regional, and distant progression. Currently, the seventh edition of the American Joint Committee on Cancer (AJCC), Tumor-nodes-metastasis (TNM) system is used for bladder cancer staging (Table 80.3).

Table 80.2 Classification of the transitional cell neoplasms of the bladder

Normal
Flat lesions
Flat hyperplasia
Flat lesions with atypia
Reactive (inflammatory) atypia
Atypia of unknown significance
Dysplasia (low grade intraurothelial neoplasia)
Carcinoma in situ (high-grade intraurothelial neoplasia)
Papillary lesions
Papillary hyperplasia
Papillary neoplasms
Papilloma
Papillary urothelial neoplasm of low malignant potential
Papillary carcinoma, low grade
Papillary carcinoma, high grade

Following an episode of gross haematuria, UUT–UCC is most commonly diagnosed and staged by the combination of endoscopic inspection, biopsy of the abnormal tissue, and radiographic imaging. Similarly to bladder cancer, imaging for UUT–UCC is important for proper local, regional, and distant staging. Renal pelvis and ureteral tumors are also staged based on the AJCC TNM classification system (Table 80.4).

80.2 Prognostic Factors

Papillary nonmuscle invasive tumors of the lower and upper urinary tract may either recur or progress during a patient's lifetime. The number of tumors initially diagnosed, the maximum diameter of the tumor, the T-category and the grade of the tumor, the existence of concomitant carcinoma in situ, and the history of prior recurrence are the major prognostic factors used to predict recurrence and/or progression of these tumors. Tumor stage and grade, presence of lymph vascular invasion, and lymph node status are important prognostic factors associated with oncologic outcome in patients with muscle invasive bladder cancer and UUT–UCC.

Table 80.3 Bladder cancer TNM staging system

Primary tumor (T)	Tx	Primary cannot be assessed
	T0	No evidence of primary tumor
	Ta	Noninvasive papillary tumor
	Tis	Carcinoma in situ
	T1	Tumor invades subepithelial connective tissue
	T2	Tumor invades muscle
	pT2a	Tumor invades superficial muscle layer (inner half)
	pT2b	Tumor invades deep muscle (outer half)
	T3	Tumor invades perivesical tissue
	pT3a	Tumor invades perivesical tissue microscopically
	pT3b	Tumor invades perivesical tissue macroscopically (extravesical mass)
	T4	Tumor invades any of the following: prostate, uterus, vagina, pelvic wall, and abdominal wall
	T4a	Tumor invades prostate, uterus, and vagina
	T4b	Tumor invades pelvic wall, abdominal wall
Regional lymph nodes (N)	Nx	Regional lymph nodes cannot be assessed
	N0	No regional lymph node metastases
	N1	Metastasis in a single lymph node, 2 cm or less in greater dimension
	N2	Metastasis in a single lymph node, more than 2 cm but not more than 5 cm in greatest dimension; or multiple lymph nodes, none more than 5 cm in greatest dimension
	N3	Metastasis in a lymph node, more than 5 cm in greatest dimension
Distant metastasis (M)	Mx	Distant metastasis cannot be assessed
	M0	No distant metastases
	M1	Distant metastasis

80.3 Indication and Dilemmas of Imaging in Urothelial Cancer: The Urologist Perspective

The most common clinical presentation of urothelial carcinoma is painless macroscopic hematuria. Radiological imaging is the first and one of the most crucial steps in the patient's work-up. Radiology may clarify the diagnosis but also may provide the clinician with valuable information regarding the grade and stage of the disease. Modern cross-sectional imaging such as multidetector computer tomography and magnetic resonance may further improve staging and grading of urothelial cancer.

80.4 Imaging and Diagnosis

Ultrasound (US) examination of the urinary tract is a noninvasive, readily available, inexpensive and radiation-free diagnostic tool, which is often used as the first imaging modality for patients presenting with hematuria. With respect to bladder cancer diagnosis, transabdominal US has a specificity of 99 % in the expense of a lower sensitivity of 63 %. Factors that may increase sensitivity are the improvement of the spatial resolution, soft tissue contrast, and volumetric coverage of US technique. The major drawback of US is the fact that it is operator dependent. It would be interesting to know whether other approaches such as the transrectal

Table 80.4 UUT-UCC cancer TNM staging system

Primary tumor (T)	
Tx	Primary tumor cannot be assessed
T0	No evidence of primary tumor
Ta	Papillary noninvasive carcinoma
Tis	Carcinoma in situ
T1	Tumor invades subepithelial connective tissue
T2	Tumor invades the muscularis
T3- renal pelvis only	Tumor invades beyond muscularis into peripelvic fat or the renal parenchyma
T3- ureter only	Tumor invades beyond muscularis into periureteric fat
T4	Tumor invades adjacent organs, or through the kidney into the perinephric fat
Regional lymph nodes (N)	
Nx	Regional lymph nodes cannot be assessed
N0	No regional lymph node metastases
N1	Metastasis in a single lymph node, 2 cm or less in greater dimension
N2	Metastasis in a single lymph node, more than 2 cm but not more than 5 cm in greatest dimension; or multiple lymph nodes, none more than 5 cm in greatest dimension
N3	Metastasis in a lymph node, more than 5 cm in greatest dimension
Distant metastasis (M)	
M0	No distant metastases
M1	Distant metastasis
Stage groups	
Stage 0a	Ta N0 M0
Stage 0is	Tis N0 M0
Stage I	T1 N0 M0
Stage II	T2 N0 M0
Stage III	T3 N0 M0
	T4 N0 M0
Stage IV	Any T N1-3 M0
	Any T Any N M1

or transvaginal US, would add into the diagnostic accuracy of the method [11, 12].

Regarding the upper urinary tract, the diagnostic accuracy of US is lower as it is depended on the size of the lesion and on the existence of concomitant obstruction of the collecting system. The later creates an anechoic background and increases the acoustic difference between normal and pathologic features leading to a better diagnosis. Still, US is considered as an invalid method for diagnosing tumors located into the ureter [7].

Intravenous urography (IVU) has a limited role in the diagnosis of bladder tumors. This is mainly due to the fact that its sensitivity for small tumors and carcinoma in situ is very low. Filling defects of the upper tract are highly suspicious of urothelial tumors. However, conventional IVU is no longer indicated as a routine exam for diagnosing upper tract urothelial carcinoma [7]. It has been replaced by computed tomography (CT) scan [7].

Multidetector computed tomography (MDCT) is currently not recommended for bladder tumor diagnosis during the initial evaluation of a painless hematuria, as it cannot adequately replace cystoscopy and biopsy. However, multiplanar and volume MDCT techniques by filling the bladder through a catheter with air or contrast may allow for an inside virtual view of the bladder. Compared to conventional cystoscopy, virtual cystoscopy has shown 95 and 87 % sensitivity and specificity in identifying bladder lesions [13]. It remains to see whether further advancements in this technique may eventually replace conventional cystoscopy.

MDCT is a valuable tool for diagnosing upper urinary tract tumors. The sensitivity and specificity of MDCT when used for UUT–UCC diagnosis vary from 40 to 96 and 40 to 99 %, respectively. Accuracy depends on tumor morphology and size. Papillary lesions of 5–10 mm in size are extremely difficult to miss with MDCT. Papillary lesions <3 mm and flat lesions are more difficult to detect [14–16]. As MDCT is regularly used in patients with macroscopic hematuria with a negative cystoscopy, it is important for the clinician to order for a properly designed study. In this chapter, technical details regarding the appropriate protocol with timely asked images before and after the injection of contrast will be underlined.

Magnetic resonance imaging (MRI) has several advantages over CT. It is the primary option in assessing patients with allergy and lacks radiation exposure [17]. However, it is also not recommended as a first line imaging for the patient who presents with painless macroscopic hematuria. The role of MRI in detecting UUT–UCC is similar to MDCT. Newer technology such as MR urography (MRU) performed with modern MR scanners provides the clinician with high-quality images of the kidney, ureter, and bladder. These images are coming on a three dimensional (3D) gradient-echo sequence during a single breath hold of the patient. Still a disadvantage of the method is the inability to detect small filling defects in a nondilated collecting system. This is mainly due to the lower spatial resolution of MRI as compared to CT scan. Urologists should be aware of the advantages and disadvantages of these methods when they order for them.

80.5 Imaging and Staging/Grading

80.5.1 T-Staging/Grading

Transabdominal US has a limited role in tumor staging. It is of interest whether endoluminal US, either transurethral or transureteric, may differentiate Ta from T1 disease or T1 from T2 disease. Although there is some evidence showing high correlation with tumor stage, these techniques are invasive and should still be considered as experimental [7, 9]. IVU does not provide any direct information for tumor stage and grade [7]. In contrast, MDCT urography has increased sensitivity in staging transitional cell carcinoma. The accuracy of the MDCT in determining extravesical tumor extension varies from 55 to 92 % [18]. Stranding and haziness of the perivesicular fat are highly indicative of a T3b stage [15]. However, the same findings may be related to a recent transurethral resection of the bladder tumor. The clinician should be in close collaboration with the radiologist in order to define the proper timing for imaging and to clarify the findings.

Based on the water content differences of various tissues and MRI's multiplanar capability magnetic resonance is an ideal method to differentiate enhancing extravesical tumor from postoperative stranding and normal perivesicular fat. Again, the urologist should be capable of understanding the technology behind his order. It should be ideal to inform the radiologist about the clinical problem he is searching. For example, T3b disease is better seen when the radiologist performs postcontrast imaging at an early phase (20–70 s delay) of a T1-weighted imaging. Similarly, T1 or T2 imaging at a later phase may differentiate the invasion within the muscular layers. Overall staging accuracy of MRI ranges between 73 and 96 % [17]. Newer modalities such as the application of diffused-weighted images (DWI) may further improve the accuracy of staging. Furthermore, advances in DWI may be able not only to differentiate normal parenchyma from neoplastic processes but determine also the histologic type of the tumor.

80.5.2 N and M Staging

MDCT is a valuable tool for detecting lymph node and distant metastases. The method shows a diverse specificity for staging lymphadenopathy in primary tumors of the bladder and upper urinary tract ranging from 55 to 92 % [18]. Conventional MRI was not proved to be superior to MDCT [19]. We believe that criteria other than the absolute size of the lymph node are needed to increase these rates. This is mainly due to the fact that normal-sized lymph nodes can be affected by the cancer as well as that lymph nodes can be enlarged by benign pathology. Another important question is whether the same criteria of positivity should be used for pelvic as well as abdominal lymph nodes. The application of lymphotropic contrast agents has demonstrated improved sensitivity to conventional MRI in distinguishing malignant from benign lymphadenopathy [20]. Although it was introduced over a decade ago, it has not been established into clinical practice. Similarly, there is no evidence supporting routine use of positron emission tomography (PET) scan in nodal staging of bladder cancer [21].

Discovery of distant metastases is extremely important in patients' management as it changes the treatment approach from surgical to conservative, in means of chemotherapy. MDCT and MRI are also indicated to detect tumor spread to other distant organs such as the liver and lung. When bladder muscle invasion is documented M-staging with the above techniques is recommended prior to decision making. Other sites of metastases such as bone and brain are rare and imaging is performed only when symptoms indicate such an involvement. MRI is the preferred method as it is more sensitive and specific to bone scan in detecting bone metastases [22].

80.6 Imaging and Follow-up

The follow-up of nonmuscle invasive bladder tumors is based on regular cystoscopies. Currently, there is no noninvasive method that could replace endoscopy. There is a lot of evidence showing that US has a lower sensitivity compared to cystoscopy when these methods are used for patient follow-up. IVU is no longer included in the follow-up protocols of patients with bladder cancer [7]. Periodical evaluation of the upper urinary tract should be performed with the use of MDCT or MRI for the aforementioned reasons. In the cases that the kidney is spared, UUT–UCC should be closely followed up with ureterorenoscopies. MDCT and MRI are also

Table 80.5 Suggestions for imaging follow-up based on initial tumor staging after cystectomy

Procedures	Months after cystectomy								
<pT1	3	6	12	18	24	30	36	48	60
Ultrasound kidneys	x								
CT/MRI thorax and abdomen plus UUT			x		x		x	x	x
pT2									
Ultrasound kidneys	x								
CT/MRI thorax and abdomen plus UUT		x	x	x	x		x	x	x
>pT3 or N+									
Ultrasound kidneys	x								
CT/MRI thorax and abdomen plus UUT		x	x	x	x	x	x	x	x

Table 80.6 Imaging rating for urothelial carcinoma with, or without, cystectomy

Radiological procedure	Rating scale[a]	Comments relative	Relative radiation level
X ray chest	4		Minimum
CT urography	8		High
X ray abdomen loopogram	5	In patients with an ileal loop postcystectomy	Medium
X-ray intravenous urography	5	Utilization of intravenous urography has continued to decline with the increasingly widespread use of CT urography	Medium
MR imaging abdomen and pelvis without and with contrast	7	See ESUR guidelines on contrast media version7.0	None
CT abdomen and pelvis with contrast	1	Appropriate if CT urography is not available. Visceral/nodal status evaluated during CT	High
CT chest with contrast	5	Performed if chest X ray is equivocal	Medium
US pelvis (bladder)	3		None
FDG-PET whole body indicated for suspected or nodal metastasis	2	Indicated for suspected nodal or distant metastasis	High

After 5 years of follow-up, oncological surveillance can be stopped and surveillance continued with functional surveillance

[a] 1 is least appropriate; 9 is most appropriate

indicated to exclude local and distant advancement of the disease. Surveillance of the upper urinary tract with cross-sectional imaging is also recommended for those patients who undergo radical cystectomy for muscle invasive bladder cancer. Pathologic T2 and T3 or N+ disease after radical cystectomy should be followed with MDCT and/or MRI every 6 months postoperatively for 2 years and annually thereafter for at least 5 years [23]. Table 80.5 shows the European Association of Urology (EAU) guidelines for follow-up imaging after cystectomy. EAU has recently rated the appropriateness of imaging for urothelial carcinoma with or without cystectomy (Table 80.6).

80.7 Conclusion

Radiologic imaging plays an important role in the detection, differential diagnosis staging and follow-up of urothelial cancer. Despite significant advancements, it has not been able to replace invasive diagnostic procedures such as cystoscopy and ureteroscopy. Modern imaging is undoubtedly a valuable tool in the diagnosis of upper tract urothelial cancer and certainly has replaced conventional IVU. Significant evolution in imaging technology provides the urologist with an increased armamentarium for more accurate staging of urothelial cancer fact which may alter treatment strategies.

References

1. Munoz JJ, Ellison LM (2000) Upper tract urothelial neoplasms: incidence and survival during the last 2 decades. J Urol 164:1523–1525
2. Ploeg M, Aben KK, Kiemeney LA (2009) The present and future burden of urinary bladder cancer in the world. World J Urol 27:289–293
3. Hall MC, Womack S, Sagalowsky AI et al (1998) Prognostic factors, recurrence, and survival in transitional cell carcinoma of the upper urinary tract: a 30-year experience in 252 patients. Urology 52:594–601
4. Margulis V, Shariat SF, Matin SF et al (2009) Outcomes of radical nephroureterectomy: a series from the Upper Tract Urothelial Carcinoma Collaboration. Cancer 115:1224–1233
5. Olgac S, Mazumdar M, Dalbagni G, Reuter VE (2004) Urothelial carcinoma of the renal pelvis: a

clinicopathologic study of 130 cases. Am J Surg Pathol 28:1545–1552
6. Ferlay J, Randi G, Bosetti C et al (2008) Declining mortality from bladder cancer in Europe. BJU Int 101:11–19
7. Babjuk M, Oosterlinck W, Sylvester R, Kaasinen E, Bohle A, Palou-Redorta M, Roupret M (2011) EAU Guidelines on non-muscle-invasive urothelial carcinoma of the bladder, the 2011 update. Eur Urol 59:997–1008
8. Stenzl A, Cowan NC, De Santis M, Kuczyk MA, Merseburger AS, Ribal MJ, Sherif A, Witjes JA (2011) Treatment of muscle-invasive and metastatic bladder cancer: update of the EAU Guidelines. Eur Urol 59:1009–1018
9. Roupret M, Zigeuner R, Palou J, Boehle A, Kaasimen E, Sylvester R, Babjuk M, Oosterlinck W (2011) European Guidelines for the diagnosis and management of upper urinary tract urothelial cell carcinomas: 2011 update. Eur Urol 59:584–594
10. Eble JN, Sauter G, Epstein JI (eds) et al (2004). Pathology and genetics of tumours of the urinary system and male genital organs. IARC press, Lyon, France
11. Datta S, Allen G, Evans R et al (2002) Urinary tract ultrasonography in the evaluation of haematuria: a report of over 1,000 cases. Ann Roy Coll Surg Engl 84(3):203–205
12. Dibb M, Noble D, Peh Y et al (2001) Ultrasonographic analysis of bladder tumors. J Clin Imag 25416–25420
13. Kim JK, Ahn HJ, Park T et al (2002) Virtual cystoscopy of the contrast filled bladder in patients with gross haematuria. Am J Roentgenol 179:763–768
14. Dillman JR, Caoili EM, Cohan RH et al (2008) Detection of upper tract urothelial neoplasms: sensitivity of axial, coronal reformatted, and curved-planar reformatted image-types utilizing 16-row multi-detector CT urography. Abdom Imaging 33:707–716
15. Wang LJ, Wong YC, Chuang CK, Huang CC, Pang ST (2009) Diagnostic accuracy of transitional cell carcinoma on multidetector computerized tomography urography in patients with gross haematuria. J Urol 181:524–531
16. Wang LJ, Wong YC, Huang CC et al (2010) Multidetector computerized tomography urography is more accurate than excretory urography for diagnosing transitional cell carcinoma of the upper urinary tract in adults with haematuria. J Urol 183:48–55
17. Tekes A, Kamel I, Imam K et al (2003) MR Imaging features of transitional cell carcinoma of the urinary bladder. Am J Roentgenol 180(3):771–777
18. Kundra V, Silverman PM (2003) Imaging in oncology from the University of Texas M. D. Anderson Cancer Center. Imaging in the diagnosis, staging, and follow-up of cancer of the urinary bladder. AJR Am J Roentgenol 180(4):1045–1054
19. Sobin L, Wittekind C (eds) (1997) TNM classification of malignant tumours. Wiley-Liss, Baltimore, MD
20. Harisnghani M, Barentsz J, Hahn P et al (2003) Noninvasive detectino of clinically occult lymph-node metastases in prostate cancer. N Engl J Med 348:2491–2499
21. Swinnen G, Maes A, Pottel H et al (2010) FDG-PET/CT for the preoperative lymph node staging of invasive bladder cancer. Eur Urol 57(4):641–647
22. Schmidt GP, Schoenberg SO, Reiser MF et al (2005) Whole-body MR imaging of bone marrow. Eur J Radiol 55(1):33–40
23. Stenzl A, Witjes JA, Compérat E, Cowan NC, De Santis M, Kuczyk M, Lebret T, Ribal MJ, Sherif A (2011) Guidelines on bladder cancer muscle-invasive and metastatic http://www.uroweb.org/gls/pdf/07_Bladder%20Cancer_LR%20II.pdf

81 US Findings in Urothelial Cancer

Ioannis A. Tsitouridis and Georgios E. Glataganas

81.1 Renal Pelvis Urothelial Cancer

Transitional cell carcinoma (TCC) is the most common neoplasm of the urinary collecting system. In the upper tract, the tumor in the majority of the cases is located in the renal sinus.

The ultrasound findings of the TCC of the renal pelvis varied depended on: (a) if the neoplasm is flat or pedunculated, (b) the size of neoplasm in accordance to the quantity of fluid in the rest of the renal pelvis, (c) the effects upon the calyces causing obstructive hydronephrosis, and (d) the intralesion procedures such as hemorrhage, rupture, and dislocation of a part of the lesion.

In the majority of cases, the lesion is hypoechoic or isoechoic relative to the surrounding renal parenchyma but when it is hemorrhagic or high grade, echo texture occasionally changes to a mixed pattern (Figs. 81.1, 81.2, 81.3, 81.4, and 81.5).

Complete invasion of renal pelvis and renal calyces disappears the central echotexture of the kidney (faceless kidney), (Fig. 81.6).

The tumor may extend to the renal cortex and although it is infiltrative, it can cause focal distortion of renal margins.

It is essential for characterization to rule out renal adenoma, squamous cell carcinoma, renal cell carcinoma which invade the renal sinus, blood clot, and fungus ball. The real problem in the diagnosis of TCC with ultrasound is to rule out blood thrombus from hemorrhage.

Ultrasound already plays a complementary role in the evaluation of renal pelvis urothelial cancer in patients with renal impairment or iodinated contrast allergy, but at present US is the primary imaging method for patients with hematuria to assess the underlying pathology.

81.2 Bladder Urothelial Cancer

Bladder tumor appears on ultrasound as echo-poor lesion, although it steads as echogenic lesion in contrast to anechoic fluid into the bladder. The bladder wall is more echogenic than the tumor, thus permitting a clear distinction between lesion and bladder wall, leading to early detection of a superficial lesion and early invasion into the interior layers of bladder wall (Figs. 81.7, 81.8).

Ultrasound difficulty includes deeper invasion of the bladder wall, accurate evaluation of bladder neck region, inability to assess invasion of surrounding structures, and accurate staging of lymph nodes status.

I. A. Tsitouridis (✉) · G. E. Glataganas
Department of Radiology, General Hospital Papageorgiou, Thessaloniki, Ring Road Thessaloniki Efkarpia, 685111, Thessaloniki, Greece
e-mail: tsitouridis.1@gmail.com

G. E. Glataganas
e-mail: gialim@hol.gr

A. D. Gouliamos et al. (eds.), *Imaging in Clinical Oncology*,
DOI: 10.1007/978-88-470-5385-4_81, © Springer-Verlag Italia 2014

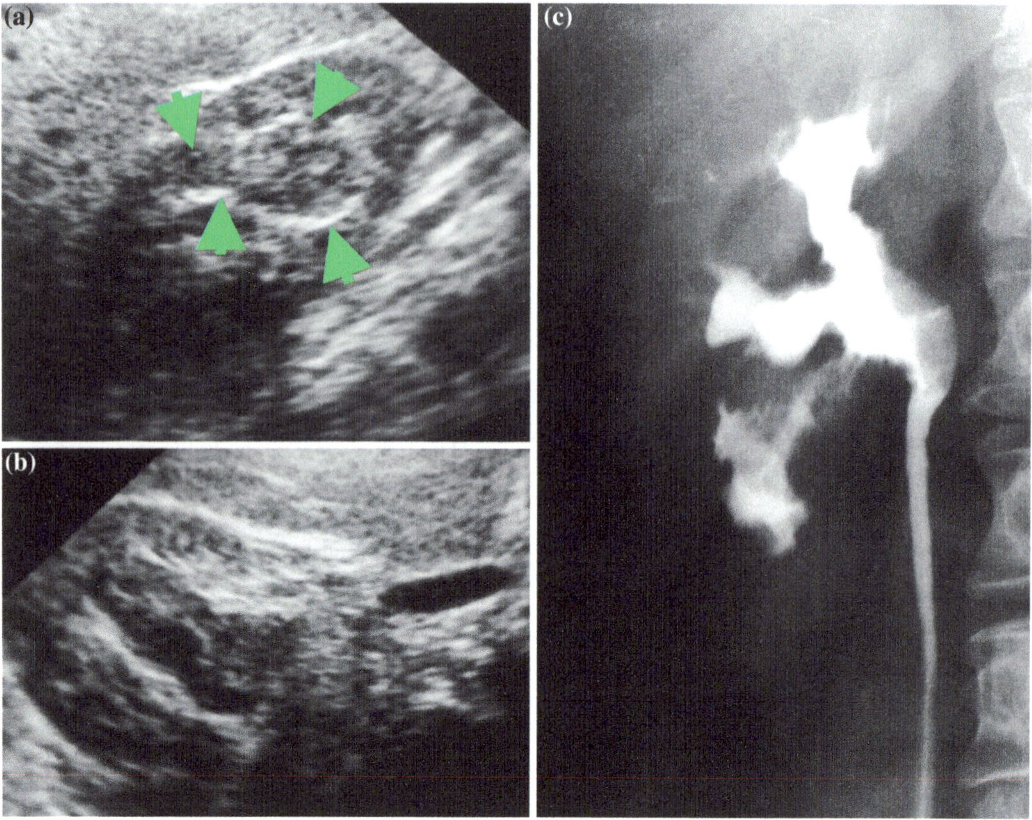

Fig. 81.1 **a**, **b** Sagittal and axial *gray-scale* sonograms which reveal an urothelial cancer in the calyces of the lower renal pole (*arrows*). **c** The corresponding intravenous pyelogram (*arrows*)

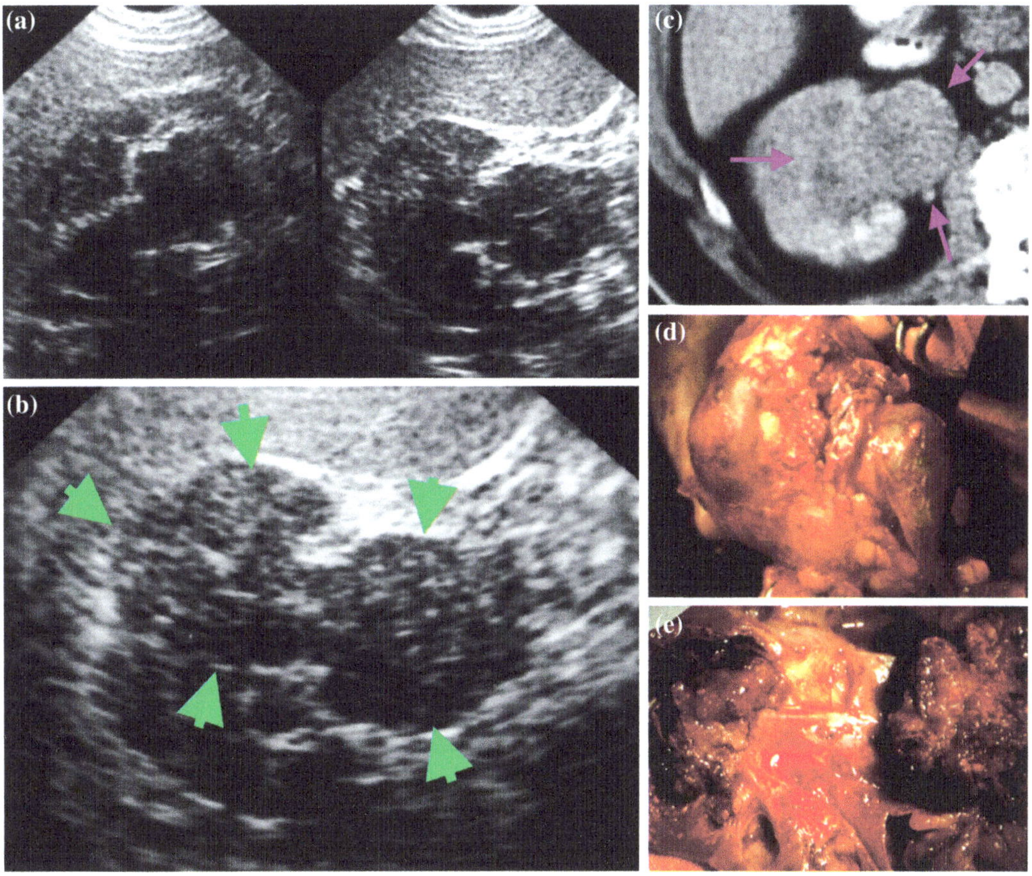

(a) (b) (c) (d) (e)

Fig. 81.2 **a**, **b** Sagittal and axial *gray-scale* sonograms which reveal an urothelial carcinoma of the *right* renal pelvis. The carcinoma extended into the neighboring renal cortical parenchyma (*arrows*). **c** Axial CT scan which reveals the hypodence urothelial tumor (*arrows*). **d**, **e** The photograph of the surgical specimen of the renal pelvis and the tumor extension into the renal parenchyma

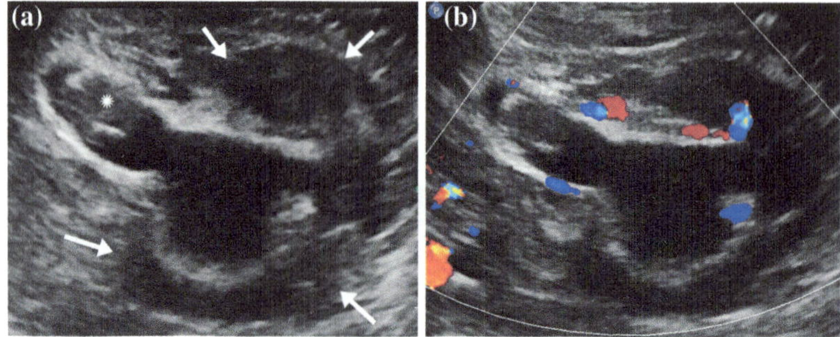

Fig. 81.3 **a**, **b** Axial *gray scale* and *color* Doppler sonograms of the *left* kidney (*arrows*) which reveal in a nondepended location of the pelvis an urothelial cancer (*asterisk*)

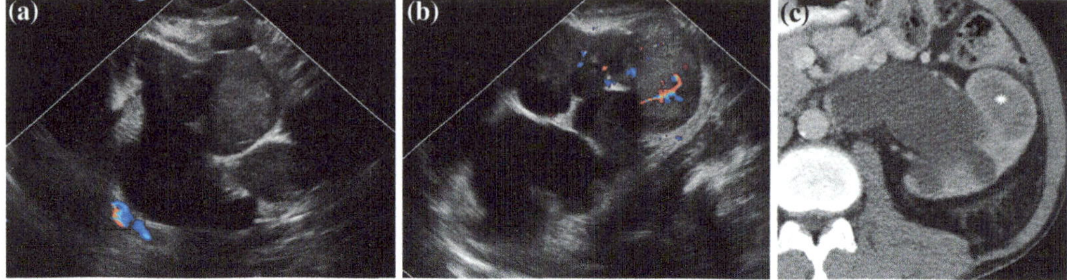

Fig. 81.4 **a**, **b** Oblique sagittal *color* Doppler sonograms of the *left* kidney which reveal urothelial cancer invasion in the renal pelvis (*arrows*) and intracalyceal neoplastic extension (*asterisk*). **c** Axial CT scan which shows the dilatation of the pelvis and the intracalyceal tumor (*asterisk*)

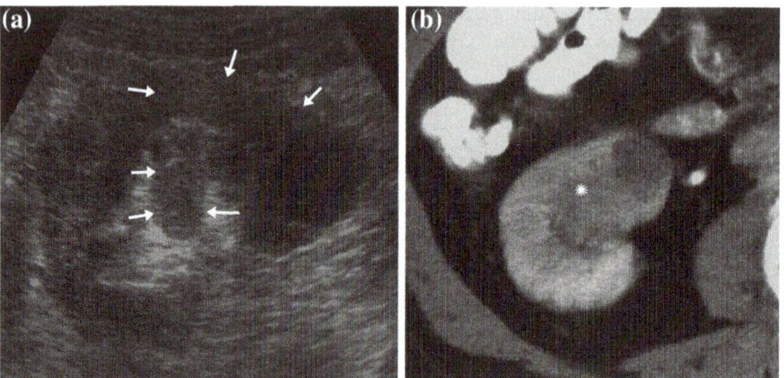

Fig. 81.5 **a** Oblique axial *gray-scale* sonogram of the *right* kidney, which reveals intracalyceal urothelial cancer with cortical invasion. **b** Axial CT scan which reveals the extension of the urothelial cancer (*asterisk*)

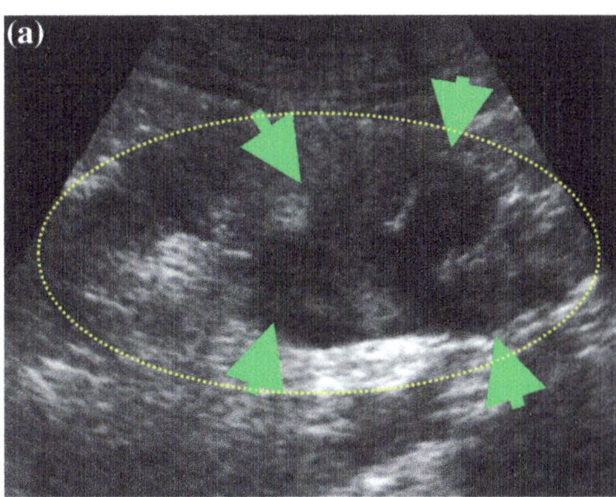

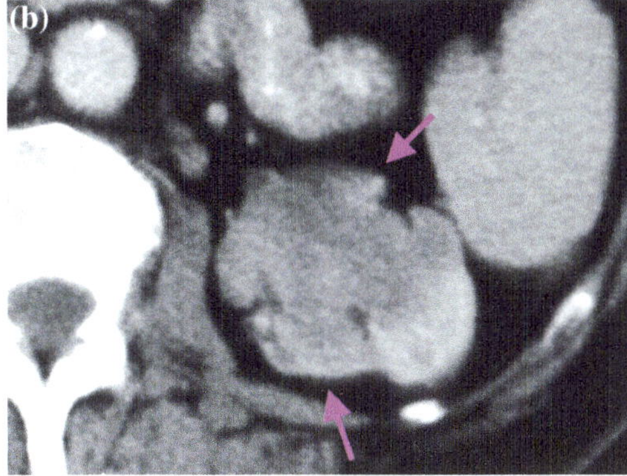

Fig. 81.6 **a** Sagittal *gray-scale* sonogram of the *left* kidney which reveals intracalyceal urothelial cancer with complete invasion of the renal parenchyma obliterating the renal sinus (faceless kidney). **b** Axial CT scan shows a soft tissue mass (*arrows*) filling the *left* renal pelvis

Intravesical ultrasound exam reduces the problem of visualization because of acoustic shadow production behind the air-containing bowel loops. The accuracy of intravesical ultrasound ranges between 62 and 92 % [1].

As in all endo-ultrasound techniques, the penetration is not good enough for evaluation of the surrounding structures but is very accurate for local staging, superficial localized lesion, and early tumor detection.

Transrectal US is the method of choice for sonographic approach of the region of bladder trigone, but the disadvantage of difficult approach of bladder dome and anterior bladder wall makes the method only occasionally to be used.

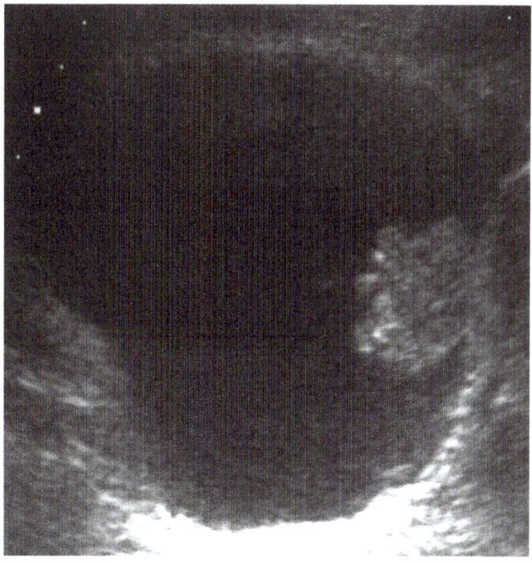

Fig. 81.7 Urothelial cancer of the bladder with papillary configuration in the *left* lateral wall (*echogenic line*)

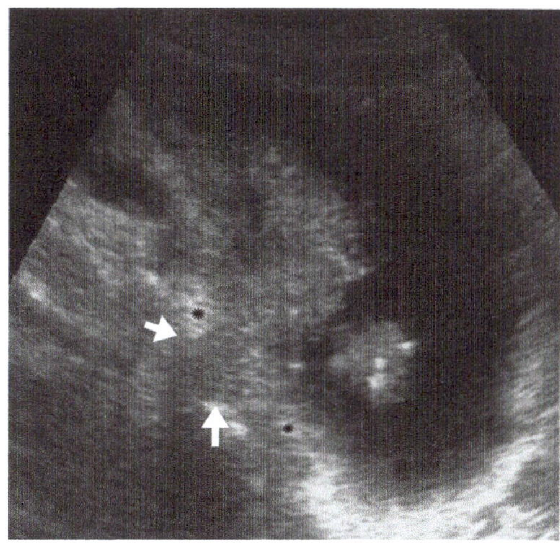

Fig. 81.8 Urothelial cancer of the bladder with papillary configuration in the *right* lateral wall with extravesical invasion (*arrows*), (focal obliteration of the *echogenic line* of the wall-*asterisk*)

Reference

1. Abu-Yousef NN, Narayana AS, Franken EA, Brown RC (1984) Urinary bladder tumors studied by cystosonography. Radiology 153:220–226

82 CT and MRI Findings in Urothelial Cancer

Fotios D. Laspas

82.1 Introduction

Urothelial cancer is commonly multifocal and characterized by a high incidence of metachronous tumors. Although the evaluation of the urinary bladder may be performed with direct visualization using cystoscopy, the tumors in the upper urinary tract are mainly diagnosed using imaging methods. Moreover, imaging modalities play an important role in the staging and surveillance of urothelial cancer. Computed tomography (CT) urography is the preferred imaging modality for the evaluation of hematuria, the detection and staging of urothelial cancer. Magnetic resonance imaging (MRI) can be considered for appropriate indications, as the case of compromised renal function, severe iodinated contrast allergy, or pregnancy (to whom radiation exposure is better to be avoided), although it is considered superior to CT in demonstrating the extent of bladder wall invasion [1].

82.2 Diagnosis

Early detection of bladder cancer is important, since superficial tumors typically carry a good prognosis. CT urography has a reported sensitivity and specificity of over 90 % for the diagnosis of bladder malignancies in patients with hematuria [2]. Despite these encouraging results, flat lesions and lesions at the bladder base adjacent to the prostate gland, particularly in patients with benign prostatic hypertrophy may be undetectable with CT urography; thus, cystoscopy remains as the primary diagnostic modality for the work up of the lower urinary tract. However, tumors may arise in bladder diverticula (Fig. 82.1). These lesions are often not evident on cystoscopy and cross-sectional imaging may be necessary for diagnosis [1]. Moreover, as previously mentioned, urothelial cancer is commonly multifocal. Approximately, 2–3 % of patient with bladder cancer will have concomitant upper track disease [3]. Thus, a thorough evaluation of the upper urinary track is important in these patients.

CT urography is the gold standard for exploration of the upper urinary tract with reported sensitivity and specificity of 93.5 and 94.8 % for the detection of urothelial cancer [4] (Fig. 82.2). MRI is infrequently used in the primary investigation of upper tract urothelial cancer. The detection rate of MRI urography is 75 % for tumors <2 cm and the method is indicated in patients who cannot be subjected to a CT urography [5].

82.3 Staging

In bladder cancer, the important question of local staging is whether there is muscle invasion,

F. D. Laspas (✉)
CT&MRI Department, "Hygeia" Hospital,
4, Erythrou Stavrou Str. & Kifisias Av,
15123, Marousi, Athens, Attica, Greece
e-mail: fotisdimi@yahoo.gr

A. D. Gouliamos et al. (eds.), *Imaging in Clinical Oncology*,
DOI: 10.1007/978-88-470-5385-4_82, © Springer-Verlag Italia 2014

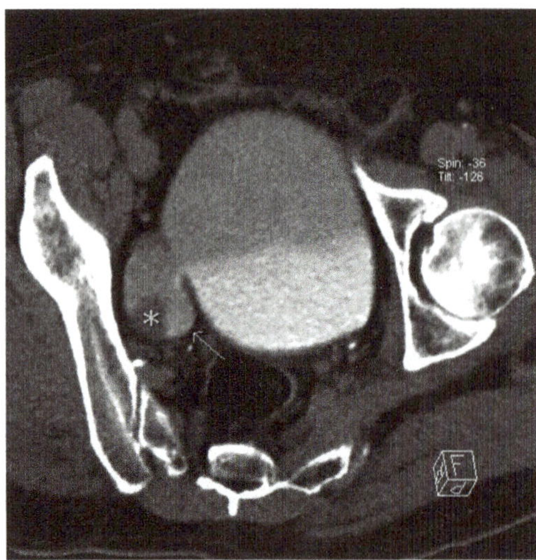

Fig. 82.1 Multiplanar reconstruction (MPR) CT image shows a soft tissue mass (*asterisk*) in a bladder diverticulum (*arrow*) in 68-year-old man

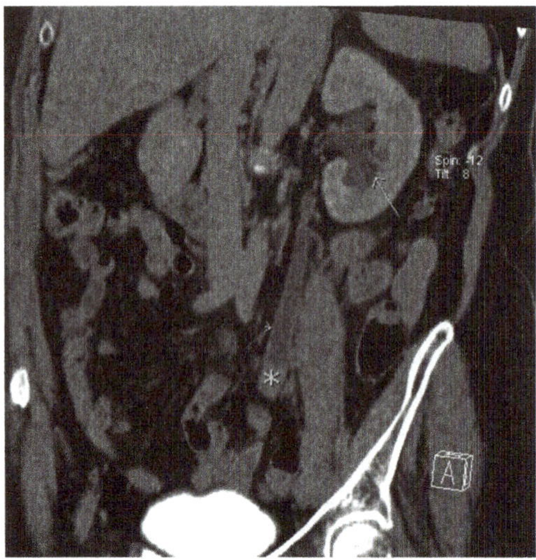

Fig. 82.2 Coronal multiplanar reconstruction (MPR) CT urography scan of 69-year-old patient shows dilatation of the left pelvicalyceal system (*long arrow*) and proximal ureter (*short arrow*) due to obstruction by midureteric transitional cell carcinoma (*asterisk*)

as patients with superficial cancer, which is confined to the mucosa and lamina propria, are often treated with transurethral resection, while patients with muscle-invasive cancer are treated with cystectomy. Cystoscopy and biopsy are the standard of reference for local staging of lower tract urothelial cancer. CT technique is unable to demonstrate the various bladder wall layers accurately; thereby, its accuracy in the T staging of bladder cancer is seriously limited [6]. However, MRI provides superior soft tissue resolution compared with CT and allows occasionally detection of muscle-invasive disease [2]. The detrusor muscle is low in signal on T2-weighted images, while the signal intensity of tumors is typically intermediate. In patients with stage T2b disease, the hypointense band (muscle) is interrupted by the tumor [2]. Both CT and MRI cannot detect microscopic invasion of perivesical fat (stage T3a) [7]. In patients with invasive bladder cancer (Fig. 82.3), the goal of CT or MR imaging is to detect T3b disease or higher, which may help to stratify patients into those who might benefit from neoadjuvant chemotherapy before definitive cystectomy and those who should undergo radiotherapy rather than radical surgery [7]. For local staging of bladder tumors, the role of a multiparametric MRI approach with conventional and functional sequences (diffusion-weighted images and dynamic contrast material techniques) is evolving and has not yet been fully established. It is important to mention that if imaging is done after transurethral biopsy or resection, perivesical fat stranding is often seen and it is difficult to discriminate postprocedure reactions from

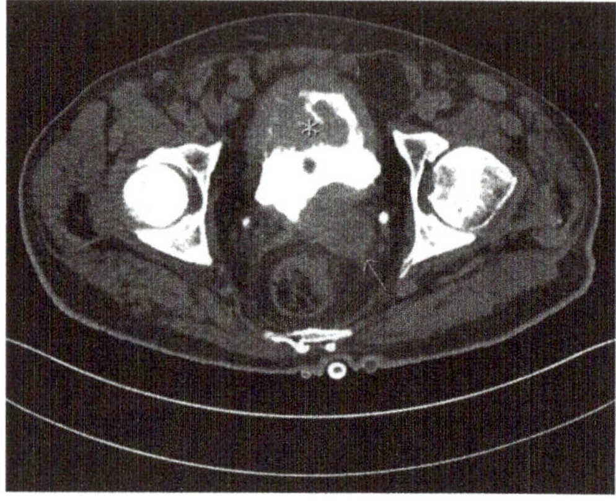

Fig. 82.3 Invasive urothelial carcinoma in a 74-year-old man. CT urography scan shows extensive irregular bladder wall thickening (compatible with primary tumor), a tumor (*asterisk*) on the right anterior lateral wall of the bladder, and extravesical tumor spread involving the left seminal vesicle (*arrow*)

extravesicular extension [8]. Hence, imaging for local staging is best to be performed before biopsy or transurethral resection.

Cross-sectional imaging (mainly CT) is now routinely employed in the surgical planning of patient with upper urinary tract urothelial cancer. CT can demonstrate extension into the peripelvic or periureteric fat. Although CT does not permit distinction between T1 and T2 tumors, it does allow discrimination of early stage disease confined to the collecting system wall from locally advanced tumors [9]. In early stage pelvicalyceal tumors (T1 or T2 disease), a fat plane or a layer of contrast medium separates the mass from the renal parenchyma (Fig. 82.4). Increased peripelvic fat attenuation and abnormal enhancement of the adjacent parenchyma are signs of a T3 tumor [10]. Unlike in renal cell cancer, invasion of the renal vein or inferior vena cava is seen rarely. As with CT, MRI can determine intra- and extra-renal local extension of tumor and has been shown to allow accurate local staging of tumors larger than 2 cm [9]. Therefore, it offers an alternative staging modality in patients who cannot be subjected to a CT.

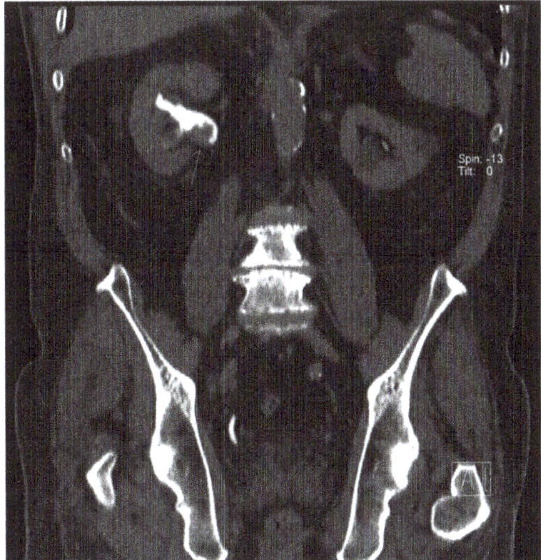

Fig. 82.4 Coronal multiplanar reconstruction (MPR) CT image shows a mass (*arrow*) as filling defect in the right renal pelvis. A fat plane separates the mass from the renal parenchyma in keeping with early stage pelvicalyceal tumor

Both CT and MRI are effective in detection of nodal (short-axis diameter larger than 1 cm) and hematogenous metastases of urothelial cancer. Either of these findings is critical, because it has profound implications for treatment planning. Using size criteria for detecting lymphatic spread has known limitations as small lymph nodes may contain tumor and enlarged lymph nodes may be reactive. CT and MRI show similar rates of accuracy for nodal staging. Distant metastases most commonly occur to the lungs, liver, bones, and brain. Both CT and MRI are sensitive techniques for the detection of liver metastases. Concerning hematogenous spread to lungs, CT is the ideal method, although chest radiography can be sufficient in low risk patients. Brain imaging (CT or MRI) and bone scanning are generally performed only in the presence of symptoms and signs suggesting disease at these sites.

82.4 Follow-up Evaluation

The hallmark of urothelial cancer is the high rate of recurrence and strict follow-up of these patients after treatment is mandatory. Nearly 2–4 % of patients with bladder cancer develop upper tract urothelial cancer, while 30–40 and 2–6 % of patients with upper tract urothelial cancer develop bladder or contralateral collecting system recurrence, respectively [3]. Cystoscopy, urine cytology, and imaging of the upper tract are usually performed in order to identify metachronous tumors early enough for curative therapies. Other sites of disease recurrence (especially in the case of invasive tumors) are lymph nodes, liver, and lungs. Common practices include routine cross-sectional imaging of the abdomen and pelvis and periodic chest evaluation (with CT or radiography), while CT of the head and bone scanning are performed in the event of symptoms.

82.5 Conclusion

Technical advances of multidetector CT and MRI allow these modalities to be useful adjuncts to cystoscopic evaluation by providing critical information about the diagnosis, staging, and surveillance of patients with urothelial cancer. Therefore, cross-sectional imaging plays a crucial role in directing clinical management of these patients.

References

1. Mouli S, Casalino DD, Nikolaidis P (2012) Imaging features of common and uncommon bladder neoplasms. Radiol Clin North Am 50(2):301–316
2. Verma S, Rajesh A, Prasad SR, Gaitonde K, Lall CG, Mouraviev V, Aeron G, Bracken RB, Sandrasegaran K (2012) Urinary bladder cancer: role of MR imaging. Radiographics 32(2):371–387
3. Lee EK, Dickstein RJ, Kamta AM (2011) Imaging of urothelial cancers: what the urologist needs to know. AJR 196(6):1249–1254
4. Jinzaki M, Matsumoto K, Kikuchi E, Sato K, Horiguchi Y, Nishiwaki Y, Silverman SG (2011) Comparison of CT urography and excretory urography in the detection and localization of urothelial carcinoma of the upper urinary tract. AJR 196(5):1102–1109
5. Rouprêt M, Zigeuner R, Palou J, Boehle A, Kaasinen E, Sylvester R, Babjuk M, Oosterlinck W (2011) European guidelines for the diagnosis and management of upper urinary tract urothelial cell carcinomas: 2011 update. Eur Urol 59(4):584–594
6. Vikram R, Sandler CM, Ng CS (2009) Imaging and staging of transitional cell carcinoma: part 1, lower urinary tract. AJR 192(6):1481–1487
7. Cowan NC, Crew JP (2010) Imaging bladder cancer. Curr Opin Urol 20(5):409–413
8. Bostrom PJ, van Rhijn BW, Fleshner N, Finelli A, Jewett M, Thoms J, Hanna S, Kuk C, Zlotta AR (2010) Staging and staging errors in bladder cancer. Eur Urol suppl 9:2–9
9. Browne RF, Meehan CP, Colville J, Power R, Torreggiani WC (2005) Transitional cell carcinoma of the upper urinary tract: spectrum of imaging findings. Radiographics 25(6):1609–1627
10. Vikram R, Sandler CM, Ng CS (2009) Imaging and staging of transitional cell carcinoma: part 2, upper urinary tract. AJR 192(6):1488–1493

83 Clinical Implications of Urothelial Cancer

Gerasimos J. Alivizatos

83.1 Diagnosis-Staging

For non-muscle invasive bladder cancer (Ta, T1 and CIS) ultrasonography (US) is the first method used to investigate the anatomy of the bladder and the upper urinary tract. Intravenous urography has been used for decades and today CT urography is being used with increased frequency. CT urography is the gold standard for exploration of the upper urinary tract with reported sensitivity and specificity of 93.5 and 94.8 % for the detection of urothelial cancer. MRI is infrequently used in the primary investigation of upper tract urothelial cancer. The detection rate of MRI urography is 75 % for tumours <2 cm and the method is indicated in patients who cannot be subjected to a CT urography. Muscle invasive bladder cancer is first being evaluated with US and intravenous urography but CT and MRI scans are used for TNM classification. PET/CT scans do not offer additional information and should not be used [1, 2].

83.2 Follow-up Strategies

Imaging plays an important role in the follow-up of patients with urothelial cell cancers. The investigations used include chest X-ray, CT urography and both CT and MRI are effective in detection of nodal (short-axis diameter larger than 1 cm) and hematogenous metastases of urothelial cancer. PET scans can be used for the evaluation of suspected nodal metastasis as well [1, 2].

References

1. Babjuk M, Oosterlinck W, Sylvester R, Kaasinen E, Bohle A, Palou-Redorta M, Roupret M (2011) EAU Guidelines on non-muscle-invasive urothelial carcinoma of the bladder (the 2011 update). Eur Urol 59:997–1008
2. Swinnen G, Maes A, Pottel H et al (2010) FDG-PET/CT for the preoperative lymph node staging of invasive bladder cancer. Eur Urol 57(4):641–647

G. J. Alivizatos (✉)
3rd Urological Department, HYGEIA Hospital,
Erythrou Stavrou 4, 15123, Athens, Greece
e-mail: gali@hol.gr

A. D. Gouliamos et al. (eds.), *Imaging in Clinical Oncology*,
DOI: 10.1007/978-88-470-5385-4_83, © Springer-Verlag Italia 2014

84 Introduction to Testicular Cancer

Gerasimos J. Alivizatos and Pavlos A. Pavlakis

Cancer of the testis is relatively uncommon, accounting for 1–1.5 % of male neoplasms and 5 % of all urological tumours in general [1]. However, several epidemiological features of testicular cancer are particularly striking, including the peak incidence in young men and the rising incidence over the last 50 years in young whites. Within the developed countries, 3–10 new cases per 100,000 males/per year have been reported. In the United States, testicular cancer is one of the most common malignancies in the age rate of 20–40, and the second most common cancer after leukemia among males aged 15 to 19 years [2] .

Epidemiological risk factors for the development of testicular tumors include a history of cryptorchidism or undescended testis, Klinefelter's syndrome, familial history of testicular tumors, infertility and the presence of a tumor in the contralateral testicle [3].

New advances in imaging, tumor markers, and the introduction of cisplatin-based chemotherapy have improved survival from 10 % in the 1970s to more than 90 % today [4].

In this chapter all contributors deal with the recent advances in various new imaging techniques and it is important to understand what is being offered today with these new applications since some of these inovations might help the clinicians in improving the survival of our patients and their quality of life.

G. J. Alivizatos (✉) · P. A. Pavlakis
3rd Urological Department, Hygeia Hospital,
Erythrou Stavrou 4, Athens, 15123, Greece
e-mail: gali@hol.gr

84.1 Pathological Classification

Since there are many different histological variations within this group of tumors it is important to clarify the various subtypes [5] .

1. Germ cell tumours (90–95 %)
   Intratubular germ cell neoplasia, unclassified type (IGCNU)
   Seminoma (including cases with syncytiotrophoblastic cells)
   Spermatocytic seminoma (mention if there is sarcomatous component)
   Embryonal carcinoma
   Yolk sac tumour
   Choriocarcinoma
   Teratoma (mature, immature, with malignant component)
   Tumours with more than one histological type (specify percentage of individual components).
2. Sex cord/gonadal stromal tumours
   Leydig cell tumour
   Malignant Leydig cell tumour
   Sertoli cell tumour
   lipid-rich variant
   sclerosing
   large cell calcifying
   Malignant Sertoli cell tumour

A. D. Gouliamos et al. (eds.), *Imaging in Clinical Oncology*,
DOI: 10.1007/978-88-470-5385-4_84, © Springer-Verlag Italia 2014

Granulosa cell tumour
- adult type

juvenile type
Thecoma/fibroma group of tumours
Other sex cord/gonadal stromal tumours
- incompletely differentiated

mixed
Tumours containing germ cell and sex cord/ gonadal stromal (gonadoblastoma).

3. Miscellaneous non-specific stromal tumours
Ovarian epithelial tumours
Tumours of the collecting ducts and rete testis
Tumours (benign and malignant) of non-specific stroma.

84.2 Clinical Examination

The physical examination of the testes is best performed with the patient standing and the urologist seated facing him.

The most common presentation of a testicular tumor is that of a painless mass but in 25 % of the cases scrotal pain might be present as well. During the clinical examination, firstly the affected and then the normal contralateral testis must be examined, noting size and consistency.With palpation, testicular or extratesticular masses can be found. Atrophy of the affected or contralateral testis is common, particularly in patients with a history of cryptorchidism. Any firm area within the testis is suggestive of malignancy and should prompt further investigations [6] .

A hydrocele may accompany a testicular cancer and impair the examiner's ability to evaluate the testis. In this case, scrotal ultrasonography to evaluate the testis is warranted. The patient should also be examined for any evidence of palpable abdominal mass or tenderness, inguinal lymphadenopathy (particularly if he has had prior inguinal or scrotal surgery), gynecomastia, and supraclavicular lymphadenopathy; and auscultation of the chest should be done in a search for intrathoracic disease.

Orchioepidymitis can also confuse the diagnostic procedure and in some cases might delay the proper diagnosis.

84.3 TNM Classification

The TNM classification of testicular cancer is done according to the guide lines of the International Union against Cancer (UICC) published in 2009 [7].

pT Primary tumour
pTX Primary tumour cannot be assessed
pT0 No evidence of primary tumour (e.g. histological scar in testis)
pTis Intratubular germ cell neoplasia (testicular intraepithelial neoplasia)
pT1 Tumour limited to testis and epididymis without vascular/lymphatic invasion: tumour may invade tunica albuginea but not tunica vaginalis
pT2 Tumour limited to testis and epididymis with vascular/lymphatic invasion, or tumour extending through tunica albuginea with involvement of tunica vaginalis
pT3 Tumour invades spermatic cord with or without vascular/lymphatic invasion
pT4 Tumour invades scrotum with or without vascular/lymphatic invasion
N Regional lymph nodes clinical
NX Regional lymph nodes cannot be assessed
N0 No regional lymph node metastasis
N1 Metastasis with a lymph node mass 2 cm or less in greatest dimension or multiple lymph nodes, none more than 2 cm in greatest dimension
N2 Metastasis with a lymph node mass more than 2 cm but not more than 5 cm in greatest dimension, or multiple lymph nodes, any one mass more than 2 cm but not more than 5 cm in greatest dimension
N3 Metastasis with a lymph node mass more than 5 cm in greatest dimension
pN Pathological
pNX Regional lymph nodes cannot be assessed
pN0 No regional lymph node metastasis
pN1 Metastasis with a lymph node mass 2 cm or less in greatest dimension and 5 or fewer positive nodes, none more than 2 cm in greatest dimension
pN2 Metastasis with a lymph node mass more than 2 cm but not more than 5 cm in greatest

dimension; or more than 5 nodes positive, none more than 5 cm; or evidence or extra nodal
extension of tumour

pN3 Metastasis with a lymph node mass more than 5 cm in greatest dimension

M Distant metastasis

MX Distant metastasis cannot be assessed

M0 No distant metastasis

M1 Distant metastasis

M1a Non-regional lymph node(s) or lung

M1b Other sites

S Serum tumour markers

Sx Serum marker studies not available or not performed

S0 Serum marker study levels within normal limits

The International Germ Cell Cancer Collaborative Group (IGCCCG) introduced a prognostic based staging system for metastatic germ cell cancer in which histology, location of the primary tumor, location of metastases and prechemotherapy marker levels have been incorporated as prognostic factors (Table 84.1) [8].

84.4 Imaging Dilemmas in Testicular Cancer

Imaging modalities play an important role in every step from diagnosis to follow up after treatment and their impact in the decision making is of great value.

84.4.1 Imaging and Diagnosis

Scrotal ultrasound (S/U) is the standard diagnostic procedure to explore the presence of a testicular mass [9]. It is an important tool also in those cases where physical examination is limited either by pain or by a hydrocele.

S/U should also be performed in those cases where a retroperitoneal mass is found or when serum tumor markers (chorionic gonadotrophin alfa fetoprotein) are elevated. One question that remains open is the accuracy by which a

Table 84.1 Prognostic-based staging system for metastatic germ cell cancer (international germ cell cancer collaborative group)

Good-prognosis group
Non-seminoma (56 % of cases)
5-year PFS 89 %
5-year survival 92 %
All of the following criteria:
• Testis/retroperitoneal primary
• No non-pulmonary visceral metastases
• AFP < 1,000 ng/mL
• hCG < 5,000 IU/L (1,000 ng/mL)
• LDH < 1.5 × ULN
Seminoma (90 % of cases)
5-year PFS 82 %
5-year survival 86 %
All of the following criteria:
• Any primary site
• No non-pulmonary visceral metastases
• Normal AFP
• Any hCG
• Any LDH
Intermediate prognosis group
Non-seminoma (28 % of cases)
5 years PFS 75 %
5-year survival 80 %
• Testis/retroperitoneal primary
• No non-pulmonary visceral metastases
• AFP 1,000–10,000 ng/mL or
• hCG 5,000–50,000 IU/L or
• LDH 1.5–10 x ULN
Seminoma (10 % of cases)
5-year PFS 67 %
5-year survival 72 %
Any of the following criteria:
• Any primary site
• Non-pulmonary visceral metastases
• Normal AFP
• Any hCG
• Any LDH
Poor prognosis group
Non-seminoma (16 % of cases)

(continued)

Table 84.1 (continued)

Good-prognosis group
5-year PFS 41 %
5-year survival 48 %
Any of the following criteria:
• Mediastinal primary
• Non-pulmonary visceral metastases
• AFP > 10,000 ng/mL or
• hCG > 50,000 IU/L (10,000 ng/mL) or
• LDH > 10 × ULN
Seminoma
No patients classified as poor prognosis

*Pre-chemotherapy serum tumour markers should be assessed immediately prior to the administration of chemotherapy (same day)
PFS progression-free survival; *AFP* alpha-fetoprotein; *hCG* human chorionic gonadotrophin
LDH lactate dehydrogenase

radiologist can give information upon the differential diagnosis between a seminoma and a non seminomatous germ cell tumour.

There are a few cases when a suspicious lesion in ultrasound examination is not a tumour and a urologist would like to know what other investigation could offer more information after the U/S in order to avoid removing a testis with a benign lesion.

Magnetic resonance imaging (MRI) has also been used for the diagnosis of testicular cancer but it should be explained why an expensive diagnostic procedure can be justified and if it is recommended in every case [10].

84.4.2 Imaging and Staging

U/S exam does not provide accurate information for staging and the American Joint Committee on Cancer (AJCC) recommends radiologic investigation of the chest, the abdomen and the pelvis. Rarely, if any peculiar symptoms are present the status of the brain and the skeleton has to be checked as well.

The lymph nodes that have to be evaluated are the retroperitoneal the supraclavicular and the mediastinal nodes. All these groups of nodes are being assessed with CT scans which offer a sensitivity of 70–80 % [11]. One issue that still remains is the definition of an abnormal node. The cut off value of 1 cm is being used but it has been shown that with this value 20–40 % of metastasis are missed. With smaller cut off values sensitivity improves but specificity worsens. MRI has been used as well but it seems that it does not offer any clear advantages to CT scans and therefore it's routine use is not recommended [12]. In cases were intravenous contrast can be harmfull, MRI is indicated.

PET scans have also been studied as an initial tool for staging of testicular cancer but it's use in the initial staging procedure does not add any valuable extra information after a CT scan and therefore is not recommended [13].

Examination of the liver is being performed with the abdominal CT scan but it is the only organ that can be checked thoroughly with an ultrasound examination as well.

84.4.3 Imaging and Follow Up

After termination of the selected treatment option (surveillance, lymph node dissection, chemtherapy or radiation), restaging is being performed with physical examination, measurment of serum tumour markers and imaging that includes mainly chest X-rays and abdomino-pelvic CT scans. The recommended follow up shedule depends on the histology of the tumor and on the stage of the disease when the diagnosis was first established. CT scans reveal wether chemotherapy influences the size of the affected nodes. A common problem in metastatic testicular cancer is the evaluation of residual lymph masses after chemotherapy. If tumor cells are still present within the residual masses, surgical removal is mandatory [14]. If the residual masses are fibrotic tissue, observation can be recommended but again the histology of the tumor and the size of the residual nodes influence the decisions taken by oncologists and urologists. CT scans cannot distinguish viable tumor from fibrotic tissue and therefore PET scans can, in some cases, give an answer to such dilemmas [15]. Surgical removal of these residual masses need skilled surgeons and should be performed in highly specialized centers. In many situations vascular surgeons have to be recruited as well since the aorta and the vena cava can be traumatized.It is therefore of outmost importance to know in advance if these operations are necessary or not and when they are planned a group of experts must collaborate in order to achieve good results [16].

84.5 Conclusions

In this chapter all the contributors will analyze the latest developments of all imaging modalities that are used today in order to offer the correct information to urologists and oncologists who treat men with testicular cancer. Correct information leads to correct decisions upon further chemotherapy and upon surgical procedures and all these difficult decisions have the purpose to avoid unnecessary therapies that might hamper the quality of life of our patients.

References

1. La Vecchia C, Bosetti C, Lucchini F et al (2010) Cancer Mortality in Europe, 2000–2004, and an overview of trends since 1995. Ann Oncol 21(6): 1323–1360
2. Cancer Incidence in Five Continents (2007) vol IX. Curado MP, Edwards B, Shin R, et al (eds) IARC Scientific, Publication No. 160
3. Mannuel H, Mitikiri N, Khan M et al (2012) Testicular germ cell tumors: biology and clinical update. Curr Opin Oncol 24(3):266–271
4. Tummala M, Hussain A (2008) Recent developments in germ cell tumors. Curr Opin Oncol 20(3):287–293
5. Albers P, Albercht W, Algaba F et al (2011) EAU guidelines on testicular cancer: 2011 update. Eur Urol 60(2):304–319
6. Morarles-Barrera R, Valverde C, Rodon J et al (2010) Bilateral testicular germ cell tumors: a single hospital experience. Clin Trans Oncol 12(4): 299–302
7. Fleming J, Cooper J, Henson D et al (1997) Testis. In American joint committee on cancer staging manual, 5th edn Philadelfia, Lippincot-Raven
8. International Germ Cell Collaborative Group (1997) International germ cell consensus classification: a prognostic factor based staging system for metastatic germ cell cancers. J Clin Oncol 15(2):594–603
9. Kim W, Rosen MA, Langer JE et al (2007) US-MR Imaging correlation in pathologic conditions of the scrotum. Radiographics 27(5):1239–1253
10. Cassidy FH, Ishioka KM, McMahon CJ et al (2010) MR imaging of scrotal tumors and pseudotumors. Radiographics 30(3):665–683
11. Husband JE, Barrett A, Peckham MJ (1981) Evaluation of computed tomography in the management of testicular teratoma. Br J Urol 53(2): 179–183
12. Ellis JH, Blies JR, Kopecky KK et al (1984) Comparison of NMR and CT imaging in the evaluation of metastatic retroperitoneal lymphadenopathy from testicular carcinoma. J Comput Assist Tomogr 8(4):709–719
13. Oechsle K, Hartmann M, Brenner W, et al (2008) German multicenter positron emission tomography study group. 18F Fluorodeoxyglucose positron emission tomography in nonseminomatous germ cell tumors after chemotherapy: the German multicenter positron emission tomography study group. J Clin Oncol 20;26(36):5930–5
14. Winter C, Pfister D, Busch J et al (2012) Residual tumor size and IGCCCG risk classification predict additional vascular procedures in patients with germ cell tumors and residual tumor resection: a multicenter analysis of the German testicular cancer study group. Eur Urol 61(2):403–409
15. De Santis M, Becherer A, Bokemeyer C et al (2004) Pont J. 2–18fluoro-deoxy-D-glucose positron emission tomography is a reliable predictor for viable tumor in postchemotherapy seminoma: an update of the prospective multicentric SEMPET trial. J Clin Oncol 22(6):1034–1039
16. Daneshmand S, Albers P, Fossa A et al (2012) Contemporary management of postchemotherapy testis cancer. Eur Urol 62(5):867–876

85 US Findings in Testicular Cancer

Ioannis A. Tsitouridis and Georgios E. Glataganas

Testicular tumors are a heterogeneous group of neoplasms in which the sonographic findings represent very closed to their histologic nature.

Seminomas are more homogeneous with clearly defined margins and internal septa. Nonseminomatous tumors have more heterogenous appearance.

Ultrasound (US) is the initial imaging and also the method of choice in the evaluation of testicular tumors, with a sensitivity almost 100 %, but the histologic type of tumor is very difficult to be determined with high accuracy from the sonographic findings only (1).

The indications for sonographic exam in the evaluation of a testicular tumor include:

(a) The evaluation of palpable intratesticular mass
(b) The evaluation of a testis with increased size
(c) The detection for a tumor under the presentation of hydrocele, hematocele, trauma, or infection
(d) The detection for underlying tumor in patients with microlithiasis
(e) The evaluation of a burned out testicular tumor in cases of extragonadal tumor
(f) The evaluation of the testis in cases of polysystemic neoplasia.

Seminomas are hypoechoic tumors, with clearly defined margins, homogeneous, with internal echogenic septa. Over 10 % of seminomas contain cystic elements which represent tumor necrotic areas or dilatation of the rete testis due to obstruction from the tumor (Figs. 85.1, 85.2).

Color Doppler US usually reveals rich internal vasculature in seminomas, although tumors smaller than 1.6 cm can usually reveal low vascularity [1].

Nonseminomatous testicular tumors have a heterogeneous pattern of echoes distribution due to necrosis, calcification, hemorrhage, and fibrosis. Like in seminomas, the cystic elements represent tumor necrosis or dilatation of the rete testis and only in teratomas are true epithelial cysts. At Color Doppler US of the solid part of these tumors usually reveals rich internal vasculature (Fig. 85.3) [2].

In recent years, real-time sonoelastography is used to add informations to the conventional ultrasound for testicular tumor characterization (Fig. 85.4).

All the large-sized testicular tumors reveal reduced elasticity (hard lesions) with a sensitivity of 100 %, specificity 81 %, and accuracy 94 % [3].

Although some small-sized malignant lesions may preserve its elasticity, in the majority of the cases (87.5 %) they behave as hard lesions.

I. A. Tsitouridis (✉) · G. E. Glataganas
Department of Radiology, General Hospital Papageorglou, Thessaloniki, Ring Road Thessaloniki-Efkarpia, Thessaloniki, 685111, Greece
e-mail: tsitouridis.1@gmail.com

G. E. Glataganas
e-mail: gialim@hol.gr

A. D. Gouliamos et al. (eds.), *Imaging in Clinical Oncology*,
DOI: 10.1007/978-88-470-5385-4_85, © Springer-Verlag Italia 2014

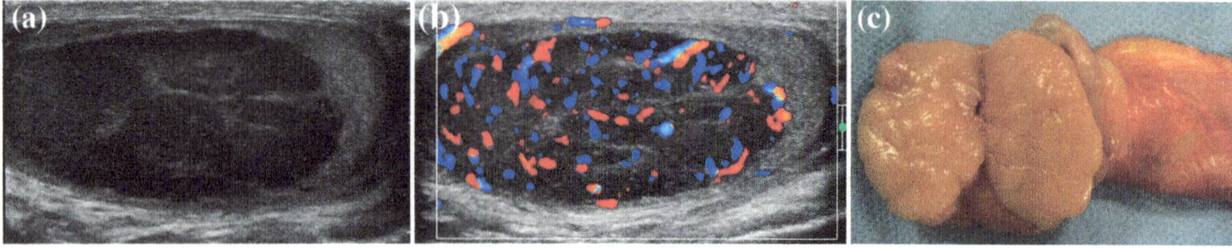

Fig. 85.1 **a** Sagittal *gray-scale* sonogram which reveals a seminoma in the *right* testis, hypoechoic with internal septa (*echogenic lines*) with rich vascularity (**b**). **c** Photograph of the surgical specimen

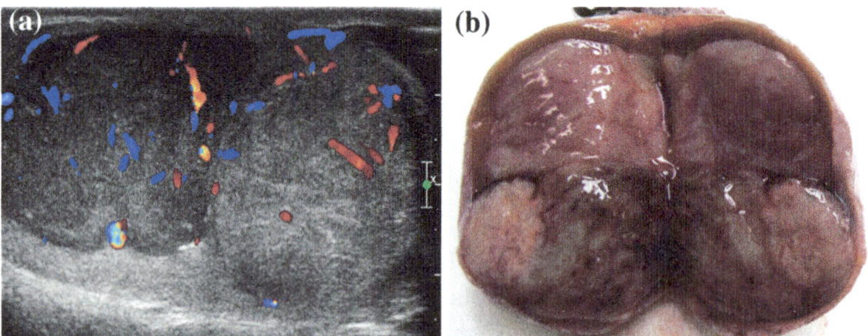

Fig. 85.2 **a** Sagittal color doppler sonogram of the right testis. There are two large nodules of seminomas and only little normal testicular tissue. **b** Macroscopic view of the seminomatous nodules and the small peripheral normal testicular tissue

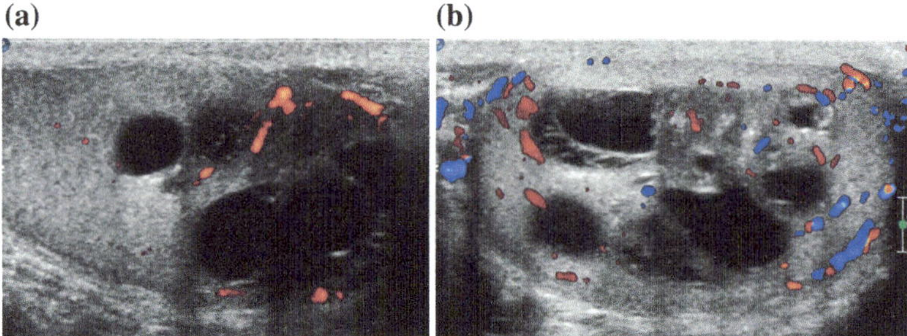

Fig. 85.3 **a, b** Sagittal color doppler sonogram of the left testis which reveals a mixed nonseminomatous tumor (teratoma and embryonic carcinoma). There are true teratomatous cystic lesions in the tumor

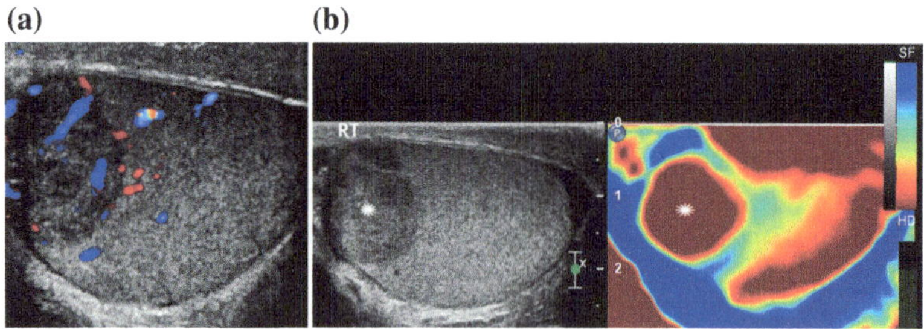

Fig. 85.4 **a** Sagittal color doppler sonogram of the *left* testis which reveals a seminoma with rich vascularity in the upper testicular pole. **b** Elastography of the left testis reveals that seminoma (*asterisk*) is a hard lesion (*red*) in comparison to the normal testicular parenchyma

In the small-sized testicular nodules sonoelastography reveal lower sensitivity (87 %), increased specificity (98.2 %), and lower accuracy (95 %), [3].

US has a limited role in the staging and follow-up of patients with testicular tumor. US has usually two indications in the staging procedure:

(a) Complementary to MRI evaluation of invasion of tunica albuginea, tunica vaginalis, and spermatic cord,

(b) US is used to evaluate the other testis for a second tumor, because danger for a second tumor in the other testis is 2–5 % for the first 15 years, especially in patients with seminomas under the age of 30 years [4].

References

1. Andipa E, Liberopoulos K, Asvestis C (2004) Magnetic resonance imaging and ultrasound evaluation of penile and testicular masses. World J Urol 22: 382–391
2. Sohaib SA, Koh DM, Husband JE (2008) The role of imaging in the diagnosis staging and management of testicular cancer. AJR 191:387–395
3. Goddi A, Sacchi A, Magistretti G, Almolla J, Salvadore M (2012) Real –time tissue elastography for testicular lesion assessment. Eur Radiol 22: 721–730
4. Krege S, Beyer J, Souchon R et al (2008) European consensus conference on diagnosis and treatment of germ cell cancer: a report of the second meeting of the European germ gell cancer consensus group. Eur Urol 53:478–513

CT and MRI Findings in Testicular Cancer

86

Fotios D. Laspas

86.1 Introduction

Ultrasonography (US) remains the primary imaging method for detecting testicular masses. Magnetic Resonance Imaging (MRI) of the scrotum is an efficient diagnostic tool, but it is usually used when the US findings are equivocal. Computed Tomography (CT) is the standard imaging modality for the staging and follow-up evaluation of testicular tumors, while MRI may be helpful in patients with an inconclusive CT study.

86.2 Diagnosis

In general, the diagnosis of testicular cancer is made pathologically at surgery. The US is the imaging method of choice for confirming the presence of a testicular mass which has been detected in clinical examination. MRI is mainly used as a problem solving tool. The diagnostic accuracy of MRI in the preoperative characterization of malignant testicular tumors is higher than 96 % [1].

The differentiation of seminomatous from nonseminomatous testicular neoplasms is clinically important as treatment and prognosis differ between the two tumor types. MRI may be helpful in the histologic subtyping of testicular cancer [2], but this has little clinical value because orchidectomy is mandatory for primary treatment.

On MRI, seminomas are usually well defined and homogeneous and appear as hypointense lesions within the high-signal normal testicular parenchyma on T2-weighted images (Fig. 86.1). On the other hand, nonseminomatous tumors are typically more heterogeneous masses on both T1-weighted and T2-weighted images, with areas of hemorrhage or necrosis showing heterogeneous enhancement after intravenous gadolinium administration.

86.3 Staging

Once the diagnosis of testicular cancer has been established, assessment of disease extent must be performed. The TNM staging system is mainly used [3]. MRI seems to be more efficient than US in evaluation of local tumor extension, but it is of little significance as every patient with a testicular cancer must undergo orchidectomy and thus the histological analysis of the specimen is taken into account in determining the T stage (postoperative T staging) [4].

Testicular cancer lymphatic spread follows the testicular veins to paraaortic lymph nodes up to the level of the renal hila reflecting the retroperitoneal embryological origin of the testis [5]. Lymph nodes in the aortocaval chain at the

F. D. Laspas (✉)
CT&MRI Department, Hygeia Hospital,
4, Erythrou Stavrou Str. & Kifisias Av., 15123,
Marousi, Athens, Attica, Greece
e-mail: fotisdimi@yahoo.gr

A. D. Gouliamos et al. (eds.), *Imaging in Clinical Oncology*,
DOI: 10.1007/978-88-470-5385-4_86, © Springer-Verlag Italia 2014

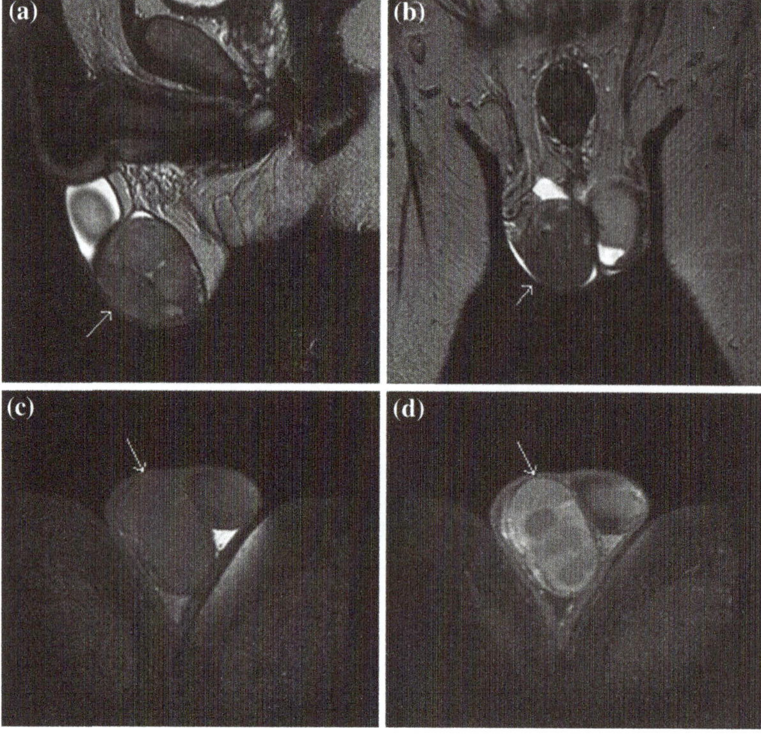

Fig. 86.1 29-year-old man with seminoma of right testicle. Sagittal (**a**) and coronal (**b**) T2-weighted MR images show multinodular right testicular lesion (*arrow*) of low signal intensity compared with normal testicular parenchyma. Transverse T1-weighted MR images before (**c**) and after (**d**) gadolinium administration show enhancement of the mass (*arrow*)

level of the second lumbar vertebral body are considered as the primary sites of spread for right-sided tumors, while left-sided tumors typically spread to lymph nodes left paraaortic nodal group just below the left renal vein. Isolated contralateral nodal metastases (without the presence of the ipsilateral nodes) are uncommon. Moreover, metastases to the pelvic and inguinal lymph nodes are also rare in the absence of bulky retroperitoneal disease or previous scrotal or inguinal surgery (because the normal lymphatic drainage pathways are disrupted by surgery) [5]. Mediastinal nodal involvement may also occur in patients with metastatic retroperitoneal lymph nodes. Hematogenous spread most commonly occurs to the lungs. Other common sites of disseminated disease include the brain, bones, and liver, although essentially any organ may be involved mainly in the setting of advanced disease [6].

Multidetector CT (MDCT) remains the most widely available and primary imaging modality for testicular cancer staging. Metastatic lymphadenopathy varies in size from small lymph nodes to bulky masses (Fig. 86.2). On CT, nodal masses from seminoma frequently appear of soft tissue attenuation, whereas retroperitoneal masses from nonseminomatous tumors tend to be heterogeneous in density, with areas of cystic change and soft tissue elements [6]. In large volume disease, the diagnosis of metastatic lymphadenopathy is readily made, however, the assessment of small-volume metastatic disease (which is critical for patient staging and management) is often inaccurate, as a substantial proportion of lymph nodes with microscopic invasion are not enlarged to an abnormal size. Taking the standard lymph node size criterion (short axis diameter larger than 1 cm), the CT specificity for retroperitoneal metastatic lymphadenopathy is high (up to 100 %), however, its sensitivity is low (ranges from 24 to 78 %) [4, 7]. MRI is comparable to CT for detecting lymph nodes [8] and has the same limitation of using size criteria (inability to detect microscopic invasion in normal-sized lymph nodes and differentiate malignant from reactive lymphadenopathy). Therefore, MRI is proposed as an alternative method for retroperitoneal nodal evaluation, especially in young adults to whom

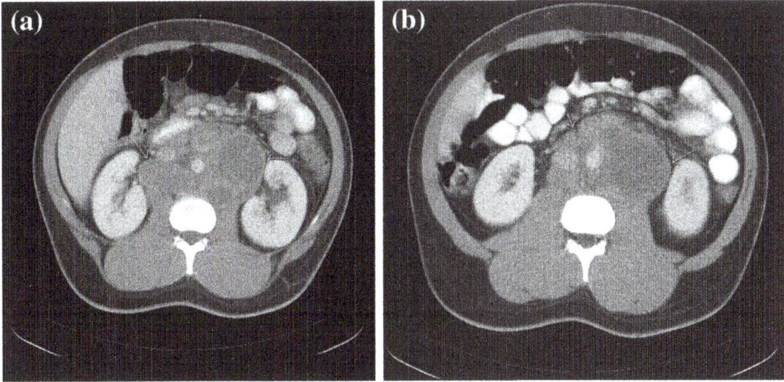

Fig. 86.2 24-year-old man with metastatic nonseminomatous germ cell tumor. CT images (**a**, **b**) show a large heterogeneous retroperitoneal nodal mass (*arrows*)

radiation exposure should be avoided. Moreover, new MRI techniques such as lymphotropic nanoparticle-enhanced MRI are being explored in detecting lymph node metastasis [9].

MDCT is the most useful imaging method for assessing metastatic disease in the chest, abdomen, and pelvis. Concerning hematogenous spread to lungs, CT is the ideal method. For the detection of liver metastases, MRI is a sensitive technique; however, it is used as problem solving tool when CT findings are inconclusive. Brain imaging (CT or MRI) and bone scanning are generally performed only in the presence of symptoms suggesting disease at these sites and in patients with multiple metastases and poor prognosis. Concerning cerebral metastases, MRI is more sensitive for the detection of smaller lesions than CT.

86.4 Follow-up Evaluation—Response to Therapy

Another important use of radiologic imaging is for early detection of tumor recurrence. In testicular cancer, recurrence mainly occurs in the retroperitoneal lymph nodes and within the first year after orchidectomy [4]. Early detection of tumor relapse is clinically important because it is associated with a very high survival rate after treatment. CT remains the mainstay of imaging in the follow-up protocols. Some authors still recommend that chest radiography can be sufficient for assessment of the lung, especially in low-risk groups of metastatic disease, despite, the fact that it is far less sensitive than chest CT. Brain imaging is indicated in cases where there is clinical suspicion of brain metastases. The abdominopelvic MRI is mainly used when iodinated contrast agent is contraindicated, such as in the cases of compromised renal function and severe allergy. However, abdominopelvic MRI could be used as an alternative method for the assessment of abdominal metastatic disease in order to reduce radiation exposure. The frequency of monitoring varies depending on the type of the tumor, stage, and initial treatment. As the relapses mainly occur within the first year after orchidectomy, follow-up should be more intensive in the first year.

CT is the primary imaging method for monitoring the response to therapy, mainly by measuring the change in size of metastases. Reduction in the size of metastases shows a response to the treatment, while increase in the size or appearance of new lesions indicates progression of the disease. However, a retroperitoneal persistent nodal mass frequently remains after therapy. The observation of retroperitoneal residual mass does not always indicate the presence of viable tumor cells, as this residual mass after therapy may consist of only fibrotic and necrotic tissues. It is impossible to distinguish necrotic remnants from residual vital tumor tissue preoperatively. PET is more accurate than conventional imaging modalities for assessing the success of treatment in the presence of residual masses, especially in pure seminoma [10].

86.5 Conclusion

For diagnosis of testicular cancer, US confirms the presence of a testicular tumor, while MRI is a valuable problem solving tool. CT is the standard imaging technique for staging, monitoring during treatment, and follow-up of patients with testicular cancer, although other imaging methods (chest radiograph, MRI, and PET) are also helpful playing a supportive role.

References

1. Tsili AC, Argyropoulou MI, Giannakis D et al (2010) MRI in the characterization and local staging of testicular neoplasms. AJR 194(3):682–689
2. Tsili AC, Tsampoulas C, Giannakopoulos X et al (2007) MRI in the histologic characterization of testicular neoplasms. AJR 189(6):331–337
3. Albers P, Albrecht W, Algaba F, et al (2011) European association of urology. EAU guidelines on testicular cancer: 2011 update. Eur Urol 60(2):304–19
4. Brunereau L, Bruyère F, Linassier C et al (2012) The role of imaging in staging and monitoring testicular cancer. Diagn Interv Imaging 93(4):310–318
5. Paño B, Sebastià C, Buñesch L et al (2011) Pathways of lymphatic spread in male urogenital pelvic malignancies. Radiographics 31(1):135–160
6. Sohaib SA, Koh DM, Husband JE (2008) The role of imaging in the diagnosis, staging, and management of testicular cancer. AJR 191(2):387–395
7. Dalal PU, Sohaib SA, Huddart R (2006) Imaging of testicular germ cell tumours. Cancer Imaging 6:124–134
8. Sohaib SA, Koh DM, Barbachano Y et al (2009) Prospective assessment of MRI for imaging retroperitoneal metastases from testicular germ cell tumours. Clin Radiol 64(4):362–367
9. Hilton S (2009) Contemporary radiological imaging of testicular cancer. BJU Int 104:1339–1345
10. Becherer A (2011) PET in testicular cancer. Methods Mol Biol 727:225–241

87 PET/CT Findings in Testicular Cancer

Chariklia D. Giannopoulou

Positron emission tomography (PET), in combination with computed tomography (CT), (PET/CT) has been used in the last decade in germ cell testicular cancer, tackling conventional imaging shortcomings and diagnostic controversies, such as accurate initial staging of early stage patients, post-chemotherapy residual mass characterization, workup of patients with rising tumor markers and negative or equivocal conventional imaging and predicting response to treatment.

A glucose analogue, ^{18}F-fluoro-2-deoxy-D-glucose (FDG), is the most commonly used PET tracer in testicular cancer. In general, increased FDG tumor uptake is due to the increased number of glucose transport molecules and the increased activity of hexokinase isoenzymes, making FDG a probe for imaging tumor metabolism, aggressiveness, and viability. FDG-PET/CT provides functional information about the metabolical activity of disease sites, and especially about viability in residual masses that cannot be correctly predicted by anatomical, conventional imaging.

Non-FDG PET tracers have also been used in testicular germ cell tumors (CGTs) such as 39-deoxy-39-18F-fluorothymidine (18F-FLT)—a probe for imaging cellular proliferation—[1] and radio-labeled integrins [2].

Seminomatous germ cell tumors (SGCT), including their metastases, show high FDG uptake, and express significantly greater FDG avidity than non-seminomatous germ cell tumors (NSGCT), whereas mature teratomas have low FDG uptake [3].

False-positive findings are due the fact that FDG is not a tumor-specific tracer; normal and benign cells may also accumulate it. Apart from the normal distribution (brain, kidneys, and bladder) sites of inflammation, granulomata, and tissues in certain other non-malignant conditions may concentrate FDG. Post-radiotherapy inflammatory reactions, as well as post-chemotherapy metabolic flare may also be responsible for non-specific FDG uptake resulting in false-positive studies.

On the other hand, false-negative findings may be due to lesion's size (foci smaller than 1 cm are at the limits of systems' resolution), to tissue histology for a mature differentiated teratoma has low FDG uptake, or to short time elapsed after chemotherapy.

It is evident that special care should be taken about the timing of PET/CT that should be performed not earlier than 6 weeks post chemotherapy, in order to obtain maximum accuracy.

C. D. Giannopoulou (✉)
Nuclear Medicine Department, Evangelismos Hospital, Ipsilandou 75–77, 10676 Athens, Greece
e-mail: harisg@otenet.gr

A. D. Gouliamos et al. (eds.), *Imaging in Clinical Oncology*,
DOI: 10.1007/978-88-470-5385-4_87, © Springer-Verlag Italia 2014

87.1 Initial Staging: Early Detection of Micro-Metastases

There is not enough evidence supporting the value of FDG-PET in the staging at presentation of patients with either SGCTs or NSGCTs.

The predictive value of FDG-PET at the initial staging of patients with clinical stage I/II GCTs has been a question of dispute, as it affects patients' management, i.e., the selection of surveillance against primary retroperitoneal lymphadenectomy for NSGCTs, or surveillance versus radiation therapy for SGCTs.

CT is the established method of staging patients with SGCTs. However, the great percentage of false-negative CT results—due to its inability to detect microscopic metastases in approximately 30 % of patients—hampers the accurate diagnosis of early stage disease, and the correct differentiation of stage I from stage IIA NSGCT patients [4].

Anatomical imaging (CT) findings are solely based on lymph node (LN) size and morphology, whereas FDG uptake reflects the metabolical LN status: relatively small LNs may harbor active disease and enlarged LNs may be reactive. Another PET advantage over CT, improving PET sensitivity, is standard whole-body scanning covering areas that are not routinely scanned by CT. On the other hand, PET resolution of about 10 mm may limit sensitivity for the detection of small volume disease; however, newer PET/CT systems may achieve a resolution of 5 mm or less.

FDG-PET/CT could be useful for small-volume metastatic disease diagnosis in patients with early stage II NSGCT and inconclusive conventional imaging studies.

In a recently published paper from a German multicentre trial, studying the predicting value of FDG-PET in primary staging of retroperitoneal LN metastases in patients with newly diagnosed early stage NSGC, the PPV and NPV of FDG–PET were 95 and 78 %, while for CT, PPV and NPV were 87 and 67 %, respectively. The authors concluded that FDG–PET as a primary staging tool for NSGCT yielded slightly better results than CT and that false-negative findings were more frequent with CT, rendering FDG–PET mostly useful as a diagnostic tool in case of inconclusive CT scan [5]. These results are in keeping with those of previous studies [6].

However, an earlier UK study of patients with clinical stage I NSGCT examining the ability of FDG PET to identify patients without occult metastatic disease was stopped prematurely, because of the high number of FDG–PET false-negatives: Of 88 patients with negative PET scans, 33 patients relapsed with an estimated one-year relapse-free rate of 63.3 % [7].

Concluding, although FDG-PET/CT does not have an distinctive role in staging of patients with SGCTs or NSGCTs, it could be useful for small-volume metastatic disease diagnosis in patients with early stage II NSGCT and inconclusive conventional imaging studies.

87.2 Response to Treatment Assessment. Residual Mass Characterization

Assessing residual disease after treatment in both seminoma and nonseminomatous germ cell tumors of the testis is of great importance in patients' management, as it contributes to patient selection for surgical resection, especially those with masses greater than 1 cm.

87.3 Seminomatous GCTs

After seminoma resection, patients with seminomatous testicular GCTs are generally followed up with CT. Surveillance using serum tumor markers is unreliable, because of its limited sensitivity—only 30 % of seminoma relapses are marker positive [8].

In patients with post-chemotherapy residual masses, FDG-PET due to its ability to differentiate between necrosis/fibrosis and residual or recurrent viable tumor has been proved sensitive as well as specific for detecting recurrent disease

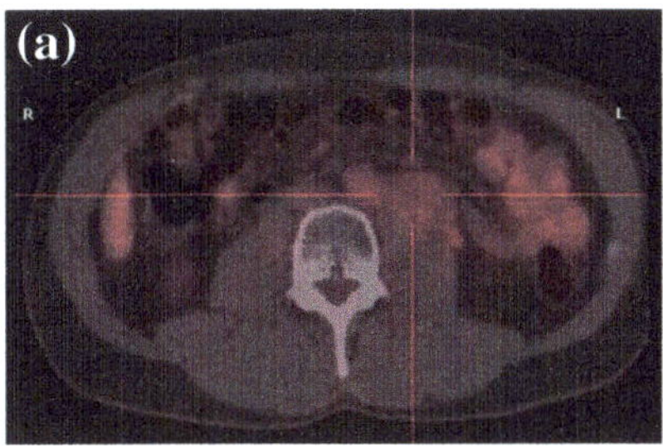

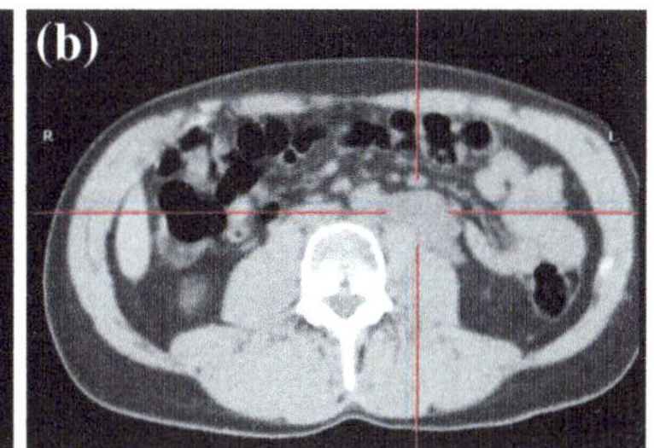

Fig. 87.1 **a** FDG-PET/CT, axial fused image showing residual retroperitoneal mass without increased FDG uptake, in a patient with seminoma, 2 months after the completion of chemotherapy. This is a true negative study, as there was no evidence of active disease after 3 years of follow-up. **b** Corresponding CT axial image

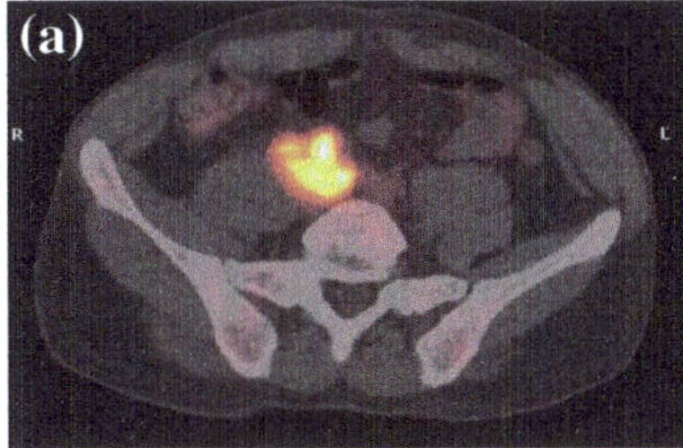

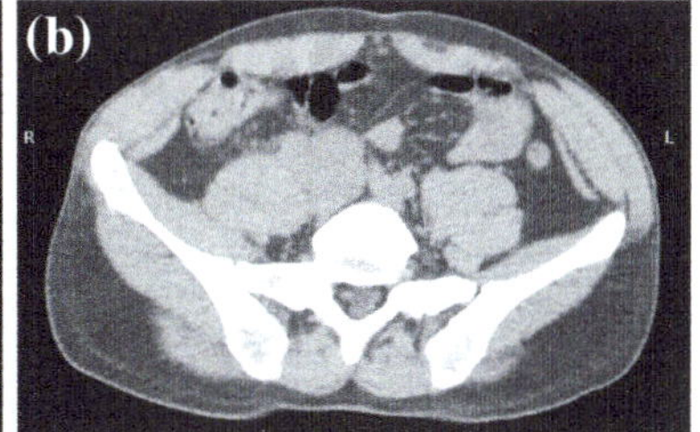

Fig. 87.2 **a** FDG-PET/CT, axial fused image of a 56-year-old patient with IIb seminoma, 7 weeks after first-line chemotherapy completion, showing intense FDG uptake in the residual retroperitoneal mass. After surgery, histology revealed viable tumor in the resected mass. **b** Corresponding CT axial image

and selecting those patients who could thereafter be treated surgically (Figs. 87.1, 87.2).

In a large, prospective, multicenter trial [9], FDG-PET was performed in 51 patients with metastatic seminoma and post-chemotherapy residual masses greater than 1 cm, detected by CT. FDG-PET findings were correlated with the histological findings as to tumor viability, or to clinical or radiological (CT) evidence of progressive disease. In that study it was shown that FDG-PET can identify viable tumor with a specificity of 100 %, a sensitivity of 80 %, a positive predictive value of 100 %, and a negative predictive value of 96 %, versus CT's respective values of 74 % specificity, 70 % sensitivity, 37 % positive predictive value, and 92 % negative predictive value. The authors conclude that FDG-PET performed within 4–12 weeks after chemotherapy, can accurately predict viable residual tumor. In patients with residual lesions greater than 3 cm and negative FDG-PET, surgery can be omitted, whereas if PET is positive, residual lesions, even smaller than 3 cm, can be considered as harboring viable tumor, hence surgery can be of benefit [9].

These results are in keeping with a prospective study in 48 patients with metastatic seminoma and CT-documented residual mass after chemotherapy, investigating whether FDG PET predicts viable tumor. FDG-PET had sensitivity and specificity of 80 and 100 %, respectively, compared with CT sensitivity and specificity being both 73 %. In conclusion, in patients with post-chemotherapy seminoma residuals, a positive PET is highly predictive for the presence of viable tumor. A negative PET scan can accurately exclude disease in lesions ≥3 cm, with a slightly higher sensitivity than CT, thus contributing to avoid unnecessary additional treatment for these patients [10].

In a recent study by Hintz, the ability of FDG-PET for predicting residual tumor viability was evaluated in 20 patients with seminoma following chemotherapy for advanced disease.

Histopathological findings were correlated with PET results. All patients with viable tumor were identified correctly by FDG-PET. No false-negative results were observed, but nine patients had false-positive PET results. FDG-PET had an overall sensitivity of 100 % and specificity of 47 % in detecting residual viable tumor [11].

In conclusion, in patients with post-chemotherapy seminoma residuals, a positive PET is strong indicator of residual active—viable tumor regardless of lesion size. A negative PET scan can accurately exclude disease in lesions ≥3 cm. In order to enhance specificity, reducing the incidence of false-positive results, the PET scan should be performed at least 6 weeks after the completion of chemotherapy.

In keeping with international guidelines [12–14] *PET-CT study is recommended in the post chemotherapy management of pure seminoma patients in order to assess whether residual viable tumor is present. In patients with a residual mass >3 cm, normal levels of serum markers and negative PET, no further treatment is needed and close surveillance is recommended. If PET scan is positive, surgical resection should be considered.*

87.4 Nonseminomatous Germ Cell Tumors

Most patients (70 %) with advanced metastatic NSGCT will show complete response to first-line chemotherapy, with subsequent normal serum markers and mass disappearance. In the rest 30 %, who show partial response to treatment with negative marker levels and persistent residual masses, the major imaging diagnostic challenge is to differentiate, in a, noninvasive way, between fibrosis or necrosis, that occurs in approximately half of those patients, from either mature or immature teratomas—that have to be operated upon as they are chemotherapy resistant, tend to grow, and undergo malignant transformation—or viable/active disease.

FDG-PET cannot reliably distinguish mature teratoma from benign residual mass, because mature teratoma has low FDG uptake and cannot be differentiated from fibrotic or necrotic tissue (Fig. 87.3). In a prospective multicenter study of 121 patients with stage IIC or III NSGCT, with histological confirmation [15], FDG-PET predicted correctly tumor viability with a 56 % accuracy, comparable to CT accuracy (55 %). Sensitivity and specificity of FDG-PET were 70 and 48 %. With viable carcinoma as the unique malignant finding, the negative predictive value was 83 % for FDG-PET. Authors conclude that this trial demonstrated that FDG-PET cannot add a clear clinical benefit to the standard diagnostic procedures—CT and serum tumor markers—in the prediction of tumor viability in residual masses.

However, in a previous prospective study, Kollmannsberger et al. [16] demonstrated that FDG-PET could correctly characterize residual masses with a specificity of 92 % and a sensitivity of 59 % in a high-risk population of 45

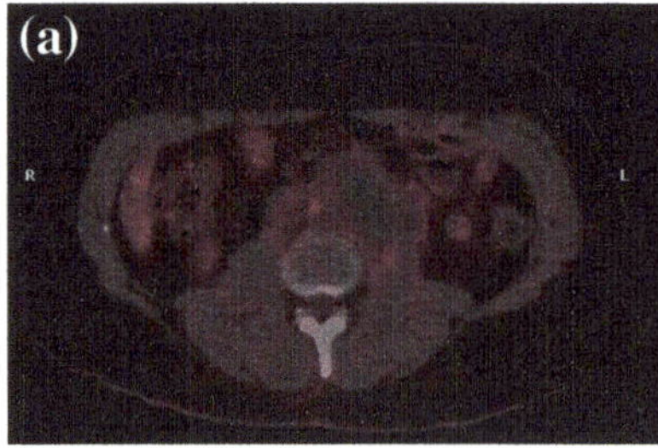

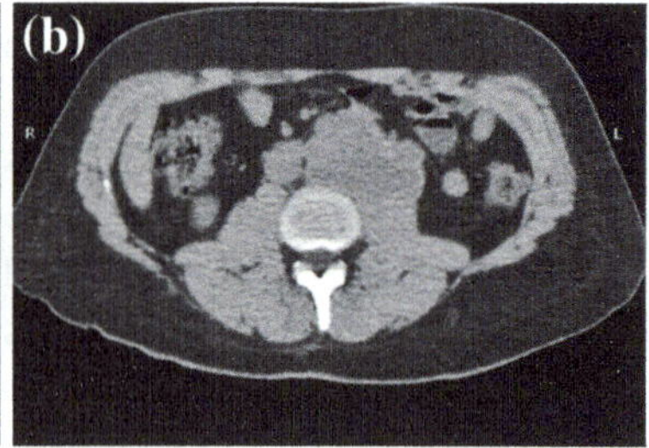

Fig. 87.3 a FDG-PET/CT, axial fused image of a 34-year-old patient with mixed nonsemonomatous germ cell tumor, 40 days after the completion of cisplatin-based combination chemotherapy. There is no increased FDG uptake noted in the residual retroperitoneal masses shown on corresponding CT axial image (**b**). This is a false-negative study: after surgery, histology revealed mature cystic teratoma in the resected masses

patients with nonseminomatous germ cell tumors, concluding that positive PET is highly predictive for the presence of viable carcinoma.

Possibly, FDG-PET could contribute in defining the lesions worth operating, i.e., those with high FDG uptake most likely to harbor viable tumor, in patients with multiple residual masses.

In conclusion FDG-PET has no clear additional role in predicting residual mass histology in patients with advanced metastatic NSGCT after the completion of chemotherapy.

References

1. Pfannenberg C, Aschoff P, Dittmann H et al (2010) PET/CT with 18F-FLT: does it improve the therapeutic management of metastatic germ cell tumors? J Nucl Med 51:845–853
2. Aide N, Briand M, Bohn P et al (2011) $\alpha v\beta 3$ imaging can accurately distinguish between mature teratoma and necrosis in 18F-FDG-negative residual masses after treatment of non-seminomatous testicular cancer: a preclinical study. Eur J Nucl Med Mol Imaging 38:323–333
3. Vela A, Deslandes E, Vera P et al (1999) The management of residual masses after chemotherapy in metastatic seminoma. BJU Int 83:649–653
4. Hilton S, Herr HW, Teitcher JB (1997) CT detection of retroperitoneal lymph node metastases in patients with clinical stage I testicular nonseminomatous germ cell cancer: assessment of size and distribution criteria. Am J Roentgenol 169:521–525
5. De Wit M, Brenner W, Hartmann M et al (2008) 18F-FDG–PET in clinical stage I/II non-seminomatous germ cell tumours: results of the German multicentre trial. Ann Oncol 19:1619–1623
6. Lassen U, Daugaard G, Eigtved A et al (2003) Whole-body FDG-PET in patients with stage I non-seminomatous germ cell tumours. Eur J Nucl Med 30:396–402
7. Huddart RA, O'Doherty MJ, Padhani A et al (2007) 18 fluorodeoxyglucose positron emission tomography in the prediction of relapse in patients with high-risk, clinical stage I nonseminomatous germ cell tumors: preliminary report of MRC trial TE22–the NCRI testis tumour clinical study group. J Clin Oncol 25:3090–3095
8. Sohaib SA, Koh D, Husband JE et al (2008) The role of imaging in the diagnosis, staging and management of testicular cancer. Am J Roentgenol 191:387–395
9. De Santis M, Becherer A, Bokemeyer C et al (2004) 2–18fluoro-deoxy-D-glucose Positron Emission Tomography Is a Reliable Predictor for Viable Tumor in Postchemotherapy Seminoma: An Update of the Prospective Multicentric SEMPET Trial. J Clin Oncol 22:1034–1039
10. Becherer A, De Santis M, Karanikas G et al (2005) FDG PET is superior to CT in the prediction of viable tumour in post-chemotherapy seminoma residuals. Eur J Radiol 54:284–288
11. Hinz S, Schrader M, Kempkensteffen C et al (2008) The role of positron emission tomography in the evaluation of residual masses after chemotherapy for advanced stage seminoma. J Urol 179:936–940
12. Motzer RJ, Agarwal N, Beard C et al (2012) Testicular cancer clinical practice guidelines in oncology. J Natl Compr Canc Netw 10:502–535
13. Schmoll HJ, Jordan K, Huddart R et al (2010) Testicular seminoma: ESMO clinical practice guidelines for diagnosis, treatment and follow-up. Ann Oncol 21(S5):140–146
14. Warde P, Huddart R, Bolton D et al (2011) Management of localized seminoma, stage I-II: SIU/ICUD consensus meeting on germ cell tumors GCT shanghai 2009. Urology 78:S435–S443
15. Oechsle K, Hartmann M, Brenner W et al (2008) Positron emission tomography in nonseminomatous germ cell tumors after chemotherapy: the German multicenter positron emission tomography study group. J Clin Oncol 26:5930–5935
16. Kollmannsberger C, Oechsle K, Dohmen B et al (2002) Prospective comparison of [18F] fluorodeoxyglucose positron emission tomography with conventional assessment by computed tomography scans and serum tumour markers for the evaluation of residual masses in patients with nonseminomatous germ cell carcinoma. Cancer 94:2353–2362

88 Clinical Implications in Testicular Cancer

Gerasimos J. Alivizatos and Pavlos A. Pavlakis

88.1 Diagnosis-Staging

Diagnosis of testicular tumors is performed with ultrasonography (US). MRI of the scrotum has higher sensitivity and specificity than US but should be used in ambiguous cases only. Nodal metastases in the abdomen and in the thorax are performed mainly with CT scans. MRI scans have been used as well and can be helpful in some cases (ambiguous CT findings, allergy to contrast materials) but its wide use in the staging procedure is not justified. PET scans are also not recommended in the staging procedure of testicular cancer [1].

88.2 Follow-up Strategies

Follow-up after treatment is being performed with tumor markers and imaging modalities. CT scans are used to evaluate lymph nodes and PET scans are used as well. The main role of FDG-PET, however, lies in the characterization of postchemotherapy residual masses, due to its ability to differentiate between necrosis/fibrosis and residual or recurrent viable tumor. In this context PET-CT study is recommended in the postchemotherapy management of pure seminoma patients in order to assess whether residual viable tumor is present. In nonseminomatous germ cell tumors of the testis, however, FDG-PET should be used with caution, as it cannot differentiate between mature teratoma and fibrosis [2].

References

1. Winter C, Pfister D, Busch J et al (2012) Residual tumor size and IGCCCG risk classification predict additional vascular procedures in patients with germ cell tumors and residual tumor resection: a multicenter analysis of the German Testicular Cancer Study Group. Eur Urol 61(2):403–409
2. Daneshmand S, Albers P, Fossa A et al (2012) Contemporary management of post chemotherapy testis cancer. Eur Urol 62(5):867–876

G. J. Alivizatos (✉) · P. A. Pavlakis
3rd Urological Department, Hygeia Hospital,
Erythrou Stavrou 4, 15123, Athens, Greece
e-mail: gali@hol.gr

A. D. Gouliamos et al. (eds.), *Imaging in Clinical Oncology*,
DOI: 10.1007/978-88-470-5385-4_88, © Springer-Verlag Italia 2014

Introduction to Prostate Cancer

89

Gerasimos J. Alivizatos and Pavlos A. Pavlakis

Prostate cancer (PCa) is the most common malignancy in the Western World accounting for almost 15 % of all diagnosed male cancers and approximately 5 % in undeveloped countries [1]. It is calculated that a man in developed countries has a 16 % of lifetime risk of being diagnosed with PCa and a 2.57 % risk of dying from this disease [2]. Therefore PCa is one of the most important medical problems among men and the cost of treating this cancer is rising dramatically. In the United States it was estimated that only for PCa in 2009, the amount of money spent was $11.9 billions [3]. This accelerating cost is caused by the introduction of new diagnostic tools (MRI, PET) and new therapeutic options (daVinci robotic radical prostatectomy and new novel chemotherapeutic and immunotherapeutic agents).

Epidemiological risk factors for PCa development include increasing age, animal fat consumption, ethnic origin, and a family history.

In this chapter all contributors present the latest developments in PCa imaging from diagnosis to local and distant staging and in the follow-up period. It is important to see if with these innovations it is possible to prevent unnecessary biopsies and to offer more precise information that will enhance the proper selection of the best therapeutic option.

89.1 Classification

About 95 % of prostatic carcinomas are adenocarcinomas. Squamous cell carcinoma and other types such as signet-ring carcinoma, transitional carcinoma, neuroendocrine carcinoma, or sarcoma are the remaining 5 %.

The grading of prostatic adenocarcinoma is being performed according to the ISUP 2005 Gleason score [4].

The TNM classification used today worldwide is presented in Table 89.1 [5].

Another classification in which prognostic factors are included (TNM stage, PSA, and Gleason score) is presented in the latest version of the Guidelines of the European Association of Urology upon PCa and this classification is presented in Table 89.2 [6].

89.2 Screening

The most debated controversy of PCa is the issue of screening. The introduction of screening based on the combination of digital rectal examination (DRE) and serum prostate specific antigen (PSA) testing has increased the opportunity for earlier diagnosis at lower stages of the disease. There is no doubt that all the cases of PCa do not belong in one entity. There are cases

G. J. Alivizatos (✉) · P. A. Pavlakis
3rd Urological Department Hygeia Hospital,
Erythrou Stavrou 4, 15123 Athens, Greece
e-mail: gali@hol.gr

A. D. Gouliamos et al. (eds.), *Imaging in Clinical Oncology*,
DOI: 10.1007/978-88-470-5385-4_89, © Springer-Verlag Italia 2014

Table 89.1 Tumor node metastasis (TNM) classification of PCa

T—Primary tumor
TX primary tumor cannot be assessed
T0 no evidence of primary tumor
T1 clinically inapparent tumor not palpable or visible by imaging
T1a tumor incidental histological finding in 5 % or less of tissue resected
T1b tumor incidental histological finding in more than 5 % of tissue resected
T1c tumor identified by needle biopsy (e.g., because of elevated prostate-specific antigen [PSA] level)
T2 tumor confined within the prostate
T2a tumor involves one half of one lobe or less
T2b tumor involves more than half of one lobe, but not both lobes
T2c tumor involves both lobes
T3 tumor extends through the prostatic capsule
T3a extracapsular extension (unilateral or bilateral) including microscopic bladder neck
Involvement
T3b tumor invades seminal vesicle(s)
T4 tumor is fixed or invades adjacent structures other than seminal vesicles: external sphincter, rectum, levator muscles, and/or pelvic wall
N—regional lymph nodes
NX regional lymph nodes cannot be assessed
N0 no regional lymph node metastasis
N1 regional lymph node metastasis
M—distant metastasis
MX distant metastasis cannot be assessed
M0 no distant metastasis
M1 distant metastasis
M1a non-regional lymph node(s)
M1b bone(s)
M1c other

Table 89.2 Prognostic grouping

Group I	T1a-c N0 M0 PSA < 10 Gleason < 6
	PSA < 10 Gleason < 6
Group IIA	T1a-c N0 M0 PSA < 20 Gleason 7
	T1a-c N0 M0 PSA > 10 < 20 Gleason < 6
	T2a, b N0 M0 PSA < 20 Gleason < 7
Group IIb	T2c N0 M0 any PSA any Gleason
	T1-2 N0 M0 PSA > 20 any Gleason
	T1-2 N0 M0 any PSA Gleason > 8
Group III	T3a, b N0 M0 any PSA any Gleason
Group IV	T4 N0 M0 any PSA any Gleason
	Any T N1 M0 any PSA any Gleason
	Any T any N M1 Any PSA any Gleason

of aggressive tumors that need prompt therapy and cases with indolent behavior. The problem is that today it is difficult to distinguish these two subgroups and therefore overdiagnosis leads to overtreatment. The most reliable studies published upon screening are the European randomized study of screening for prostate cancer (ERSPC) and the prostate, lung, colorectal, and ovarian study (PLCO) [7, 8]. The PLCO study did not justify screening but has been criticized for a high contamination rate in the control arm. The ERSPC did achieve a mortality reduction rate by 20 % but with a considerable harm such as unnecessary biopsies, overdiagnosis and overtreatment. In simple numbers this study showed that in order to prevent one death from PCa, 1,410 men had to be screened and 48 additional cases had to be treated. From the results of this study the European Association of Urology, the American Urological Association, the American Cancer Society, and the National Comprehensive Cancer Network have updated their recommendations regarding PCa screening [9] but massive widespread screening is not justified even today. It is believed that the correct way to proceed today with the issue of screening is to inform our patients about the existing dilemmas and explain in detail the pros and cons of every decision taken from PSA measurement to aggressive therapy. Therefore, a shared path with our patients is advisable and we have to remember that every decision is individualized and risk factors such as age, comorbidity, family history, and ethnicity should influence our strategy [9].

89.3 Imaging Dilemmas in Prostate Cancer

89.3.1 Imaging and Diagnosis

After a DRE of the prostate (DRE) and a PSA measurement the urologists decides to proceed with a transrectal ultrasonography of the prostate (TRUS) and a prostatic biopsy. TRUS is today the most important tool in the diagnostic process since all prostatic biopsies are performed under TRUS guidance. Its widespread use is due to the fact that it is rapid, effective, and radiation free. The classic picture of a tumor is that of a hypoechoic lession in the peripheral zone. Unfortunately there are many isoechoic and hyperechoic tumors as well and therefore during the past 15 years continuous innovations are being reported. The development of contrast agents have contributed in three- and four-dimensional resolution images, in contrast-enhanced ultrasonography and in sonoelastography [10].

Recently, MRI has been used as a diagnostic tool but it still remains an expensive modality with questionable results.

89.4 Imaging and Clinical Staging

89.4.1 T-Staging

The local extension of the tumor is typically performed with DRE, with PSA measurements and with TRUS. DRE was the principal method of PCa staging, however it has a limited value due to interobserver error and depends upon clinical experience. Therefore, it has been shown that it can underestimate the extension of the tumor. PSA measurement depends upon the size of the tumor, its differentiation, and upon the stage of the disease. Used alone it cannot predict accurately the stage of the tumor but in combination with DRE and the Gleason score it can offer more accurate predictions [11].

TRUS remains as the most common tool for local staging but its ability to distinguish between intraprostatic to extraprostatic disease is still limited. Color doppler images and contrast agents have been tried in an effort to improve the sensitivity of this diagnostic modality [12]. The identification of seminal vesicle infiltration still remains a challenge for TRUS and therefore it is safer to take separate biopsies from the vesicles during the biopsy procedure.

The utility of MRI as a staging tool has also been evaluated. Endorectal coil has been tested and lately MR spectroscopic imaging and positron emission tomography (PET) have been tried for the accurate local staging and experts in these fields have been invited to present in separate chapters the latest developments in these expensive but promising tools.

A practical problem from the urological point of view is the proper timing of implementing these technologies. Since it is impossible to ask for MRI and PET scans before the prostatic biopsy the question is how accurate images do we get after the biopsy, when 12–20 cores have been taken. Local inflammation and hemorrhage caused by the biopsy gun might influence the quality of the images and lead to overstaging. There is also no consensus upon the time interval that has to be allowed between the biopsy and the next radiological scan.

The fact is that from a clinical point of view, an urologist has to decide wether to perform surgery to his patient or to refer him for local radiotherapy and this decision depends strongly on the accuracy of the information provided by the imaging modalities and therefore every new innovation is always welcome.

89.4.2 N and M: Staging

Lymph nodes and distant metastases are being evaluated mainly with chest X-rays, with bone scans, and with CT scans.

N—Staging before surgery can be evaluated with CT scans which can identify enlarged nodes. Of course, it is not clear what is the definition of an enlarged node but the threshold of 1 cm has been commonly used.

A common question urologists face in everyday practice is when to ask for CT scans, in cases diagnosed with local PCa. It seems that low PSA values (<20 ng/ml) and tumors with Gleason score up to 6 do not need further abdominal investigations since the chance of metastases is very low [13]. Nomograms in which the PSA values and Gleason scores are used to help identifying cases with low risk for nodal involvement are commonly used [14].

MRI has been used as well to search for pathological nodes, but it is still debatable if this expensive imaging technique adds valuable information compared to a CT scan. PET scans and PET/CT scans have also been tried in many protocols but the radiologists have to convince with hard evidence that the addition of these modalities offer information that might change the decision making.

Urologists still perform lymph node dissection for proper N-staging but surgery comes at a latter phase when clinical staging has convinced the surgeon that lymph nodes are free from metastases.

Bone lesions are identified best by bone scintigraphy and again it is not mandatory to ask for this examination in low-risk patients.

The EAU 2011 guidelines offer a table—summary for staging of PCa (Table 89.3).

89.5 Imaging and Follow-up

Follow-up of men who have been treated for PCa is being performed with PSA measurements. If biochemical relapse occurs the question is to identify the site of the relapse in order to select further treatment. If we can identify local relapse after a radical prostatectomy, local radiotherapy can be offered as another option and cryotherapy has been suggested after radiotherapy relapse.

Transrectal ultrasonography and biopsy at the bladder-urethra anastomosis has been suggested in order to confirm local reoccurrence after biochemical relapse in men who underwent radical prostatectomy.

Bone scans are used during the follow-up period when PSA rises after the implementation of a definitive treatment or when symptoms from the skeleton arise.

CT and MRI scans have been used as well but the identification of the site of tumor relapse with these modalities is not very accurate. Recently, PET scans have been used for such situations and in some cases they might offer some answers [15].

Table 89.3 Staging of PCa—recommendations (EAU 2011 guidelines) [6]

Local staging (T-staging) of PCa should be based on magnetic resonance (MR) imaging. Further information is provided by the number and sites of positive prostate biopsies, the tumor grade and the level of serum PSA
For local staging TRUS should not be used since it has low sensitivity and a tendency to understage PCa
Lymph node status (N-staging) need only be assessed when potentially curative treatment is planned
Patients with stage T2 or less, PSA < 20 ng/mL and a Gleason score <6 have a lower than 10 % likelihood of having node metastases and can be spared nodal evaluation
In clinically localized PCa, staging must be done by pelvic lymph node dissection since it presents the only reliable staging method, given the significant limitations of preoperative imaging in the detection of small metastases (<5 mm)
Skeletal metastasis (M-staging) is best assessed by bone scan. This may not be indicated in asymptomatic patients if the serum PSA level is <20 ng/mL in the presence of well or moderately differentiated tumors
In equivocal cases, 11C-choline-, 18F-flouride-PET/CT or whole body MRI are an option

89.6 Conclusions

Imaging modalities play a crucial role in the diagnosis, in staging, and in the follow-up period of treatment in patients with PCa. Overdiagnosis and overtreatment is a major problem and until the biological characteristics of the aggressive tumors that need treatment are identified, screening cannot be advocated. New imaging technologies (MRI, PET scans) are being tested and in some cases they do offer extra information to the clinicians. The goal of every urologist is to intervene when he believes that he will improve the survival of his patients without hampering the quality of their lives.

References

1. Center MM, Jemal A, Lortet-Tieulent J et al (2012) International variation in prostate cancer incidence and mortality rates. Eur Urol 61(6):1079–1092
2. Jemal A, Bray F, Center MM et al (2011) Global cancer statistics, 2008. CA Cancer J Clin 61:69–90
3. Centers of Medicare and Medicaid Services (2009) National health expenditure fact sheet. US Department of Health and Human Services, Baltimore
4. Epstein JI, Allsbrook WC Jr, Amin MB et al (2005) ISUP grading committee. The 2005 international society of urologic pathology (ISUP) consensus conference on gleason grading of prostatic Carcinoma. Am J Surg Pathol 29(9):1228–1242
5. Sobin LH, Gospodariwicz M, Wittekind C (eds) (2009) TNM classification of malignant tumours. UICC international union against cancer, 7th edn. Wiley, New York, pp 243–248
6. Heidenreich A, Bellmunt J, Bolla M et al (2011) EAU guidelines on prostate cancer. Part 1: screening, diagnosis, and treatment of clinically localised disease. Eur Urol 59(1):61–71
7. Schröder FH, Hugosson J, Roobol MJ et al (2009) Screening and prostate-cancer mortality in a randomized European study. N Engl J Med 360(13):1320–1328
8. Andriole GL, Crawford ED, Grubb RL 3rd et al (2009) Mortality results from a randomized prostate-cancer screening trial. N Engl J Med 360(13):1310–1319
9. Xiaoye Z, Albertsen P, Andriole G et al (2012) Risk based prostate cancer screening. Eur Urol 61(4):652–661
10. Gravas S, Mamoulakis Ch, Rioja J et al (2009) Advances in ultrasound technology in oncologic urology. Urol Clin N Am 36(2):133–145
11. Partin AW, Mangold LA, Lamm DM et al (2001) Contemporary update of the prostate cancer staging nomograms (Partin tables) for the new millennium. Urology 58(6):843–848
12. Pinto F, Totaro A, Palermo G et al (2012) Imaging in prostate cancer staging: present role and future perspectives. Urol Int 88(2):125–136
13. Cagiannos I, Karakiewicz P, Eastham JA et al (2003) A preoperative nomogram identifying decreased risk of positive pelvic lymph nodes in patients with prostate cancer. J Urol 170(5):1798–1803
14. Haese A, Epstein JI, Huland H et al (2002) Validation of a biopsy-based pathologic algorithm for predicting lymph node metastases in patients with clinically localized prostate carcinoma. Cancer 95(5):1016–1021
15. Castellucci P, Fuccio C, Rubello D et al (2011) Is there a role for C-choline PET/CT in the early detection of metastatic disease in surgically treated prostate cancer patients with a mild PSA increase <1.5 ng/ml? Eur J Nucl Med Mol Imaging 38(1):55–63

Endorectal Ultrasound and Prostate Cancer

90

George P. Zacharopoulos

In the early days the prostate was evaluated for cancer by a simple digital rectal examination, and a blind biopsy was performed in order to obtain a tissue diagnosis. The rapid evolution of the ultrasound technology offers a better way to evaluate the prostate, and biopsy techniques have been developed using ultrasound guidance only. Two ultrasound-guided methods are currently in use, the Endorectal or transrectal ultrasound (TRUS) and, in selected cases the Transperineal.

90.1 Gray-Scale TRUS

The "classic" sonographic finding of prostate cancer, the hypoechoic lesion in the peripheral zone was initially described using TRUS (Fig. 90.1).

Nowadays most patients diagnosed with prostate cancer have no palpable abnormality or specific sonographic findings. The visualization provided by the new higher resolution transducers, coupled with the ability to direct the biopsy needle into various regions of interest (Fig. 90.2) and to provide uniform spatial separation of the areas to be sampled, has helped to make TRUS-guided prostate biopsy a standard technique in the diagnosis of prostate cancer.

The normal prostate has a uniform echo pattern. The transitional zone surrounds the urethral zone and extends from the ejaculatory ducts proximally and is surrounded by the fibromuscular band. It presents a mixed echotexture usually due to different grades of benign prostatic hyperplasia. Especially in young men the transitional zone accounts for a small percentage of the gland while these changes in older men due to benign prostatic hypertrophy, can increase considerably causing compression and relative atrophy of the peripheral zone. The peripheral zone extends from the posterolateral aspect of the prostate from the base to the apex and has a very homogeneous echotexture which differentiates and gives clear boundaries from the transitional zone (Fig. 90.3).

There is no clear distinction between central and transitional zone. The seminal vesicles are detected at the base of the bladder and normally are hypoechoic in comparison to the prostatic gland.

Most of prostate cancers arise from the peripheral zone. The initially typical finding described for cancer, the hypoechoic lesion in the peripheral zone of the prostate, however, is also described for noncancer lesions such as focal prostatitis, granulomatous prostatitis, focal atrophy, and for prostatic infarcts leading the sensitivity and specificity of the method to very low percentages. Malignancy is found in only 17–57 % of hypoechoic lesions [1]. Furthermore

G. P. Zacharopoulos (✉)
Department of Diagnostic Ultrasound, Hygeia Hospital, 4 Erythrou Stavrou Street, 15123, Maroussi, Greece
e-mail: g.zacharopoulos@hygeia.gr

A. D. Gouliamos et al. (eds.), *Imaging in Clinical Oncology*,
DOI: 10.1007/978-88-470-5385-4_90, © Springer-Verlag Italia 2014

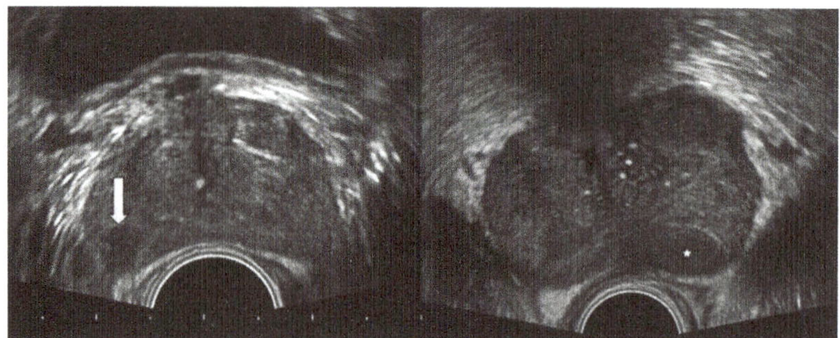

Fig. 90.1 The typical hypoechoic lesion of the prostate peripheral zone. *White arrow* Focal lesion. *Asterisk* Diffuse lesion

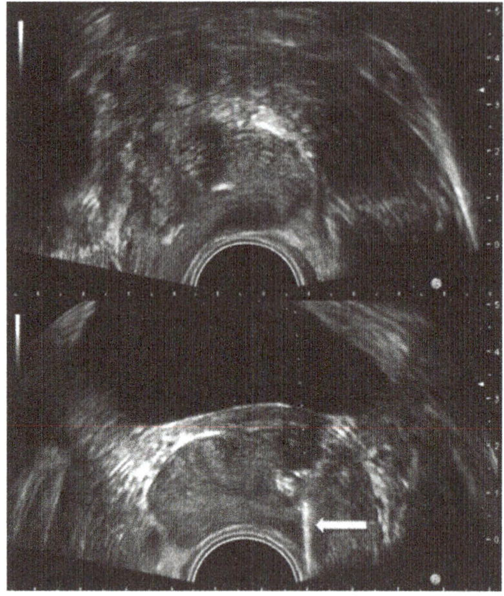

Fig. 90.2 The standard TRUS guided prostate biopsy. The *dotted line* represents the course of the biopsy needle (*white arrow*)

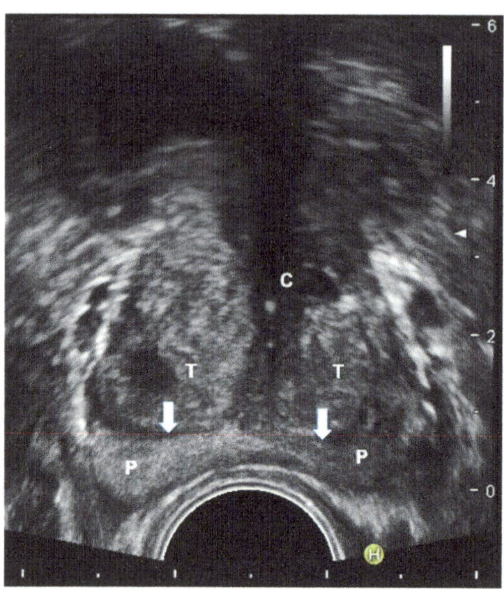

Fig. 90.3 The sonographic illustration of the prostate zonal anatomy. *P* peripheral zone. *T* transitisonal zone. *C* central, periurethral zone. *White arrows* indicate the clear-cut boundaries between transitional and peripheral zone

prostate cancer detection rate is reported to be 25.5 % with a hypoechoic lesion and 25.4 % without a hypoechoic lesion [2].

This has led to the potential use of additional imaging tools such as Gray-scale 3D ultrasound, color Doppler imaging, intravenous contrast agent administration, and the use of most recently introduced elastographic techniques in order to increase both sensitivity and specificity of the method.

90.2 3D Gray-Scale Ultrasound

Gray-scale 3D ultrasound has yielded so far no better sensitivity and specificity rates as compared to 2D TRUS (2D 74 and 52 %, 3D 85 and 41 %). However, it is claimed that this method may identify tumor extracapsular extension with a sensitivity of 84 % and specificity of 96 % [3].

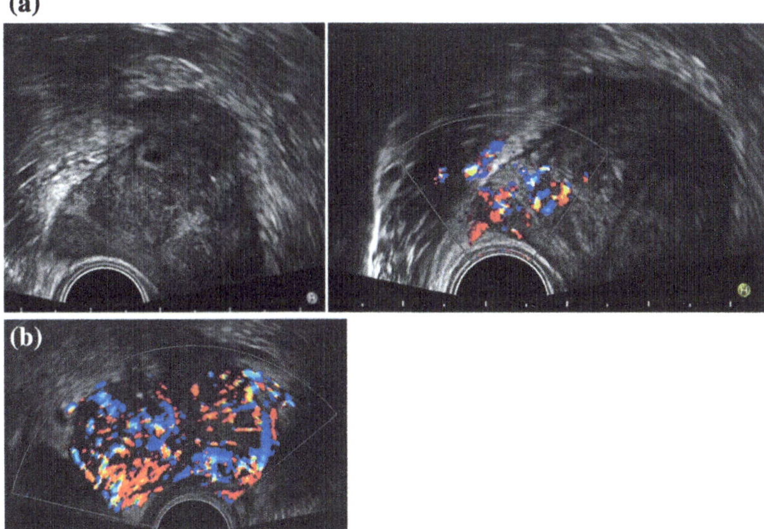

Fig. 90.4 *Color* doppler ultrasound of the prostate. **a** Hypervascularity of a peripheral zone focal hypoechoic lesion. In this patient the diagnosis was focal prostatitis. **b** Hypervascularity of the whole gland in a case of clinically silent diffuse prostatitis

90.3 Doppler Ultrasound

Doppler ultrasound has a limited ability to display small, deep, and low volume-flow blood vessels, such as those of the prostate. Furthermore, the utility of color Doppler ultrasound rests only on the theory that tumors in general, and prostate tumors in particular, have different blood flow characteristics from the surrounding normal tissue (Fig. 90.4a).

Some investigators have studied the enhancement of Doppler imaging results with the administration of a PDE-5 inhibitor [4].

The latest literature, however, fails to support that this technique has being superior to traditional gray-scale imaging in the diagnosis of prostate cancer [5].

During the TRUS-guided prostate biopsy, Color Doppler may provide considerable assistance in depicting the hypervascular appearance of the gland in cases of clinically silent inflammations (Fig. 90.4b).

90.4 Contrast-Enhanced Ultrasound

The addition of intravenous contrast agents has been used to promote vascular visualization. The initial aim was to explore whether the use of sonographic contrast agents could enhance the visualization of neovascularity associated with prostatic cancer. Also this method proved to be time and cost increasing with poor additional results so far.

90.5 Elastography

As prostate cancer is stiffer than the normal prostatic tissue especially in the peripheral zone, elastographic methods were soon developed in order to delineate better than b-mode imaging and if possible depict foci of isoechoic prostatic cancer that were previously undetected [6].

Currently, there are two types of ultrasound elastography in clinical use for imaging the prostate. Compression elastography and shear wave elastography.

Compression elastography shows the relative tissue stiffness or displacement (strain) in response to an external applied force. The image is produced after the comparison of multiple signals acquired before and after compression using specialized software calculating the relative difference in tissue movement from two superimposed images estimating the relative tissue deformation. The deformation measurements are then depicted on a new image the elastogram on which the stiffer areas are coded

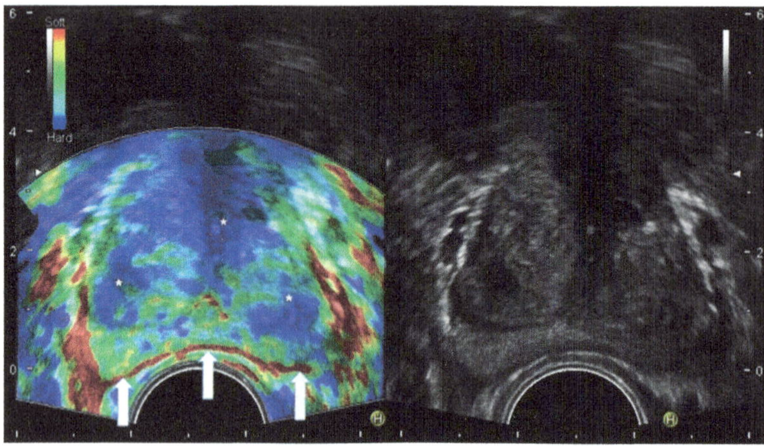

Fig. 90.5 Normal prostatic elastogram. Notice the *green color coding* of the peripheral zone with *blue foci* <5 mm. *Asterisks* transitional zone *dark blue areas* at typical periurethral and peripheral sites representing areas of focal hyperplasia. *White arrows* normal intact capsule rim sign coded in *red color*

as dark blue and the soft areas red with intermediate stiffness coded as green areas.

The elastographic appearance of the normal prostate includes heterogeneous depiction of the transitional zone with prevalence of the green areas, however, small foci of dark blue areas can be present probably due to foci of focal hyperplasia. In benign prostatic hyperplasia these dark blue areas can be numerous and increase in size especially in the peripheral areas of the transitional zone as well in the periurethral zone. However, in both cases the prostatic capsule is depicted in green and red and in the peripheral zone there are no dark blue areas greater than 5 mm in diameter (Fig. 90.5).

Strain elastography tends to be very specific for suspicious hypoechoic lesions in the peripheral zone. Thus, faint or ambiguous hypoechoic lesions can be characterized as benign with code scale between green and red (focal prostatitis, granulomatous prostatitis, infarct, focal atrophy, etc.). Suspicious cancer lesions are depicted in dark blue. Furthermore the involvement of the prostatic capsule can be assessed in the areas adjacent to the cancer lesion, a fact that increases the final role of the prostatic elastography as can give better information for the staging of prostatic cancer (Fig. 90.6a and b).

The method already includes a 3D volume rendering that can provide a more detailed assessment of the cancer lesions valuable for surgical planning.

A recent study has shown that elastographic guided biopsies yielded cancer detection rate of 21.3 % and systematic biopsies 19.1 %. On a per patient basis the sensitivity was 74 % and specificity 60 % [7]. With elastography, targeted obtained biopsies were considerably less than those taken with the systematic approach.

Another study has shown a per patient sensitivity and specificity of 91.7 and 86.8 %, respectively. The corresponding values per core sample were 72.5 and 100 % [6].

The second elastographic technique in clinical use is the Shear Wave Elastography. In this technique the elasticity is displayed differently using a color coded image superimposed on a B-mode image. Thus, stiffer tissues are coded in red and softer tissues in blue. The image obtained using a conventional ultrasound probe is refreshed in real-time without the need of any external compression by the user (Fig. 90.7).

The fact that ultrasound wave is generated automatically by the ultrasound transducer is claimed that allows a user independent image which is reproducible meanwhile also the real-

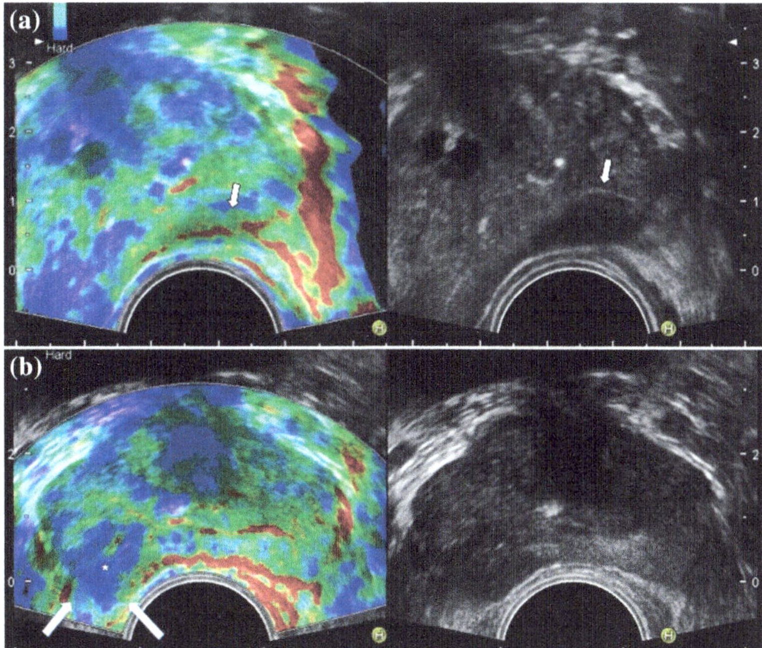

Fig. 90.6 **a** Elastogram of a peripheral zone hypoechoic focal lesion. It presents with soft *green* and *red color pattern*. At biopsy it was a focal prostatitis lesion. **b** Elastogram of a peripheral zone hypoechoic lesion. It shows a hard *dark blue pattern* (*asterisk*). Notice the missing red capsule sign due to capsule invasion (*white arrows*). The lesion was prostatic carcinoma with extracapsular extension

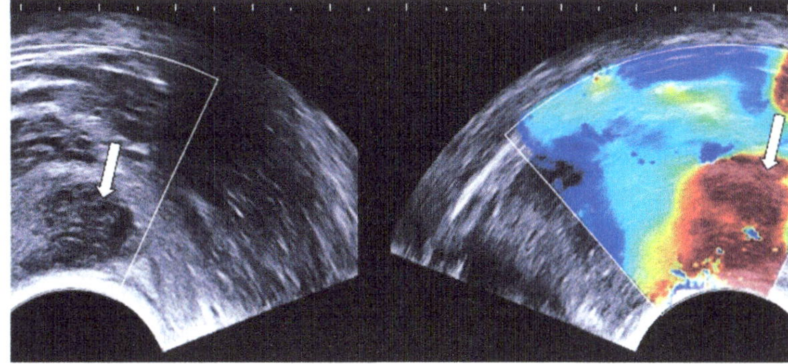

Fig. 90.7 Shear wave elastogram of a peripheral zone hypoechoic lesion. The *red color pattern* corresponds to a hard neoplastic focus. The shear wave force was measured at 42.4 kPa

time scanning of this method can reduce both complexity and duration of the elastographic examination in comparison to the compression elastography examination [8].

However, both the above-mentioned elastographic methods are ultrasound examinations that still require training, and have a learning curve, which does not differ before mastering the technique.

Both methods, however, are not yet established for routine use, yet they look very promising and can give valuable information.

Expecting to improve accuracy of diagnosis for prostate lesions, and possibly reduce biopsy cores guiding ideally the biopsy nevertheless finally taking part also for staging the prostate cancer.

The current state-of-the-art TRUS probe is a high-resolution probe, imaging the prostate in real time and capable of performing all the new techniques, including 3D color Doppler, use of enhancing microbubbles, and the latest elastographic imaging techniques. In the ultrasound probe an appropriate single use adapter is fitted that accepts the needle of a biopsy gun, thus allowing multiple cores of tissue to be obtained.

90.6 Prostate Biopsy

An abnormal digital rectal examination is still the absolute indication for prostate biopsy independently of the patient's PSA value. It includes a well-delineated nodule, a focal induration, a diffusely hard prostate, and prostate asymmetry.

Nowadays, however, the most common indication for prostatic biopsy is elevated serum PSA. PSA levels greater than 4 ng/mL is the cutoff in order to consider biopsy. However, age-adjusted normal PSA values are available, a rising PSA over time may also be an indication for biopsy especially in high-risk groups. Informed consent is signed before biopsy, which outlines especially the complications of the procedure. The complications of the TRUS biopsy are rare and include hematuria, rectal bleeding, and septicemia.

The preparation includes an enema 2 hours before the procedure or a formal bowel preparation the day before.

The administration of prophylactic antibiotics 1 day before and 4 day after is standard procedure. Special care is needed for patients with valvular disease (parenteral antibiotics) and for patients on anticoagulants or antiplatelet drugs which have to be discontinued.

Regarding anaesthesia many institutions perform different methods, including use of intrarectal lidocaine, and injection of a solution of 1 % xylocaine along the neurovascular bundles. In our institution we use mild sedation in the presence of anaesthesiologist.

A DRE is performed prior to biopsy confirming the appropriate bowel preparation as well the absence of rectal pathology that could contraindicate the insertion of the ultrasound probe. At the same time with the DRE there is a confirmation of possible palpable prostatic abnormalities.

After the insertion of the probe a thorough ultrasound examination is performed including both seminal vesicles. The prostatic volume is assessed performing the appropriate measurements and special care is taken to identify hypoechoic or hyperechoic lesions at the peripheral zone.

Compression elastography is then performed in order to evaluate the elastic properties of the peripheral zone and of the capsule.

Having all the parameters we then proceed with obtaining the core biopsies using an 18G needle.

90.7 Optimization of Prostatic Biopsy

In 1989 was introduced the systematic sextant biopsy by Hodge et al. [9]. This technique was recommended based on patients with positive DRE. Since then most men who are undergoing prostatic biopsy do not have any palpable lesion or a hypoechoic lesion in the peripheral zone. Thus, several investigators suggested modifications of this method as there could be underestimation of the incidence of cancer. Currently, there are several proposed protocols that suggest increasing the number of cores and extending also the sampling fields of the prostate.

Eskew et al. suggested a 5-region biopsy method in which cores are obtained in addition to the standard sextant biopsies from the far lateral peripheral zone and from midline. By obtaining at least 13 cores, or 18 cores in glands greater than 50 g, the authors reported a significant increase in cancer detection over sextant biopsies [10].

More recent evidence, however, support that biopsy sampling should include cores from the parasagittal base and apex, the inferior anterior horn, the midline peripheral zone, and the anterior transitional zone as these additional cores increase cancer detection.

Although the ideal number of cores is not clear yet we cannot underestimate the impact of prostatic volume on prostate biopsy technique and the role of the inclusion of the transitional zone especially in second biopsy cases.

According to the authors' experience, we perform a 12 core biopsy including six peripheral zone four transitional zone and two apical cores as a first prostatic biopsy. The peripheral zone cores are taken after elastographic evaluation in an effort to enhance systematic biopsy by targeted sampling. On a second biopsy the number cores should increase taking always in consideration prostatic volume and the increased morbidity and also the increased risk of overdiagnosing foci of micro tumors that do not need treatment. The negative second biopsy does not exclude completely the presence of cancer thus if there is a strong clinical suspicion a saturation biopsy is indicated transperinealy.

90.8 Conclusion

TRUS, with the ability of guided biopsy of the prostate, remains the gold standard for the depiction of prostatic cancer.

A considerable number of improvements, over the past 15 years, have increased the detection accuracy of prostatic cancer.

Extensive imaging studies are still needed to establish the exact role of each one of the newer techniques.

However, it is obvious that we may expect less need for systematic biopsies in the future.

Ultrasound may also provide better information on preoperative local staging

References

1. Engelbrecht MR, Barentsz JO, Jager GJ et al (2000) Prostate cancers tagging using imaging. BJU Int 86(Suppl 1):123–134
2. Onur R, Littrup PJ, Pontes JE, Bianco FJ Jr (2004) Contemporary impact of transrectal ultrasound lesions for prostate cancer detection. J Urol 172:512–514
3. Mitterberger M, Pinggera GM, Pallwein L et al (2007) The value of three-dimensional transrectal ultrasonography in staging prostate cancer. BJU Int 100:47–50
4. Morelli G, Pagni R, Mariani C et al (2011) Results of vardenafil mediated power Doppler ultrasound, contrast enhanced ultrasound and systematic random biopsies to detect prostate cancer. J Urol 185:2126–2131
5. Smeenge M, de la Rosette JJ, Wijkstra H (2012) Current status of transrectal ultrasound techniques in prostate cancer. Curr Opin Urol 22(4):297–302. Review
6. Kapoor A, Kapoor A, Mahajan G et al (2011) Real-time elastography in the detection of prostate cancer in patients with raised PSA level. Ultrasound MedBiol 37:1374–1381
7. Aigner F, Pallwein L, Junker D et al (2010) Value of real-time elastography targeted biopsy for prostate cancer detection in men with prostate specific antigen 1.25 ng/ml or greater and 4.00 ng/ml or less. J Urol 184:913–917
8. Correas J, Khairoune A, Tissier A et al (2011) Transrectal quantitative shear wave elastrography: application to prostate cancer: a feasibility study. Poster ECR, Radiol Congr. doi:10.1594/ecr2011/C-1748
9. Hodge KK, McNeal JE, Terris MK et al (1989) Random systematic versus directed ultrasound guided transrectal core biopsies of the prostate. J Urol 142:71–75
10. Eskew LA, Applewhite JC, McCullough DL (1999) Update of the 5 region prostate biopsy method: the durability of a decreased false negative rate of prostate biopsy. Proc Annu Meet Am Urol Assoc 1249:324

MRI in Prostate Cancer

91

Nikolaos V. Kritikos

MR imaging of the prostate emerged as a new diagnostic tool for the study of prostate cancer in the mid-1980 s. Ever since new MR techniques have evolved making MR prostate imaging a promising modality for detecting and staging of the prostate tumors. Basic morphologic sequences (T1-weighted (T1W) and T2-weighted (T2W)) in combination with recent advances which include functional and physiologic MR imaging techniques allow a more sophisticated approach of the prostate cancer, adding new information beyond the traditional morphologic assessment. In addition, the quality of the performed MRI exams of the prostate is essentially improved using new imaging unit hardware and software. Another era of advance is the development of MR-compatible devices, allowing invasive procedures as targeted prostate biopsy to be performed.

91.1 MR Prostate Anatomy

MRI is the better prostate imaging modality to delineate the normal prostate anatomy . T1W images are not so helpful in this prospective, since prostate gland appears with homogeneously intermediate signal intensity. T1W images are useful though to evaluate the contour of the prostate gland, and the periprostatic tissues as the neurovascular bundle. Also T1W sequences are helpful to evaluate the prostate gland after biopsy, revealing high signal intensity focus due to post-biopsy hemorrhage. T2W sequences are much more sensitive in depicting the prostate zone anatomy. In T2W images peripheral zone has high signal intensity in comparison with central zone which appears with intermediate signal intensity. Central zone is usually heterogenous due to presence of benign prostatic hyperplasia. The contour of the prostate gland is also clearly delineated by T2W images. The fibromuscular layer which represents the pseudo capsule of the gland appears as low intensity rim, in contrast with the high signal intensity of the periprostatic fat (Fig. 91.1).

Neurovascular bundles are identified as foci of low signal intensity posterolateral to the capsule, vas deferens and seminal vesicles appear with high signal intensity while anterior fibromuscular stroma has low signal intensity. Distal prostatic urethra can be identified as a low signal intensity ring.

91.2 Anatomic Imaging and Prostate Cancer

Prostate cancer has typically low signal intensity in T2W images in contrast to the normal high signal intensity of the peripheral zone. The signal intensity of prostate cancer may be variable

N. V. Kritikos (✉)
Director of Imaging Department, Mitera Hospital, Marias Polydouri 4, Agios Stefanos, 14565 Attica, Greece
e-mail: nikkr68@yahoo.gr

A. D. Gouliamos et al. (eds.), *Imaging in Clinical Oncology*,
DOI: 10.1007/978-88-470-5385-4_91, © Springer-Verlag Italia 2014

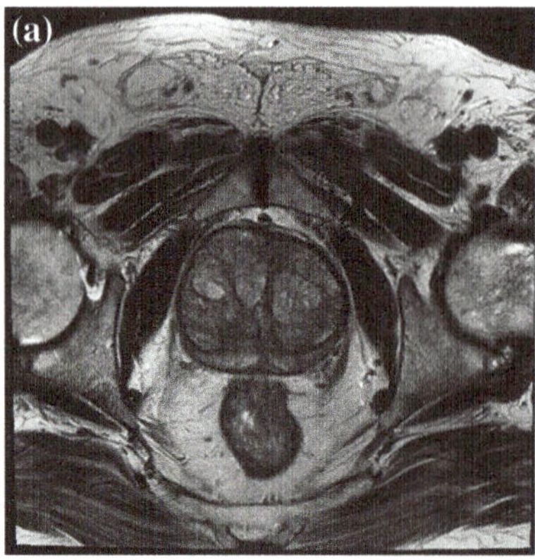

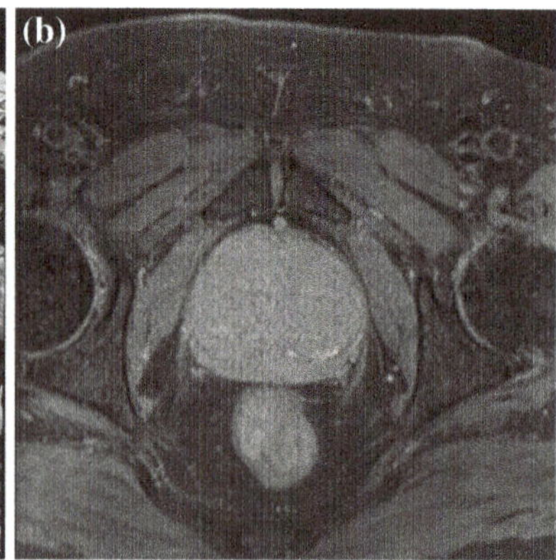

Fig. 91.1 Normal anatomy of the prostate gland obtained at 3.0T. **a** Axial T2W image shows high signal intensity normal peripheral zone which is sharply defined by the central zone and (**b**) axial T1W fat-saturated image shows no difference in signal intensity between peripheral and central zone

though depending upon the growth pattern, density, and the Gleason score. High grade prostate tumors appear with higher signal intensity than lower grade cancers in T2W images. Also dense cancers use to appear with lower signal intensity that those who grow thinly.

Unfortunately the *diagnosis* of the prostate cancer of the peripheral zone is not always straightforward. There are prostate tumors with signal intensity similar to the high signal intensity peripheral zone. Also many benign conditions mimic cancer. Inflammation, scars, hemorrhage, effects of radiation or hormonal therapy may also have low signal intensity inconspicuous from prostatic cancer.

Signal heterogeneity of the central zone poses additional difficulties in the interpretation of MR images of the prostate since the stromal type of benign prostatic hyperplasia has low signal intensity similar to the prostate cancer. Findings that may support the diagnosis of cancer are lack of the low intensity rim usually seen in case of benign prostatic hyperplasia, homogenous low signal intensity, ill-defined margins, lenticular shape, low signal intensity of the retroprostatic fat, and fibromuscular stroma invasion.

T2W images, despite the aforementioned limitations is the basic tool to detect extracapsular extension (ECE) of prostate cancer. Findings which predict local advanced disease are bulging prostatic contour, irregular margin, direct breach of the capsule, capsular retraction, obliteration of the rectoprostatic angle, asymmetry, or encasement of the neurovascular bundle. In case of *seminal vesicles invasion* (SVI) findings include enlarged low signal seminal vesicles, obliteration of the angle between prostate and seminal vesicles, and direct extension. Irregular contour of the prostate gland, low signal intensity of the retroprostatic fat, and direct breach of the capsule are the criteria with the highest sensitivity while the specificity is high for all of the above mentioned.

Assessment of ECE and SVI in case of prostate cancer is crucial to determine the proper therapeutic approach, since ECE and SV invasion are very important prognostic factors for recurrence after radical prostatectomy. Patients with advanced local disease by the means of ECE and SV invasion have overall worse prognosis since there is greater risk of a positive surgical margin and increased incidence of lymph node metastasis.

A lot of studies have been performed to evaluate the sensitivity and specificity of MRI morphological imaging to detect prostate cancer. Results have shown a wide variation with sensitivity to range between 57 and 84 % and specificity between 50 and 94 %. In a similar way, sensitivity and specificity of T2W prostate imaging to access extra capsular extension, and SVI invasion vary from 13 to 95 %, 49 to

97 % and 23 to 78 %, 81 to 99 %, correspondingly [1, 2].

T2W imaging is used to depict intrapelvic disease beyond prostate gland pathology. Lymph node involvement in prostate cancer patients is a question since assessing node size and morphology to predict lymph node neoplastic disease is inaccurate. Normal-sized lymph nodes may hide metastatic disease impossible to reveal using only morphologic criteria.

Conclusively, there are a lot of limitations assessing intra prostate cancer probable extra capsular extension and lymph node involvement using only anatomic MR images.

The conventional opinion that limitations in detecting and localizing intraprostatic cancer are not important since the major question to be answered is extracapsular extension is overwhelmed by new concepts in treatment of prostate cancer patients. Application of minimally invasive treatments requires additional information as exact localization of clinically important lesion (index lesion) in multicentric prostate cancer as well as information about tumor biological aggressiveness.

91.3 Functional Prostate MR Imaging

Tremendous advance in technology has allowed important improvement in MR prostate imaging adding in conventional morphologic study functional and metabolic information.

91.4 Dynamic Contrast-Enhanced MR Imaging

Dynamic contrast-enhanced imaging is a new promising technique based upon the alterations in vascularity of prostate cancer by means of angiogenesis and vasculogenesis.

Hypoxia in cancerous tissue provokes building of neovessels from already normal existing vessels or formation of new blood vessels de novo. These changes in case of prostate cancer are much more pronounced than those related with benign conditions as prostatitis or *benign prostatic hyperplasia.*

Tumor angiogenesis influence microvascular blood flow, surface area, and permeability via production of angiogenic factors. Such factors as vascular endothelial growth factor and vascular permeability factor lead to the formation of a disorganized vascular bed with weak walls and increased permeability.

Prostate cancer has higher mean vessel density (number of vessels per unit area) compared with normal prostatic tissue which is related to patient prognosis by means of local recurrence or metastatic disease.

Dynamic contrast-enhanced imaging includes fast T1W sequences acquired after intravenous injection of low-molecular-weighted gadolinium chelate. These fast sequences are more suitable for tissue characterization than slower ones but suffer from low spatial resolution.

The choice for the technique to be used is patient-tailored and depends upon the desired sensitivity, time of acquisitions, and area of coverage must be emphasized though that fast sequences allow a more sophisticated diagnostic approach by estimating different pharmacokinetic enhancement parameters.

At this time it is generally acceptable that optimal spatial and temporal resolution can be achieved by obtaining dynamic images every 5 s for a period of 5 min.

Prostate cancer is a highly vascularized tumor, so in contrast-enhanced MRI images has increased uptake and fast wash out of contrast media in comparison with the normal prostatic tissue.

Quantitative analysis of the contrast media uptake of prostate cancer in T1W contrast-enhanced images, and subsequent changes in T1W signal intensity are more conventional and easy to use in clinical practice. Semi-quantitative analysis incorporate time signal intensity parameters as outset time, mean gradient, time to peak enhancement, magnitude of peak enhancement, and wash out (Fig. 91.2).

The rate of enhancement reflects the alterations in neovessel volume and permeability, so that prostate cancer has typically rapid wash out

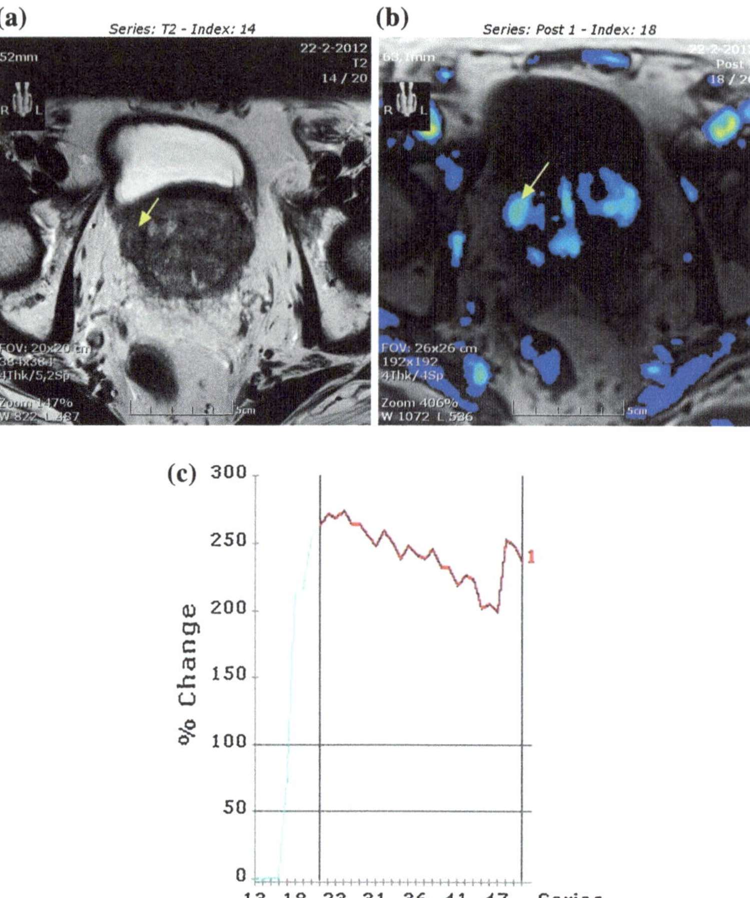

Fig. 91.2 Prostate cancer in 65-year-old man with a Gleason Score 3 + 3. **a** Axial T2W image shows low signal intensity focus in the *right side* of the peripheral zone. **b** *Color-map* and kinetic *curve* from dynamic contrast-enhanced MR images show rapid wash-in of contrast media in the corresponding lesion on T2W images

(especially high grade cancers) and also higher peak enhancement in comparison with normal prostate tissue or benign disease.

Estimating the time amount of early arterial enhancement is a fast and simple way to study the distribution of contrast media in the suspicious lesion. However, suffers from high intra-observers variability, and is very difficult to standardize the method.

Quantitative analysis of dynamic contrast enhancement MRI images is based upon the estimation of distribution of contrast media molecules between vascular and extravascular spaces. For this to be done DCE MR imaging uses complicated mathematical models named pharmacokinetic tracer kinetic compartmental models (TKCM). One of the most often used TKCM models is four compartment Toft's model which includes extracellular-extravascular space, intravascular blood plasma compartments and whole body intravascular and extravascular space, calculating basic parameters as k-trans (related to the permeability of the vessels) k-ep (reverse reflex rate constant between extracellular and vascular space), and volume fraction (ve). K-trans is the most important parameter to be estimated.

Nowadays there are several software programs in use, so that the aforementioned model-based parameters can be reproduced in parametric color maps, which can be overlaid in anatomic images.

Quantitative analysis though most complicated has the advantage that is more standardized method, independent of technical issues as far as sequences, and parameters are concerned.

Dynamic contrast-enhanced MR imaging has several limitations. At first precise evaluation of small-sized prostate cancers (volume <5 ml) is difficult because of partial volume effect.

Also, low Gleason Score cancers may not have the expected hemodynamic features already described. Localization of prostate cancer in central gland poses additional difficulties. Stromal type of benign prostate hyperplasia may be hypervascular and have identical enhancement to prostate cancer. Prostatitis in the peripheral gland because of the hemodynamic alterations due to inflammation may also be indistinguishable from prostate cancer. Motion of the surrounding organs as rectum and bladder is a common source of error leading to poor resolution of DCE MR images. Even if MR prostate scan is performed as recommended (6–8 weeks after biopsy) residual hemorrhage can be the source of false negative or false positive results. Finally, DCE MR imaging needs to be more standardized since many investigators use different acquisition times and methods of analysis.

DCE imaging has unsatisfactory specificity and sensitivity in detection and localization of prostate cancer when used alone (74–96 % and 46–96 %, respectively) [2].

Although its undoubtable shortcomings, DCE imaging has a great potential to provide valuable information in detection, localization, and staging of prostate cancer, especially when it is combined with anatomic imaging and other functional methods as MR Spectroscopy and Diffusion imaging.

91.5 Diffusion-Weighted Imaging

Diffusion-Weighted imaging is relatively new imaging technique based upon the different speed of motion distribution (Brownian motion) of water in intracellular and extracellular space. Cellular proliferation in cancerous tissue leads to reduction of extracellular space so that the amount of water molecules is reduced and restricted to intracellular space. Except alterations in cellular density, also cell membrane integrity is impaired so that diffusion-weighted images which reflect these changes can yield valuable information about the functional status and the microenvironment of tissues making possible to differentiate benign from malignant tissue.

Obtaining diffusion-weighted images is achieved using gradient echo planar sequences with different b-values where b-value is defined as the diffusion gradient value. B-value is the basic parameter to influence diagnostic accuracy of diffusion-weighted sequences. When b-value is increased diffusion sensitivity is increased. The prolonged time acquisition in high b-value diffusion images results in reduced image quality and signal to noise ratio (SNR). In lower b-values, the spatial resolution is better, and the signal to noise ratio is increased but accuracy of acquired images is reduced since low b-value diffusion imaging reflects also the tissue perfusion. Classically two series of traced diffusion images are acquired using 0 and 1,000 b-values in prostate imaging. Diffusion images are used to produce the second component of the diffusion study, apparent diffusion coefficient (ADC) map. ADC is the basic MRI measurable diffusion biomarker which represents both diffusion and capillary perfusion. Low ADC reflects restricted water molecular motion and so reduced diffusion.

In normal prostatic gland ADC is variable depending upon the anatomic zone which is examined. This is explained by means of different tissue composition in peripheral and central gland. Fibrous tissue in stromal type of benign prostatic hyperplasia is responsible for the low ADCs acquired. In a similar manner muscular tissue in anterior fibromuscular stroma leads to reduced diffusion. In contrary prostatic intraepithelial neoplasia have average higher ADCs as normal peripheral zone. In younger patients interpretation of diffusion images in central zone is more straightforward while in

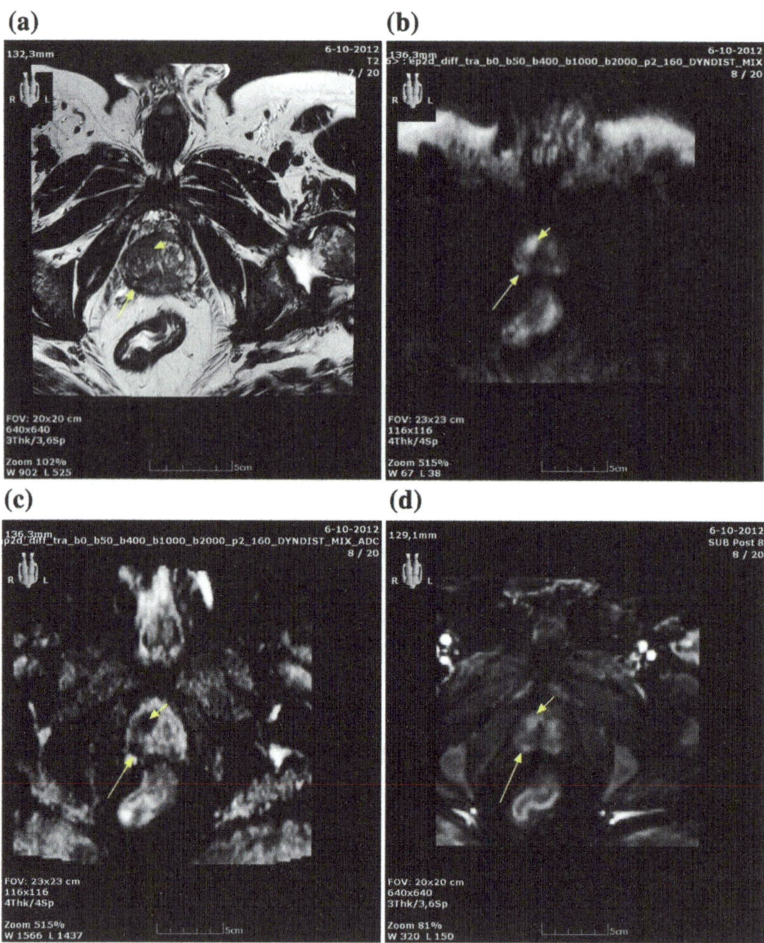

Fig. 91.3 Multifocal prostate cancer in 68-year-old man with a Gleason Score 4 + 4. Axial T2W image shows a low signal intensity lesion located in the *right side* of the central gland with ill-defined margins (erased charcoal sign) and second smaller one in the *right side* of the prostate apex (**a**). Axial diffusion image (**b**) obtained with b-value 2,000 and apparent diffusion coefficient map (**c**) show high–signal intensity and low ADC of the lesion, respectively. (**d**) Raw dynamic contrast-enhanced image shows increased uptake of contrast media

elderly additional difficulty poses the abundant fibrous tissue.

Prostatic cancer ADCs are clearly related with Gleason Score. Poorly differentiated prostate cancers have lower mean ADC because of the severe damage of architecture of the prostate gland, increased cell density, and restricted extracellular space. In contrary well-differentiated prostate cancers may show similar mean ADCs to normal prostatic tissue. Heterogeneity of prostate cancer is an important misleading factor in interpretation of diffusion MR prostate images since in the same lesion may coexist components with different Gleason score and correspondingly with different mean ADCs. Sparse prostate cancers even of high grade may show high ADCs due to the interposition of normal prostatic tissue (Fig. 91.3).

Diffusion-weighted imaging seems to have a better performance in cases of postbiopsy hemorrhage in comparison with T2W imaging even in foci of hemorrhage conventionally show lower mean ADCs than normal peripheral zone.

Many studies have been performed in order to define threshold ADCs for malignancy with poor results. There is a lot of variability in acquired diffusion-weighted images among variable centers since different MR systems acquisition parameters and magnetic field strengths are used. The overall sensitivity and specificity reported in the literature reflect this variation (54–94 % and 61–100 %, respectively) [3].

Diffusion MR imaging is valuable technique most easy to use between other functional methods since it is very fast and without need of contrast media injection. Additionally, diffusion imaging is able to provide great contrast between cancerous and normal prostatic tissue.

There are though several shortcomings of the method. Images acquired with high b-values are very helpful in localizing prostate cancer but suffer from low in plane spatial resolution cause of the low signal to noise ration even in high field strength magnets. Diffusion imaging is very susceptible to magnetic field in homogeneities and motion artifacts. Periprostatic fat is responsible for chemical shift artifacts while the variations in magnetic susceptibility in air tissue and bone tissue interfaces may cause severe distortions of the images. Improvement in image quality and overcoming of these artifacts can be achieved using fast sequences and parallel imaging.

In spite of its limitations diffusion imaging especially in combination with anatomic imaging and other functional techniques can be used not only in localization and detection but also in evaluation of aggressiveness of prostate cancer and can improve the overall sensitivity and specificity of multiparametric prostate study.

91.6 MR Spectroscopy

MR spectroscopy of the prostate is the third component of multiparametric study based upon the chemical shift phenomenon and providing metabolic information about the prostate cancer. The whole prostate gland is examined and is subdivided into multiple voxels. MR spectra are measured in each voxel, reflecting different resonance frequencies analogous to the amount of specific metabolites. These unique resonance frequencies or chemical shift are expressed in parts per million (ppm). Chemical shift of tetramethylsilume in heavy water is used as null point. Measured spectra are used to produce parametric maps.

Prostate spectra reflect basic anatomic and metabolic features of prostatic tissue and are closely related to the glandular –stromal tissue analogy. High concentration of citrate is expected in peripheral zone due to its rich glandular content. In contrary central gland is poor to glandular tissue. Dominance of stromal component leads to poor citrate levels. For the same reason citrate levels are reduced in anterior fibromuscular band.

Prostate cancer has typically decreased citrate and increased choline levels.

Variations in MR spectra because of complex prostate anatomy and also the fact that data acquired does not correspond to absolute concentration of metabolites are overcomed by using metabolic ratios. Conventionally, interpretation of MR spectra includes choline to citrate ratio (Fig. 91.4).

A well-established scoring system for standardization of metabolic rations has been revised by Jung et al. [4].

The suggested scoring system focuses on spectral data acquired from the peripheral zone of the prostate gland (lately the scoring system

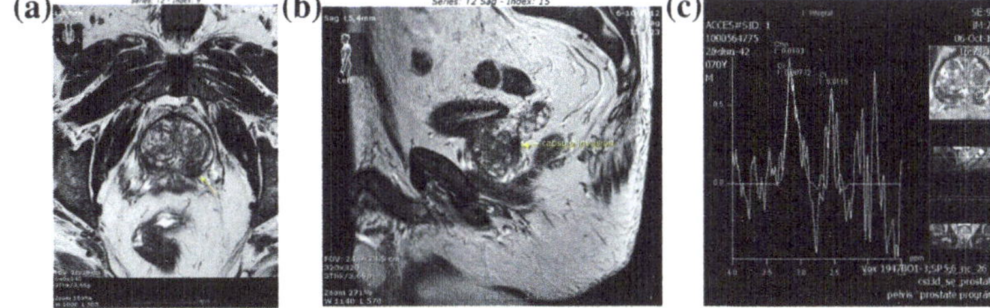

Fig. 91.4 Prostate cancer in 70-year-old patient with a Gleason Score 3 + 4. **a** Axial T2W image shows a low signal intensity lesion in the *left side* of the apex with budging of the prostate contour. **b** Sagittal T2W image shows clearly extracapsular extension and invasion of the adjacent seminal vesicle (**c**) MR spectra of the aforementioned lesion typical for prostate cancer

has been revised taking into account information about metabolic ratios of lesions in central gland). A five point MR spectroscopic scale is defined by the alterations of metabolic ratios of the suspicious lesion in comparison with the mean standard deviation. Score 1 lesion have metabolic ration less than 1SD above the mean, score 2 less than 2SD, score 3 less than 3SD, score 4 less than 4SD, and score 5 more than 4SD. Lesions which assigned with score 1 and 2 are considered to be benign. Score 3, 4, 5 are classified as equivocal, possibly malignant, and probably malignant correspondingly.

There are several technical issues in clinical application of MR spectroscopy. Motion artifacts can be a significant source of error in interpreting MR spectroscopy images. Susceptibility artifacts because of the air in nearby rectum may reduce the quality of acquired MR spectra. To avoid partial volume phenomenon effects the operator must have a thoughtful and time-consuming approach in planning the exam. Homogeneity of the magnetic field over the examined area is necessary in order to acquire high quality images. Also concern about avoiding interference of periprostatic tissue must be taken since the high fluid signal intensity of seminal vesicles for example may lead to false positive results. MR spectroscopy is the most demanding functional method by means of complicated and time consuming post processing of the acquired data despite the advance in software. The operator who will perform the MR spectroscopy must be well trained and experienced so that diagnostic good quality images are achieved.

Besides the technical problems inherent difficulty in MR spectroscopy diagnostic performance is due to the different tissue composition of the prostatic gland zones and also in benign disease. Stromal type of benign prostatic hyperplasia use to have low levels of citrate and polyamines so can mimic prostate cancer. For these reasons localization of prostate cancer in central gland may be extremely problematic. Sparse cancers intermixed with normal prostatic tissue may exhibit confusing metabolic ratios while the same problem of diagnostic accuracy may be encountered in case of mucinogenic prostate cancers. Such type of prostate cancer use to have high signal intensity in T2W images and false negative MR spectra because of the low density of the cancerous cells. Evaluation of small-sized cancers poses additional difficulty because of overlapping of spectral signal intensities from the adjacent normal prostatic tissue. Glandular elements show high levels of citrate and high signal intensity in T2Wimages, so that MR spectra of small neoplastic lesions may be distorted. Acute prostatitis may also mimic cancer in MR spectroscopy so that co-evaluation of anatomic images and clinical and laboratory findings is required for the correct diagnosis to be done. Postbiopsy hemorrhage causes severe local magnetic field distortion along with MR spectral degradation so is highly recommended MR spectroscopy to be performed at least 6–8 weeks after biopsy.

MR spectroscopy is undoubtedly a powerful diagnostic tool in the assessment of prostate cancer though difficult in clinical practice because of technical issues.

Reported sensitivity and specificity of the method in several studies ranges from 77 to 81 % and 46 to 61 %, correspondingly [5]. The sensitivity and specificity aforementioned may greatly improve when MR spectroscopy is used in combination with morphological imaging and other functional techniques.

91.7 MR Lymphography

Diffusion-weighted imaging has been used for evaluation of lymph nodes in case of prostate cancer with promising results. Metastatic lymph nodes conventionally have density and subsequently restricted diffusion in contrary with reactive lymph nodes. Widespread adoption of diffusion imaging in this era is not established. Major shortcomings are the lack of standardization of the technique and the fact that inflammatory lymph nodes may show ADCs similar to the metastatic ones.

MR lymphography is an emerging tool performed with the use of ultrasmall superparamagnetic iron oxide particles(USPIO). These particles also known as ferumoxtran 10 are engulfed from macrophages found in normal lymph nodes. Metastatic lymph nodes because of their architectural distortion do not uptake the contrast media and this result in bright signal in T2 gradient images while normal lymph nodes appear dark.

In a similar way to diffusion imaging for benign lymph node disease may yield misleading results in MR lymphography: Reduced uptake ferumoxtran-10 is reasonably expected in inflammatory lymph nodes with central necrosis.

Spatial resolution of MR images is another parameter not to allow detecting of minimally invaded lymph nodes leading to false negative results.

MR lymphography with USPIO though not yet commercially available and despite its shortcomings is a promising technique with high sensitivity and specificity (90 and 98 % correspondingly) [6].

91.8 MR Imaging-Guided Biopsy

MR imaging is generally accepted that provides more detailed information about prostate anatomy and is the most accurate modality for detection and localization of prostate cancer. An interesting and hopeful technique taking advantage of MR imaging high spatial resolution is MR-guided biopsy of suspicious lesions. Technological advancement has allowed use of MR-compatible devices which overcome the restrictions of MRI unit environment so that MR imaging-guided biopsies can be implemented. At least two functional methods are highly recommended to be performed for localization of the prostate tumor before biopsy. Planning software programs which are available contribute significantly to the success of the procedure allowing accurate placement of needle guide.

Complications of the method are not severe and include pain, hematuria, and urinary infection.

Duration of MRI-guided biopsy (lasting even 2 hours) is a possible disadvantage.

The reported *detection rate* of prostate cancer in several studies with MR-guided biopsy ranges from 38 to 59 % [7].

New evaluating techniques include fused MR imaging and transrectal U/S-guided biopsy and robotically assisted MR-guided biopsy.

At present, clinical application of MR-guided prostate biopsy is limited in cases of patients who are highly suspicious for cancer after repeated negative U/S-guided biopsies.

91.9 Role of MR Imaging in *Post-treatment Prostate Cancer* and in Tumor Recurrence

Therapeutic choices for prostatic cancer include prostatectomy, androgen deprivation therapy, and localized treatment options as radiation therapy (high dose external beam or brachytherapy), cryosurgery, photodynamic therapy, and high-intensity focus ultrasound. Local extent of tumor, tumor aggressiveness, and distant metastases or lymphadenopathy is critical in order to decide the optional treatment of each patient as mentioned previously in this chapter. MR imaging may substantially help not only in pro-treatment evaluation of prostate cancer but also in diagnostic approach of recurrence and post-treatment changes.

Radiation induces architectural distortion of the prostate gland because of atrophy and fibrosis resulting in diffuse decreased signal intensity and blurriness of normal zone anatomy. In that way morphological imaging seems to be incapable to differentiate residual tumor from irradiated gland both of them appearing with low signal intensity in T2W images. Sensitivity and specificity of anatomic imaging can be increased when used in combination with diffusion imaging since cancerous foci continue to show low ADCs in contrast with adjacent parenchyma. Dynamic contrast enhancement imaging is an alternative method to be performed, depicting fast uptake of contrast media by residual tumor in contrast with normal parenchyma which appears usually hypovascular. Because of post radiation atrophy MR spectra analysis of irradiated prostate cancer seems to be less helpful. Metabolic alterations in normal tissue reflect in decreased levels of citrate and increased level of choline in a similar way to the metabolic profile of cancerous tissue. Assessment of MR spectra peaks though may be indicative of residual tumor or not, since glandular atrophy is expected to cause low metabolite peaks.

Morphological assessment after focused ultrasound therapy and cryotherapy has the same limitations as those mentioned above, concerned postradiation diagnostic difficulty in prostate cancer. Decreased signal intensity of normal gland in T2W sequences, resembles that of cancer as soon as the initial edema found in immediately post-therapeutic period has subsided. Performance of diffusion-weighted imaging is quite as good as in post radiated gland, limited by low signal intensity of sub sequential fibrosis of normal prostate. Dynamic contrast imaging and MR spectroscopy have shortcoming especially in case of cryotherapy because of post treatment cell necrosis. Dynamic contrast-enhanced imaging though has a great potential in differentiation benign from malignant tissue after ultrasound therapy when the misleading inflammatory changes found at the outset of therapy are not any long present.

T2W images is the workhorse in evaluation of recurrence tumor after radical prostatectomy. Initial enthusiasm has been mediated because of the many false positive results due to prostatic tissue and seminal vesicle remnants, scars, and hemorrhage. Reported sensitivity and specificity ranges from 48 to 61 % and 52 to 82 % respectively [8]. However, T2W imaging remains a basic tool with increased accuracy when evaluated in combination with one or more functional methods. Dynamic contrast MR imaging by semi-quantitative analysis seems to be a quite accurate method to differentiate cancer recurrence from benign disease or postoperative changes. Conventionally, cancerous tissue enhances more and faster than benign disease. MR spectroscopy have been performed supplementary to dynamic contrast imaging in a few studies till now based upon the choline to citrate ratio, in assessment of tumor recurrence after radical prostatectomy.

Androgen deprivation therapy is an alternative treatment for advanced prostate cancer. MR imaging is of limited clinical usefulness in this era. Acquired data includes T2W morphology of the gland and metabolic profile by MR spectroscopy. Normal tissue shows higher signal intensity than cancer in T2W imaging and also metabolic atrophy in comparison with residual tumor. MR findings though are variable depend upon the type and duration of therapy.

Conclusively, MR anatomic together with functional imaging can provide valuable information in case of suspected biochemical or clinical recurrence of prostate cancer. Proper interpretation of MRI findings requires good knowledge of the limitation and shortcomings of the method.

91.10 MRI Prostate Imaging: Present and Future

A new landscape in prostate cancer imaging has risen in past years. High field (3T) MR scanners allow advanced MR techniques to be performed more accurately taking benefit from higher spatial and temporal resolution and high SNR. Ability to acquire high quality images without usage of *endorectal coils* in high field strength scanners is very important since many patients would either wise avoid performing the exam. Conventionally is preferable to use endorectal coil for MR prostate imaging also in 3T scanners to take full advantage of the high SNR.

Incorporation of new techniques (dynamic contrast-enhanced, imaging, diffusion imaging, and MR spectroscopy) adds a lot of valuable information to conventional and anatomic imaging improving overall the performance of the method. Detection, localization, staging, evaluation of cancer recurrence can be better achieved combining anatomic images with one or more functional techniques.

Recently, guidelines for multiparametric MR imaging have been published by European society of Urogenital Radiology to set the correct indications for the optimal protocol to be used [9].

According to the aforementioned *guidelines* MR imaging in low risk patients as defined by National Comprehensive Cancer Network is helpful to assess the extent of intraprostatic disease. In intermediate risk patients indications of MR imaging include local staging and extraprostatic disease extension. High risk patients benefit from MR imaging by means of revealing nodal or skeletal disease.

Additional a PI-RADS scoring system is suggested where every parameter is scored on a five point scale though criteria for assigning score in each parameter are not generally accepted.

Despite the undoubtful advance, there are a lot of challenges to confront with in MR imaging. Technical issues have to be solved in order to overcome inherent limitations of functional sequences (artifacts, low spatial and temporal resolution, complicated post processing software, and lack of standardization).

Variable biological signatures of prostate cancer require a deeply sophisticated approach taking into account MR imaging together with other biomarker and clinical data so that the best treatment choice will be done for a given clinical situation.

Finally, new promising techniques as MR lymphography and MR-guided biopsy have to further evolve to become clinically applicable and gain a widespread acceptance.

References

1. Oto A, Kayhan A, Jiang Y et al (2010) Prostate cancer: differentiation of central gland cancer form benign prostatic hyperplasia by using diffusion-weighted and dynamic contrast-enhanced MR imaging. Radiology 217:715–723
2. Sadha V, Baris T, Naira M et al (2012) Overview of dynamic contrast-enhanced MRI in prostate cancer diagnosis and management. AJR 198:1277–1288
3. Woodfield C, Tung G, Grand D et al (2010) Diffusion weighted MRI of peripheral zone prostate cancer: comparison of tumor apparent diffusion coefficient with Gleason score and percentage of tumor on core biopsy. AJR 194:316–322
4. Jung JA, Coakley FV, Vigneron PB et al (2004) Prostate depiction at endorectal MR spectroscopic imaging: investigation of a standardized evaluation system. Radiology 233:701–708
5. Young Jun C, Jeong Kon K, Namkug K et al (2007) Functional MR imaging of prostate cancer. Radiology 27:63–75
6. Heesakkers RA, Hövels AM, Jager GJ et al (2008) MRI with a lymph-node-specific contrast agent as an alternative to CT scan and lymph-node dissection in patients with prostate cancer: a prospective multicohort study. Lancet Oncol 9(9):850–856
7. Yacob H Jo, Sad Verma, Moultan S Jo et al (2012) Imaging guided prostate biopsy: conventional and emerging techniques. Radiographics 32:819–837
8. De Visscherc P, De Meerleer G, Fütterer J, Villeirs G (2010) Role of MRI in follow-up after local therapy for prostate carcinoma. AJR 194:1427–1433
9. Ho Barentsa, Richenberq J, Clements R et al (2012) ESUR prostate MR guidelines 2012. Eur Radiol 22(4):746–747

92 Nuclear Medicine Findings in Prostate Cancer

Lida N. Gogou

92.1 Initial Staging

Bone scintigraphy is a highly sensitive imaging procedure for detecting bone metastases but it is often nonspecific. Positive findings may be related also to degenerative joint disease or to benign bone disease such as skeletal trauma or Paget's disease.

It is particularly important in high-risk primary staging before radical prostatectomy or radiation therapy to assess the patient's burden of the disease to evaluate prognosis and efficacy of specific treatment [1, 2].

Bone Scintigraphy (B.S) offers the advantage of providing whole body examination. The most commonly used tracer for imaging the skeleton is methylene diphosphonate (MDP) labeled with Technetium 99 m (Tc-99 m).

From the early eighties, it was described that patients found initially to have an abnormal bone scan had a mortality rate at 2 years of approximately 45 % compared with 20 % for those with a normal scan. For preoperative management bone scan is not required in asymptomatic patients or where PSA levels are below 10 ng/ml, whereas, in symptomatic patients with bone pain and low or increased PSA the bone scan is recommended. In a large analysis, bone metastases were found in less 1 % at patients with PSA < 20 ng/ml and negative predictive value was 99.7 %. Spine is the most common site for metastases. As the diagnostic accuracy of planar BS is low, SPECT and SPECT/CT procedures are proposed for imaging.

SPECT/CT has optimized the use of planar BS with an improved sensitivity range of 87–92 %, specificity of about 91 %, a positive predictive value of 82 %, a negative predictive value of 94 % and accuracy of 90 %. Recently Even-Sapir [3] with multi field of view (FOV) SPECT reported sensitivity 92 % (over 62 % for planar images) in patient based analysis and from 39 to 71 % in a lesion based analysis (Fig. 92.1a, b).

PET/CT is a modern imaging modality that offers several unique advantages compared with other imaging techniques. The purpose of combining CT and PET systems in a single scanner (PET/CT) offers the precise anatomical localization of regions (and lesions) identified on the PET tracer uptake images. Fluorine-18-Fluorodeoxyglucose (^{18}F FDG) is the most commonly used positron emission tomography (PET) radiotracer for oncology. But ^{18}F FDG is of limited value in Prostate cancer due to low FDG avidity of most Prostate cancer cells, and to the often small volume of the primary tumor (micro carcinoma). In addition urinary activity limits pelvic evaluation and increased uptake in benign prostatic hyperplasia. The majority of primary prostate tumors (81 %) present low FDG uptake [3].

The average SUV (a semiquantitive index) was 4.5 ± 1.4 for prostate cancer, compared to 4.1 ± 1.0 for benign tissue. Nevertheless, the overall clinical experience with ^{18}F FDG in

L. N. Gogou (✉)
16, Taygetou st, P.Psychico, 15452 Athens, Greece
e-mail: lidagogou@yahoo.com

A. D. Gouliamos et al. (eds.), *Imaging in Clinical Oncology*,
DOI: 10.1007/978-88-470-5385-4_92, © Springer-Verlag Italia 2014

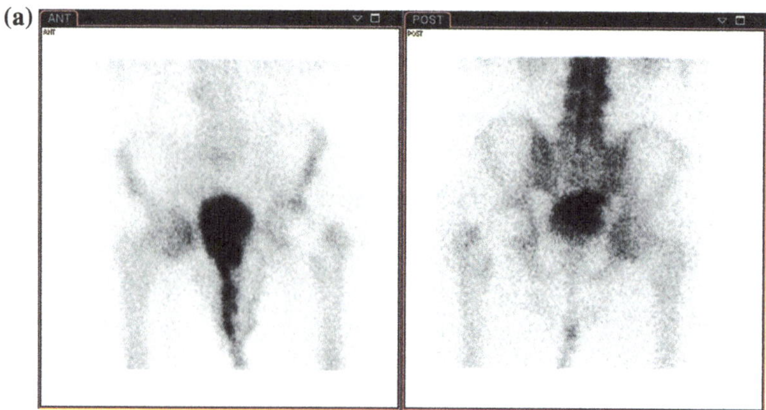

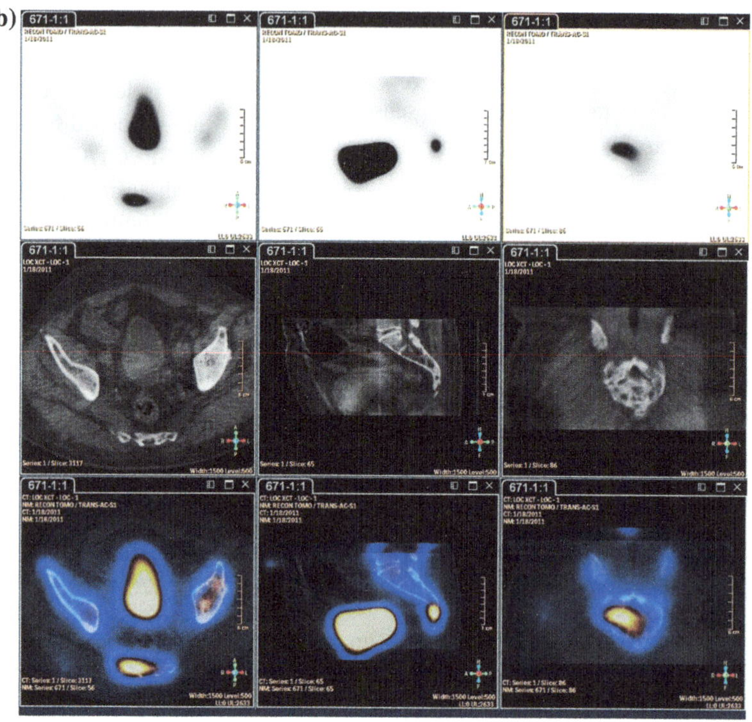

Fig. 92.1 **a** Staging of prostate Ca (Gl = 8, PSA = 55 ng/ml) Tc-99 m MDP—bone scan: Pelvis (*normal static view*) **b** SPECT/CT imaging revealed a bone metastasis in the sacrum

Prostate cancer suffers from heterogeneity in published studies with regard to the clinical phase of the disease, the relatively small numbers of patients and the variability and limitations in the validation criteria.

^{18}F FDG is insensitive for staging pelvic lymph nodes prior surgery and presents lower sensitivity than bone scintigraphy for the detection of active bone metastases. Shreve et al. [4] reported sensitivity only 62 % for bone metastases and a positive predictive value of 98 %. In predominantly sclerotic bone metastases FDG is less accurate and such lesions show lower tracer uptake than lytic bone metastases. FDG uptake is higher in tumors with higher Gleason scores (>7) and close correlation between increased PSA and PSA velocity levels has been shown in some clinical studies [5]. ^{18}F Fluoride a pure bone seeking substance may provide a more sensitive "conventional" bone scan and is superior for FDG non avid tumors. Comparative studies by Even-Sapir [3] were performed in patients with either localized high risk or metastatic Prostate cancer. The sensitivity and specificity of ^{18}F

Fluoride PET/CT was 100 % and 100 %, respectively (versus 70 and 57 % for planar BS) and authors concluded that ^{18}F Fluoride PET/CT is highly sensitive and specific imaging modality for the detection of bone metastases in high risk Prostate cancer patients (with Gleason > 8, PSA >20 ng/ml, or nonspecific sclerotic lesion on CT).

Other PET tracers used to study primary Prostate cancer include ^{11}C and ^{18}F labeled Choline derivative and ^{11}C Acetate. Both Choline and Acetate are key components of the lipid synthesis pathways and Choline uptake seems to be a marker of cell proliferation in Prostate cancer. The major advantage of the two tracers (over FDG) is the negligible renal excretion of tracer for better visualization of the prostate bed and regional pelvic lymph nodes. The major obstacle for routine use is the short life of ^{11}C and the age-related physiologic accumulation of ^{11}C Acetate.

^{18}F Fluoromethyl Choline (FCH) has the advantage of a longer half-life (T½ = 110 min) compared with ^{11}C Choline (T½ = 20 min) and early dynamic imaging by using coregistered CT data can be performed.

But FCH PET/CT imaging seems to have a limited value for initial staging of prostate cancer. Schmid et al. [6] published that FCH is not appropriate for initial T staging due to the limited spatial resolution of PET that does not enable the assessment of capsular infiltration, which in turns defines T3 tumors.

Husarik et al. [7] demonstrated that SUV_{max} values in metastatic lymph nodes (mean 5.04) and in bone metastases (mean 6.3) at initial staging were higher than those of subcutaneous fat (mean 0.2) or physiological uptake in bone of lumbar spine (mean 1.3). The possibility to enhance the detection rate of bone metastases on FCH PET/CT is late imaging at 65–200 min post injection, because the accumulation in bone metastases on late imaging rises compared to early imaging. To note that late imaging has no influence in lymph node metastases uptake.

FCH PET/CT can be helpful to guide biopsy if a patient has persistent elevated PSA levels and the biopsies remain negative for tumor. One major limitation of FCH PET/CT for initial staging is the general inability of PET imaging to detect micrometastases [7]. The identification of occult lymph node metastases appears to have an impact on the outcome of patients with Prostate cancer because these patients show significantly increased risk of recurrence or death (Fig. 92.2).

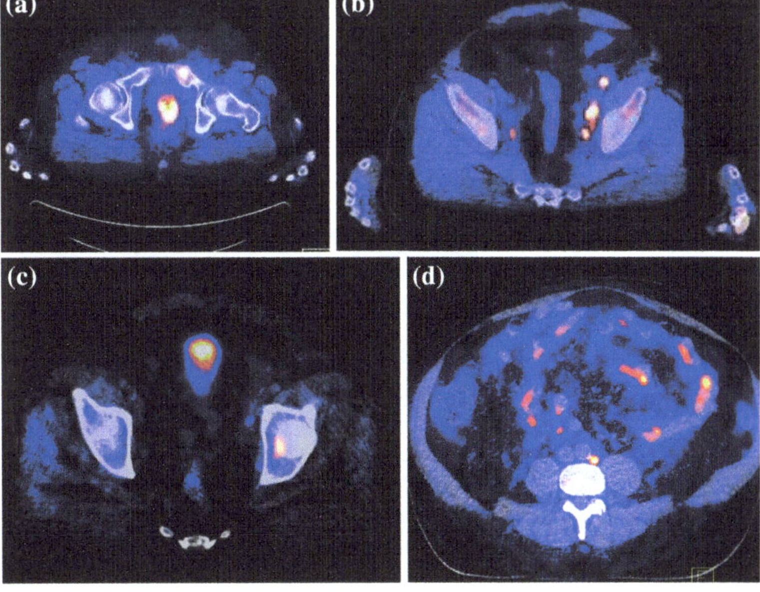

Fig. 92.2 Prostate cancer: (Gl = 7, PSA = 42 ng/ml-) Initial staging 18F FCH: lesion of the prostate (on the *left* SUVmax = 11, 7) Pubic (SUVmax = 10, 5) + L. Acetabulum (SUVmax = 6, 7) bone metastases, Inter + Ext Iliac LN (SUVmax = 11, 0) and paraortic LN (SUVmax = 4) metastases

92.2 Restaging

Bone scans remain the most common examination requested in patients suspected of having new skeletal metastases, usually in the setting of new bone symptoms or increasing PSA levels. The pattern of increasing PSA levels correlates with positive bone scan independently of other clinical variables.

In patients with confirmed metastatic disease, serial scans are often used to assess the extent of bone involvement and the effectiveness of therapy. As patients with prostate cancer with bone metastases often survive for a number of years, the bone scan provides a convenient method to monitor the disease over time.

Caution must be used in early assessment of bone metastases response to treatment due to the flare phenomenon, which is seen in some patients within the first 6 months after hormonal manipulation, whether via administered drugs or orchiectomy, and is associated with good prognosis [8]. It is important than clinicians appreciate that decisions to change or discontinue therapy should not be made until there is convincing clinical radiographic and scintigraphic evidence of metastatic disease progression. Patients with a flare phenomenon seen on bone scan, it might be valuable to exploit the high sensitivity and specificity of ^{18}F Fluoride PET/CT.

In a follow-up study FDG PET/CT has potential value when PSA > 4 ng/ml or increases > 0.2 ng/ml per month, in advanced or untreated cancer, in negative bone/scan and in equivocal pelvic CT findings. It is known that ^{18}F FDG PET/CT has poor accuracy for differencing local recurrence and scar. However is more likely to detect distant metastases (Fig. 92.3).

The detection rate of metastases by FDG PET/CT is highly depended on the level of the serum PSA and on the rate of change of the serum PSA level over time (PSA velocity). FDG PET detected lymph node metastases in 50 % of patients with PSA greater than 4 ng/ml or PSA vel greater than 0.2 ng/ml/month. The low detection rate of metastases by FDG PET/CT in patients with low PSA (or low PSA vel) may indicate that the incidence of metastasis is low in this group of patients. Or it may mean that there exists a small tumors burden which is below the spacial resolution of PET or that the tumor has a low glycolytic rate which is below the metabolic resolution of FDG PET.

Schoder et al. [9] reported sensitivity 79 % and specificity 66 % for PSA levels > 2.4 ng/ml. The same author [10] presented that overall FDG PET detects local or systemic disease in 31 % of patients with PSA relapse. PET/CT is superior to CT but inferior to MRI for detection of recurrence in the prostate bed. ^{11}C Acetate may also be useful in the detection of tumor recurrence in some patients treated previously with prostatectomy or radiation, with lesion dectability of 75 % and false positive rate of up to 15 %.

Choline PET imaging plays a more relevant role in the detection of Prostate relapse. Choline PET shows higher specificity and higher accuracy compared to all conventional imaging

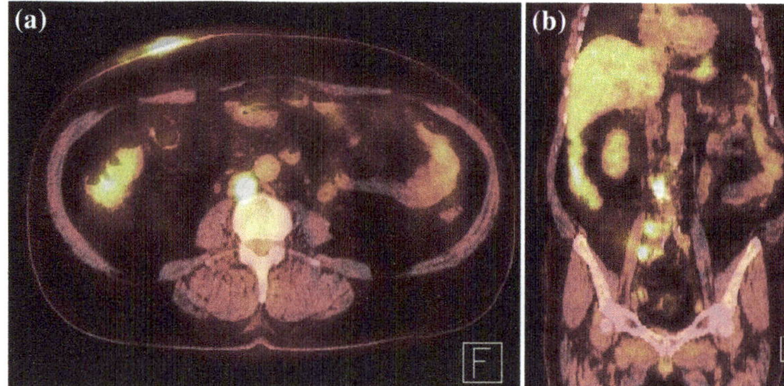

Fig. 92.3 Restaging of prostate cancer, 4y post prostatectomy and hormotherapy (Gl = 8, PSA = 80 ng/ml) ^{18}F FDG PET/CT: shows metastatic paraortic LN (SUVmax = 6, 0)

methods. Choline PET imaging, supplying a whole body tomography exam, has the major advantage of detecting local and distant metastases, within a single session, with a good accuracy. However, patient criteria still have to be defined. The exact threshold of serum PSA, the influence of medication (e.g., testosterone deprivation) and PSA kinetics are important factors on PET/CT detection. In particular, patients with high risk of distant metastases or those susceptible to second surgery and/or radiation therapy could benefit the most from early identification of the site of recurrence. The accuracy of conventional imaging modalities in detecting lymph nodes is low. Molecular imaging, particular Choline PET/CT represents the more accurate exam to stage high risk Prostate cancer and it is useful in staging patients with biochemical relapse, in particular when PSA kinetics is high or PSA levels are more than 2 ngr/ml [11, 12].

In biochemical recurrence imaging with ^{18}F FCH PET/CT seems to be higher among patients with higher PSA at the time of recurrence, shorter PSA dt (PSA duplication time) or higher initial Gleason grade [13].

Cimitan et al. [14] found positive FCH scans in 54 patients examined for rising PSA post radical prostatectomy, radical radiotherapy or while on hormones. All patients with PSA > 4 ng/ml and initial Gleason > 7 had positive scans, but rarely positive (3/38) among patients with PSA < 4 ng/ml. Pelosi et al. [15] noted an overall detection rate of 42.9 % in patients with rising PSA post-prostatectomy and demonstrated an increase in positive ^{18}F FCH scans, with higher PSA at recurrence (20 % at PSA < 1 ng/ml, 44 % at PSA 1–5 ng/ml and 82 % at PSA > 5 ng/ml).

Husarik et al. [7] found FCH imaging reliable for detection of PSA recurrence > 2 ng/ml with good sensitivity 83–87 %, moderate sensitivity (70–75 %) for PSA recurrence < 2 ng/ml and for small lymph mode metastases (<1 cm) with minimal FCH uptake. Langsteger et al. [16] noted the higher specifity of FCH compared with ^{18}F Fluoride (96 vs. 91 %) and the better accuracy levels (95 vs. 98 %).

The overall sensitivity for detecting any recurrence with FCH imaging at PSA levels 2–5 ng/ml seems to be acceptable (>80 %) but the sensitivity decreases for PSA levels < 2–5 ng/ml (about 50 %). Known that insolated local recurrence is more likely at lower PSA levels and these recurrences may be more difficult to detect [17, 18].

92.3 Therapy Response

^{18}F FDG PET may have a limited role in assessing treatment response to chemotherapy in hormone resistant disease and also in monitoring anti androgenic treatment. Early changes in glucose metabolism could enable monitoring metabolic changes in Prostate tumors after treatment in advanced disease with aggressive Prostate cancer [19].

Recently Mc Carthy et al. [20] examined prospectively 26 patients with castrate-resistant Prostate cancer and ^{18}F FCH PET/CT imaging was compared with standard imaging (bone scan or CT) for monitoring treatment. In FCH PET/CT 81 % of the detected lesions are concordant and 19 % are discordant after a 2 years follow-up.

False positive results were related to inflammatory lymph nodes and false negative to sclerotic metastases and iliac metastases post radiation therapy. FCH imaging presented 96 % sensitivity, 96 % specificity, 99 % PPV, 81 % NPV, and 96 % accuracy for the detection of bone and soft tissue metastases in castrate-resistant patients.

Radiotherapy dose escalation to the whole Prostate has been associated with improved disease control and together with higher gastrointestinal and genitourinary toxicity.

^{11}Choline and ^{18}F-FCH PET/CT may be useful for defining dominant intra prostatic lesion ($d > 5$ mm) for local salvage therapy, for any pelvic lesion in recurrence stage for salvage therapy and also guiding dose escalation [21].

In patients treated with stereotactic body radiation therapy 3 years overall survival was 92 %.

The androgen receptor plays an important role in the growth and proliferation of Prostate cancer as well as modulation of androgen status. ^{18}F FDHT is a radiolabeled analog of dihydrotestosterone. Preliminary studies reported that ^{18}F FDHT may be useful in monitoring treatment response [22].

92.4 Conclusion

In Prostate cancer imaging techniques could be useful for staging of primary disease, restaging after PSA relapse, detection of metastatic lesions and predicting the aggressiveness of the disease.

In Nuclear Medicine imaging common techniques using bone scan with Tc-99 m MDP (planar and SPECT/CT), Positron Emission Tomography imaging added supplementary value with the new agents as ^{18}F FDG and ^{18}F Fluoride.

Advanced technology with coregistiation of CT or MRI images with SPECT or PET, improvements in imaging cameras, image reconstruction algorithms have improved the quality of images. Also development of new tracers as ^{11}C Choline, ^{18}F Choline, and radiolabeled androgen-receptor binding compounds with higher selectivity and rapid localization promise a greater staging, restaging and treatment monitoring of Prostate Cancer.

References

1. Beheshti M, Langsteger W, Fogelman I (2009) Prostate cancer: role of SPECT and PET in imaging bone metastases. Sem. Nucl Med 39:396–407
2. Krasnow AZ, Hellman RS, Timins ME (1997) Diagnostic bone scanning in ongology. Sem Nucl Med 27:107–141
3. Even-Sapir E, Metser U, Mishani E et al (2006) The detection of bone metastases in patients with high risk prostate cancer: Tc-99 m MDP planar bone scintigraphy, single and multi-field of view SPECT, F-18-Fluoride PET and F-18-Fluoride PET/CT. J. Nucl Med 47:287–297
4. Shreve PD, Grossman HB, Gross MD et al (1996) Metastatic prostate concer: initial findings of PET with 2 deoxy-2 (^{18}F) fluoro-D-glucose. Radiology 199:751–756
5. Langsteger W, Heinisch M, Fogelman I (2006) The role of fluorodeoxyglucose, ^{18}F-Dihydroxy – phenylalanine, ^{18}F- Choline and ^{18}F-Fluoride in bone imaging with emphasis on prostate and bone. Sem Nucl Med 36:73–92
6. Schmid DT, John H, Zweifel R et al (2005) Fluorocholine PET/CT in patients with prostate concer: initial experience. Radiology 235:623–628
7. Husarik D, Mirabell R, Dubs M et al (2008) Evalution of 18F Choline PET/CT for staging and restaging of prostate cancer. Eur J Med Mol Imaging 35:253–263
8. Cook GJ, Fogelman I (2001) The role of nuclear medicine in monitoring treatment in skeletal malignancy. Sem Nucl Med 31:206–211
9. Schoder H, Larson SM (2004) Position emission tomography for prostate, bladder and renal cancer. Sem Nucl Med 34(4):274–292
10. Schoder H, Herrmann K, Gonen M et al (2005) 2-F-18-Fluoro-2 deoxyglucose position emission tomography for the detection of disease in patients with prostate specific antigen relapses after radical prostatectomy. Clin Cancer Res 11(3):4761–4769
11. Skanjeti A, Pelosi E (2011) Lymph node staging with Choline PET/CT in patients with prostate cancer: a review I. SRN Oncol 219064:1–6
12. Picchio M, Briganti A, Fanti S et al (2011) The role of choline positron emission tomography/computer tomography in the management of patients with prostate specific antigen progression after radical treatment of prostate cancer. Eur Urol 59(1):51–60
13. Fuccio C, Rubello D, Castellucci P et al (2011) Choline PET/CT for prostate cancer: main clinical applications. Eur J Radiol 80(2):50–56
14. Cimitan M, Bertolus R, Morassant S et al (2006) ^{18}F Fluoro Choline PET/CT imaging for the detection of recurrent prostate cancer at PSA relapse: experience in 100 consecutive patients. Eur J Nucl Med Mol Imag 33:1387–1398
15. Pelosi E, Arena V, Skanjeti A et al (2008) Role of whole body ^{18}F Choline PET/CT in disease detection in patients with biochemical relapse after radical treatment for prostate cancer. Radiol Med 113:895–905
16. Langsteger W, Balogova S, Huched V et al (2011) ^{18}F Fluorocholine and Sodium Fluoride ^{18}F PET/CT in the detection of prostate cancer: prospective comparison of diagnostic performance determine by masked reading. Q J Med Imaging 55:448–457
17. Bauman G, Belhocine T, Kovacs M et al (2012) ^{18}F Fluorocholine for prostate cancer imaging: a systemic review of the literature. Prostate Cancer Prostatic Dis 15:45–55
18. Picchio M, Giovannini E, Messa C (2011) The role of PET /computer tomography scan in the management of prostate cancer. Curr Opin Urol 21(3):230–236

19. Jadvar H (2011) Prostate cancer: PET with ^{18}F FDG, ^{18}F or ^{11}C Acetate and ^{18}F or ^{11}C Choline J. Nucl Med 52:81–89
20. Mc Carthy M, Siew T, Campbell A et al (2011) F-Fluoromethycholine (FCH) PET imaging in patients with castration-resistant prostate cancer: prospective comparison with standard imaging. Eur J Nucl Med Mol Imag 38:14–22
21. Picchio M, Giovannini E, Crivellaro C et al (2010) Clinical evidence on PET/CT for radiation planning in prostate cancer. Radiother Oncol 96(3):347–350
22. Larson SM, Morris M, Gunther I et al (2004) Tumor localization of 16 beta ^{18}F-Fluoro 5 alpha-dihydrotestosterone versus ^{18}F FDG in patients with aggressive metastatic prostate cancer. J Nucl Med 45:366–367

93 Clinical Implications of Prostate Cancer

Gerasimos J. Alivizatos and Pavlos A. Pavlakis

93.1 Diagnosis-Staging

Transurethral ultrasound (TRUS)-guided biopsies is the best method to diagnose prostatic carcinoma and a minimum of 8–12 biopsy cores are recommended depending on the size of the gland. TRUS offers information for local staging (T staging) as well but due to its low sensitivity MRI images can offer valuable information. The evaluation of pelvic lymph nodes (N staging) is done with CT scans but small metastases cannot be identified with preoperative imaging technology and therefore lymph node surgical dissection is still needed in cases where the Gleason score is >6 or when the PSA value is >20 ng/ml. Skeletal metastases (M staging) are best evaluated with bone scans. In ambiguous cases where dilemmas arise C-choline-, F-flouride-PET/CT, and whole body MRI have been offered as an alternative option but these modalities should not be used routinely in everyday practice [1, 2].

93.2 Follow-Up Strategies

TRUS and biopsy have been used to detect local recurrence but it is recommended only if it will change the treatment decision and if a palpable lesion is present. Metastatic sites can be detected with CT or MRI scans and with bone scans. These modalities should not be used routinely in patients with stable low PSA values and will offer information when symptoms become present or when the PSA value exceeds the level of 20 ng/ml. For the identification of local recurrence after radical prostatectomy endorectal MRI has been used but it is not recommended in every case. PET/CT has been examined in patients with biochemical relapse after definitive treatment (radical prostatectomy and local radiation) and it has been shown that metastases can be identified. The capacity of this modality to identify metastatic sites is influenced by the PSA level, PSA velocity and by PSA doubling time. With PSA values <1 ng/ml, the assistance of PET/CT is questioned [1, 2].

References

1. Heidenreich A, Bellmunt J, Bolla M et al (2011) EAU guidelines on prostate cancer. Part 1: screening, diagnosis, and treatment of clinically localised disease. Eur Urol 59(1):61–71
2. Pinto F, Totaro A, Palermo G et al (2012) Imaging in prostate cancer staging: present role and future perspectives. Urol Int 88(2):125–136

G. J. Alivizatos (✉) · P. A. Pavlakis
3rd Urological Department, Hygeia Hospital,
Erythrou Stavrou 4, 15123 Athens, Greece
e-mail: gali@hol.gr

A. D. Gouliamos et al. (eds.), *Imaging in Clinical Oncology*,
DOI: 10.1007/978-88-470-5385-4_93, © Springer-Verlag Italia 2014

Part XII
Melanoma

Introduction to Melanoma

94

Dimitrios I. Bafaloukos

Cutaneous melanoma is the most widely metastasizing neoplastic disease, with the least predictable pattern of spread. The incidence of melanoma worldwide has increased, by average of 2.5 % per year, a rate higher than any other malignancy. In the USA, the lifetime risk for developing melanoma has increased from 1:1,500 in 1930 to 1:75 in 2000. The current lifetime risk for developing the disease in Australia is 1 in 25 [1]. Melanoma confined to the epidermis is effectively curable, and thin lesions carry a 98 % 5-year survival rate. However, patients with primary tumors of >4 mm thickness have a <50 % survival rate. Nearly 50 % of patients are at risk for reccurence, which is most common in the years immediately after diagnosis [2]. An estimated 20 % of all fist recurrences occur locally, 50 % occur in the regional lymph nodes, and 30 % arise at distant sites [3]. The median survival for disseminated disease is just 7–9 months, but now with the use of B-RAF inhibitors and biological agents shows a trend to surpass the 12 months.

Despite the known benefits of early detection of recurrence, no evidence-based surveillance guidelines exist and clinical patterns vary widely. Thus, it is important to define optimal follow-up strategies, including the most effective imaging techniques and evaluation intervals, assuming that early diagnosis, detection of metastases and prediction of response are beneficial and crucial for the patients.

References

1. Rigel DS, Friedman RJ, Kopf AW (1996) The incidence of malignant melanoma in the United States: issues as we approach the 21st century. J Am Acad Dermatol, 34(5 Pt 1):839–847
2. Leiter U, Meier F, Garbe SB (2004) The natural course of cutaneous melanoma. J Surg Oncol 86(4):172–178
3. Benvenuto-Andrade C, Oseitutu A, Agero AL, Marghoob AA (2005) Cutaneous melanoma: surveillance of patients for recurrence and new primary melanomas. Dermatol Ther 18(6):423–435

D. I. Bafaloukos (✉)
Metropolitan Hospital, E. Makariou 9—E. Venizelou 1, 18547 N. Faliro, Greece
e-mail: dimmp@otenet.gr

A. D. Gouliamos et al. (eds.), *Imaging in Clinical Oncology*,
DOI: 10.1007/978-88-470-5385-4_94, © Springer-Verlag Italia 2014

95 Imaging Findings in Melanoma

Roxani D. Efthymiadou

Cutaneous melanoma is the most serious type of skin cancer. Its incidence has increased rapidly during the past few decades probably due to the increased ultraviolet radiation exposure but also to the earlier and more accurate diagnosis. Melanoma is an aggressive disease which may spread almost to any organ of the body. It has been well established that early detection and accurate staging are of critical value for the appropriate treatment and patient's prognosis. Unfortunately, in many cases the lesions are detected late. The most common metastatic sides are the lungs, the liver, and central nervous system (CNS) [1].

The role of imaging modalities in staging of melanoma is extremely important. Imaging studies include plain radiographs, ultrasound (US), computed tomography (CT), magnetic tomography, lymphoscintigraphy, bone scan, and PET-CT.

The role of plain chest radiograph (CXR) is controversial. In daily practice CXR is mainly obtained for follow-up of cases of nonmetastatic melanoma. Although it is an inexpensive method with low radiation exposure, it is not recommended for patients with metastatic lung disease because of the low sensitivity of this procedure [2]. The low sensitivity is related with the usually very small size of the pulmonary metastases. Furthermore, many studies found no positive results among patients with asymptomatic localized disease who underwent CXR. In these patients, CXR proved to be not a cost-effective examination. On the other side, investigators support that CXR should be used as a widely available, low-cost and noninvasive imaging procedure. As a general rule routine CXR is not recommended in asymptomatic patients with node-negative melanoma.

CT is the method of choice for staging of patients with melanoma, especially in TNM stage III or in recurrence of the disease [3]. The role of the procedure in the evaluation of asymptomatic patients with stage I or II remains controversial because of the high incidence of false positive findings and the low detection rate.

The new-generation multidetector scanners provide detailed high quality images with less artifacts in a really very short time. CT scans are performed pre and post intravenous contrast administration, during the arterial and the portal venous phase. Metastases of melanoma are usually hyperdense, so they are well detected in precontrast images. Intravenous contrast medium should be avoided in allergic patients and also in cases with renal failure in order to protect kidneys from further renal damage. CT must be also avoided in pregnants and if possible in young population, because of the radiation exposure. US and MRI could be alternative choices in such cases. According to large

R. D. Efthymiadou (✉)
CT, MRI and PET-CT Department, Hygeia Hospital, Pittakou 21, Nea Ionia, 14231 Attiki, Greece
e-mail: r.efthimiadi@hygeia.gr

A. D. Gouliamos et al. (eds.), *Imaging in Clinical Oncology*,
DOI: 10.1007/978-88-470-5385-4_95, © Springer-Verlag Italia 2014

studies, CT demonstrated sensitivity 58–75 % and specificity 70–76 % [4].

CT of the chest is the main imaging method for evaluating lung metastases which are very common in melanoma but also for detecting pleural or pericardial effusion or lymphadenopathy at the mediastinum and the axillae. As large autopsy series demonstrated, chest involvement was found in 70 % of patients with melanoma. Respiratory failure due to lung metastatic disease is the main cause of death from melanoma [3, 4]. Multidetector CT of the lungs may reveal very small pulmonary nodules which cannot be detected with any other imaging procedure. The lung foci vary in size; they usually are in the range of 1–2 cm but they may also be very small, even less than 5 mm or very big, even more than 5 cm (Fig. 95.1). Metastatic disease at the lungs may have the type of lymphangitic spread which also can be detected by CT even in early stages. The method is performed post intravenous contrast administration mainly for evaluating enlarged lymph nodes at the mediastinum which usually accompany lung lesions. Occasionally, mediastinal lympadenopathy is the initial imaging finding of the disease. A pericardial effusion may be present as melanoma metastasizes at the heart more often than any other tumor. Secondary deposits may be found not only to the pericardium but even to the myocardium and sometimes they are big enough to be recognized at CT images [4]. CT of the chest may also reveal secondary deposits at the bones and the soft tissue as the muscles and the subcutaneous fat (Fig. 95.2). Melanoma metastasizes to the breast more frequently than any other cancer. The lesions appear as single or multiple, well-defined noncalcified soft tissue masses.

Melanoma may metastasize to any organ of the abdomen as the liver, the spleen, the kidneys, the adrenals, the pancreas, the gall bladder, and the gastrointestinal tract [1, 4]. Oral contrast administration is necessary for an adequate opacification of the bowel. Intravenous contrast medium administration is also necessary in order to separate lymph nodes from the vessels and to obtain a detailed evaluation of the parenchymatous organs. Multiphase CT of the abdomen is the procedure of choice for detecting metastases at the liver and the spleen. Hepatic and splenic metastases are related to the stage of the disease. In large autopsy series, secondary deposits at the liver were found in 58 % of patients. As prereferred, oral and intravenous contrast administration are necessary for an adequate evaluation. Hepatic metastases may vary in size, shape, and density. They may be single or multiple, partly calcified, necrotic, or hemorrhagic, and they may enhance in a homogeneous, inhomogeneous, or ring-like pattern. Their size may vary from a few mm to more than 12 cm. The detailed anatomic study of the liver provided by CT and MRI is of critical importance for patients with metastatic

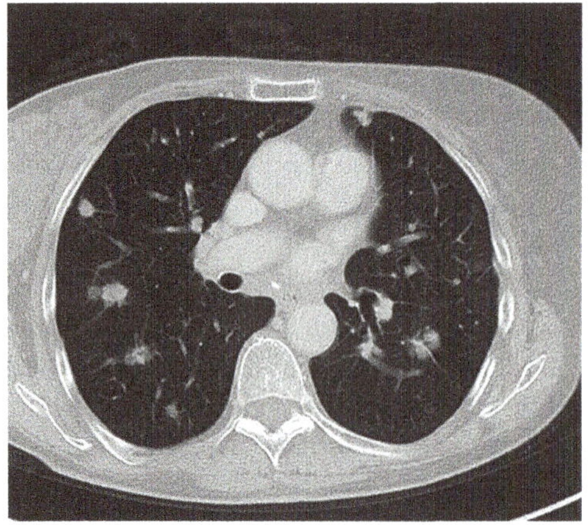

Fig. 95.1 CT of the chest: multiple ill-defined nodular lesions at both lungs in metastatic melanoma

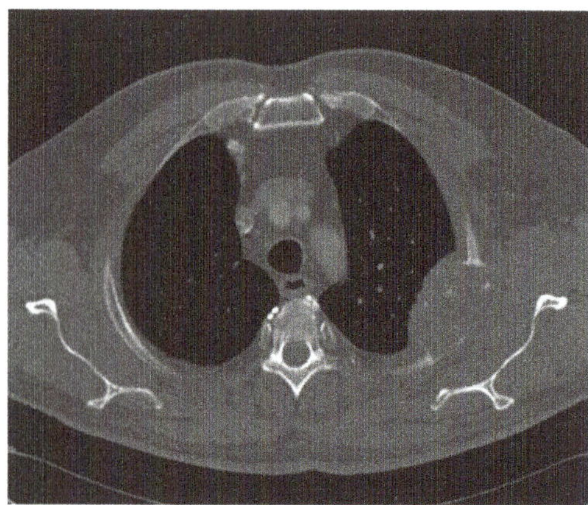

Fig. 95.2 CT of the chest: osteolytic metastasis from melanoma at the 6th left rib

disease who could benefit from surgery or ablation, in order to exclude any other unexpected foci of the disease [3].

Although splenic metastases are generally rare in patients with cancer, melanoma, and ovarian carcinoma are the two most frequently spreading at the spleen neoplasms [4]. Splenic secondary deposits are found at almost 30 % of patients with melanoma. Typically, they appear as single or multiple low-density lesions, usually solid, variable in size, better revealed in contrast enhanced images. Rarely they take the form of cystic or target like lesions.

Gastrointestinal spread of melanoma is found in 4.4 % of patients, may be present anywhere from the mouth to the anus but is most frequent in the small bowel. Imaging studies used to detect these metastases are CT of the abdomen and the pelvis, follow-through of the small bowel, and enteroclysis. Gastrointestinal spread may cause symptoms like pain, nausea, vomiting, etc. but may also be detected in the routine investigation in asymptomatic patients. The metastatic lesions on CT mimic primary or metastatic adenocarcinoma or even lymphoma. Ulcerating lesions can provoke complications as acute abdomen or seeding of the peritoneum. Metastases on the small bowel can be small or large, single or multiple. It is interesting that even patients with multiple secondary deposits may have no symptoms. Metastases to the large bowel are rare and occur as large and usually ulcerating tumors. Mesenteric spread appears as soft tissue mass at the mesentery or the omentum. Although rare, metastases of melanoma to the gall bladder are the most frequent metastases at this organ as they account for more than 50 % of all secondary deposits at it [3, 4].

Secondary deposits may be observed at the kidneys and the adrenals mainly at cases with widespread metastatic disease. In autopsy series renal metastases were found in 35 % of patients with melanoma. On CT scans, metastatic deposits appear as single or multiple, usually bilateral lesions, best revealed at post contrast images. They may be solid with inhomogeneous density or cystic like lesions with peripheral enhancement. In many studies, metastases in the perirenal and pararenal spaces were described [4].

Adrenal metastases were found in up to 50 % of patients with melanoma in autopsy series. The secondary deposits may vary in size and appearance. They may be unilateral or bilateral, round or oblong with a maximum diameter in the range of 4–6 cm [4].

Nodal involvement is very common in melanoma. The evaluation of lymph node metastases revealed by CT is based on size criteria for every nodal group all over the body. Therefore, CT is insensitive for the detection of small metastases to the lymph nodes [3, 4]. On the other hand, the procedure may be complicated by false positive findings as the enlarged lymph nodes detected by CT may not be metastatic: they may be reactive or inflammatory. In the evaluation of nodal involvement, other imaging modalities as lymphoscintigraphy and PET-CT may have the initial role.

Involvement of musculoskeletal system is common in metastatic melanoma. Secondary deposits may be found at the bones, the muscles, and the subcutaneous tissue all over the body. A lesion at the skin or the subcutaneous fat may be the initial sign of metastatic spread. Subcutaneous nodules surrounded by fat are a frequent finding in melanoma. They may represent a secondary deposit or even the primary tumor and can be easily detected on CT scans [1, 3]. The subcutaneous nodules can extend to the muscles or to the skin as an ulcerating lesion. Muscle metastases are relatively rare. Their typical appearance on CT is that of a hyperdense relative to muscle lesion. They may be single or multiple. Intravenous contrast medium administration permits a better definition of the tumor's borders.

Although rare, bone metastases may be the initial finding of spread of the disease. They have a poor prognosis with an average survival not more than a few months after their diagnosis. They are typically lytic and may be accompanied with soft tissue mass. Periosteal reaction is not common. Most metastatic bone lesions are found in the axial skeleton (almost 80 % of them, according to a study, and specifically 35 % in the ribs). CT scans may reveal bone metastatic lesions and the surrounding if existed soft tissue mass, all over the body, in the initial staging and the restaging of patients with melanoma [3]. The examination can be completed with three-dimensional (3D) reconstructed images, in order to provide the clinician more anatomic information. Bone scanning, MRI, and PET-CT are imaging procedures that may also be used in the evaluation of bone lesions.

Melanoma metastases at the CNS are very common. In fact, melanoma is the third after lung and breast cancer mostly metastasizing to the brain tumor. According to autopsy data, 49–73 % of patients with widespread disease have cerebral metastases. Brain metastases carry a very grave prognosis, with a median survival of 4 months after the diagnosis and correspond to the second cause of death after lung involvement in patients with melanoma. On CT images brain metastases are detected as single or usually multiple lesions which may be hyperdense on noncontrast images and enhance homogenously or in a ring-like pattern after intravenous contrast administration. They can be infra- or supratentorial and in most cases are surrounded by edema. Cerebral lesions are more common than cerebellar. Rarely, CT images may demonstrate nodal subependymal lesions, meningeal spread, or even metastases at the choroid plexus. MRI permits a more sensitive and detailed evaluation of CNS in patients with melanoma [5].

US has not been widely used in staging of patients with melanoma. Its role may be complementary in selected cases. US can be performed in order to evaluate node beds that drain the primary site before sentinel node biopsy (SNL). This technique is based on the ability of the method to detect morphological changes in metastatic lymph nodes. Nodes with loss of the normal fatty appearance of their hilum can be selected for fine needle aspiration. Although US cannot replace SNL it may be used in some cases to detect spread of the disease to the lymph nodes. The sensitivity of US for the detection of nodal metastasis is up to 82 % with a positive predictive value of 52 % [6]. High frequency US is a useful imaging procedure for the evaluation of superficial nodes as the cervical or the inguinal nodes but not efficient enough for deeper nodes like the axillary, the iliac, and the mesenteric. US may be used as an alternative imaging method when CT the method of choice for staging melanoma in daily practice should be avoided like in young population, pregnants, and patients with renal failure or with allergy to iodinated contrast. In such cases US may be useful mainly for the evaluation of the abdomen and pelvis, the superficial nodes, and the soft tissue. Hepatic or splenic metastases typically appear as single or multiple, of various size, hypoechoic lesions, which in sometimes may be heterogeneous due to hemorrhagic elements. US is useful to distinguish a cystic renal lesion from a solid one (more suspicious to be malignant) but also to detect possible secondary deposits to the gall bladder: focal mucosal thickening or polypoid lesions larger than 7 mm are suspicious to be malignant. Echocardiography is the imaging method of choice for detecting a pericardial effusion, quantifying its volume, and evaluating its hemodynamic effects. Although US is not the initial imaging procedure for staging melanoma its role is under estimation. Further large studies are needed to confirm the cost-effectiveness of the method and to determine the specific patient population that can get profit.

The role of magnetic resonance imaging (MRI) in staging of melanoma is mainly complementary to CT, especially for the evaluation of the brain, the spinal canal, the musculoskeletal system, the anatomical structures of the head and neck and the parenchymatous organs of the abdomen and the pelvis. The total accuracy of MRI for the detection of metastatic disease range from 77 to 79 %.

MRI is more sensitive compared to the other imaging methods to identify secondary deposits to the CNS [7]. Particularly, in patients with melanoma MRI is more sensitive than CT in the evaluation of the brain and the spinal cord. Although CT is the initial imaging method in staging of melanoma, MRI of the CNS should be performed in patients with symptoms and normal CT scan or in cases of uncertain findings, where a further and more detailed evaluation is needed. Brain metastases of melanoma may have a wide range of appearances in MRI images. Metastases with the typical melanotic pattern demonstrate high signal intensity on T1—weighted images and low signal intensity on T2—weighted images, due to the contained melanin and blood products (Fig. 95.3). In the amelanotic pattern the metastases appear hypointense or isointense to the cortex on T1 images and hyperintense to isointense on T2 images. Except their typical melanotic and amelanotic patterns, brain secondary deposits may also have other types of appearances which mainly are related with the amount of the melanin and of the products of hemorrhage that they contain. Melanoma metastases may be extremely small, so that they can easily be mistaken for vessels or artifacts. As they are characterized by rapid growth, a close follow-up should be useful in order to detect them. Rarely, brain metastases may be milliary, located at the cortex or the subcortical white matter, or even they can be subependymal appearing as nodular periventricular areas with marked enhancement after intravenous contrast material administration. Although rare, meningeal involvement can be found in metastatic melanoma. The spread is more frequent in leptomeninges than in the dura and it is better demonstrated in contrast enhanced T1—weighed images. Metastases at the choroid plexus are uncommon and they are usually observed in patients who have additional cerebral or meningeal metastases. They have variable signal intensity on T1 and T2 images and frequently demonstrate heterogeneous enhancement.

Except its obvious value in staging, MRI of the brain is also used for planning and monitoring gamma-knife therapy in patients with metastatic melanoma.

MRI is the imaging method of choice for the evaluation of the spinal canal. Intramedullary or meningeal secondary deposits are uncommon and are related as the cerebral metastases with a grave prognosis. They are better recognized at T1 post contrast images as enhanced lesions along the spinal cord or the cauda equina.

MRI is a useful procedure for a further investigation of focal lesions at the parenchymatous organs of the abdomen in order to differentiate benign from malignants entities. On MRI, hepatic metastases appear as areas with low signal intensity in T1 images and moderately high on T2 images while hemangiomas typically have very high signal intensity (they are very bright) on T2 images and a characteristic pattern of enhancement on post contrast T1 images (Fig. 95.4a, b).

MRI is an imaging modality with excellent results in the evaluation of bones and soft tissue. MRI may reveal signs of bone metastases much more earlier than CT as it has high sensitivity in evaluating marrow abnormalities but the specificity of the method is relatively low.

MRI is the best imaging modality for evaluating secondary deposits (which are uncommon) at the anatomical structures of the head as the orbits, the muscles, and the subcutaneous fat but also of the neck as the pharynx and the parotid glands [5].

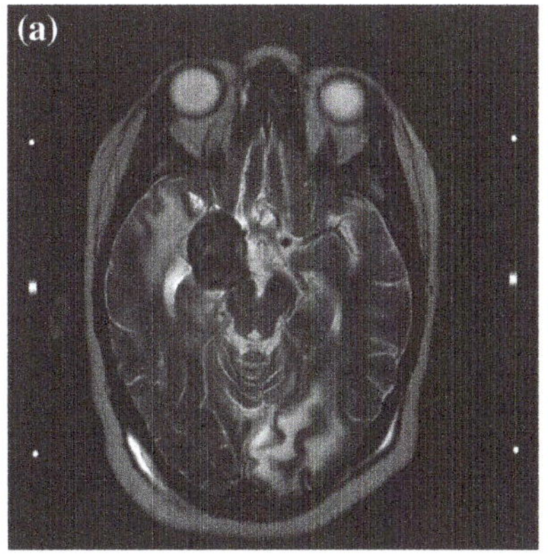

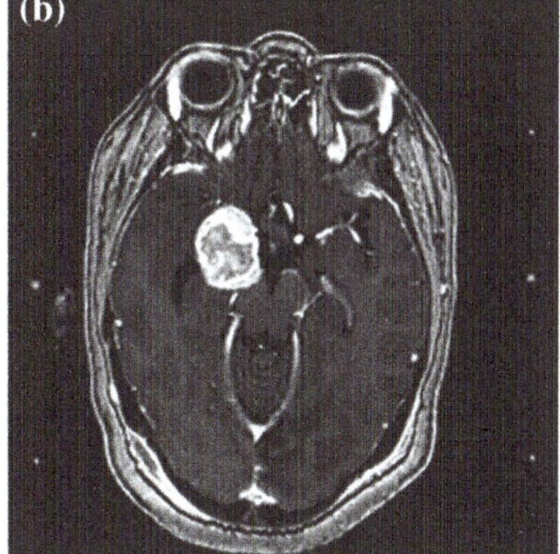

Fig. 95.3 MRI: melanotic pattern of brain metastasis in patient with melanoma on T2 (**a**) and T1p/c (**b**) images

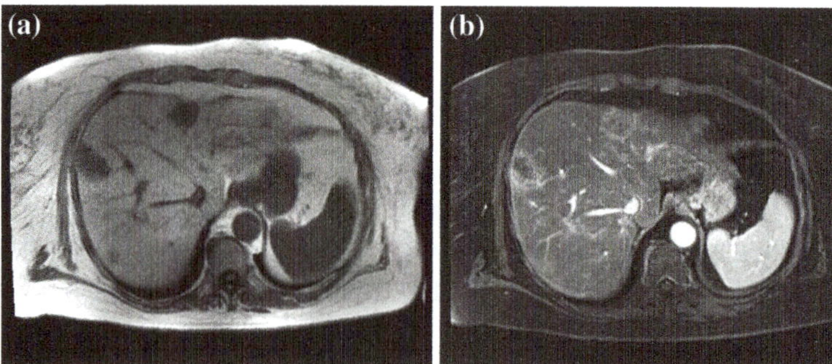

Fig. 95.4 Hepatic metastases on T1 (**a**) and T1 spir p/c (**b**) images in patient with metastatic melanoma

Complementary to the anatomical information provided by radiological imaging procedures, nuclear medicine techniques play essential role in management of patients with melanoma providing functional information.

Bone scan is a simple, widely used procedure for screening the whole skeleton for secondary deposits. The method can identify osteoblastic activity at the site of metastasis months earlier than the plain films but cannot detect purely lytic lesions with no activity of osteoblasts. Bone scan is not recommended for routine staging of patients in melanoma because of the low specificity of the method and the fact that the bone metastases are not frequent in the early stage of the disease. However, bone scanning is recommended in symptomatic patients as the patients with bone pain, when plain radiographs or even CT scans are negative.

Lymphoscintigraphy is a nuclear medicine technique that demonstrates the pattern of lymphatic drainage to the sentinel lymph node (SLN), the first node receiving the lymph drainage from the primary neoplastic lesion before involving other nodes (Fig. 95.5). After intradermal injection or the radioactive tracer close to the primary tumor, the SLN is detected in most patients within 10–30 min with the use or gamma camera with single-photon emission computed tomography (SPECT) or with SPECT-CT. At the time of surgery a hand-hell gamma camera is used. If the sentinel node (SN) is negative for metastatic involvement, it is very likely that the rest regional nodes are also negative. The biopsy of SNL can play critical value for the management and the prognosis of the patient with melanoma. Although the features of the primary tumor are very significant for the staging and the prognosis, the status of SLN seems to be the most important prognostic factor in intermediate thickness melanoma. The method, if performed by experienced stuff, has less than 5 % false negative findings [2, 3]. The radiation dose of lymphoscintigraphy is very low, as very small amount of radioactivity is injected and the CT, if added to SPECT, is of low-dose technique. Lymphoscintigraphy and SLN biopsy are indicated for the initial staging of clinically node-negative cases of melanoma and also for the patients being at risk for regional node spread upon the histological features of the primary lesion. For stage IA disease with adverse histological characteristics, stage IB and stage II disease, SLN biopsy is recommended.

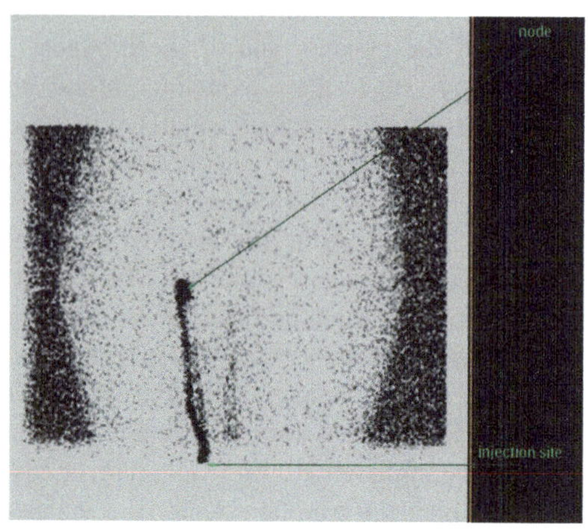

Fig. 95.5 Lymphoscintigraphy: sentinel lymph node at the right inguinal area from a primary site at the right femur

During the past few years, PET-CT has become a strong imaging tool for the evaluation of many malignancies. PET-CT is a fused method which combines in one single modality the detailed anatomical information provided by CT with the functional information provided by positron emission tomography (PET). The radiotracer used for PET is 18F-FGD, which is glucose labeled with 18F. 18F-FDG is trapped at cancer cells because they have increased metabolic activity and exclusively use glucose as a source of energy. Malignant melanoma is typically FDG avid disease as most deposits even the small ones appear strongly hypermetabolic with very elevated standard uptake value (SUV) measurements (Figs. 95.6a, b). As many studies have shown, PET-CT is more accurate in the management of patients with melanoma than CT, MRI, or PET alone. The sensitivity of the method is higher compared to CT and MRI. PET-CT is strongly recommended for the evaluation of stage III or IV melanoma, with a sensitivity of 98 %, specificity 94 %, and accuracy 96 % [8]. Compared to MRI, PET-CT is more accurate in N staging and in the detection of subcutaneous and skin metastases while MRI is more sensitive in the evaluation of the liver, the bones, and the brain and the spinal canal [7]. According to a retrospective study of patients with all stages of melanoma (I–IV) and different time points in course of the disease [9], PET-CT turned out to be more accurate than CT in N and in M initial staging with an overall accuracy of 97 %, while the accuracy of CT was 79 %. PET-CT revealed much more visceral and nonvisceral metastases than CT alone and led to change patients' management in more than 35 % of them [8]. PET-CT is also valuable for restaging and detecting recurrent melanoma. As a whole body procedure PET-CT demonstrates the total extent of the disease but may also reveal unexpected findings (Figs. 95.7a, b). It is also an excellent imaging tool to clarify equivocal findings on conventional imaging. False positive results may be due to brown fat, post therapeutic changes (recent surgery or radiotherapy), normal activity in the bowel, the myocardium and the collecting urinary system, inflammation (infection or granulomatous disease), benign tumors as

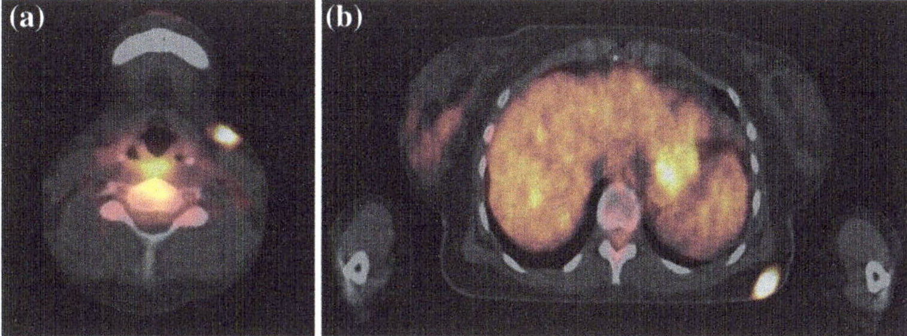

Fig. 95.6 **a** Fused PET-CT image: subtly enlarged hypermetabolic submandibular lymph node in metastatic melanoma, **b** Fused PET-CT image: hypermetabolic melanoma deposit at the subcutaneous fat

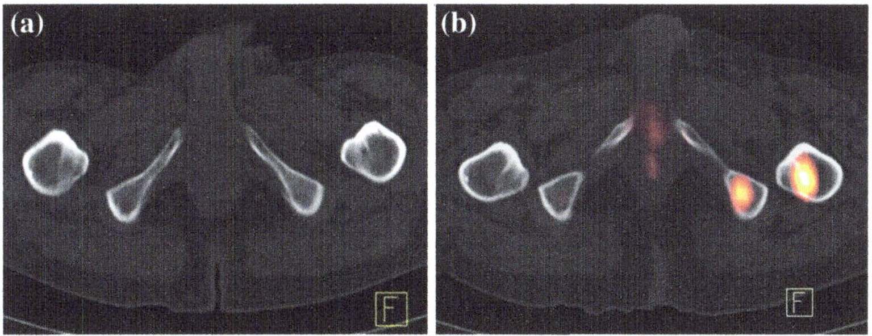

Fig. 95.7 Metastases from cutaneous melanoma at the left ischium and at the left femur on PET-CT images (**b**), not obvious on CT (**a**)

adenomas and attenuation artifacts. False negative findings conclude very small lung nodules (<8 mm) which may be FDG-negative even if they are metastatic. CT of the lungs remains the imaging method of choice for detection and follow-up for such small lung lesions. PET-CT cannot replace SN procedure in the early stages of the disease (stages I–II) for the detection of micrometastasis. However, FDG-PET-CT could replace conventional imaging in stage III and IV metastatic melanoma except of the evaluation of the brain (MRI provides better estimation) and of the lungs (CT remains the method of choice). Besides its high cost, studies have shown that PET-CT if properly used is a cost-effective method [9, 10].

As above described, today, the clinicians have in their disposal a variety of imaging procedures for the initial staging, restaging and follow-up of patients with melanoma. The information provided by imaging is of critical significance for the patient's management and prognosis.

References

1. King DM (2004) Imaging of metastatic melanoma. J HK Coll Radiol 7:66–69
2. Meyers MO, Yeh JJ, Frank J et al (2009) Method of detection of initial recurrence of stage II/III cutaneous melanoma: analysis of the utility of follow-up staging. Ann Surg Oncol 16(4):941
3. Mohr P, Eggermont AM, Hauschild A et al (2009) Staging of cutaneous melanoma. Ann Oncol 20(suppl 6):vi14–21
4. Fishman EK, Kuhlman JE, Schuchter LM et al (1990) CT of malignant melanoma in the chest, abdomen, and musculoskeletal system. Radiographics 10(4):603
5. Escott EJ (2001) A variety of appearances of malignant melanoma in the head: a review. RadioGraphics 21:625–639
6. Voit C, Van Akkooi AC, Schäfer-Hesterberg G et al (2010) Ultrasound morphology criteria predict metastatic disease of the sentinel nodes in patients with melanoma. J Clin Oncol 28(5):847
7. Pfannenberg C, Aschoff P, Schanz S et al (2007) Prospective comparison of 18F-fluorodeoxyglucose positron emission tomography/computed tomography and whole-body magnetic resonance imaging in staging of advanced malignant melanoma. Eur J Cancer 43(3):557
8. Strobel K, Dummer R, Husarik DB et al (2007) High-risk melanoma: accuracy of FDG PET/CT with added CT morphologic information for detection of metastases. Radiology 244(2):566
9. Reinhardt MJ, Joe AY, Jaeger U, Huber A et al (2006) Diagnostic performance of whole body dual modality 18F-FDG PET/CT imaging for N- and M-staging of malignant melanoma: experience with 250 consecutive patients. J Clin Oncol 24(7):1178
10. Jiménez-Requena F, Delgado-Bolton RC, Fernández-Pérez C et al (2010) Meta-analysis of the performance of (18)F-FDG PET in cutaneous melanoma. Eur J Nucl Med Mol Imaging 37(2):284

Clinical Implications of Melanoma

96

Dimitrios I. Bafaloukos

Cutaneous malignant melanoma has a predilection for young adults. Early stage disease is curable with surgery.

The majority of patients at first metastatic relapse have disease confined to a single organ. However, it should be remembered that the disease can be widely disseminated, with any number and combination of metastatic sites potentially being involved.

The skin imaging is crucial for the early detection of the disease. There is a real need for non-invasive techniques for in vivo imaging of skin. There are many different techniques that are in use in the clinic, aiding in diagnosis of early melanomas (dermoscopy, confocal laser scanning microscopy, high frequency ultrasound, positron emission tomography, magnetic resonance imaging) [1]. However, while these modalities are useful in the evaluation of superficial spreading skin cancers, they are not able to image at depth, which is very important, so that, there remains a critical need for a high-resolution technique to answer the question of whether tumors have invaded through the basement membrane.

Anyway, following diagnosis, accurate disease staging is important for appropriate treatment planning. The use of routine chest X-ray for screening of early-stage melanoma is controversial. Ultrasound, CT and MRI, all have the ability to identify nodal and distant metastases, but there is general agreement that their routine use for asymptomatic patients with melanoma is not indicated [2]. The use of radionuclide studies in the form of sentinel node localization is, however, quiet widely practiced and may limit invasive elective regional lymph node dissection to those who are shown to have involved sentinel nodes [3].

The clinical implications of PET using FDG in the management of patients with melanoma are significant. PET has been shown to have a strong role in detection of metastatic disease. FDG-PET can highlight metastases at unusual sites that are easily missed with conventional imaging modalities. It is more sensitive than CT for detection of metastatic lesions in skin, lymph nodes, and abdomen, but it has limitations in detection of early-stage disease, small lung nodules and brain metastases. For the brain metastases MRI of the brain is the more sensitive method. FDG-PET also, cannot replace sentinel node biopsy, which is much more sensitive in detecting microscopic lymph node metastases [4].

During melanoma follow up, patients are clinically monitored, including the "skin-self examination", in order to detect a relapse and to recognize additional skin tumors, especially secondary melanomas, as early as possible. However, it is unknown if this policy leads to improve survival rates.

D. I. Bafaloukos (✉)
Metropolitan Hospital, E. Makariou 9—E. Venizelou 1, 18547 N. Faliro, Greece
e-mail: dimmp@otenet.gr

A. D. Gouliamos et al. (eds.), *Imaging in Clinical Oncology*,
DOI: 10.1007/978-88-470-5385-4_96, © Springer-Verlag Italia 2014

There is currently no consensus on the frequency of follow-up and the use of imaging techniques. In recent series, most relapses have been detected by the patients themselves, questioning the usefulness and cost-effectiveness of F/U visits every 3 months during the first 3 years and every 6–12 months thereafter. Increased intervals between controls may reduce false positive findings and suffice for psychological support of the patients.

Since patients with a thin primary melanoma have only a small risk of relapse, routine imaging techniques are definitively not necessary for this patient population. In high risk patients, ultrasound of lymph nodes, CT or whole body PET/PET-CT scan may lead to an earlier diagnosis of regional or systemic relapses.

However, an impact of radiological exams upon survival has not been demonstrated. Regarding brain, MRI should be done in suspicious or symptomatic patients [5].

In conclusion the explosion of imaging techniques and the close cooperation of many specialties have lead to better staging, early detection of surgically respectable recurrent disease and metastases and the selection of the most appropriate therapies for patients with melanoma.

References

1. Smith L, MacNeil S (2011) State of the art in non-invasive imaging of cutaneous melanoma. Skin Res Technol 17:257–269
2. King DM (2004) Imaging of metastatic melanoma. JKH Coll Radiol 7:66–69
3. Wagner JD, Davidson D, Coleman JJ et al (1999) Lymph node tumor volumes in patients undergoing sentinel lymph node biopsy for cutaneous melanoma. Ann Surg Oncol 6:398–404
4. Kumar R, Alavi A (2005) Clinical applications of fluorodeoxyglucose-positron emission tomography in the management of malignant melanoma. Curr Opin Oncol 17(2):154–159
5. Dummer R, Hauschild A, Pentheroudakis G (2009) Cutaneous malignant melanoma: ESMO clinical recommendations for diagnosis, treatment and follow-up. Ann Oncol 20(Sup 4):129–131

Index

A. D. Gouliamos et al. (eds.), *Imaging in Clinical Oncology*,
DOI: 10.1007/978-88-470-5385-4, © Springer-Verlag Italia 2014

Lightning Source UK Ltd.
Milton Keynes UK
UKOW07n1704221215

265230UK00004B/36/P